GW01216920

BSAVA Manual of Small Animal Cardiorespiratory Medicine and Surgery

Edited by

FILTON Copy

Virginia Luis Fuentes

MA VetMB CertVR DVC MRCVS
Department of Veterinary Medicine and Surgery
College of Veterinary Medicine
University of Missouri at Columbia
Clydesdale Hall
Columbia, MO 65211, USA

and

Simon Swift

MA VetMB CertSAC MRCVS
Langdale Veterinary Hospital
Cheadle Hulme, Cheshire SK8 5LU

Published by:

British Small Animal Veterinary Association
Kingsley House, Church Lane
Shurdington, Cheltenham
GL51 5TQ, United Kingdom

A Company Limited by Guarantee in England.
Registered Company No. 2837793.
Registered as a Charity.

A catalogue record for this book is available from the British Library

ISBN 0 905214 33 1

Typeset by: Fusion Design, Fordingbridge, Hampshire, UK

Printed by: Lookers, Upton, Poole, Dorset, UK

Other Manuals

Other titles in the BSAVA Manuals series:

Manual of Anaesthesia for Small Animal Practice
Manual of Canine and Feline Gastroenterology
Manual of Canine and Feline Nephrology and Urology
Manual of Companion Animal Nutrition and Feeding
Manual of Canine Behaviour
Manual of Exotic Pets
Manual of Feline Behaviour
Manual of Ornamental Fish
Manual of Psittacine Birds
Manual of Raptors, Pigeons and Waterfowl
Manual of Reptiles
Manual of Small Animal Arthrology
Manual of Small Animal Clinical Pathology
Manual of Small Animal Dentistry, 2nd edition
Manual of Small Animal Dermatology
Manual of Small Animal Diagnostic Imaging
Manual of Small Animal Endocrinology, 2nd edition
Manual of Small Animal Fracture Repair and Management
Manual of Small Animal Neurology, 2nd edition
Manual of Small Animal Oncology
Manual of Small Animal Ophthalmology
Manual of Small Animal Reproduction and Neonatology

Contents

Contributors

Dawn Merton Boothe DVM PhD DipACVIM DipACVCP
Department of Veterinary Physiology & Pharmacology,Texas A & M University,
College of Veterinary Medicine, College Station,TX 77843, USA

Janice McIntosh Bright DVM
Department of Clinical Science, Colorado State University, 300 West Drake Road,
Fort Collins, CO 80523, USA

Serena E. Brownlie BVM&S PhD CertSAC MRCVS
Broadacres, Bedford Road, Little Houghton, Northampton NN7 1AW

R. Eddie Clutton BVSc DVA DipECVA MRCVS
Department of Veterinary Clinical Studies, Royal (Dick) School of Veterinary Studies,
University of Edinburgh, Easter Bush Veterinary centre, Easter Bush, Midlothian EH25 9RG

Malcolm A. Cobb MA VetMB PhD DVC MRCVS
Leo Animal Health, Longwick Road, Princes Risborough, Bucks HP27 9RR

Brendan Corcoran MVB PhD DipPharm MRCVS
Department of Clinical Studies, Royal (Dick) School of Veterinary Studies, University of Edinburgh,
Summerhall, Edinburgh EH9 1QH

Peter G.G. Darke BVSc PhD DVR DVC DipECVIM MRCVS
Department of Veterinary Clinical Studies, Royal (Dick) School of Veterinary Studies,
University of Edinburgh, Summerhall, Edinburgh EH9 1QH

Joanna Dukes McEwan BVMS MVM DVC MRCVS
Department of Veterinary Clinical Studies, Royal (Dick) School of Veterinary Studies,
University of Edinburgh, Summerhall, Edinburgh EH9 1QH

J. David Fowler DVM MVSc DipACVS
Department of Veterinary Anaesthesiology, Radiology & Surgery, Western College of
Veterinary Medicine, University of Saskatchewan, Saskatoon, Canada S7N 5B4

Anne French MVB DVC MRCVS
Department of Veterinary Clinical Studies, Royal (Dick) School of Veterinary Studies,
University of Edinburgh, Summerhall, Edinburgh EH9 1QH

John Grandage BVetMed MA DVR MRCVS
Department of Anatomy, University of Cambridge, Downing Street, Cambridge CB2 3DY

Michael E. Herrtage MA BVSc DVR DVD DSAM MRCVS
Department of Clinical Veterinary Medicine, University of Cambridge, Madingley Road,
Cambridge CB3 0ES

Barbara M. Kirby BS RN DVM MS DACVS DECVS
Department of Veterinary Clinical Studies, Royal (Dick) School of Veterinary Studies,
University of Edinburgh, Summerhall, Edinburgh EH9 1QH

Linda Lew DVM MSc DipACVS
VCA Franklin Park Animal Hospital, 9846 West Grand Avenue, Franklin Park, IL 60131, USA

Christopher J.L.Little BVMS PhD CertSAC MRCVS
Animal Health Product Development, Pfizer Ltd, Ramsgate Road, Sandwich, Kent CT13 9NJ

Virginia Luis Fuentes MA VetMB CertVR DVC MRCVS
Department of Veterinary Medicine and Surgery, College of Veterinary Medicine,
University of Missouri at Columbia, Clydesdale Hall, Columbia, MO 65211, USA

Mike Martin MVB DVC MRCVS
Veterinary Cardiorespiratory Centre, 43 Waverley Road, Kenilworth, Warwickshire CV8 1JL

Brendan C. McKiernan DVM DipACVIM
Denver Veterinary Specialists, Wheat Ridge Animal Hospital, 3695 Kipling Street, Wheat Ridge,
CO 80033, USA

Elizabeth A.C. Munro MA VetMB DVR MRCVS
Department of Veterinary Clinical Studies, Royal (Dick) School of Veterinary Studies,
University of Edinburgh, Summerhall, Edinburgh EH9 1QH

Pamela J. Murison BVMS CertVA MRCVS
Department of Veterinary Clinical Studies, Royal (Dick) School of Veterinary Studies,
Easter Bush Veterinary Centre, Easter Bush, Midlothian EH 25 9RG

Claire J.A. Spackman DVM MSc DipACVS MRCVS
College of Veterinary Medicine, Mississippi State University, Mississippi State, MS 39762, USA

Richard A. Squires BVSc PhD DVR DipACVIM DipECVIM MRCVS
Centre for Companion Animal Health, Massey University, Palmerston North, New Zealand

Rebecca L. Stepien DVM MS DipACVIM
School of Veterinary Medicine, University of Wisconsin - Madison, 2015 Linden Drive West,
Madison, WI 53706, USA

Martin Sullivan BVMS PhD DVR DipECVDI MRCVS
Department of Veterinary Clinical Studies, University of Glasgow Veterinary School, Bearsden Road,
Bearsden, Glasgow G61 1QH

Richard A.S. White BVetMed PhD DSAS DVR DipACVS DipECVS FRCVS
Department of Clinical Veterinary Medicine, University of Cambridge, Madingley Road,
Cambridge CB3 0ES

Robert N. White BSc BVetMed CertVA DipECVS MRCVS
Davies White, Manor Farm Business Park, Higham Gobion, Hitchin, Herts SG5 3HR

Paul R. Wotton BVSc PhD DVC MRCVS
University of Bristol, Department of Clinical Veterinary Science, Langford House, Langford,
Bristol BS40 5DU

Foreword

This manual marks another milestone in the history of BSAVA publications, being the longest yet. The Editors are to be congratulated on their choice of contributors, who bring an international approach to the book and ensure that the knowledge contained therein is as up to date as possible. Although there are more than 30 authors included in the book, the Editors have succeeded in achieving a consistency of approach to all aspects of the subject. The revolution in printing technology has enabled them to make full use of colour in the illustrations.

There are four main sections, the general introduction, clinical problems, therapy, and finally surgical techniques. Each section follows a consistent line of progression through the thorax and respiratory tree.

This manual brings together the different disciplines in a problem solving approach to cardiorespiratory medicine and surgery. A particularly pleasing feature is the inclusion of anaesthetic problems and techniques in conjunction with the surgical techniques for which anaesthesia is required. Other facets of anaesthesia are to be found in conjunction with treatment protocols of heart failure and techniques for bronchoscopy. This mirrors the diagnostic problems faced by veterinary surgeons in the consulting room and I am sure that this manual will be considered as invaluable an aid to the busy practitioner as others in the series.

J.F.R. Hird MA BVSc DVA DipECVA MRCVS
BSAVA President 1998-99

Preface

There has been an explosion of interest and knowledge in the fields of small animal cardiac and respiratory disease. The use of ultrasound has revolutionized our approach to cardiac disease, allowing many diagnoses to be reached non-invasively. Our pharmaceutical armoury is ever expanding, permitting more effective treatment modalities. This has been paralleled by advances in surgery, and a new wave of interest in respiratory disease. It became apparent that there was a growing need for a BSAVA publication to cover this area, and this manual is the result. We are much indebted to Bryden Stanley for her invaluable assistance in planning this manual and contacting prospective authors.

In Part One, the first three chapters provide basic information on the underlying pathophysiological mechanisms, which are essential to a proper understanding of cardiac and respiratory disease. After discussion on the approach to a clinical case and basic investigative tests, specialized techniques are described in Chapter 6. Part Two covers clinical problems, initially in a problem-oriented approach before discussing specific areas. Part Three provides a guide to therapy and Part Four gives an update on the surgical techniques currently available.

As with all manuals, we have tried to keep the emphasis on what is relevant for the clinician. We are grateful to Vicki Martin for her help with the illustrations and Aart van der Woude for his enhancement of the radiographs in chapters 5, 13, 16 and 18. We would also like to thank Marion Jowett for her cajoling and encouragement in the final stages. Above all we would like to thank the many authors for their hard work and patience; the style and emphasis of the chapters reflect the range and depth of their experience.

This book has been long in gestation but we are sure the wait was worthwhile. We hope that you will find it stimulating to read, and invaluable in your day-to-day work.

Virginia Luis Fuentes
Simon Swift

August 1998

PART ONE

Introduction and Overview

An Anatomical Background

John Grandage

AN ALPHABETICAL TOUR THROUGH THE LARYNX AND CHEST

This introductory account takes a personal tour through the larynx and chest, highlighting topics that appeal, that may have been inadequately covered or whose significance may have been underestimated in standard works. There is not the space here for detailed descriptions. For that sort of information the comprehensive accounts listed under literature below should be consulted.

Aditus laryngis

This is the proper name for the entrance to the larynx. It is an orifice with a complex shape that marks the boundary between the pharynx and the laryngeal vestibule (Figure 1.1). An endotracheal tube must therefore navigate the aditus, the vestibule, the rima glottidis and the infraglottic cavity in traversing the larynx to reach the trachea. The aditus itself is roughly horizontal in a standing dog whereas the rima glottidis is inclined at about 45 degrees. Because the cranial parts of the larynx project upwards from the pharyngeal floor, the aditus is surrounded by a gutter of pharyngeal mucous membrane, the piriform recesses laterally and the vallecula rostrally. The margin of the aditus is covered in mucous membrane that stretches from the epiglottis to the cuneiform and corniculate processes via the ary-epiglottic folds. The apex of the epiglottis may rest on the roof of the soft palate or slip beneath it. During panting, the epiglottis oscillates up and down above and below the soft palate, so that incoming air is drawn in through the nose while outgoing air flows out through the mouth.

Arteries

Arteries of the chest are asymmetrical (Figure 1.2). Because the aorta develops from the fourth left aortic arch:

- The left subclavian sprouts directly off the aorta, while the right comes off the brachiocephalic artery
- The right intercostal arteries are longer than those on the left because they have to traverse the width of the vertebrae
- The recurrent laryngeal nerves wind round different vessels on each side – the ligamentum arteriosum on the left, and the right subclavian on the right
- The oesophagus and trachea pass on the right side of the aorta.

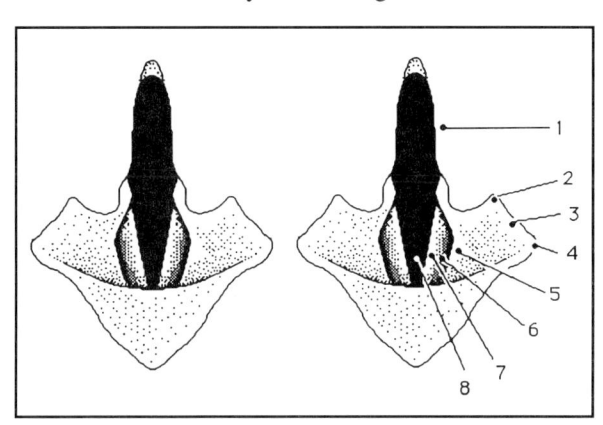

Figure 1.1: The aditus laryngis and its contents. Its margin is supported by the corniculate (1) and cuneiform (2) processes of the arytenoid cartilage from which the ary-epiglottic fold (3) stretches to the lateral margin of the epiglottis (4). The aditus opens into the vestibule, within which is the vestibular fold (5) which flanks the cranial border of the laryngeal ventricle (6) and the vocal fold (7) which forms the ventral boundary to the rima glottidis (8).

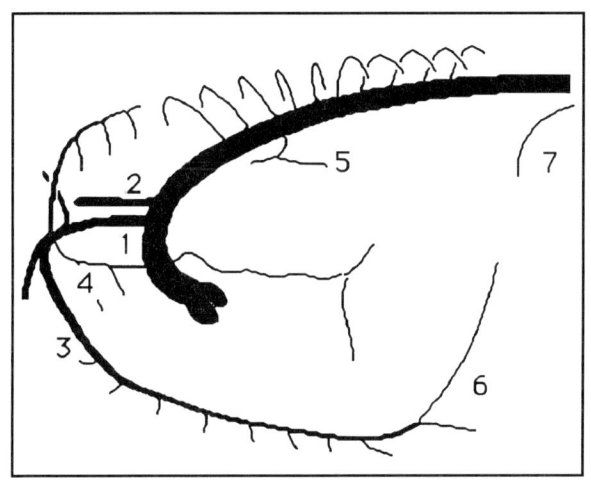

Figure 1.2: The main arteries of the chest viewed from the left: the brachiocephalic (1), left subclavian (2), internal thoracic (3), pericardiophrenic (4), broncho-oesophageal (5), musculophrenic (6), and phrenic branch of the phrenico-abdominal (7).

Breed and species variations

Apart from size, the most obvious differences appear to be in proportions. Deep-chested hounds have elongated hearts, and more obviously three-lobed diaphragms. Dachshunds have wide tracheas and the relative development of the costal cartilages tends to be disproportionately large in chondrodystrophoid breeds. Boxers' costal cartilages show complex calcification patterns. In cats, the heart is more inclined and the diaphragm more caudal.

Bronchial tree

The bulk of the lung is made up of bronchial tree and pulmonary vessels (Figure 1.3). The generations of branches are: trachea, principal bronchi, lobar bronchi, segmental bronchi, several generations of unnamed bronchi, bronchioles (characterized by the absence of cartilage, mucous glands and a typical diameter of

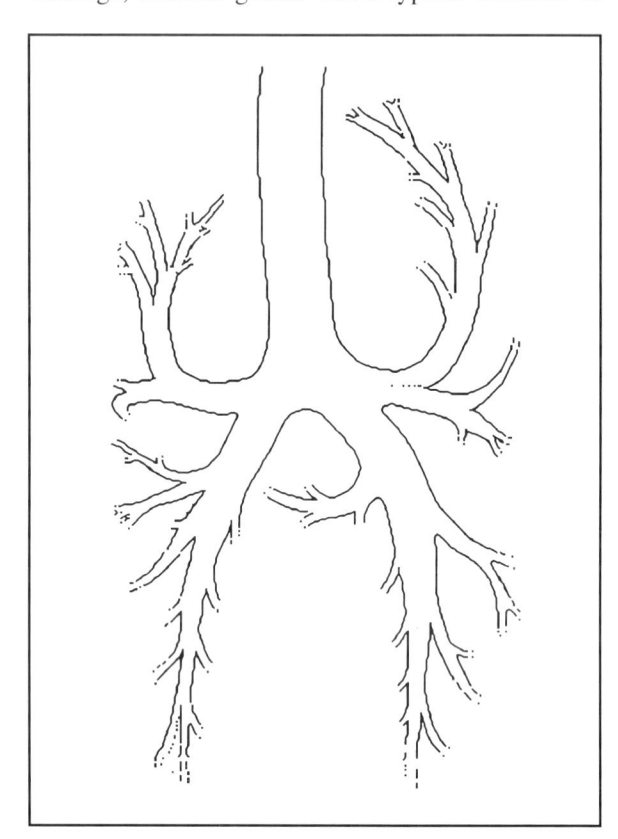

Figure 1.3: The bronchial tree of the dog (dorsal view). Right and left principal bronchi, divide into cranial and caudal lobar bronchi on the left, and cranial, middle, caudal and accessory lobar bronchi on the right. The left cranial lobe is partly subdivided by an incomplete fissure into cranial and caudal parts. End-on lobar bronchi account for the black dot on radiographs at the base of the heart.

about 1 mm or smaller), terminal bronchioles, respiratory bronchioles, alveolar ducts, acini, alveolar sacs and alveoli.

The lung is one of the few organs with a dual circulation, bronchial and pulmonary, with the tree nourished by its own bronchial arteries, vessels given off the broncho-oesophageal artery.

Cardiac notches

The chest is tapered, with insufficient room for both the heart and the lungs in the cramped quarters of its ventral part. The lungs insinuate (or are sucked) between heart and chest wall as far as they can, but there always remains a small window, the cardiac notch, where the heart and its wrappings are pressed directly against the chest wall (Figure 1.4). The notch is significant because it is where access can be gained to the heart for ultrasound scans and direct injection, and where the pleural and pericardial cavities can be tapped without the danger of lung puncture.

Textbooks usually specify precise boundaries to the cardiac notches but this is misleading and even dangerous. Cardiac notches are of inconstant form, location and size. Variations are caused by the state of respiration, the shape of the thorax, and the posture of the animal. They are naturally larger during expiration when the ribs are compressed, in deep-chested dogs and on the dependent side of the animal. While the notch is always present close to the midline, access here is complicated by the presence of the internal thoracic vessels that run a few millimetres from the midline.

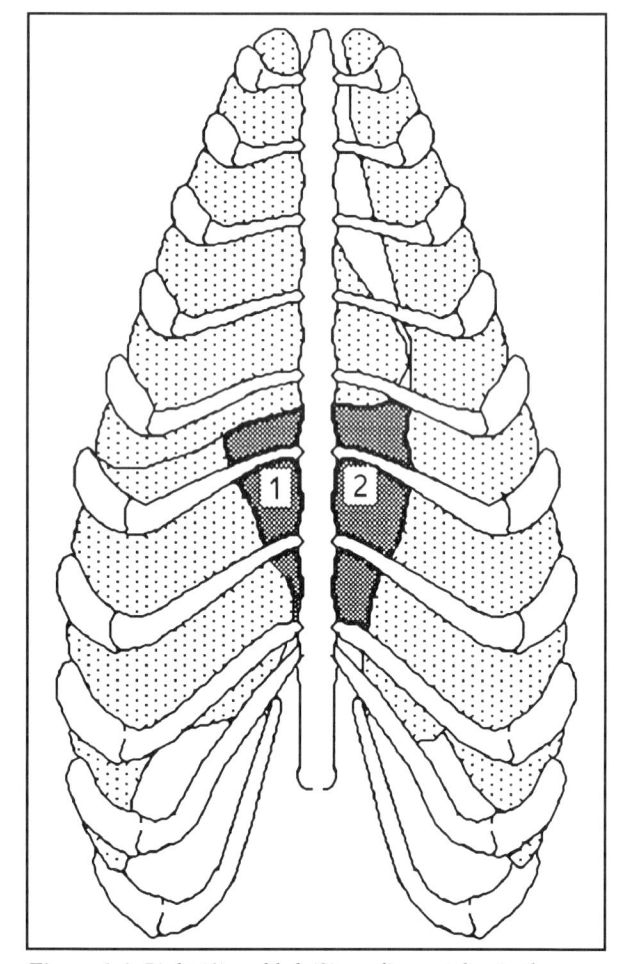

Figure 1.4: Right (1) and left (2) cardiac notches in the inflated exposed lungs of a dog cadaver (ventral view). Their size, shape and position vary according to posture, respiration and other factors (see text).

Caudal vena cava

This vessel is the key to much thoracic topography. It pierces the diaphragm in the middle of the central tendon of the right half of the diaphragm, far from the aorta with which it subsequently has a much closer relationship. It is not an isolated tube, but rides atop a flimsy fold of pleura, the plica venae cavae. The fold sweeps up from near the sternal floor and helps form a deep pleural recess caudal to the heart in which the accessory lobe of the lung resides.

Costal arch

The costal arch is formed by the costal cartilages of the asternal ribs uniting with each other by means of fibrous tissue. The fibrous joints (syndesmoses) allow the cartilages to roll over one another. The last pair of ribs are floating and their short costal cartilages do not contribute to the costal arch.

Costal cartilages

These calcify early, especially the middle members of the series, and most show extensive signs of ossification by 6 months. The portion adjacent to the costochondral junction is the least calcified and may be incised without difficulty. The ribs themselves grow from their distal ends and are easily palpable even in normal animals, but especially in the young and spectacularly in animals with certain growth disorders.

Diaphragm

Radiographs and abdominal inspection fail to give a true impression of the form of the diaphragm (Figure 1.5). It is cup-shaped rather than saucer-shaped with most of the

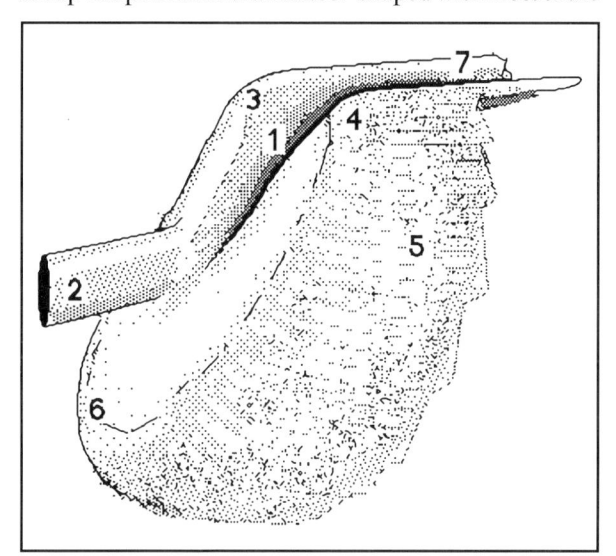

Figure 1.5: The diaphragm of the dog viewed from the left and from the cranial aspect. Note the depth of the median fissure (1), the eccentric position of the vena cava (2), how the dependent crus (in this case the right (3)) sags forward in front of the upper one (left crus (4)) and how a large part of the muscular part (5) lies against the thoracic wall rather than the lung. The cupola (6) reaches about the sixth or seventh rib in most species; the boundary of the lumbo-diaphragmatic recess (7) is more variable.

walls of the cup being muscular and pressed against the sides of the chest while only the floor of the cup, which is partly tendinous, faces the basal surface of the lungs. A deep median fissure plunges into the dorsal half of the diaphragm, and subdivides it into two distinct lobes dorsally and one ventrally. The caudal parts of the oesophagus and aorta are lodged in the fissure whose muscular walls make up the so-called crura of the diaphragm. The crura taper off into tendons that insert on the bodies of the 3rd and 4th lumbar vertebrae.

Unfortunately, there is no official Nomina Anatomica Veterinaria (NAV) term for each of the dorsal halves of the diaphragm, so they are variously called dorsal lobes, crura, or hemidiaphragms. Here, we will use the words right and left crura in a broader sense than simply the lumbar components, to include the whole of the dorsal parts, and the word cupola to refer to the whole of the dome-shaped ventral part. The positions of the two crura and cupola are particularly sensitive to the posture of the animal. The flimsy bag-like nature of the diaphragm means it is unable to hold the abdominal viscera in a firm way. Rather, the diaphragm bulges and sags like a sack of potatoes, the lowest portion perhaps two centimetres further forward than the upper portion. A dog lying on its right side has the right crus lowermost and pushed furthest forward, while a dog on its left has the left crus so disposed. The cupola of the diaphragm lies reasonably close to its sternal attachment.

Fat

Fat accumulates in the chest particularly between the transverse thoracic muscle and the sternum, over and beneath the intercostal muscles and within the mediastinum, especially the cranial mediastinum. It can cause the heart to elevate.

Gravity

Gravity has a greater influence on the anatomy of the thoracic organs than on the anatomy of any other region. Always consider whether a particular organ may sink, sag, fill, inflate or float. It is because the apex of the heart is free to swing in its pericardial sac that the prone position is favoured for radiography.

Heart surfaces

Because of the ambiguity caused by the physiological 'left side of the heart' (referring to the left atrium and left ventricle), the surface of the heart seen from the left hand side has recently been designated the 'auricular' surface, because only from this view are both left and right auricles visible. From a right-sided vantage, the heart surface is referred to as the 'atrial' surface, because both atria (and neither auricle) are visible.

Intercostal nerves

Intercostal nerves run for the most part between the pleura and the deep surface of the internal intercostal muscle close to the caudal border of the ribs but separated from them by the intercostal vessels. They are mixed sensory/motor nerves that give off lateral and ventral cutaneous branches.

Intercostal spaces

Fibre direction of the intercostal muscles is similar to the abdominal obliques – the external ones coursing caudoventrally, the internal cranioventrally. The two layers are easily separable. The internal intercostal can also be lifted from the underlying costal pleura. While it continues to be claimed that the external muscle is inspiratory and the internal is expiratory, there is evidence that both are active in both phases of respiration.

Laryngeal cartilages

The signet ring-shaped cricoid is the firm chassis of the larynx (Figure 1.6). From its sides, the 'U'-shaped thyroid hangs by each arm of the 'U' so that it can swing like a visor, pulled down by the cricothyroid muscle and up by several muscles and ligaments. Most complicated of all are the paired 'W'-shaped arytenoids that owe their complex shape to the fusion of the arytenoid proper with the corniculate and cuneiform processes. Each arytenoid swivels on the cricoid, like a knob on a radio, via a joint on the caudal arm of the 'W'. As the two ventral arms of the 'W' swivel, they tow the ends of the paired vestibular and vocal folds in and out. The remaining two dorsal arms of the W form the cuneiform and corniculate processes which flank the entrance to the larynx (see aditus laryngis).

The flexible parts of the laryngeal skeleton, the epiglottis and the corniculate and cuneiform processes, are made of elastic cartilage, the more rigid parts of hyaline cartilage that is frequently calcified.

Laryngeal muscles

Two groups of muscles are specifically associated with the larynx (Figure 1.7). A superficial group of extrinsic muscles arise from it and stretch elsewhere,

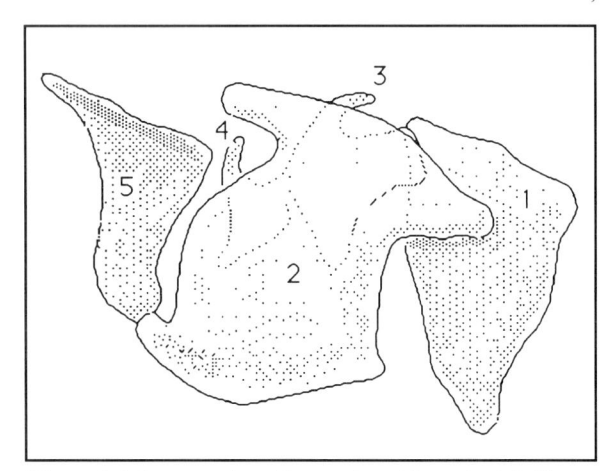

Figure 1.6: Laryngeal cartilages viewed from the left. The cricoid (1), thyroid (2) and epiglottic (5) cartilages are unpaired. The arytenoid cartilages are paired and bear corniculate (3) and cuneiform (4) processes.

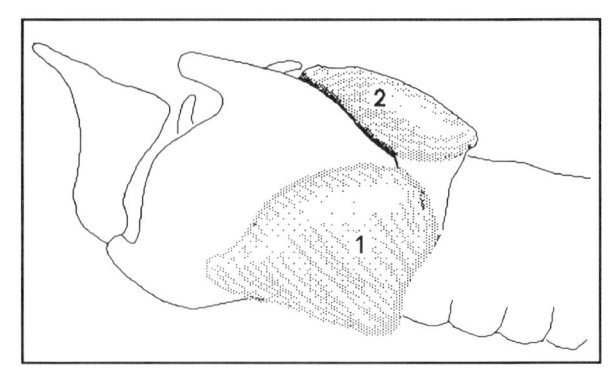

Figure 1.7: Some laryngeal muscles viewed from the left. The cricothyroid (1) and dorsal cricoarytenoid (2) are visible as soon as the pharyngeal constrictors are removed. The deeper lateral cricoarytenoid and the vocal and vestibular subdivisions of the thyroarytenoid lie deep to the thyroid cartilage.

and a deeper intrinsic group move individual cartilages in relation to each other. In addition, because the hyoid bones are so intimately associated with the larynx, any of the intrinsic and extrinsic hyoid muscles are also likely to affect the larynx; they are not discussed here.

The extrinsic muscles include:

- The most caudal of the pharyngeal constrictors (thyropharyngeus and cricopharyngeus) which form inverted U-shaped hoops over the dorsum of the larynx and whose relaxation and constriction conclude the act of swallowing
- The sternothyroid which runs with the more superficial sternohyoid and is concerned with pulling the larynx caudally
- The muscles uniting the larynx to the hyoid (the thyrohyoid and hyoepiglotticus) concerned with tilting the larynx upwards or depressing the epiglottis, respectively.

Most of the intrinsic muscles serve to guard the airway by adducting the vocal and vestibular folds. They lie sandwiched between the mucous membrane and the cartilages, and consist of the thyroarytenoid (and its vocal and vestibular subdivisions), and the lateral cricoarytenoid. A single pair of abductors of the vocal folds, the dorsal cricoarytenoid, lies atop the larynx where it is accessible. The cricothyroid serves to stretch the vocal folds by lowering the thyroid.

Laryngeal nerves

The larynx is supplied by two pairs of vagal nerves. The recurrent laryngeal nerves are given off inside the chest, loop around the right subclavian on the right and the ligamentum arteriosum on the left, and run back up the neck on the dorsolateral part of the trachea until they reach the larynx, where they change their name to the caudal laryngeal nerves. They slip between the dorsal cricoarytenoid muscle and the cricopharyngeus to supply all the muscles except the cricothyroid. Each anastomoses with the internal branch of the cranial laryngeal nerve of that side.

The cranial laryngeal nerve itself is given off the vagus early in its course (from the distal ganglion). It divides into an external branch, which runs over the pharyngeal constrictors to innervate the cricothyroid muscle, and an internal branch, which plunges into the larynx immediately caudal to the hyopharyngeus then round the cranial border of the thyroid cartilage to reach the laryngeal mucous membrane.

Laryngeal ventricles
The entrances to these chambers lie cranial to the vocal folds and caudal to the vestibular folds. They are capacious enough to stand out clearly on radiographs.

Literature
Several significant anatomical texts have been published since 1990. Only these and not the surgical or radiological literature will be covered (bibliographic details at the end of the chapter). The new edition of Evans (1993) remains the finest description of dog anatomy. There is also a vast atlas by Anderson and Anderson (1994) that assembles many scattered but fine illustrations of dog anatomy. Colour photographic atlases are now fashionable. An introductory atlas by Boyd (1992) includes ultrasound. The atlas by Done and Stickland (1994) is in their dissection series, and that by Budras *et al.* (1993) is in the surgical series. There is a genuinely veterinary anatomy of cats by Hudson and Hamilton (1993), and a cat dissection guide by Rosenzweig (1990). Endoscopic and/or ultrasound information is in the works of Barr (1990), Tams (1990), Brearley *et al.* (1991), and Feeney *et al.* (1991). A splendid text illustrating in line drawings all of the official NAV terms is at last available (Schaller *et al.*, 1992).

Lung fissures
Deep fissures extend to the hilus of the lungs and are thought to help the lung to accommodate the changing shape of the thorax associated with spinal and diaphragmatic movements (Figure 1.8). The left lung has a single interlobar fissure and an incomplete intralobar fissure that subdivides the cranial lobe into cranial and caudal parts. The right lung has three interlobar fissures subdividing the cranial, middle, caudal and accessory lobes. All the fissures are obliquely disposed, so that they are rarely seen on radiographs of normal lungs, although they do become conspicuous when thickened or when the pleural cavity is filled with fluid. The form of the fissures is quite variable so that in some dogs, the cranial lobe seems to overlap the middle, whereas in others the middle seems to overlap the cranial. Intrapleural pressure declines as one proceeds deeper into the fissures.

Lungs
The right lung is substantially larger than the left. Its cranial lobe wraps around the heart and is supported by a curving bronchus and companion pulmonary vessels which contrast distinctly on radiographs with the straighter lobar bronchus of the cranial lobe of the left lung. The impressions in the lung surface described with such affection in anatomy texts collapse with the lung when the chest is opened but do reappear when the lung is inflated. One impression often overlooked but visible on radiographs is the deep groove that is evident in the apical part of the cranial lobe where the internal thoracic artery dives ventrally towards the sternum from its subclavian parent.

The lungs vary a great deal according to posture. The dependent lung is not only hypostatically congested but is compressed by the heavy heart and bulging diaphragm; in contrast the upper lung (or upper parts of the lung) is better ventilated and expanded.

Lymph nodes
There are surprisingly few inside the dog thorax (Figure 1.9). A single lymphocentre for the viscera lies at the tracheal bifurcation made up of the large, constant, right, left and middle tracheobronchial nodes. The parietal lymphocentres have inconstant nodes. A small cluster of two or three nodes may be found in the cranial mediastinum close to any of the great vessels found there; at least one sternal node, sometimes serving both sides is found between the internal thoracic vessels and the sternum; an intercostal node is rarely seen high in the middle of the chest wall.

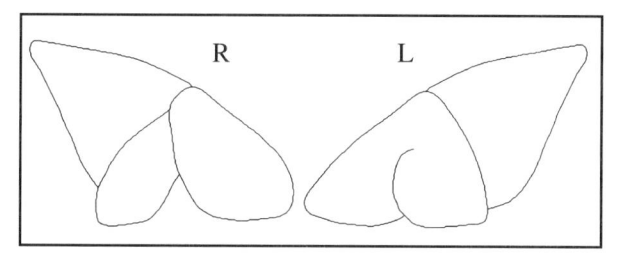

Figure 1.8: The fissures of the dog's lungs. These are the most typical though variations are common.

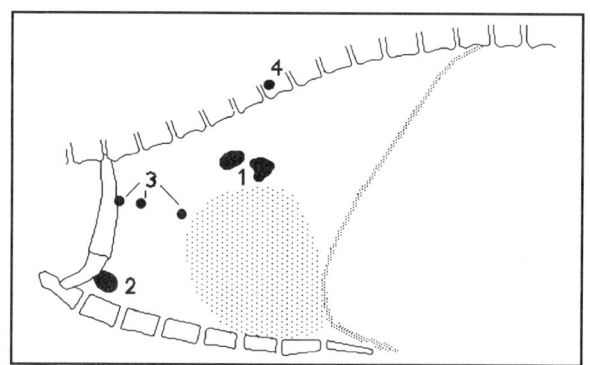

Figure 1.9: Lymph nodes of the dog's chest. The cluster of about three tracheobronchial nodes (1) at the tracheal bifurcation is the most constant, the sternal (2) pretty constant, the cranial mediastinal variable (3) and the intercostal (4) rarely present.

Mediastinum

The mediastinum is the partition dividing the thorax. It is sometimes claimed to be a space or a potential space, but it is not - it is a thing. It is composed of two sheets of pleura and whatever structures happen to be sandwiched by these sheets - oesophagus, heart, aorta, trachea, thymus, azygos vein, thoracic duct, lymph nodes. Being a partition, it can become filled with air as in pneumomediastinum; in some regions (such as caudally), it is delicate, so flimsy in fact that the slightest trauma can fenestrate it - any pneumothorax is then, automatically, bilateral.

Muscles

In addition to the muscles of the thoracic wall, there are some within the thorax itself (Figure 1.10). The longus colli encroaches into the chest running as far caudally as the 6th thoracic vertebra. The transverse thoracic muscle bridges a shallow fat-laden suprasternal space in which the internal thoracic vessels run. The quadratus lumborum encroaches on the caudal part of the chest too, arising from the bodies of the last three thoracic vertebrae. It does not attract attention because it is concealed by the diaphragmatic crura, but in cats it is seen on most lateral radiographs because of the more caudal disposition of the diaphragm (see also diaphragm, intercostal muscles).

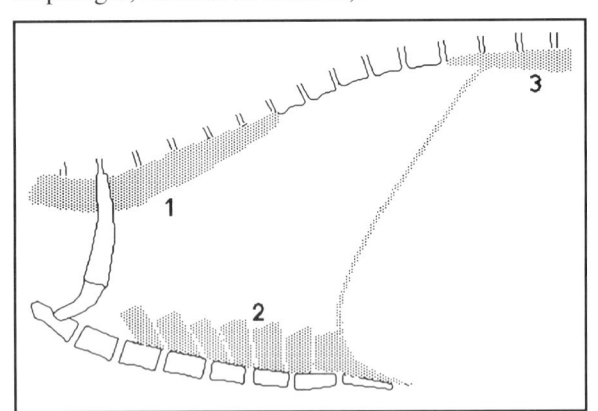

Figure 1.10: Muscles of the dog's chest in addition to the diaphragm and intercostals: longus colli (1), transverse thoracic (2) and quadratus lumborum (3).

Oesophagus

The oesophagus is curiously inconspicuous on radiographs due to its tapered, laterally-flattened form within the mediastinum. It is sometimes seen as a gas-filled loop drooping around the thoracic inlet to one side of the trachea. Anaesthetized dogs that have spent a long time in left lateral recumbency often reveal an inflated oesophagus due to regurgitation of fundic stomach gas. It is nourished by four or five vessels arranged in series:

- Near its pharyngeal origin by branches of the cranial thyroid arteries (off the carotids)
- In the caudal cervical region by the left caudal thyroid artery (off the brachiocephalic)
- In the cranial thorax by the broncho-oesophageal arteries (off the aorta)
- In the caudal thorax by the oesophageal branch (off the left gastric)
- It is innervated by successive branches of the vagus (pharyngo-oesophageal, recurrent laryngeal and dorsal and ventral branches).

Pericardium

The several layers classically ascribed to the pericardium give the impression of a series of tough bags, one after another, that hold the heart securely. This is misleading. If a lung is lifted, the heart can be seen lolling within a single, flimsy, roomy bag that is not much of a tether. The bag has to be capacious to accommodate an organ that may be variably filled. Only when the heart is seriously dilated or the pericardial sac itself is abnormally filled with fluid is the bag under any real tension. When a dog lies on its side, the heart falls away to the dependent side. When there is pneumothorax, the absence of tension within the pleural sac allows the pericardium to fall far away (making the heart appear to rise on lateral radiographs).

The single membranous bag which makes up the de facto pericardium consists strictly of a veil of fibrous tissue (the fibrous pericardium) sandwiched between glistening serous layers (the mediastinal pleura laterally and the parietal serous pericardium deeply). It is separated from the heart by the pericardial cavity. The surface of the heart itself, the epicardium, is made up of an adherent skin, perhaps unfortunately referred to as the visceral layer of serous pericardium. The serous membrane of the epicardium and lining to the pericardial sac are only in continuity around the great vessels.

While most of the pericardial cavity ends blindly around the base of the heart, a slender passageway exists that forms a bridge between left and right sides. The bridge, the transverse sinus of the pericardium, is lodged between the great arteries and the pulmonary veins and is a legacy of the folding of the original heart tube.

Phrenic nerves

From cervical nerves five, six and seven, these arise on the deep side of the roots of the brachial plexus. On the left side, the nerve courses in the mediastinum over the atria; on the right, it runs a similar course until it reaches the caudal vena cava when it runs in the plica venae cavae. The nerve's proximity to the heart means it may, rarely, be stimulated by the heart so that each breath and heart beat are synchronous.

Pleural recesses

These are a key to understanding the functional anatomy of the chest (Figure 1.11). The lungs can be pictured as having been vacuum-packed in an oversized bag of cling film, the film representing the parietal pleura. Parts of the film extend as a collapsed double fold well

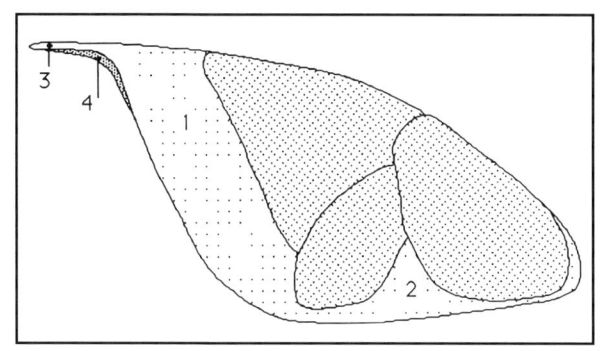

Figure 1.11: The pleural recesses of the dog's chest extend beyond the sharp borders of the lungs. The costo-diaphragmatic (1) is the largest and the costomediastinal (2) includes the region of the cardiac notches. The lumbodiaphragmatic (3) and mediastinodiaphragmatic (4) recesses are less accessible but still capacious.

beyond the sharp edges of the lungs. The empty spaces within these parts of the film represent the pleural recesses. The sharp edges of the lungs are made up of the basal and ventral borders, and pleural recesses lie adjacent to both. The largest is the so-called costodiaphragmatic (or phrenicocostal) pleural recess that extends beyond the basal border of the lung in a band just cranial to the costal arch, about 5 cm wide in an average dog. As a simplified rule of thumb, this recess extends in a curved line from the elbow to the origin of the last rib of a standing dog. The recess continues to follow the basal border of the lung dorsally and then medially in a huge arch, changing its name as it goes to the lumbodiaphragmatic and mediastino-diaphragmatic recesses, respectively. A more varied and restricted recess lies on the floor of the chest adjacent to the ventral border of the lung – the costomediastinal recess – the one that corresponds to the cardiac notch.

During inspiration, the recesses are partly effaced as their walls of parietal pleura are peeled apart through the action of the diaphragm or the drawing forwards of the ribs. Once the parietal pleura is separated, the sharp borders of the lungs expand to fill the newly available space; the remaining recess is smaller. The recesses are never normally totally obliterated, though they get close to it during pneumothorax and hydrothorax when air or fluid can accumulate within them. Pleural re-cesses are important for ultrasound examination be-cause they provide a window for the probe, and for surgical access to the pleural cavity without endanger-ing the lung.

Pulmonary arteries

Despite the low pressure in these vessels and their thin walls, they still look like arteries, with creamy surfaces and round cross-sectional appearance (Figure 1.12).

Pulmonary ligaments

These short webs of pleura stretch horizontally from the caudal mediastinum to the caudal lobes of the lungs

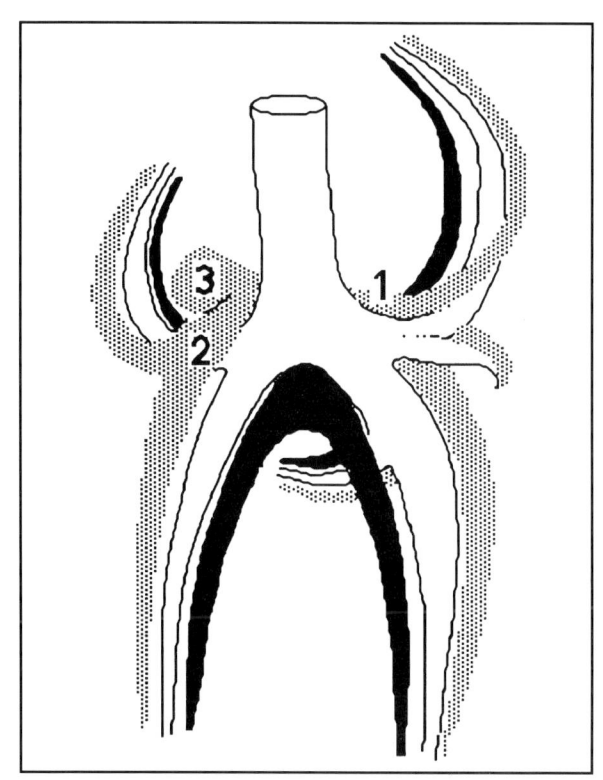

Figure 1.12: Right (1) and left (2) pulmonary arteries arise from a common pulmonary trunk (3). Their branches mostly lie on the lateral side of their companion bronchi whereas the veins (black) lie on the medial side.

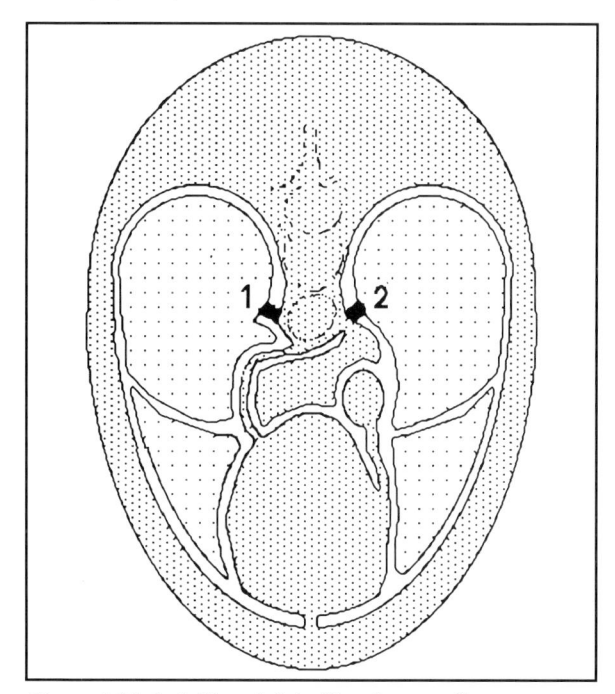

Figure 1.13: Left (1) and right (2) pulmonary ligaments stretch from the caudal mediastinum to the medial surfaces of the caudal lobes of the lungs.

(Figure 1.13). They are the pulmonary equivalents of the intestinal mesenteries which, by tethering the cau-dal lobes, prevent them from rotating. They extend caudally from where the principal bronchi enter the hilus and may interfere with surgical exposure of the caudal mediastinum.

Pulmonary veins

Pulmonary veins, unlike their arterial counterparts, have no independent course within the chest; they pursue their whole course within the lung itself and open directly into the left atrium. Their terminal portions can be partly seen on the medial surface of the lungs where the parenchyme is unable to conceal them totally. In general the veins run on the medial sides of the corresponding bronchi except at the periphery where they run an interlobular course (See Pulmonary arteries).

Rima glottidis

The nostrils and the glottal cleft are the narrowest parts of the upper airway. The walls of the glottis are firm dorsally because of their cartilaginous support (the vocal processes of the arytenoids) but flexible ventrally where the mucous membrane overlies the vocalis muscle and vocal ligament. The cleft itself is mostly rhomboidal and usually widens slightly during inspiration and closes slightly during expiration, but of course can close off totally to a vertical slit. The laryngeal ventricles lie immediately cranial to the rima.

Stellate ganglion

This, officially the cervicothoracic ganglion, together with its neighbour, the middle cervical ganglion, is the largest focus of autonomic nerves in the body (Figure 1.14). The stellate ganglion is a sympathetic ganglion found high in the chest resting on the longus colli muscle beneath ribs one and two at the cranial end of the sympathetic chain. It communicates with the middle cervical ganglion via one (or more) branches that wrap around the subclavian artery – the ansa subclavia. The vagosympathetic trunk divides at the middle cervical into mostly sympathetic components going to the stellate ganglion and vagal components coursing towards the oesophagus. Several cardiac autonomic nerves arise from around and between the two ganglia. Accordingly, they mostly run in the cranial mediastinum obliquely caudoventrally over the trachea and oesophagus to reach the heart.

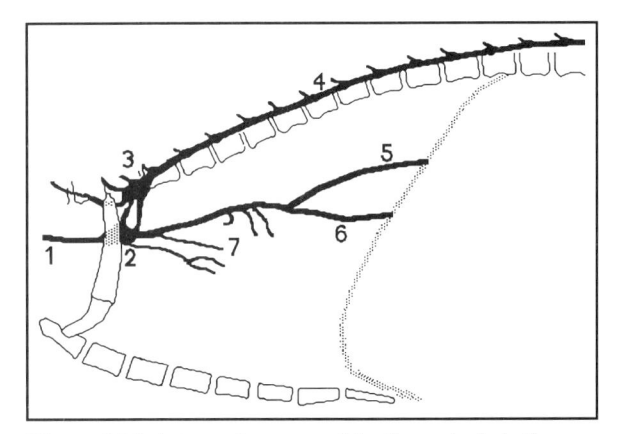

Figure 1.14: Autonomic nerves of the thorax include the vagosympathetic trunk (1), the middle cervical ganglion (2), the stellate ganglion (3), the sympathetic chain (4), the dorsal (5) and ventral (6) vagus, and the cardiac nerves (7).

Thoracic duct and other lymphatics

An hour or two after a fatty meal, the thoracic duct is a conspicuous white vessel, but at other times it is quite hard to locate, being pale and collapsed (Figure 1.15). The course of lymphatics follows a general rather than a strict pattern and it is false to say precisely where a vessel will lie or where it will terminate. With this proviso, we can say that the thoracic duct typically arises from the cisterna chyli between the diaphragmatic crura and runs between the aorta and the azygos vein until it reaches the precardiac mediastinum where it slips over to the left. From there it runs, often in a plexiform pattern, forwards to the great veins at the thoracic inlet, usually terminating in the left jugular near its junction with the cranial vena cava; alternative terminations should always be considered. The vessel is often seen running just ventral to the longus colli muscle.

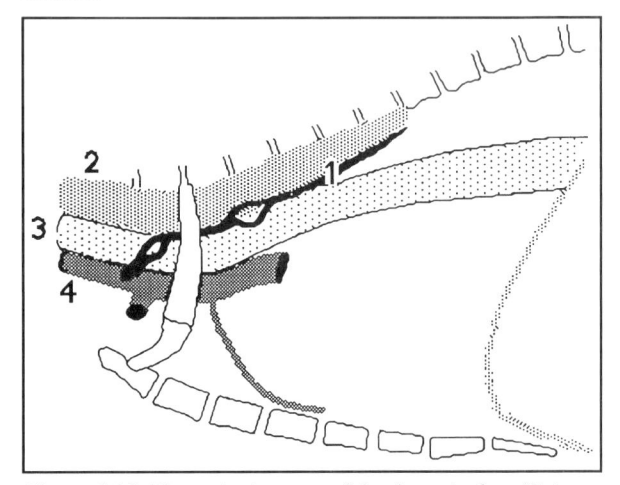

Figure 1.15: The typical course of the thoracic duct (1) in the cranial mediastinum, ventral to the longus colli (2), dorsal to the oesophagus (3), before running into one or other of the great veins (4) at the thoracic inlet.

Valves

Heart valves lie in a plane that passes through the shoulder joints, with the pulmonary lying in the third intercostal space, the aortic and right AV in the fourth and the mitral in the fifth. While it may appeal to listen at these specific sites for the sounds generated by the particular valve of interest, other factors are important too. Posture, respiratory phase and the interposition of the lungs means that we do not always hear valves the loudest when the stethoscope is placed closest to them.

Vascular rings

The series of paired aortic arches are laid down when puppy embryos are only about 4 mm long (already nearly 3 weeks old) and it is little wonder that one or other channel sometimes develops preferentially over another. Essentially, in normal mammals, the right ventral aorta disintegrates leaving the oesophagus room to expand to the right. The commonest anomalies involve a retention of the right aortic arch so that the oesophagus and trachea now pass on its left hand

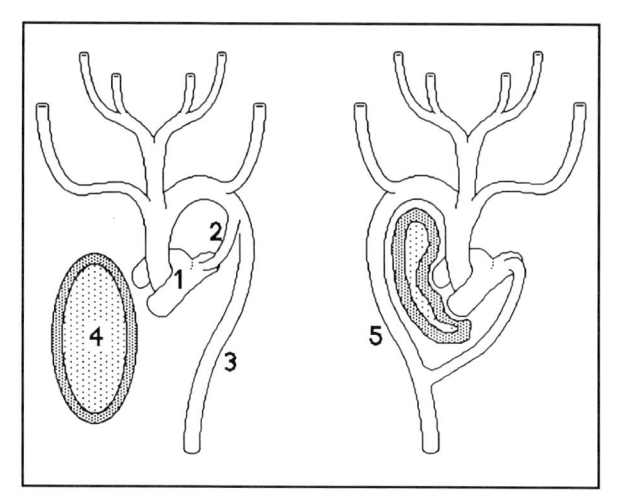

Figure 1.16: The normal arrangement of pulmonary trunk (1), ductus arteriosus (2) , aorta (3), and oesophagus (4) (left) and the situation with a persistent right aortic arch (5) (right).

surface. This is dangerous because the pulmonary trunk and its ductus arteriosus still arise from the left, thus forming a complete ring of tissue around the oesophagus and trachea (Figure 1.16).

Veins

The venous patterns of the thorax bear only a distant correlation with the arterial ones. The cranial vena cava is formed from paired brachiocephalic veins which in turn are formed from the union of external jugular and subclavian veins. The paired internal thoracic veins unite to form a common trunk that drains into the vena cava. The azygos vein (the right one in the dog) not only drains the chest but also the vertebral

canal, and, accordingly it can act as a normal alternative route for venous return from the abdomen. It is also incriminated in some portosystemic shunts. It passes to the right of the aorta and can make an impression on the inflated oesophagus seen on radiographs. The caval veins are valve-free. Whereas the aorta and oesophagus each pass through a slippery hiatus in the diaphragm, the caudal vena cava is intimately bound to the central tendon of the diaphragm at the foramen venae cavae. Two flattened ribbon-like phrenic veins drain into it at this point.

REFERENCES

Anderson W and Anderson BG (1994) *Atlas of Canine Anatomy.* Lea and Febiger, Waverley, Baltimore

Barr F (1990) *Diagnostic Ultrasound in the Dog and Cat.* Blackwell, Oxford

Boyd JS (1992) *A Colour Atlas of Clinical Anatomy of the Dog and Cat*, pp. 200; 327 figs. Wolfe Publishing Ltd, London

Brearley MJ, Cooper JE and Sullivan M (1991) *A Colour Atlas of Small Animal Endoscopy.* Wolfe Publications Ltd, London

Budras KD, Fricke W, Henschel E and Poulsen-Mautrup C (1993) *Anatomy of the Dog, an Illustrated Text*, 3rd edn, pp. 224. Wolfe Publishing Ltd, London

Done S and Stickland N (1994) *Colour Atlas of Veterinary Anatomy of the Dog and Cat*, pp. 504; 750 figs. Wolfe Publishing Ltd, London

Evans HE (1993) *Miller's Anatomy of the Dog*, 3rd edn, pp. 1113. Saunders, Philadelphia

Feeney DA, Fletcher TF and Hardy RM (1991) *Atlas of Correlative Imaging Anatomy of the Normal Dog*, pp 382. Saunders, Philadelphia

Hudson LC and Hamilton WP (1993) *Atlas of Feline Anatomy for Veterinarians.* Saunders, Philadelphia

Rosenzweig LJ (1990) *Anatomy of the Cat: Text and Dissection Guide*, pp. 347. WCB International, Seaford, Victoria

Schaller O (ed) (1992) *Illustrated Veterinary Anatomical Nomenclature.* Ferdinand Enke Verlag, Stuttgart

Tams TR (ed) (1990) *Small Animal Endoscopy.* CV Mosby, St Louis.

The Pathophysiology of Respiratory Disease

Brendan Corcoran

INTRODUCTION

The function of the respiratory system is to allow interaction between the circulation and the atmosphere facilitating the transport of oxygen into and carbon dioxide out of the systemic circulation. Basically, this process involves two physiological mechanisms: the mechanical movement of air through the airways to and from the alveolar surface; and the movement of gases across the alveolar–capillary interface. In terms of physiology, both these mechanisms are essentially separate and operate using different physiological mechanisms. However, there are additional physiological systems, including baroreceptors, chemoreceptors and respiratory neural networks, which allow an interaction between both, and pathological changes affecting one will result in changes in the physiological response of the other.

MECHANICS OF AIR MOVEMENT IN THE RESPIRATORY SYSTEM

Air movement during the respiratory cycle

The movement of air in and out of the lungs is determined by the mechanical properties of the conducting airways, the lung parenchyma and the chest wall (rib cage and diaphragm). The neural control of respiration is very complicated and a detailed description is not necessary in this chapter. Suffice it to say that neural activation of the muscles of respiration initiates the inspiratory part of the respiratory cycle.

At the end-expiratory point, the resting lung volume is the functional residual capacity (FRC) and the pleural pressure is marginally negative relevant to atmospheric pressure (Figure 2.1). As inspiration begins, with contraction of the diaphragm (phrenic nerve activation), pleural pressure becomes more negative than atmosphere and air is drawn into the airways and lung. This procedure continues until the desired tidal volume is achieved or the limits of lung and chest wall expansion are reached. During normal breathing, expansion of the lung activates lung stretch receptors which suppress inspiratory drive.

In the dog and cat, there is no end-inspiratory pause and expiration begins immediately. Air is moved back out of the lungs by the elastic recoil of the lung and the relaxation of the chest wall. In disease situations or during strenuous exercise, recruitment of expiratory muscles will assist expiratory airflow. At the end-expiratory point, there is a short pause before the next breath.

This simple 'bellows' mechanism is extremely efficient in ventilating the lungs, but its function can be severely impaired by disease processes affecting the mechanics of the airways, lungs and chest wall.

The transmural pressure changes in the trachea should also be considered, as they are important in understanding the mechanical events in conditions such as laryngeal paralysis and tracheal collapse (see

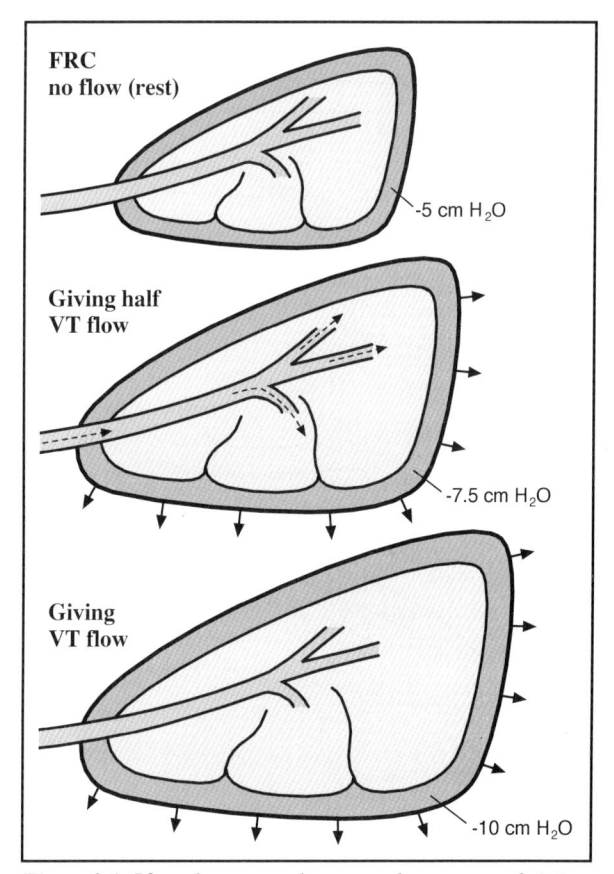

FRC
no flow (rest)

-5 cm H_2O

Giving half
VT flow

-7.5 cm H_2O

Giving
VT flow

-10 cm H_2O

Figure 2.1: Pleural pressure changes and movement of air into the lungs. VT, tidal volume; FRC, functional residual capacity.

also Equal pressure point) (Figure 2.2). On the basis of their response to transmural pressure changes, the cartilaginous airways can be divided into two segments equivalent to the extrathoracic trachea and the intrathoracic trachea and mainstem bronchi. During inspiration, the change in pleural pressure exerts a collapsing force on the extrathoracic airway while exerting retractive forces on the intrathoracic airways. The semi-rigid structure of the extrathoracic airway and the muscular control of laryngeal patency opposes this collapse, allowing inspiratory airflow. During expiration, the opposite applies. The transmural pressure across the intrathoracic airways favours collapse, while the extrathoracic airway is distended. The structure of the intrathoracic airways resists collapse and so complete expiration of the tidal volume can be achieved. In tracheal collapse and laryngeal paralysis, the mechanisms opposing the collapsing forces on the airway during inspiration and expiration are compromised resulting in inspiratory and/or expiratory airflow obstruction.

Pulmonary, airway and chest wall mechanics

The mechanical properties of the respiratory system can be divided into two areas. The static components of respiratory mechanics reflect the behaviour of the system when there is no air movement and include static compliance, elastic recoil and lung volumes. The dynamic components are concerned with mechanical behaviour of the respiratory system when there is air movement and include flow patterns (laminar and turbulent), resistance and dynamic compliance.

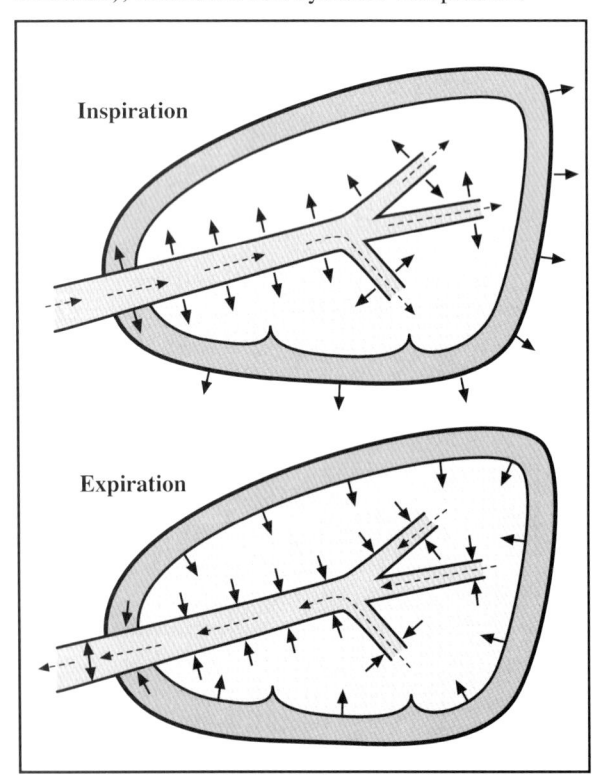

Figure 2.2: Transmural pressure changes across the intra- and extrathoracic airways during the expiratory cycle.

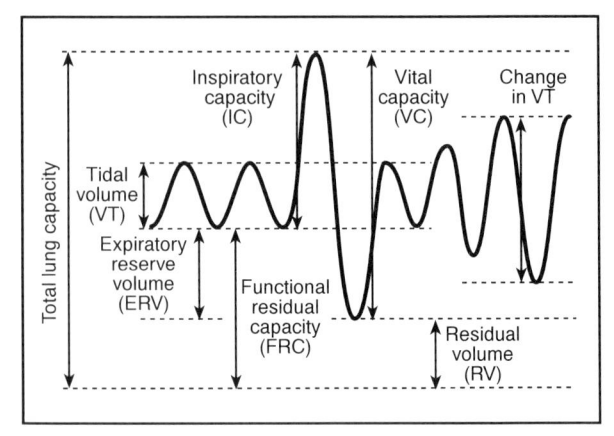

Figure 2.3: Lung volume divisions.

Lung volumes

The volume of air in the lungs is determined by the elastic properties of the lungs and chest wall, and the extent of the mechanical forces (muscular strength) the individual can achieve. The lung divisions consist of four volume divisions and two capacity divisions (Figure 2.3). At the end-expiratory point, the amount of air in the lungs is the FRC. The FRC consists of the expiratory reserve volume (ERV) and the reserve volume (RV). With an additional expiratory effort, the ERV can be expired, leaving the RV. The tidal volume (VT) is the volume inspired during quiet breathing. As oxygen requirements increase, the tidal volume can be increased to set limits determined by the ERV and the inspiratory reserve volume (IRV). The ERV and IRV are the vital capacity (VC) or the total volume range the individual can utilize. The volume limits, particularly the IRV, can be severely compromised by lung parenchymal and pleural diseases. When the IRV is reduced to such an extent that tidal volume cannot deliver adequate alveolar ventilation, the individual increases the respiratory rate in order to maintain minute volume and minute alveolar ventilation.

Static compliance

Static compliance is the relationship between volume and the pressure required to maintain that volume in the respiratory system (unit volume/unit pressure; l/cmH_2O or l/kPa). In the lung, compliance (CL) is an index of the distensibility of the lungs and is the reciprocal of elastance (Figure 2.4). A reduction in compliance equates with an increased stiffness of the lung and is classically seen in lung parenchymal diseases such as pneumonia and chronic pulmonary interstitial disease. If lung compliance is reduced the tidal volume excursion is limited and so the ability to control minute volume relies more on the respiratory rate.

The compliance of the whole respiratory system (Ctot) includes the lung (CL) and chest wall compliance (CW) and is an inverse sum relationship, such that $1/C\text{tot} = 1/CL + 1/CW$. CL and CW are of roughly equal magnitude in normal individuals. Because of

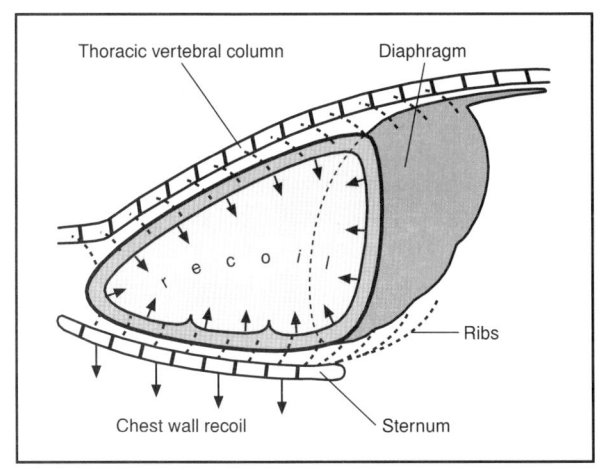

Figure 2.4: *Recoil forces on the lungs and chest wall.*

these factors, the airway pressure needed to artificially ventilate paralysed or thoracotomy patients is approximately twice normal pleural pressure.

Without the chest wall (rib cage and diaphragm), at the end of expiration the lungs would collapse due to their elastic recoil properties. The tendency of the chest wall is therefore to recoil outwards opposing the collapsing tendency of the lungs. This can be appreciated at thoracotomy, where the lungs are seen to collapse once the chest wall is opened to the atmosphere. During breathing, the compliance of the chest wall assists ventilation up to approximately 60% of vital capacity, but then opposes further lung expansion due to its elastic recoil. Conditions that alter chest wall compliance will affect lung expansion and include rib cage puncture, flail chest, diaphragmatic rupture, neuromuscular diseases, abdominal distension due to conditions such as obesity, pregnancy and gastric dilation, and chest wall obesity. Pleural effusions function to restrict lung expansion, and if the effusion is regarded as part of the chest wall, then it can be said to reduce chest wall compliance.

Respiratory resistance and dynamic compliance

Resistance is the ratio of pressure to flow ($cmH_2O/l/s$ or kPa/l/s). Dynamic compliance ($Cdyn$) is the volume change associated with the pressure difference between the end-inspiratory and end-expiratory points, and is often used as an index of peripheral airway calibre and patency. The pressure required to produce flow in the respiratory system must overcome the elastic recoil forces of the lungs and the resistance to flow through the airways. The total resistance to flow is therefore the airway's resistance (Raw) plus the lung tissue resistance. In the normal individual, the tissue resistance is low and it is the Raw that is the main determinant of total resistance. However, because the lung parenchyma exerts retractive forces on airway walls, there is a hyperbolic (non-linear) relationship between lung volume and Raw such that at low lung volumes Raw is high and decreases as the lung volume increases.

The Raw can be partitioned on the basis of the major airway sites that contribute to resistance. Up to 50% of the Raw is contributed by the upper airways, including the nasal passages, pharynx and larynx. Mouth breathing, removing the nasal component, significantly lowers this division of resistance and so is a manoeuvre commonly used during exercise or when there is severe respiratory disease. The laryngeal component of the upper airway resistance can increase dramatically with laryngeal paralysis resulting in stridor, exercise intolerance and cyanosis.

The remainder of Raw is made up of the tracheal and bronchial resistance, particularly bronchi of 2–4 mm diameter, where there are minimal amounts of cartilage but large amounts of smooth muscle. Although resistance is inversely proportional to the fourth power of the radius of the airway (Poiseuille's Law), the contribution of the smaller bronchi and bronchioles to resistance is low because of their large combined cross-sectional area.

The resistance of the airways will be altered by diseases affecting the structural rigidity of the airway (tracheal collapse), the tone of smooth muscle in the airway wall (feline asthma syndrome), extramural compression (pneumonia, neoplasia, interstitial and alveolar oedema), and accumulation of exudates in the airway lumen (chronic bronchitis, bronchopneumonia) and the thickness of the airway walls (oedema, inflammatory processes).

Dynamic opening and closing of alveoli and airways (see Static compliance)

Equal pressure point
As the lung deflates, the pleural pressure becomes more positive than airway pressure pushing air out of the lungs. Although the alveoli do not collapse due to their inherent surface tension, the airways can collapse and the point at which they collapse is close to the equal pressure point. The equal pressure point is the position within the respiratory tract where the pressures outside and inside the airway are the same. In diseases that affect the structure of the airway or the surrounding lung parenchyma, the airway may collapse during expiration. In the normal individual, dynamic compression of the airways is restricted to the non-cartilaginous airways distal to the lobar bronchi. However, if the equal pressure point moves more cranially, airway sections can collapse before the inspired tidal volume has been removed. This can result in expiratory dyspnoea and wheezing and coughing. This dynamic airway compression mechanism underlies the expiratory airflow obstruction found with tracheal collapse and pulmonary neoplasia, where the animal is breathing at normal tidal volumes, and in bronchoconstrictive diseases (e.g. feline asthma) and emphysema where hyperinflation has occurred. In these conditions there is premature closure of airways

that normally do not close during expiration (trachea and mainstem bronchi), resulting in entrapment of air and expiratory dyspnoea.

Alveolar surface tension

Considering the geometry of the lung alveoli, a very large distending pressure would be required to open collapsed alveoli. The pressure necessary to keep alveoli open would be much greater than the pressure actually achieved in the pleural space in normal individuals. To overcome this problem the alveolar surface tension is kept low by the secretion of surfactant from type II alveolar pneumocytes. This also prevents the closure of alveoli during expiration. It can therefore be appreciated that alveolar collapse associated with disease processes, either causing alveolar filling with exudates or altering surfactant production, can be difficult to reverse and areas of lung can become nonfunctional. A similar situation can also occur with prolonged recumbency or prolonged anaesthesia. In the latter case, forced lung inflation can easily be carried out, while in severe lung disease forced positive pressure ventilation can be beneficial.

AIRWAY RECEPTORS AND AIRWAY REFLEXES

Control of the pattern of breathing, bronchomotor tone and the activation of protective reflexes, such as coughing, involves reflex neural mechanisms. Although a detailed discussion of the reflexogenic control of the respiratory system is not required in this text, certain aspects of these mechanisms explain some of the clinical findings in respiratory disease.

The reflexogenic basis of coughing

Coughing is an important protective mechanism in that it permits the removal of material from the airways which cannot be removed by other lung defence mechanisms. It is particularly useful in removing accumulated mucus in inflammatory airway and lung disease, assisting the mucociliary clearance of material, expelling inhaled particulate material and protecting the airways against further inhalation of noxious material.

The cough reflex involves activation of both mechanoreceptors, which predominate in the larger airways, and chemoreceptors (irritant receptor) which are found in the medium size airways. Receptor numbers are particularly high in the larynx, the mid-trachea and at the tracheal bifurcation. Only small numbers of cough receptors are found in the smaller airways and none in the respiratory bronchioles and alveoli. Activation of the mechanoreceptors by intra- or extraluminal pressure, or of chemoreceptors by inflammatory mediators or other irritants, elicits coughing. In many cardiopulmonary diseases, such as tracheal collapse, primary neoplasia and left-sided congestive heart fail-

ure, it is extraluminal mechanical compression that is the prime cause of coughing. In diseases affecting the lower airways, such as bronchopneumonia and pulmonary/alveolar oedema, coughing is often soft and ineffectual due to the paucity of receptors at these sites. The remainder of conditions, such as acute tracheobronchitis and chronic bronchitis and asthma, elicit coughing through a combination of activation of chemoreceptors (irritants/inflammation) and mechanoreceptors (airway mucus).

The pathophysiological basis of tachypnoea and dyspnoea

The afferent input to the respiratory centres from the lung involves stretch receptors which respond to the mechanical distortion of the airways and lung parenchyma during respiration. In simple terms, braking mechanisms serve to stop inspiration and expiration at the appropriate points in the respiratory cycles. The overall response is to modify vagal and phrenic nerve output accordingly. Inspiration is controlled by the slowly adapting stretch receptors (SAR), whose activity increases as the lungs expand, while expiration is controlled by the rapidly adapting (deflation) receptors (RAR). The RAR receptors have also been called irritant receptors in the past and may have a role in the airway response to inhaled irritants, including coughing and bronchoconstriction, and initiate spontaneous deep inspirations (gasps, sighs, augmented breaths).

There is an additional group of afferent receptors which do not respond to changes in pulmonary mechanics (C-fibre afferents), but whose activity may be affected by inflammatory mediators. Activation of these receptors may cause a pulmonary chemoreflex involving bronchoconstriction, bradycardia, hypotension and rapid shallow breathing.

Apart from their potential role in controlling bronchomotor tone and coughing these receptors are involved in the altered respiratory breathing patterns seen with respiratory disease. While the respiratory response to changes in blood gases and acid-base balance with hypoxia and hypercapnia involves arterial chemoreceptors, airway and lung diseases which activate pulmonary stretch receptors may also contribute to the tachypnoea and dyspnoea seen with cardiopulmonary disease. Indeed, in the case of pulmonary thromboembolism, it is the interference with stretch receptor activity rather than the blood gas abnormalities that determines the type of breathing pattern.

PULMONARY VENTILATION

Pulmonary ventilation is the total amount of gas available to the alveoli for the transfer of oxygen and carbon dioxide. Minute ventilation is the tidal volume multiplied by the respiratory frequency. Only a proportion of the inspired air (alveolar ventilation; VA) contributes to gaseous exchange while the remainder stays in the anatomical dead space. Furthermore, of the alveolar ventilation a proportion enters inadequately perfused alveoli (even in normal subjects) and is called the physiological dead space. The anatomical and physiological dead space are roughly equal in normal individuals, but in disease the size of the physiological dead space can increase. Anatomical dead space becomes a functionally important determinant of effective alveolar ventilation when animals are connected to anaesthetic apparatus or the tidal volume is excessively low. In the latter situation, the individual may rely on rapid respiration to allow passive gas diffusion into the alveoli. In respiratory medicine alveolar hypoventilation is usually associated with upper airway obstruction, although severe pleural effusions can also be responsible. The net effect of alveolar hypoventilation is hypercapnia with acidosis and varying degrees of hypoxaemia.

Ventilation–perfusion relationships

Under ideal circumstances each alveolus would receive an equal share of the inspired air and the same amount of mixed venous blood. This would result in the optimal oxygenation of blood and the relationship between alveolar ventilation (VA) and perfusion (Q) would be 1.0. However, even in normal individuals this ideal relationship does not occur and there are differences in the VA/Q ratio in different areas of the lung. Where the VA/Q ratio deviates greatly from the normal, ventilation–perfusion mismatching (imbalance, inequality) is said to occur. If an alveolus is poorly ventilated, as with bronchopneumonia, but adequately perfused, the VA/Q is less than normal. Where there is adequate ventilation but reduced tissue perfusion, as with pulmonary thromboembolism or intrapulmonary haemorrhage, VA/Q is greater than normal. The usual situation in respiratory disease is to have areas of lung that are over-ventilated (high VA/Q) or under-ventilated (low VA/Q). VA/Q inequalities result in inefficient gas transfer, with complex effects on the removal of CO_2 from the blood and movement of O_2 across the alveolar membranes.

The mixing of blood (venous) from poorly ventilated areas of lung with properly arterialized blood lowers the overall PaO_2 causing hypoxaemia. This phenomenon is known as venous admixture. Where there are VA/Q inequalities the lungs will attempt to compensate by constricting the pulmonary arterial bed (hypoxaemic vasoconstriction) or the airways (hypercapnic bronchoconstriction) of affected regions, so reducing venous admixture. This may improve the overall respiratory gas exchange ratio (respiratory quotient; the ratio of O_2 uptake to CO_2 removal). Where severe disease is present, such manoeuvres will have very little effect. The effect of such prolonged vasoconstrictor or bronchoconstrictor effects on the function of the lung units affected is not known, but may underlie some of the lung parenchymal changes seen with chronic respiratory conditions.

Diffusion impairment

The proper transfer of gases between the pulmonary circulation and alveoli depends on a normal alveolar-capillary interface. Diseases that affect this interface result in hypoxaemia, often with normo- or hypocapnia due to increased ventilatory drive. Diffusion impairment, however, is a reasonably rare cause of blood gas abnormalities, although diffuse interstitial changes, such as with chronic pulmonary interstitial disease and interstitial oedema, are recognized causes of hypoxaemia.

Interpretation of blood gas analysis results

Hypoxaemia

The normal arterial oxygen concentration (PaO_2) is approximately 90–100 mmHg and is the most accurate indicator of respiratory function. When PaO_2 is less than 60 mmHg hypoxaemia exists and when below 30–40 mmHg clinical signs of cyanosis and central nervous system abnormalities occur. Hypoxaemia can be a consequence of alveolar hypoventilation, where concurrent hypercapnia is usually found, ventilation-perfusion mismatching and venous admixture with anatomical and physiological shunting of blood. Hypoxaemia with hypocapnia or normocapnia is often associated with pulmonary thromboembolism, where increased lung afferent nerve fibre activity, secondary to the embolism, results in tachypnoea and thereby increases the 'blow off' of CO_2.

The extent of oxygen deficit is also determined by the degree of oxygen saturation of haemoglobin and amount of dissolved oxygen in the blood, and these parameters can further complicate interpretations of hypoxaemia. At a PaO_2 of 80–90 mmHg, saturation of haemoglobin approaches 100%, but as the PaO_2 falls, the ratio of oxygenated to deoxygenated haemoglobin changes, and at PaO_2 of less than 50 mmHg, cyanosis can occur (deoxyHb > 5 g/dl). It can be readily appreciated that the tendency to develop cyanosis is greater if there is polycythaemia than anaemia. However, as PaO_2 is the easiest parameter to calculate, this is routinely used to assess the degree of respiratory impairment.

Hypercapnia and hypocapnia

The arterial CO_2 concentration ($PaCO_2$) is largely determined by ventilation, although, metabolic factors may also be involved. Since the removal of CO_2 is dependent on the partial pressure of CO_2 in the alveoli ($PACO_2$), a rise in the $PaCO_2$ reflects reduction in the removal rate of CO_2 from the alveoli. Hypercapnia therefore is associated with hypoventilation and is an indicator of alveolar minute ventilation. The rise in $PaCO_2$ will, however, stimulate respiration which can normalize the $PaCO_2$ level or even result in hypocapnia.

Hypercapnia exists where the $PaCO_2$ concentration is above 60 mmHg and is usually associated with hypoxaemia. When severe hypercapnia exists ($PaCO_2$ > 100 mmHg) respiratory depression and coma can occur. Hypocapnia is present if the $PaCO_2$ concentration is less than 15–20 mmHg and can interfere with blood flow to the central nervous system. Hypocapnia with hypoxaemia is associated with marked hyperventilation.

Differentiation of alveolar hypoventilation from VA/Q inequalities

Alveolar hypoventilation and VA/Q inequalities are the major causes of hypoxaemia and can be differentiated from each other by calculating the alveolar-arterial oxygen pressure gradient ($A–a$). The $A–a$ gradient is calculated from the formula $150 - (PaCO_2/0.8)$, with a value equal to or less than 10 mmHg occurring in normals or with alveolar hypoventilation, and an $A–a$ greater than 10 mmHg in VA/Q inequality. Respiratory failure with hypoxaemia and normo- or hypocapnia is classified as type I, and such cases will benefit from oxygen supplementation. Hypercapnic respiratory failure, typically associated with alveolar hypoventilation, is classified as type II. Oxygen supplementation should be used with care in such cases, as excess oxygen can inhibit respiratory drive, and further exacerbate the degree of alveolar hypoventilation.

AIRWAY AND LUNG PROTECTIVE MECHANISMS

Mucociliary clearance of airway mucus

The airway lining, at least in the larger airways, consists of a layer of ciliated epithelium interspersed with mucus-secreting goblet cells. The number of ciliated epithelial cells decreases in the lower airways and they are absent from the alveoli. On top of the cilia, there is a mucus blanket which entraps inhaled debris. Material from the alveoli may reach this mucus blanket because of the surface tension effects of surfactant. Using this mechanism, mucus produced in the lower airways either as fine strands or droplets can be moved to the larger airways.

Airway mucus is a complex visco-elastic material consisting of glycoproteins (mucin), lipids, carbohydrates and proteoglycans. The flow and deformation characteristics of mucus allow it to be transported by beating of the cilia on the epithelial surface. The beating cilia move the blanket of mucus in a rostral direction towards the pharynx where the material is coughed up and swallowed. Beneath the epithelium there are additional mucous glands in the submucosal layer and in disease situations the amount of mucus production may increase to assist removal of particulate debris. Where there is airway inflammation and a purulent reaction, such as bronchitis, the mucociliary mechanism will help to remove this material. In chronic bronchitis, where there is excess mucus production with increased goblet cell numbers and hyperplasia of the submucosal mucous glands, and damage to the cilia or loss of ciliated epithelium, mucus becomes trapped with resultant mucous plugging of airways. In such situations, coughing and the alveolar defence mechanisms protect the airways. In other conditions, such as acute tracheobronchitis and immotile cilia syndrome (ciliary dyskinesia), there may be ineffectual beating of the cilia. In the latter case this can result in bronchopneumonia and severe respiratory impairment.

Protective mechanisms of the lower airways and alveoli

While material present in the larger airways is removed by the mucociliary clearance mechanism, material that enters the lower airways or alveoli or is produced in response to inflammatory reactions is more effectively removed by cellular mechanisms. The alveolar epithelium consists of type I and type II pneumocytes which abut the capillary endothelium. The type II cells secrete surfactant. Interspersed between these cells are alveolar macrophages which phagocytose inhaled debris and foreign material. The macrophages re-enter the circulation and remove the material from the lung. However, in severe inflammatory diseases, macrophages may accumulate within the alveolar walls and fibroblasts may migrate to these sites resulting in alveolar fibrosis. Such changes, if unchecked, can result in permanent loss of alveoli for ventilation.

FURTHER READING

Jacobs G (1995) Cyanosis. In: *Textbook of Veterinary Internal Medicine* ed. SJ Ettinger, pp. 95–100. WB Saunders, Philadelphia
DiBartola SP and DeMorais HSA (1992) Respiratory acid–base disorders. In: *Fluid Therapy in Small Animal Practice*, ed. SP DiBartola, pp. 258–275. WB Saunders, Philadelphia

The Pathophysiology of Heart Failure

Joanna Dukes McEwan

Heart failure may be defined as circulatory failure where the heart is unable to maintain an adequate circulation for the needs of the body at normal venous pressures (Opie, 1991; Olivier, 1993).

NORMAL CARDIOVASCULAR PHYSIOLOGY

A brief review of the normal homeostatic mechanisms involved in maintaining the cardiovascular system is necessary to understand how these may become inappropriate in the heart failure patient.

Definitions

Systole is the contraction phase of the cardiac cycle.
Diastole is the relaxation phase of the cardiac cycle.
Stroke volume (SV) is the volume of blood ejected by each heart beat.
Heart rate (HR) is the number of heart beats per minute.
Cardiac output (CO) is the quantity of blood ejected by the heart into the circulation in 1 minute.

Cardiac output

Cardiac output = Stroke volume x heart rate
The four major determinants of cardiac output are:

- Heart rate
- Preload
- Afterload
- Contractility.

The *preload* is the end-diastolic volume or pressure within the left ventricle prior to systole – essentially, it is a concept to indicate the filling pressure of a ventricle.

The filling pressure determines the length to which myocardial fibres (and sarcomeres – the contractile units) are stretched. This correlates with the numbers of calcium-activated cross bridges between filaments of actin and myosin, which produce a more forceful contraction (Figure 3.1) (Knight, 1989). This is the basis of the Frank-Starling mechanism (Figure 3.2).

The Frank–Starling mechanism. Within a given

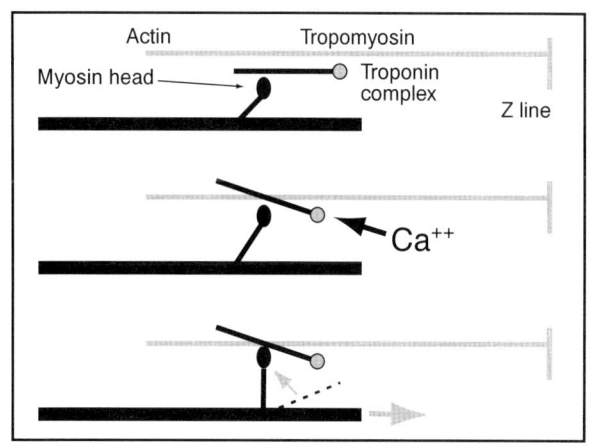

Figure 3.1: *The contractile proteins and cross-bridging.*

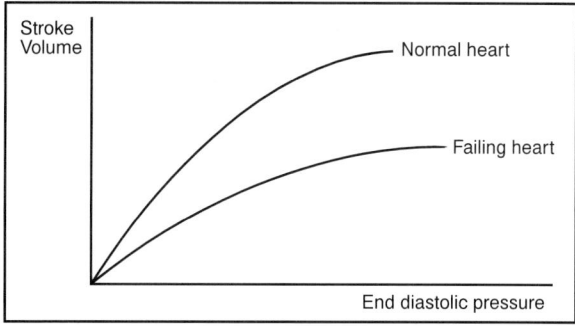

Figure 3.2: *The Frank–Starling relationship.*

range of sarcomere stretch in response to increased preload, there is a more forceful contraction, i.e. the higher the filling pressure, the higher the stroke volume. This depends on the myocardial fibres of the heart being on the ascending part of the Frank-Starling curve (Figure 3.2).

Contractility (inotropy). The contractility of a myocardial cell can be defined as the strength at which it contracts. The definition excludes resting fibre length (so the Frank-Starling mechanism) and contractility can be increased by catecholamines. Contractility occurs during systole and correlates with cytosolic calcium ion concentration.

Relaxation (lusitropy). The relaxation of a myocardial cell during diastole is not merely a passive process, but involves active uptake of calcium ions by the sarcoplasmic reticulum. It is an important process for adequate diastolic function of the myocardium.

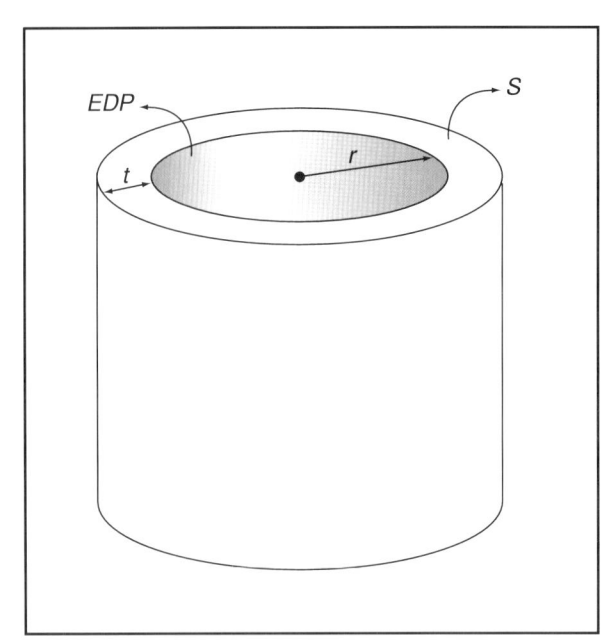

Figure 3.3: *The La Place relationship.*

The *afterload* is equivalent to the *myocardial wall stress* and is a function of the *impedance* (resistance to ejection from the particular ventricle) and the peripheral arterial resistance or *total peripheral resistance* (TPR). It is affected primarily by the intraventricular pressure and chamber size (see the La Place relationship). Often, the mean arterial pressure (MAP) is used as a measure of the left ventricular afterload in the absence of outflow tract obstruction.

The *La Place relationship* describes the physiological relationship between systolic ventricular myocardial wall stress (*S*), the intraventricular end-diastolic pressure (*EDP*), the internal radius of the ventricle (*r*) and the wall thickness of the ventricle (*t*). The ventricle can be imagined as a thick-walled cylinder for ease of understanding this illustration (Kittleson, 1988) (Figure 3.3).

$$\text{Wall stress } (S) = \frac{\text{intraventricular pressure } (EDP) \times \text{internal radius } (r)}{\text{wall thickness } (t)}$$

The relationship can be applied to either ventricle. It is important to understand how chronic anatomical adaptations to various heart diseases follow the La Place relationship; ventricular hypertrophy will help to minimize myocardial wall stress and consequently myocardial oxygen consumption.

Mean arterial pressure (MAP). This term is used as an estimate for 'average' blood pressure. It is not simply mid-way between systolic blood pressure (*SBP*) and diastolic blood pressure (*DBP*), but can be calculated from the formula:

$$MAP = DBP + (SBP–DBP)/3$$

Many indirect techniques for determining blood pressure will accurately identify this value (e.g. oscillometric technique).

The cardiac output (*CO*) and total peripheral resistance (*TPR*) are the important factors governing mean arterial pressure.

$$MAP = CO \times TPR$$

Neuroendocrine control of blood pressure and volume

The homeostatic priority of the body with regard to the cardiovascular system is to maintain mean arterial pressure.

The autonomic nervous system

Any fall in blood pressure (e.g. haemorrhage) is detected by the baroreceptors in the aortic arch and the carotid sinus. Afferent traffic via the vagus and glossopharyngeal nerves respectively causes a reflex *increase in sympathetic drive*, through the autonomic nervous system and increased catecholamine release from the adrenal medulla. Sympathetic stimulation of β_1 receptors results in increased heart rate and contractility, which increases mean arterial pressure. Stimulation of the α_1 receptors results in contraction of vascular smooth muscle. Arteriolar vasoconstriction causes an increase in mean arterial pressure, and venous vasoconstriction results in increased venous pressure and venous return to the heart, causing increased cardiac filling pressures (the preload), thereby utilizing the Frank–Starling mechanism.

The parasympathetic nervous system is dominant in the relaxed animal without heart failure; the vagal tone to the sinoatrial node is dominant, resulting in sinus arrhythmia and wandering pacemaker in the dog or an overall slower heart rate (sinus rhythm) in an unstressed cat. Some dogs (e.g. brachiocephalic breeds) with inherently high vagal tone will demonstrate first and sometimes second degree (Mobitz type I) atrioventricular block indicating the vagal influence at the atrioventricular node. If blood pressure falls, then the vagal tone decreases, with an increase in the sympathetic drive.

The balance of the autonomic nervous system is governed by the medulla oblongata in cardioinhibitory and vasomotor centres, which is a simplistic view of the complex interactions between the afferent inputs, medulla oblongata nuclei and tracts, hypothalamus and cerebellum.

The renin–angiotensin–aldosterone system (RAAS)

The juxtaglomerular apparatus of the kidneys plays an important part in the control of blood volume and blood pressure. Renin is released from this area:

- In response to adrenoceptor stimulation
- In response to reduced local perfusion (mediated through baroreceptors)
- In response to some chemoreceptors (macula densa) (Braunwald, 1992).

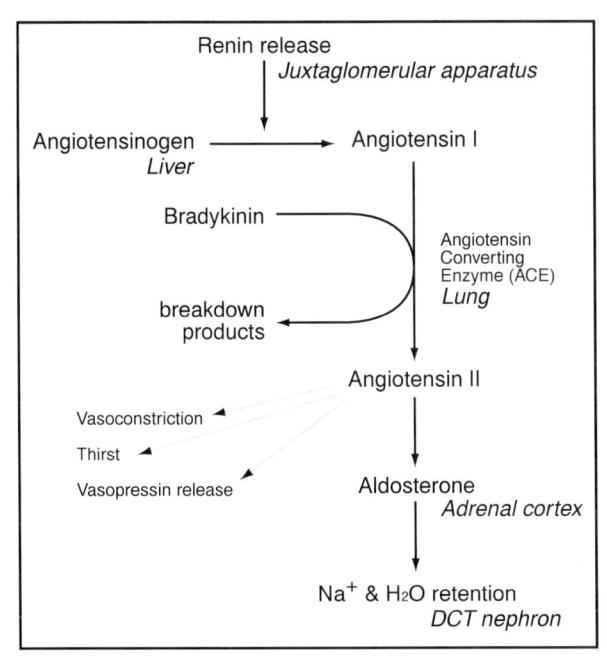

Figure 3.4: *The renin–angiotensin–aldosterone system (RAAS).*

Renin released into the circulation acts on circulating angiotensinogen (renin substrate) which is produced by the liver, to form angiotensin I. Angiotensin converting enzyme (ACE) is tissue bound and located on the luminal aspect of endothelial cells throughout the vascular system. Angiotensin converting enzyme (mainly in the lung) cleaves a dipeptide unit off the decapeptide angiotensin I to form the octapeptide, angiotensin II (Garrison and Peach, 1991) (Figure 3.4).

Angiotensin II is very active, and has a number of effects:

Vasoconstriction, which increases mean arterial pressure.

Increased synthesis and release of aldosterone from the zona glomerulosa of the adrenal cortex, with effects on the distal tubules of the nephron, resulting in *increased sodium and water retention.* Increased fluid and sodium retention increases plasma volume in order to improve diastolic filling pressures, again to utilize the Frank–Starling mechanism.

The glomerular filtration fraction is increased in the nephron through efferent arteriolar constriction and mesangial contraction (Braunwald, 1992). This increases sodium and water retention (Hamlin, 1988).

Sodium retention via a direct effect on renal tubules (Braunwald, 1992).

Increased thirst is mediated by a central nervous system action, again adding to plasma volume (Michell, 1991).

Increased synthesis and release of arginine vasopressin (AVP), otherwise known as antidiuretic hormone (ADH), via effects on the supraoptic nucleus of the hypothalamus and the neurohypophysis (posterior pituitary).

Myocardial effects: the force of contraction is increased by allowing increased entry of calcium ions through voltage sensitive channels during the plateau phase of the action potential (Garrison and Peach, 1991). *Myocardial hypertrophy* (and vascular smooth muscle hypertrophy) occurs in some species (Braunwald, 1992).

Increased noradrenaline synthesis and release throughout the autonomic nervous system, including myocardial sources (Garrison and Peach, 1991).

Increased catecholamine release from the chromaffin cells of the adrenal medulla (Garrison and Peach, 1991).

Angiotensin converting enzyme, although so-named in this setting, is actually a fairly non-specific enzyme cleaving dipeptide units off a number of substrates. *Bradykinin*, a potent vasodilator, is broken down by the same enzyme, here called kininase II (Garrison and Peach, 1991). Consequently, high angiotensin converting enzyme activity results in low naturally circulating vasodilators, helping to maintain blood pressure.

Vasopressin

This substance is released from the posterior pituitary as described previously:

- In response to angiotensin II
- By stimulation of baroreceptors by reduced CNS perfusion pressures and stimulation of chemoreceptors (Hays, 1991).

Vasopressin is a potent vasoconstrictor and high circulating levels result in increased fluid retention from the distal tubules of the nephron. Vasopressin can result in increased adrenocorticotrophic hormone secretion and cortisol levels (Garrison and Peach, 1991).

These effects together will increase volume load and mean arterial pressure. Maintenance of arterial blood pressure is *critical* for adequate perfusion of the brain and the heart. These homeostatic mechanisms are life saving in the acute hypovolaemia of haemorrhage or shock.

Atrial natriuresis factor (ANF) or atrial natriuretic peptide (ANP) is a natural antagonist to the consequences of activating the sympathetic nervous system, angiotensin II and vasopressin. ANF is released in response to atrial distension by the atrial myocytes. This occurs following restoration of normal blood pressure and circulating volume via increased cardiac output, vasoconstriction and sodium and water retention (Michell, 1991). It therefore *protects the central circulation against volume overload* (Braunwald, 1992). It also reduces tachycardia by modulating baroreceptor function (Braunwald, 1992). Levels of ANF correlate with plasma renin activity and noradrenaline concentration.

New York Heart Association classification of heart failure	
Class of heart failure	**Clinical signs**
Class 1	Evidence of heart disease on clinical examination No signs of heart failure Normal exercise capacity, unless severe strenuous exercise
Class 2	Signs of heart failure on exercise/excitement Normal at rest May or may not have radiographic evidence of cardiomegaly
Class 3	Comfortable at rest but exacerbation of signs of heart failure on minimal exertion Radiographic evidence of cardiomegaly
Class 4	Severe signs of heart failure at rest Postural compensations (orthopnoea etc.)

The International Small Animal Cardiac Health Council (ISACHC) system of heart failure classification (ISACHC, 1995)		
Class of heart failure	**Clinical signs**	
Class I	*Asymptomatic* Signs of heart disease on examination (e.g. murmur)	IA Minimal/no cardiac enlargement
	No clinical signs	IB Some cardiac enlargement present
Class II	*Mild–moderate heart failure*	Signs of cardiac failure: exercise intolerance, coughing, dyspnoea, ascites
Class III	*Advanced heart failure* Severe dyspnoea/marked ascites/hypoperfusion at rest	IIIA Home care is possible
		IIIB Hospitalization is mandatory: life-threatening pulmonary oedema/ pleural effusion

Table 3.1: Heart failure classification systems.

PATHOPHYSIOLOGY OF HEART FAILURE

It should be emphasized that heart failure is *not* the same as heart disease: a patient may have clinical evidence of heart disease (e.g. a heart murmur) which is compensated for by the above homeostatic mechanisms, often for years. Heart failure is a syndrome whereby the above homeostatic mechanisms of the heart are unable to maintain an adequate circulation for the needs of the body, or they result in excessive venous pressures.

Heart failure may be classified in a number of different ways: the presenting and clinical signs; the pathophysiology; the severity of clinical signs, giving the New York Heart Association functional classification of heart failure (Knight, 1989) or the ISACHC system of heart failure classification (ISACHC, 1995) (Table 3.1); and the anatomical basis of the heart failure.

From an anatomical basis, the cause of the heart failure can be classified by underlying disease or defect, but it is less cumbersome to subdivide into one of the divisions given below (Opie, 1991; Olivier, 1993).

Pathophysiological method of describing heart failure

- Volume overload
- Pressure overload
- Myocardial failure
- Diastolic dysfunction
- Rhythm disturbance
- High output conditions.

Volume overload

- Mitral regurgitation
- Tricuspid regurgitation
- Aortic insufficiency
- Ventricular septal defect (with left to right shunting)
- Patent ductus arteriosus.

Volume overload may be defined as a condition where one or more chambers of the heart handles a volume of blood greater than the forward stroke volume. In mitral regurgitation, the left atrium and left ventricle are volume overloaded, and the backward stroke volume (mitral regurgitation) may exceed forward stroke volume (into the aorta). As a result, the left ventricular volume is increased at the end of diastole, and the ventricle dilates. Cardiac output is maintained, nevertheless, by the Frank–Starling mechanism, as ventricular filling pressures are increased via venoconstriction and plasma volume expansion. In the long term, compensatory left ventricular eccentric hypertrophy develops, which optimizes mechanical efficiency according to the La Place relationship (Figure 3.3). Although the dilation of the left ventricle would normally result in increased left ventricular diastolic wall stress, hypertrophy of the left ventricle occurs in proportion to the left ventricular dilatation (eccentric hypertrophy) by replication of sarcomeres in series (Kittleson, 1988); this maintains myocardial wall stress within normal limits during the compensated mitral regurgitation.

Whether or not a chronic volume overloaded ventricle develops secondary myocardial failure is determined in part by the pressure of the receiving chamber. With mitral regurgitation, the left ventricle is partly pumping into a low pressure left atrium, and myocardial failure is not common. With aortic regurgitation, all the left ventricular stroke volume is into the high pressure aorta and myocardial failure commonly occurs (Braunwald, 1992). Similarly, patients with patent ductus arteriosus are more likely to develop secondary myocardial failure than those with ventricular septal defect.

Pressure overload

- Aortic stenosis
- Pulmonic stenosis
- Systemic hypertension
- Pulmonary hypertension.

A pressure overload is an increase in impedance to ventricular ejection of blood, as with any form of ventricular outflow tract obstruction. Because the relevant ventricle has to overcome the resistance to ejection of blood, systolic intraventricular pressures are increased. With a pressure overload such as aortic stenosis, the resistance to left ventricular ejection is marked, and ventricular systolic pressures will be high to overcome the increased impedance. This would result in increased systolic myocardial wall stress if the dimensions of the left ventricle remained unchanged. However, typically left ventricular hypertrophy develops, with an increase in wall thickness. This type of hypertrophy which compensates for pressure overload is concentric hypertrophy; myocardial cells become 'fatter' as sarcomeres replicate in parallel (Kittleson,

1988). Unfortunately, the coronary vasculature does not develop in proportion to the left ventricular hypertrophy and so under conditions of increased cardiac demands, the left ventricular myocardium is under considerable risk of ischaemia which may result in ectopy (ventricular arrhythmias).

Myocardial failure

- Idiopathic dilated cardiomyopathy
- Secondary to chronic volume overload
- Secondary to chronic pressure overload
- Secondary to sustained tachycardias
- Doxorubicin administration (chemotherapy)
- Taurine deficiency in cats.

In myocardial failure, the myocardial contractility is reduced, with initially normal volume and pressure loads. The cause may be known or idiopathic. Myocardial failure may be secondary to underlying heart disease, such as chronic volume overload, as well as to a variety of other causes.

Idiopathic dilated cardiomyopathy is a primary form, and underlying causes are excluded as far as possible. The clinical signs may be related to poor cardiac output (forward failure), as well as increased filling pressures (backward failure or congestive failure). There may be some eccentric myocardial hypertrophy (as the left ventricle is effectively volume overloaded), but this is not proportional to the degree of dilatation of the left ventricle: the subjective impression is of a relatively thin walled chamber.

In many cases of dilated cardiomyopathy, the left heart appears to be affected to a greater extent than the right. Obviously, the stroke volume of the left ventricle has to match that of the right ventricle, and in the early stages of myocardial failure the Frank–Starling mechanism helps to achieve this. Elevated filling pressures in the left ventricle (brought about through venoconstriction and sodium and water retention) help to increase the stroke volume – the failing left ventricle can then match the stroke volume of the relatively normal right ventricle (Levick, 1991). It is more difficult to achieve this during exercise or as left ventricular function deteriorates (Figure 3.5), and the ventricle

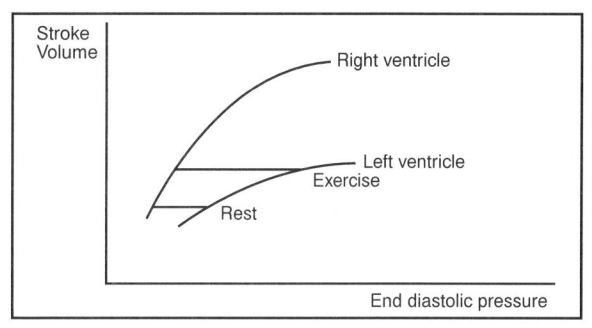

Figure 3.5: *Failing left ventricle and relatively normal right ventricle: matching stroke volumes by the Frank–Starling mechanism.*

dilates further. This is detrimental as the ventricle becomes mechanically inefficient (appreciated from the La Place relationship); this in a ventricle that can ill afford extra energy costs.

Diastolic dysfunction

The filling phase of the cardiac cycle is as important as the ejection phase. Reduced filling of the ventricle will lead to a reduced stroke volume, and elevated atrial pressures (forward and backward failure).

Diastole is more complex than systole, and consists of several phases: early passive (rapid) filling; diastasis (pause); and atrial contraction. Causes of diastolic disturbances include abnormal relaxation, abnormal chamber compliance, mechanical interference to filling, and increased heart rates.

Abnormal relaxation (lusitropy) of myocardium:

- Hypertrophic cardiomyopathy
- Myocardial ischaemia.

At the start of diastole, the rapid fall in ventricular pressure is associated with myocardial relaxation. This is an active, energy-consuming process, so relaxation may be impaired in ischaemic ventricles.

Reduced chamber compliance:

- Restrictive cardiomyopathy
- Infiltrative myocardial disease (lymphomas etc.)
- Myocardial/endocardial fibrosis
- Hypertrophic cardiomyopathy
- Pericardial disease (effusions or constrictive pericarditis).

Towards the end of diastole, ventricular filling may be reduced if the ventricle is stiff, and unable to accommodate incoming blood.

With pericardial disease, signs of right-sided failure predominate, as the right atrium and right ventricle, being low pressure systems, are more susceptible to increases in pericardial pressure and decreased compliance.

Mitral inflow obstruction:

- Mitral stenosis
- Intracardiac neoplasia.

Mechanical interference with ventricular filling can also be a cause of diastolic dysfunction.

High heart rates (including tachyarrhythmias): The diastolic period of the cardiac cycle is significantly shortened during tachycardias, which can compromise diastolic filling of the ventricles (especially the early diastolic period and diastasis). As the heart rate increases, there is increased dependence on atrial systole for ventricular filling. In tachyarrhythmias such as atrial fibrillation, the loss of atrial contraction at high heart rates can precipitate congestive failure.

Severe rhythm disturbance

Severe bradyarrhythmias and gross tachyarrhythmias may result in compromised cardiac output and reduced mean arterial pressure and signs of heart failure. Backward heart failure signs may also occur.

High output states

- Thyrotoxicosis
- Chronic severe anaemia
- Pyrexia
- Arteriovenous fistula
- Pregnancy.

Hypermetabolic or hyperkinetic states require an increased cardiac output to maintain the needs of tissue perfusion. Initial compensatory homeostatic mechanisms include increased heart rate and contractility; sodium and water retention; and vasoconstriction. Myocardial dilatation and hypertrophy may occur, and in extreme cases may even progress to heart failure. Other high output states result in reduced peripheral vascular resistance and increased venous return to the heart (preload).

'Forward' and 'backward' heart failure

It can be useful to think in terms of forward and backward failure (Table 3.2) because it helps to explain the physical signs we see of cardiac failure. However, the mechanisms involved in forward and backward failure are inextricably linked. Forward failure is the stimulus for the initiation of backward failure, and the augmentation of preload that results helps to boost cardiac output, so that chronic forward failure is rare.

Backward heart failure	Increased venous pressures	left-sided (*pulmonary oedema*)
	(Increased filling pressures)	right-sided (*ascites*)
Forward heart failure	Poor cardiac output	peracute (*syncope*)
		acute (*cardiogenic shock*)

Table 3.2: Characteristics of backward and forward heart failure.

Forward heart failure

Effects on tissues/organs: A fall in cardiac output initiates sympathetic stimulation, which results in peripheral vasoconstriction, helping to maintain mean arterial pressure. It also results in reduced organ perfusion, which may be recognized by an increased extraction of oxygen by cells to meet their metabolic requirements (reduced systemic venous partial pressure of oxygen, PvO_2). In severe tissue under-perfusion, many cells have to rely on anaerobic metabolism (PvO_2 < 21–24 mmHg/2.8–3.2 kPa) and a lactic acidosis results (Kittleson, 1988). The skin, gut, skeletal muscles and kidneys are all affected, with sometimes critical consequences for the kidneys. Reduced renal perfusion results in prerenal azotaemia which can be identified from plasma biochemistry results. Homeostatic mechanisms ensure perfusion is optimized for the critical organs, namely the brain and heart. The cerebral and coronary circulations are dependent on a minimum blood pressure for effective function, but unlike other vascular beds they are adapted to cope with reduced cardiac output by *autoregulation*. This enables the cerebral and coronary vascular resistance to *fall* in response to decreased flow. However, autoregulation is only effective with blood pressures > 50 mmHg (Levick, 1995). Cardiogenic shock may occur if homeostatic mechanisms are unable to maintain mean arterial pressure with a failing heart despite profound vasoconstriction.

If there is a sudden increase in demand for cardiac output (i.e., during exercise), the failing heart may be unable to suddenly increase output, leading to a fall in systemic arterial pressures. Metabolic vasodilation in skeletal muscle may contribute to this, and the resulting hypotension leads to inadequate cerebral and coronary perfusion (with syncope and/or arrhythmias).

Clinical recognition: The signs of syncope are discussed in Chapter 9. Signs of severe forward failure include vasoconstriction affecting the skin, extremities and muscles which are not preferentially perfused. The extremities are cold, muscles are weak and poor circulation may be appreciated from the pale mucous membranes with sluggish capillary refill and weak femoral pulse. Rectal temperature may be subnormal. Presenting signs can include fatigue, weakness and poor exercise tolerance.

Backwards heart failure

Backwards heart failure can be said to occur when elevated filling pressures are transmitted to the venous system. This is also known as *congestive cardiac failure*, where abnormal fluid accumulation may occur as oedema, ascites or pleural effusion.

Left-sided backward heart failure: (See Chapter 12). Backwards failure of the left heart leads to raised pressures in the left atrium, pulmonary veins and *pulmonary oedema*. Normal left atrial pressure in the absence of heart disease is about 4 mmHg. Should left atrial pressures slowly increase (such as with slowly progressive mitral regurgitation) then the left atrium may dilate without marked increases in pressure. Left atrial pressures as high as 40–45 mmHg may be accommodated without signs of pulmonary oedema. Pulmonary oedema is controlled in this situation by increased lymphatic drainage from the lungs (Ware and Bonagura, 1988). This appears to be more efficient from the left than the right lungs – on a dorsoventral radiograph in a patient with left-sided heart failure and mild pulmonary oedema, an interstitial infiltrate is often more obvious in the right lung fields.

If left atrial pressures suddenly increase (such as with a ruptured primary chorda tendineae of the mitral valve), then the left atrium cannot protect the pulmonary vascular bed. The pulmonary lymphatics cannot suddenly increase their drainage capacity, and dramatic pulmonary venous congestion and fulminant pulmonary oedema results.

Right-sided backward heart failure: (See Chapter 13). With increased right-sided filling pressures, raised right atrial pressures result in systemic venous congestion. This can be noted as jugular distension, but hepatomegaly, ascites and pleural effusions all suggest right-sided backward heart failure. Hepatic venous congestion may result in hepatocellular damage and raised liver enzymes, especially alanine transferase (ALT). Severe chronic venous congestion of the liver in the dog can lead to the hepatic sinusoids becoming leaky, with protein and fluid loss, and ascites. Pleural effusions may also be present with systemic venous congestion and right-sided heart failure.

Responses to heart failure

Initial responses

Maintenance of mean arterial pressure is the main homeostatic priority of the body with regard to the cardiovascular system.

A *reflex increase in sympathetic drive* is triggered by any fall in cardiac output, as a fall in blood pressure is detected by the baroreceptors.

Increased heart rate and contractility (if the myocardium is capable) results from sympathetic stimulation of β_1 receptors, producing an increase in mean arterial pressure.

Vasoconstriction is produced by stimulation of α_1 receptors via contraction of vascular smooth muscle. Arterial vasoconstriction raises mean arterial pressure, and venoconstriction increases venous pressure and venous return to the heart. Utilizing the Frank–Starling mechanism, the increased preload increases stroke volume, as long as the sick heart is still on the ascending part of the curve (Figure 3.2).

Decreased parasympathetic outflow reduces vagal tone to the heart and manifestations of this (sinus arrhythmia, etc.) will be abolished.

The *baroreceptor reflexes become blunted* in long-standing congestive heart failure, so that sympathetic outflow remains unchecked (Braunwald, 1992).

Reduced synthesis, storage and release of myocardial noradrenaline occurs later in heart failure. There is also a decrease in myocardial beta receptors, limiting the response of the myocardium to circulating catecholamines, although this is partially offset by high plasma levels of catecholamines in heart failure patients (Knight, 1989). This is known as *down-regulation* of beta receptors (Braunwald, 1992).

Intermediate (endocrine) responses to heart failure

Activation of the renin–angiotensin–aldosterone system (RAAS) resulting in:

- Vasoconstriction
- Sodium and water retention
- Myocardial hypertrophy in some cases
- Reduced levels of naturally circulating vasodilators (e.g. bradykinin).

Increased synthesis and release of arginine vasopressin has the following effects:

- Transient vasoconstriction
- Increased water retention from the distal tubules of the nephron.

Release of atrial natriuresis factor (ANF) by the atrial myocytes follows atrial distension. It is also synthesized and released by the ventricles in congestive heart failure (then known as ventricular natriuresis factor) (Braunwald, 1992). These levels are higher in acute heart failure; in more chronic settings, there is an attenuated response of myocytes and levels tend to normalize.

Thus, the classical signs of heart failure are a vicious cycle of:

- Tachycardia
- Vasoconstriction (which both increase cardiac work)
- Sodium and water retention (which may result in oedema and effusions).

These homeostatic mechanisms are obviously life saving in the acute hypovolaemia of shock or haemorrhage, but they are detrimental in a chronic setting of heart failure. The homeostatic priority of the body is to maintain mean arterial pressure, but this increases afterload. Vasodilator therapy can take advantage of this blood pressure reserve to reduce afterload and therefore the workload on the failing myocardium, so breaking the vicious cycle.

Chronic responses to heart failure

These include the structural adaptations described previously, such as eccentric or concentric hypertrophy of the left ventricular myocardium, depending upon the underlying disease. The contractile proteins also alter, with different isoenzymes of myosin depending on the underlying condition (Braunwald, 1992).

In conclusion, it can be seen that the various causes of heart failure result in a complex multisystem interaction of various mechanisms attempting to restore cardiac output. Knowledge and recognition of the pathophysiological mechanisms underlying cardiac diseases can guide the clinician to optimize treatment for each patient.

REFERENCES

Braunwald E (1992) Pathophysiology of heart failure. In: *Heart Disease. A Textbook of Cardiovascular Medicine*, ed. E Braunwald, 4th edn, p. 393. WB Saunders, Philadelphia

Garrison JC and Peach MJ (1991) Renin and angiotensin. In: *Goodman and Gilman's The Pharmacological Basis of Therapeutics*, ed. AG Gilman, TW Rall, AS Nies and P Taylor, vol 1, p. 749. McGraw-Hill, New York

Hamlin RL (1988) Pathophysiology of heart failure. In: *Canine and Feline Cardiology*, ed. PR Fox, p. 159. Churchill Livingstone, New York

Hays RM (1991) Agents affecting the renal conservation of water. In: *Goodman and Gilman's The Pharmacological Basis of Therapeutics*, ed. AG Gilman, TW Rall, AS Nies and P Taylor, vol 1, p. 732. McGraw-Hill, New York

ISACHC (1995) Recommendations for the diagnosis of heart disease and the treatment of heart failure in small animals. In: *Manual of Canine and Feline Cardiology, 2nd edn,* ed. MS Miller and LP Tilley, pp.469–502. WB Saunders, Philadelphia.

Kittleson MD (1988) Management of heart failure: concepts, therapeutic strategies and drug pharmacology. In: *Canine and Feline Cardiology*, ed. PR Fox, p. 171. Churchill Livingstone, New York

Knight DH (1989) Pathophysiology of heart failure. In: *Textbook of Veterinary Internal Medicine*, ed. SJ Ettinger, p. 899. WB Saunders, Philadelphia

Levick JR (1991) Cardiovascular responses in pathological situations. Chapter 15. In: *An Introduction to Cardiovascular Physiology*, p. 261. Butterworths, London

Levick JR (1995) Specialization in individual circulations. Chapter 13. In: *An Introduction to Cardiovascular Physiology*, 2nd edn, pp. 231-254. Butterworths, London

Michell AR (1991) Regulation of salt and water balance. *Journal of Small Animal Practice* **32**, 135

Olivier NB (1993) Pathophysiology of cardiac failure. Chapter 56. In: *Textbook of Small Animal Surgery*, ed. D Slatter, 2nd edn, vol 1, p. 826. WB Saunders, Philadelphia

Opie LH (1991) Ventricular volume overload and heart failure. Chapter 16. In: *The Heart. Physiology and Metabolism*, p. 396. Raven Press, New York

Ware WA and Bonagura JD (1988) Pulmonary oedema. Chapter 9. In: *Canine and Feline Cardiology*, ed. PR Fox, p. 205. Churchill Livingstone, New York

History and Physical Examination

Peter G.G. Darke

INTRODUCTION

The thoracic wall represents a barrier to some clinicians, creating mystique over diseases of the cardiac and respiratory systems. However, most thoracic disorders can be effectively diagnosed, and many can be successfully treated with a meticulous approach to the case.

There is a close relationship between cardiac function and pulmonary function. The lungs are liberally supplied by the circulation, and both hypoxia and pulmonary hypertension resulting from pulmonary diseases can affect the function of the heart. Similarly, cardiac failure readily causes signs of pulmonary dysfunction, through raised venous capillary pressure, reduced perfusion or frank oedema. In dogs, airway compression by the enlarged left atrium is a common complication of mitral regurgitation. Major signs of disease of either system can include dyspnoea, coughing and exercise intolerance.

As far as diseases of respiration and circulation are concerned, pet animals often show few signs of disease until failure intervenes, whereas performance in working or sporting dogs may be compromised by relatively minor disease. Dyspnoea in particular is often disregarded by owners of domestic pets until disease is advanced or even life-threatening, while coughing, often caused by relatively minor disease, is sufficiently irritating to the animal's owners as to leave them dissatisfied unless a complete cure can be achieved. Furthermore, relatively few diseases that cause coughing are immediately life-threatening, but animals showing dyspnoea should always have the diagnosis pursued aggressively, and the animal should be handled with the greatest care to avoid precipitating sudden death.

Careful history-taking and clinical examination can be very helpful in formulating an accurate diagnosis in cardiac failure, although the history and clinical findings may be much less rewarding in some cases of airway disease that cause persistent or recurrent coughing, such as chronic bronchitis.

SIGNALMENT

As in disorders involving many systems of the body, careful history-taking can pay dividends.

Type of animal

The breed, age and sex of the animal under examination can often suggest a limited range of diseases, or even a single cause. However, an experienced clinician also knows that few cases present in text-book fashion.

Age of animal

Clearly, cardiopulmonary signs in an immature animal strongly suggest the possibility of congenital disease, especially if growth is stunted. Even respiratory infections may be caused by congenital immune deficiencies. Fortunately for the alert clinician, evidence of nearly every congenital cardiac malformation can be detected as a cardiac murmur. However, other cardiac diseases such as myocarditis may also be found in immature dogs.

Conversely, every experienced small animal clinician is aware of the prevalence of neoplasia in ageing animals. This is particularly relevant to the respiratory system, with primary lung tumours rarely being found in dogs of less than 7 years old, and pulmonary metastases being common. Furthermore, mitral valve degeneration (endocardiosis) is notably prevalent in ageing small breeds of dog.

Sex

Not many cardiopulmonary diseases show a marked sexual predisposition, but cardiac disease is generally more prevalent in males than females, with the notable exception of congenital patent ductus arteriosus.

Breed

Many breeds of pure bred dog show predisposition to cardiopulmonary diseases. This knowledge can guide an informed clinician as to the likely cause of disease. For example, many congenital heart diseases are found mainly in a limited number of breeds, e.g. aortic stenosis in Boxers, Golden Retrievers, German Shepherd Dogs and Newfoundlands. Acquired dilated cardiomyopathy is found mainly in certain larger breeds of dog, e.g. Dobermanns, Old English Sheepdogs, all giant breeds and a few smaller types such as Cocker and Springer Spaniels. Similarly, some breed types are notably affected by respiratory disease, for example Yorkshire Terriers with tracheal collapse, and brachycephalic breeds with upper airway obstruction. Furthermore, airway foreign bodies are found mainly in active sporting dogs that readily run through thickets and cornfields.

Environment and lifestyle

Obviously, housebound cats are unlikely to contract respiratory infections. Likewise, it can be helpful to know whether an animal is always under close observation and supervision, or whether there may have been access to poisons (e.g. paraquat or warfarin) or road traffic. Many animals with chronic respiratory disease are obese. Conversely, most pleural effusions and congestive cardiac failure tend to cause marked cachexia.

HISTORY

As in all thorough clinical investigations, meticulous history-taking can provide vital keys to the cause of disease, even if certain features do not appear immediately relevant: for example, coughing is sometimes the most prominent clinical sign in animals with disorders such as megaoesophagus, because of aspiration pneumonia. A full history should therefore include details of alimentary function, including appetite, diet, vomiting/regurgitation, faecal consistency and pattern of defaecation. Some clients find great difficulty in discriminating between coughing and retching to vomit. The history should also include other signs that might indicate metabolic disease, such as polydipsia and state of the haircoat, as some endocrine disturbances have potent effects on cardiac function.

Naturally, details of *exercise tolerance* (in dogs), together with any episodes of weakness or *collapse* should be recorded. The precise features of any episode of collapse should be carefully ascertained. Typically, cardiac syncope occurs with excitement or exercise; the collapse may involve tonic spasm, but the animal is often flaccid, and there is usually no shaking, salivation or clonic spasm. On recovery, the animal's behaviour is usually normal, as opposed to epileptiform seizures, in which the animal is usually very active in the seizure, and often shows postictal bewilderment for some minutes or hours. Cardiac syncope is relatively rare in cats.

Details of *coughing* can include the pattern: the frequency, time and circumstances of occurrence, whether the onset of disease was sudden or insidious, and whether the frequency is increasing or decreasing. The nature of the cough should also be recorded, for example, coughing in cardiac failure or airway obstruction is often harsh, dry, wheezy and paroxysmal, and may often be brought on by excitement. Conversely, coughing in exudative pulmonary disorders tends to be softer, and it may be productive. However, in practice, these details are not usually specifically revealing. Coughing is rarely a sign of cardiac disease in cats.

Any signs of *disturbed breathing* should be evaluated: dyspnoea at exercise; previous episodes of tachypnoea; and whether there is any airway noise, for example, whistling, wheezing, sighing or rattling, that might indicate airway obstruction. Again, the pattern of this disturbance may be helpful: the frequency, progression and development should be ascertained.

Sneezing and *nasal discharge* are prominent signs of nasal disorders, but can also be seen with exudative pulmonary disease.

PHYSICAL EXAMINATION

The physical examination should also be complete and thorough. Many subtleties can be integrated to suggest a definitive diagnosis, before rushing to auscultate the thorax. For example, a diagnosis of patent ductus arteriosus can be made with confidence by an experienced cardiologist without auscultation. A prolonged thrill at the heart base, high in the left axilla, together with a hyperkinetic pulse in a young bitch, strongly suggests this diagnosis. Similarly, dyspnoea in a Dobermann with a weak rapid pulse, pale mucous membranes and slow capillary refill is consistent with dilated cardiomyopathy in this breed.

Any animal with dyspnoea should be handled with great care: disease sufficiently severe to cause dyspnoea indicates a lack of respiratory reserves, and insensitive handling of the animal can easily kill it.

Observations

The general physical condition should be noted: cardiac failure, most pleural effusions and pulmonary disorders tend to be associated with weight loss. Animals with congenital heart disease may have stunted growth. Many dogs of small breeds, however, are obese when they have chronic lower airway disease. Any signs of respiratory disease should be noted: nasal discharge, sneezing, coughing or wheezing. Ascites may indicate congestive cardiac failure, but subcutaneous oedema is seen infrequently.

The animal's posture may indicate adoption of a position of relief for dyspnoea: sternal recumbency or standing with elbows abducted, hyperventilating, with neck extended; dogs may refuse to lie down when dyspnoeic. In dyspnoea, any evidence of respiratory noise should be noted, together with whether this is inspiratory (suggesting upper respiratory obstruction) or expiratory (lower airway). Animals with chronic hyperpnoea can show barrel-chested changes.

Mucous membranes

The mucous membranes should be examined: cyanosis is a common sign of severe pulmonary alveolar or interstitial disease, pleural effusion or airway obstruction. It is relatively uncommon in cardiac failure, unless severe alveolar oedema or pleural effusion is present, or unless there is a congenital right-to-left shunt, such as tetralogy of Fallot. Pallor is more common, and is consistent with poor cardiac output, especially with severe arrhythmias or dilated cardiomyopathy. Slow capillary refill (more than 2 seconds) is also usually found in systolic failure, as opposed to anaemia, in which the capillary refill time is usually normal.

Neck and airway

The throat and neck should be palpated for swellings that might be associated with airway obstruction, oesophageal dilatation or, especially in ageing cats, thyroid tumours. The trachea should be carefully palpated throughout the neck, to provoke any cough, which will indicate its character, but also to feel for any irregularity or distortion of the airway, such as tracheal collapse. The jugular veins should be examined for distension and pulsation that may indicate right sided congestive cardiac failure. If necessary, the neck should be clipped to permit close examination, and manual pressure on the liver may cause jugular distension (hepatojugular reflux).

Thoracic palpation

The thorax should be palpated carefully for swellings, pain, rib fractures, subcutaneous emphysema or oedema. The cardiac apex beat should be felt carefully, to determine the point of maximal intensity of the heart beat, to indicate any displacement by intrathoracic masses or effusion, and to detect any thrill (vibration of turbulence in blood flow). Cardiac enlargement or hyperkinesis (e.g. in hyperthyroidism) can produce an apex beat of increased intensity, and it can be displaced or reduced by pleural effusions or masses.

Thoracic percussion

Thoracic percussion is an acquired skill: it can be practised with either a direct or indirect strike. There is a natural area of dullness in the ventral thorax over the heart, which tends to be increased in heart failure. Similarly, there is an area of dullness over the diaphragm. However, in cases of pleural effusion, a distinct line can often be appreciated between increased dullness in the ventral thorax and increased resonance in the dorsal thorax, due to the effect of lungs floating over the fluid. Coupled with muffling of heart sounds and dorsal displacement of airway sounds, this can be a strong indication of the presence of effusion. An area of dullness can also sometimes be detected over a pleural or pulmonary mass. Conversely, increased resonance can be found in severe pneumothorax.

Abdominal palpation

The presence of ascites should always alert a clinician to the possibility of congestive heart failure. In cardiac failure, the fluid is usually a modified transudate, with a moderate protein and cellular content. The abdomen should also be palpated for evidence of hepatic enlargement. Hepatomegaly is frequently found in chronic congestive failure. Pressure on the liver may accentuate jugular distension in right sided cardiac failure (hepato–jugular reflux). Dogs (particularly German Shepherd Dogs) with splenic neoplasia often present with recurrent episodes of collapse and show pallor and tachycardia, which is associated with recurrent intra-abdominal haemorrhage.

Peripheral pulse

Both femoral pulses should be palpated to determine any disparity. Loss of one or both pulses is characteristic of cats with aortic (iliac) thrombosis, but this is also occasionally encountered in dogs. Loss of one pulse may indicate unilateral thrombosis. The pulse character, rate and rhythm should be assessed. The pulse can be hyperkinetic in several disorders in which there is left ventricular overload, notably patent ductus arteriosus and aortic regurgitation. In both of these diseases, the pulse also rapidly collapses – it is a very 'sudden' pulse. The pulse can also be hyperkinetic in hyperthyroidism, some anaemias, and in bradycardias. Conversely, it is notably weakened in cardiac output failure, especially with some tachyarrhythmias, dilated cardiomyopathy, pericardial effusions and aortic stenosis, as well as in hypovolaemia. Assessment of the character of the pulse can be difficult in obese animals.

The heart rate is one of the few objective parameters of circulatory function that can readily be evaluated, and the rate should be recorded routinely. Tachycardia is almost an invariable sign of cardiac failure, although cardiac failure can also be associated with bradycardias. The pulse rate should be compared with the heart rate, preferably by simultaneous auscultation, to determine the presence of any pulse deficit, a hallmark of many arrhythmias such as atrial fibrillation and premature beats. Furthermore, in many arrhythmias there are also beat-by-beat variations in the intensity of the pulse. Not only can the presence of cardiac arrhythmias be detected from the pulse, but the precise nature of the disturbance can often also be determined.

Rectal temperature

The temperature is usually normal in most cases of cardiopulmonary disease. However, bacterial endocarditis, pyothorax or bronchopneumonia can cause persistent or recurrent pyrexia. Conversely, persistent dyspnoea can cause hypothermia.

CARDIAC AUSCULTATION

Cardiac auscultation remains one of the most effective ways by which to assess the function of the heart without recourse to further aids to diagnosis. Several aspects should be evaluated:

The *area* over which the sounds are heard. This may be increased in cardiac enlargement, decreased in the presence of pericardial or pleural effusions, or the sounds may be displaced by pleural or pulmonary masses.

The *audibility of heart sounds*. Heart sounds are generally increased in intensity in heart failure. Again, they may be muffled by the presence of effusions, tumours or widespread lung disease.

The *heart rate*. This should be compared with the pulse, for evidence of a pulse deficit in cardiac arrhythmias. Similarly, most cases of cardiac failure show tachycardia (more than about 150 beats/min in adult dogs, more than about 230 beats/min in cats). Although excitable normal dogs may show higher rates than this at the time of presentation, this tachycardia can usually be differentiated from the insistent tachycardia of heart failure which is unrelieved by periods of vagal slowing as the dog settles. Bradycardias (below 70 beats/min in dogs, less than 140 beats/min in cats) should arouse suspicion of bradyarrhythmias. In cases with a predominant escape rhythm, the rate is typically not only slow but also unusually regular.

The *cardiac rhythm*. Regular sinus rhythm is normal in cats, while sinus arrhythmia, usually synchronous with respirations, is found in most normal dogs, and this is often an indication that there is compensation for any cardiac disease. Sinus arrhythmia appears to be accentuated in many brachycephalic breeds. Disturbances in the cardiac rhythm are common in heart failure, often due to cardiac stretch in volume overload. Premature beats are often heard as a tripping in the rhythm, with a change of intensity of heart sounds, and followed by a slight pause. Missed beats are not often heard in small animals, but they can be a feature of hypertrophic cardiomyopathy in cats. Atrial fibrillation is the most common cause of a truly chaotic rhythm. This chaos is created by random arrhythmia, with variations in intensity of heart sounds and of any murmur, and loss of the second heart sound for beats that follow a very short diastolic interval. Frequent and irregular ventricular premature beats can produce similar variations. Pathological and paroxysmal tachycardias often show very sudden transitions from a normal rate to very high heart rates.

Abnormal cardiac sounds, including murmurs. Cardiac murmurs are produced by disturbed blood flow. Disturbance is favoured by an increased velocity of flow, reduced viscosity of blood and/or passage through large vessels or chambers. Blood flow is often disturbed through narrow orifices such as incompetent or stenotic valves or a septal defect, which accelerate a jet into a large chamber. However, it is well recognized that normal flow of blood of decreased viscosity will also create so-called haemic murmurs, e.g. with anaemia or hypoproteinaemia. Physiological or 'flow' murmurs can also be detected from the aortic outflow in vigorous young growing animals. Furthermore, murmurs are created not only by lesions or by increased blood velocity, but also by the dilatation or distorsion of the atrioventricular ring that takes place in cardiac enlargement. Murmurs are often therefore the *result* of heart failure, especially in dilated cardiomyopathy.

Other abnormal cardiac sounds include so-called gallop sounds (or gallop rhythms). These are often best heard over the cardiac apex, and they represent the addition of an extra sound in addition to the normal first and second sounds. This is due to the third heart sound (of passive ventricular filling – not normally heard in dogs or cats) early in diastole, or the fourth heart sound (of atrial contraction, also not normally heard in small animals) in late diastole. Gallop sounds are heard typically in volume overload of dilated cardiomyopathy or with an excessively hypertrophied ventricle (e.g. in cats with hypertrophic cardiomyopathy).

Pericardial friction sounds may also occasionally be heard in the presence of pericardial adhesions, as a scratching synchronous with heart sounds.

PULMONARY AUSCULTATION

Auscultation of the lung fields is relatively less rewarding than in some larger species. In most normal dogs and many normal cats, to-and-fro airway sounds can be heard near the base of the heart, just behind the triceps muscle. With airway obstruction, sounds may be magnified or referred to the thorax, in which case the stethoscope should be used carefully along the cervical trachea to identify the precise source of the sound. The normal airway sounds may be displaced, e.g. dorsally by pleural effusions, or to one side by pleural masses, or further accentuated by external pressure on the airway. Increased sounds from the peripheral lung field may come from small airway obstruction, in which case they are usually referred to as *wheezes*.

Normal breath sounds are poorly heard in small animals. When small airways are obstructed by exudative material, e.g. in alveolar oedema or bronchopneumonia, *crackles* may be heard, either widespread or localized. The entire lungfield should be carefully auscultated for these abnormalities. However, the severity of disease appears to correlate poorly with the extent of lung crackles in small animals.

FURTHER INVESTIGATIONS

Although much can be gained from a meticulous history and careful clinical examination, there are a number of pitfalls for the unwary. Full use should be made of aids to diagnosis.

For cardiac disease

Thoracic radiographs give a very good indication of volume load, facilitating the diagnosis of congestive heart failure (see Chapter 5i). Furthermore, angiography, which is not a particularly difficult technique, can help to identify the specific lesion in some cases. In practice it is helpful for differentiating the dilated form of cardiomyopathy from the hypertrophic form in cats. This differentiation is of considerable importance in therapy.

Electrocardiography complements radiography (see Chapter 5iii) in helping to identify chamber enlargement.

Echocardiography, increasingly available in practice, can provide a specific diagnosis for some cases, e.g. pericardial effusion, dilated cardiomyopathy, subaortic stenosis or ventricular septal defect (see Chapter 5vi). Otherwise, it may give a guide as to the origin of disease, for example, with marked right ventricular hypertrophy being found in pulmonic stenosis.

Doppler studies (Chapter 6ii) can often secure a definitive diagnosis not only as to a precise cardiac dysfunction (valve regurgitation or stenosis), but also to give a measure of the severity of disease (e.g. the pressure gradient across a valve or shunt).

Cardiac catheterization (Chapter 6iii) is otherwise required for the confirmation of many diseases. Angiography, intracardiac pressure measurements and blood gas analysis can all be carried out by this technique, but in most cases Doppler echocardiography provides a definitive diagnosis more readily.

For respiratory disease

Thoracic radiography is of prime importance. For example, this is the definitive diagnostic technique for pleural effusions and pulmonary neoplasia. Furthermore, radiographs are sensitive to alveolar pulmonary diseases such as pulmonary oedema, haemorrhage and bronchopneumonia, and are particularly of value in dyspnoeic animals. However, for interstitial disorders such as paraquat poisoning or early infiltrative neoplasia, there may be few findings. Unfortunately, also for many airway diseases that cause coughing (e.g. acute tracheobronchitis, *Oslerus (Filaroides) osleri*, chronic bronchitis), radiographs show minimal abnormalities.

Bronchoscopy is often more useful in the investigation of airway diseases which cause coughing, and/or *bronchoalveolar lavage* for culture and cytology (see Chapters 5iv and 5v).

Biochemistry and haematology are not particularly helpful in either cardiac failure or in most respiratory diseases; these provide mainly subsidiary information, apart from a few cases such as endocarditis or pyothorax, in which leucocytosis is usually found, sometimes with anaemia, and in chronic hypoxic states such as right-to-left congenital shunts, in which polycythaemia may occur (Chapter 5ii). In congestive heart failure, non-specific leucocytosis, increases in liver enzymes, decreases in plasma proteins and pre-renal azotaemia are common.

Blood gas analysis can be helpful in some cases of respiratory disease (Chapter 6i).

Cytology of effusions is essential for the diagnosis of the aetiology of pleural effusions, and lung biopsy can demonstrate the cause of some pulmonary diseases.

FURTHER READING

Darke PGG, Bonagura JD and Kelly DF (1996) *Color Atlas of Veterinary Cardiology*. Mosby-Wolfe, London

Kienle RD and Thomas WP (1995) Echocardiography. In: *Veterinary Diagnostic Ultrasound*, ed. TG Nyland and JS Mattoon, pp. 198–257. Saunders, Philadelphia

Moise NS (1989) Doppler echocardiographic evaluation of congenital heart disease. *Journal of Veterinary Internal Medicine* **3** 195–207

Diagnostic Aids

(i) Thoracic Radiology

Elizabeth A.C. Munro

INDICATIONS FOR THORACIC RADIOLOGY

There are a number of situations where radiography of the thorax is a mandatory part of the diagnostic work-up, e.g.

- Evidence of cardiac disease
- Signs of respiratory compromise
- Chronic coughing
- Abnormalities of the thoracic wall
- Screening for metastases in malignant disease
- Preceding anaesthesia in animals with evident or suspected thoracic trauma
- Swallowing disorders or vomiting for which an extrathoracic cause is not apparent.

As intrathoracic disease is not always clinically obvious, radiography may also be valuable in working up cases with vague signs such as unexplained weight loss or pyrexia. Mediastinal abnormalities in particular may be difficult to detect on clinical examination.

RADIOGRAPHIC TECHNIQUE

- *Select low mAs, high kV exposure factors*
This technique will produce a broad range of contrast providing many shades of grey, whilst enabling exposure times to be kept to a minimum and reducing movement unsharpness.

- *Collimate accurately*
The beam should be collimated from a few centimetres cranial to the first rib to just beyond the costal arch, to ensure the whole lung field is included.

- *Use a grid with large chests and high mA machines*
Although a grid will limit the effects of scatter when radiographing larger dogs (i.e. when tissue thickness exceeds 15 cm), this does require the use of significantly higher exposure factors. In machines with low mA capability, better results may be achieved if a grid is not used, to avoid lengthening the exposure time. A rare earth screen will allow exposure factors to be kept low whilst being less sensitive to scattered radiation, and can be very useful in this situation.

- *Obtain inspiratory films*
Although the exposure should in most instances be made at the point of maximum inflation of the lungs, good inspiratory radiographs can be difficult to achieve in animals with fast shallow respiration, particularly if they are obese. If the animal's condition permits, this can be overcome by intubating the animal under general anaesthesia and obtaining the radiograph when the rebreathing bag is manually squeezed to inflate the lungs. Incomplete expansion of the lungs in the anaesthetized animal may otherwise result in an overall increase in lung field density which can be mistaken for pathological change.

- *Use the same exposure factors in follow-up films*
It is vitally important when comparing chest films of the same animal taken on different occasions to ensure that the films were obtained with identical exposure factors and whenever possible at the same phase of respiration. Under these circumstances, follow-up radiography can be a very useful way to monitor progress.

STANDARD VIEWS

Dorsoventral view
In the dyspnoeic animal, the dorsoventral (DV) projection should be obtained first, in order to detect sizeable pleural effusions or pneumothorax which could cause fatal respiratory embarrassment should the animal be placed in lateral or dorsal recumbency.

The beam is centred level with the caudal border of the scapula, and care should be taken to ensure the spine and sternebrae are superimposed. In this projection the heart shape appears more constant than in the ventrodorsal (VD) view, and the vessels of the caudal lung lobes are more clearly seen.

Ventrodorsal view
The VD view is achieved by lying the animal in dorsal recumbency with the forelimbs drawn forward and the

beam centred level with the sixth rib. The lungfields appear larger, and the accessory lobe and caudal mediastinum are better visualized than in the DV view. This position will cause some compression at the heart base and is therefore best avoided in cases with cardiac or mainstem bronchial disease.

Lateral view

The forelimbs should be drawn well forward on the lateral view, and a foam wedge under the sternum is useful to correct rotation in deep chested breeds. The beam is centred over the heart. As the dependent lobe begins to collapse after a fairly short period of time, focal lesions are most visible (by virtue of the air around them) in the uppermost lung, so that both right and left lateral views should be obtained when looking for pulmonary metastases.

Other views

The standing lateral view can be valuable in seriously dyspnoeic patients. It is obtained with the patient standing alongside the radiographic cassette, which should be mounted on a stand. A horizontal beam is used to make the exposure. Oblique views are useful in the evaluation of rib tumours.

RADIOGRAPHY OF THE UPPER AIRWAY

The larynx and cervical trachea are best visualized on the lateral view with the head and neck slightly extended. Ventrodorsal and oblique views are occasionally useful in the localization of abnormalities detected on the lateral view, but are not routinely required.

Indications

- Inspiratory dyspnoea where an intrathoracic cause is not apparent
- Stridor or stertorous respiration
- Palpable mass lesions or tracheal abnormalities
- Pain on palpation of the laryngeal area
- Suspected tracheal collapse.

Normal radiographic appearance of the larynx and trachea

The larynx is a mobile structure and its position will vary, especially with swallowing. Mineralization of the laryngeal cartilages occurs as part of the ageing process in dogs, making the component parts easier to identify. The tip of the epiglottis is usually seen touching the dorsal rim of the soft palate but may also be seen ventral to the palate, or separate from it. The cricoid and thyroid cartilages, and the cuneiform parts of the arytenoid cartilages, can usually be identified. Air in the lateral ventricles may permit visualization of the vestibular folds and vocal cords (Figure 5.1). The air-

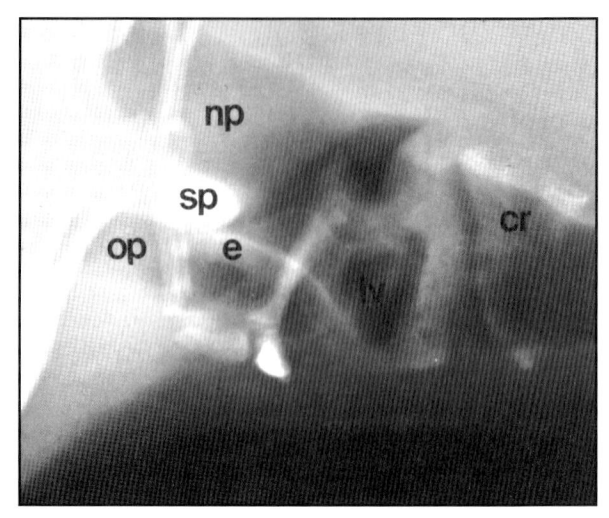

*Figure 5.1: Lateral radiograph of the upper airway of a 3-year-old Labrador Retriever. Key: **np** nasal passages, **op** oropharynx, **sp** soft palate, **e** epiglottis, **lv** lateral ventricles, **cr** cricoid cartilage. The hyoid apparatus and arytenoid cartilages may also be seen.*

filled nasopharynx, oropharyx and laryngopharynx are usually readily seen, but are less obvious in brachycephalic dogs.

Mineralization of laryngeal cartilage is minimal in cats, and they have only a laryngeal depression rather than developed lateral ventricles, so normal laryngeal anatomy is more difficult to appreciate in this species.

The normal tracheal lumen is only slightly less than that of the larynx at the level of the cricoid cartilage, and approximately three times the width of the proximal portion of the third rib. The trachea forms an increasing angle with the vertebral bodies as it runs caudally to its bifurcation, the angle being greatest in deep chested animals. It is not uncommon to see a dorsal or rightward curve in the trachea as it runs through the cranial mediastinum of normal dogs. In deep chested breeds the trachea may have a pronounced ventral dip just before the carina.

Radiographic abnormalities

The larynx

In general, radiography is a relatively insensitive means of evaluating laryngeal disorders, direct visualization at laryngoscopy often proving more rewarding. It can be of value in the detection of the following:

Soft tissue masses: Soft tissue mass lesions may produce distortion of the normal anatomy or narrowing of the airway lumen. Displacement of the larynx may arise secondarily to extrinsic masses such as enlarged retropharyngeal lymph nodes, or thyroid neoplasia.

Radiopaque foreign bodies: Items such as sewing needles are occasionally embedded in the soft tissues of the larynx.

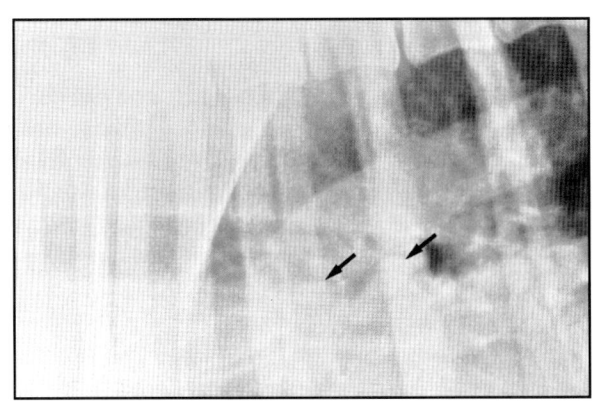

Figure 5.2: Oslerus (Filaroides) *nodules (arrows) in the caudal thoracic trachea of a 1-year-old Airedale.*

The trachea

Tracheal collapse: This may affect any part of the trachea or mainstem bronchi, with collapse at the thoracic inlet being especially frequent. The cervical trachea collapses on inspiration, and the intrathoracic trachea collapses on expiration. As this is a dynamic event it is best recognized using image intensification, but, with careful timing of exposures, it may be diagnosed with plain films. Care should be taken to identify the dorsal border of the trachea accurately at the thoracic inlet, as a false impression of tracheal collapse may be created by the ventral neck muscles and oesophagus overlying the trachea.

Tracheal narrowing: This may also rarely arise as a result of *hypoplasia*, *acquired stenosis*, or *mucosal swelling*. Nodular swellings in the caudal thoracic trachea of young dogs may be caused by the nematode *Oslerus (Filaroides) osleri*, although bronchoscopy is necessary to confirm the diagnosis (Figure 5.2).

INTERPRETATION OF THE THORACIC RADIOGRAPH

General principles

The wealth of information provided by a good quality thoracic radiograph can be intimidating unless a systematic approach to interpretation is adopted. The film should be read on a viewing box with ambient light reduced. If films are initially read wet, they should be reviewed later when drying is complete. The eye is automatically drawn towards the cardiac shadow at the centre of the film, and peripheral abnormalities are most readily overlooked. This tendency can be overcome by assessing in turn:

- Thoracic boundaries
- Pleural cavity
- Mediastinum
- Heart and great vessels
- Pulmonary parenchyma.

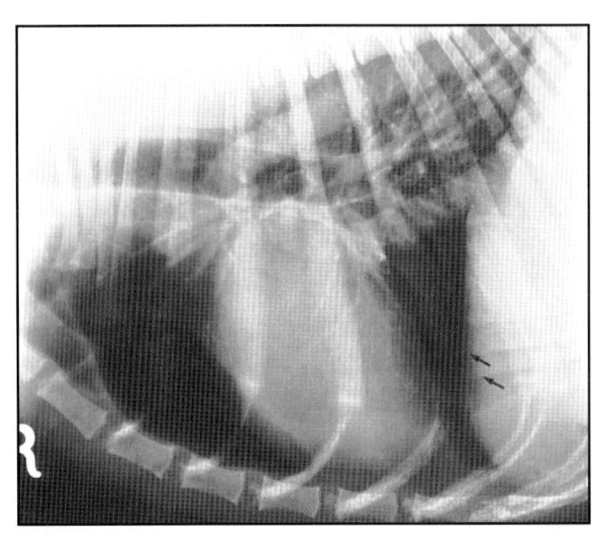

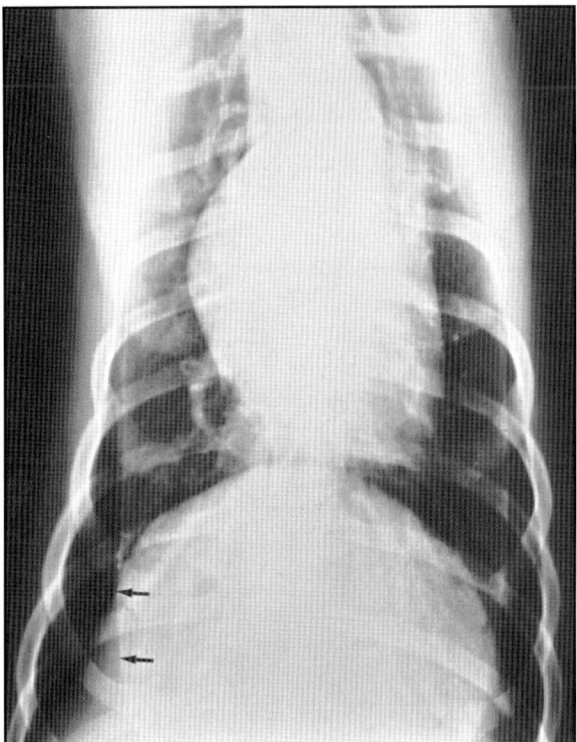

Figure 5.3: Lateral and DV thoracic radiographs of a normal 2-year-old Irish Setter. Skin folds (arrows) are most often prominent in deep chested breeds.

The differences in thoracic conformation due to breed variation in the dog are considerable, and it is useful to keep radiographs of normal animals in the viewing area for comparative purposes (Figures 5.3 and 5.4). These could include:

- A deep chested breed, e.g. Dobermann
- A barrel chested breed, e.g. Cairn
- A brachycephalic, e.g. Bulldog
- An intermediate conformation, e.g. Labrador.

In everyday practice, such a library can be quickly built up with films taken when screening for pulmonary metastatic disease.

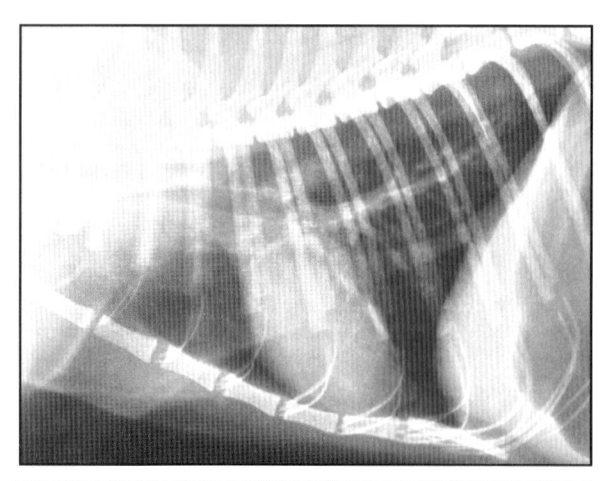

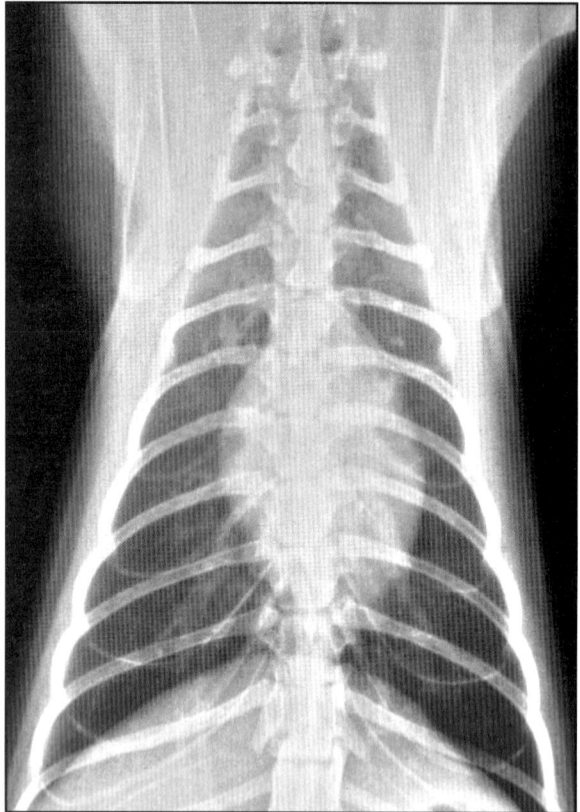

Figure 5.4: Lateral and DV thoracic radiographs of a normal cat.

The thoracic boundaries

The thorax is defined by the thoracic inlet cranially, the thoracic vertebrae dorsally, the sternebrae ventrally, the ribs laterally and the diaphragm caudally.

Body wall

The soft tissues of the body wall overlying the ribs should be examined.
Abnormalities include:

- *Accumulation of gas*: caused by penetrating wounds, gas-producing bacterial infections, subcutaneous emphysema secondary to pneumomediastinum
- *Soft tissue swelling*: caused by trauma, neoplasia, infection
- *Fat deposition*: caused by obesity.

The sternum

Sternal abnormalities caused by congenital deformities or previous trauma are common incidental findings, and can generally be dismissed as insignificant in the absence of clinical signs. There is a recognized association in the congenital abnormalities of *pectus excavatum* and *pericardioperitoneal diaphragmatic hernia*.

Osteomyelitis of the sternebrae is recognized as a reactive periosteal response and bone lysis. It is most often associated with a foreign body, or bite wound abscess. *Tumours* involving the sternebrae are uncommon, but may show a similar appearance to osteomyelitis.

The ribs

Abnormalities include the following:

Trauma: Most rib fractures are transverse (Figure 5.5). A flail segment may result if two or more ribs are fractured at more than one site, causing this section of the chest wall to be sucked inwards on inspiration, and blown outwards on expiration.

Neoplasia: The ribs are not infrequently involved in primary and metastatic neoplastic disease. Bone lysis, with or without a periosteal response, is common. With large primary tumours, the ribs on either side are pushed apart.

Generalized increased intercostal distance: This relates to the degree of thoracic expansion and is seen in *pleural effusions, pneumothorax* and diseases when *air trapping* in the lungs occurs (Figure 5.5).

Normal variants

- *Irregular, knobbly costochondral junctions* are common in dogs and can be mistaken for neoplastic nodules in the lung field
- *Curved ribs* may be found in chondrodystrophic breeds, especially the Basset Hound, which can mimic pleural effusion on the DV view.

The diaphragm

Traumatic diaphragmatic rupture is the most commonly encountered diaphragmatic abnormality. It is usually possible to make the diagnosis on plain films when abdominal contents migrate through a ventrally located tear into the thorax. When diaphragmatic rupture is suspected, the DV should be obtained first to locate which hemidiaphragm is torn. The damaged side should be lowermost on the lateral view to minimize respiratory compromise.
Features include:

- Abnormal position of the falciform fat (cats)
- Abnormal gas and fat densities within the thoracic cavity

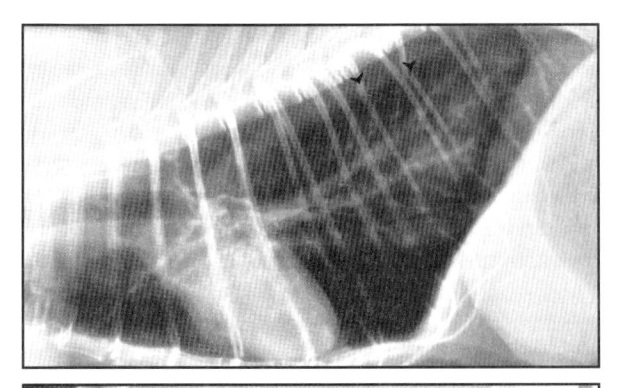

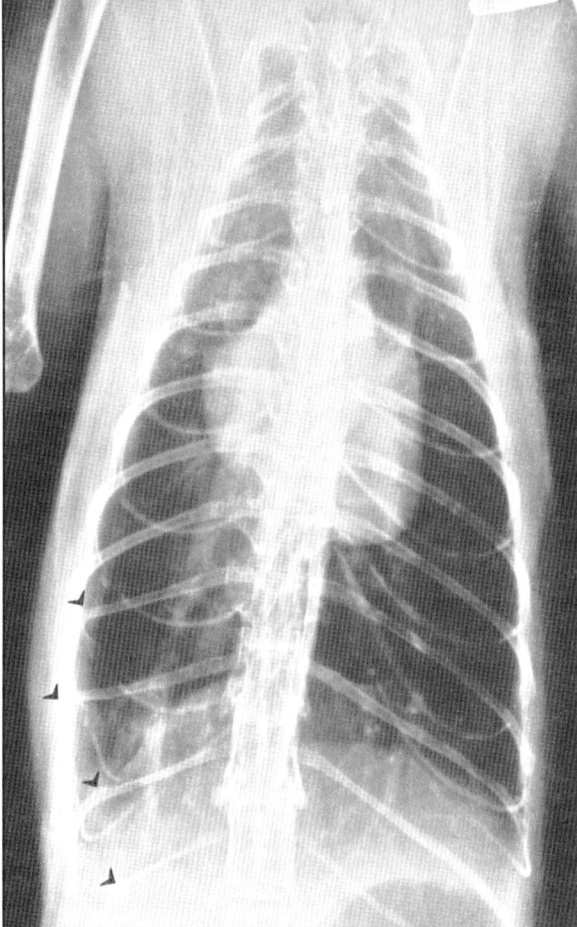

Figure 5.5: Lateral and DV views of a cat with air trapping caused by a bronchial tumour (not visible) obstructing expiration. The lung fields are overinflated, with increased intercostal distance and flattening of the diaphragm. Rib fractures (arrowheads) are also seen.

- Loss of normal diaphragmatic contours
- Reduced angle between the diaphragm and spine on the lateral view
- Cranial displacement of the gastric axis or small intestine (barium swallow may be useful).

Positive contrast coeliography can be used to confirm the diagnosis when only part of a liver lobe has herniated, which may be difficult to identify amidst the surrounding pleural effusion. A small volume (1–2 ml/kg) of a water soluble contrast medium is injected into the peritoneal cavity and the animal (cautiously!)

elevated by the hindlimbs for a minute or two to promote flow of the contrast through the defect into the pleural cavity. False negative results may still occur if the defect is plugged by viscera.

Other abnormalities of the diaphragm

Diaphragmatic masses are rare, but include granuloma secondary to migrating foreign body, neoplasia, or cyst.

The normal diaphragm is slightly *asymmetrical*, with the most cranial point on the DV or VD view lying a little to the right of mid-line. Alterations in symmetry of an intact diaphragm are usually secondary to other intrathoracic disease. Primary diaphragmatic asymmetry is seen in *unilateral phrenic nerve paralysis* or eventration (thinning of muscle mass of one hemidiaphragm).

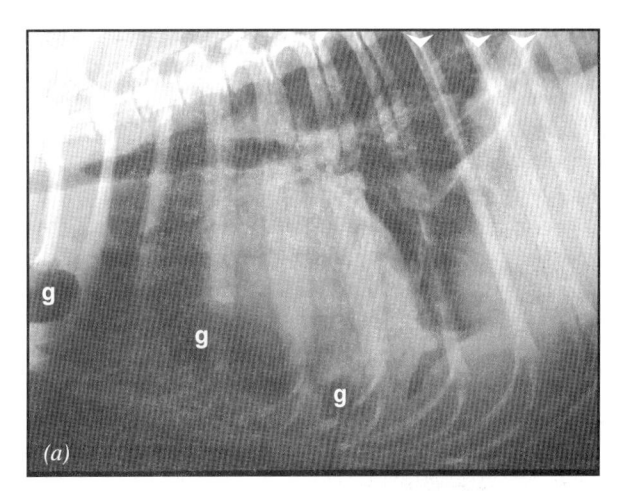

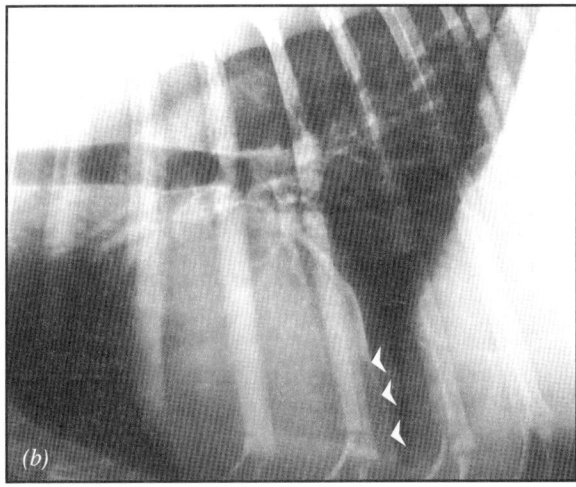

Figure 5.6: Sequential lateral radiographs of a young Flat Coat Retriever with pleural nocardiosis. (a) A moderate pleural effusion, obscuring the cardiac silhouette and diaphragmatic outline ventrally. There is also free gas within the pleural cavity, against which the dorsal borders of the caudal lung lobes are highlighted (arrowheads). Elsewhere, the free gas is in pockets (g). In this case, the pleural effusion was inflammatory, whilst the pneumothorax followed thoracocentesis and was therefore believed to be iatrogenic in origin. (b) The same dog 6 months later, by which time it was asymptomatic. There is residual pleural thickening (arrowheads). The effusion has resolved and the ventral border of the heart is now visible.

The pleural cavity

The pleural cavity represents a closed space between the parietal and visceral pleura. It is normally less than 1 mm in diameter and contains a serous fluid to reduce friction during respiratory movement. Disorders of the pleural cavity include:

- Pleural thickening
- Pleural effusions
- Pneumothorax

Pleural thickening

In older dogs, pleural thickening may result in fine pleural fissure lines delineating the lung lobes, forming a gentle arc from the periphery towards the hilus as they are struck at right angles to the X-ray beam. Pleural thickening also occurs as a result of inflammation, fibrosis or small volume pleural effusion. It may be a permanent legacy of a previous reactive effusion after the animal has become asymptomatic (Figure 5.6).

Pleural effusion

Depending on the size of the animal, volumes must exceed approximately 50-100 ml to become radiographically detectable. The mediastinum of the dog and cat is usually freely permeable with rapid equilibration of fluid in both hemithoraces. A unilateral effusion implies sealing of the mediastinum by an inflammatory process, and is common in cats with pyothorax.

Small effusions are seen as pleural fissure lines and slight retraction of the lung lobes from the thoracic wall, with blunting of the costophrenic angles, on the VD view. As the fluid builds up, the lung lobes progressively collapse to produce a typical appearance of fluid interdigitating with the individual lobes often referred to as 'scalloping'. As a result of their collapse, the lung lobes themselves become increasingly radiodense. On the lateral view, the ventral diaphragm and the cardiac apex are obscured by fluid. There is elevation of the heart from the sternum with dorsal tracheal displacement giving a false impression of cardiomegaly. This appearance can be mimicked by sternal fat beneath the heart, but as fat is less radiodense than fluid the cardiac outline may still be discerned.

In general, it is impossible to characterize the nature of the effusion on its radiographic appearance alone. Radiography should be repeated after thoracocentesis, as thoracic drainage may unmask abnormalities such as mediastinal masses, cardiomegaly or lung lobe torsions previously obscured by pleural fluid, and critical evaluation of intrathoracic structures is only possible once the effusion has been removed. Following drainage of reactive effusions with a high fibrin content, the lungs may be prevented from re-expanding to their full extent because of pleural thickening, and the lobe edges are seen to remain rounded. This appearance is referred to as *cortication*.

Pneumothorax

Free air in the pleural space is recognized as an air density of the thoracic periphery without vascular or bronchial markings. Suspicious areas should be viewed with a bright light to differentiate pneumothorax from overexposure of the lung field. The lung lobe edges can be seen retracting away from the thoracic wall, and the parenchymal density is generally greater than that of the surrounding free air. The DV view is more sensitive than the VD view in the detection of small volume pneumothorax. On the lateral view, the heart is commonly elevated from the sternum by the air. The radiograph should be scrutinized to detect an underlying cause such as rib fractures which have lacerated the lung, or cystic lesions of the lung lobes. In many cases, the source of the leakage is undetectable. As in pleural effusions, drainage is required to allow the lungs to reinflate before accurate assessment of the pulmonary parenchyma is possible.

The mediastinum

Mediastinal abnormalities are difficult to evaluate on clinical examination and thoracic radiography is important in their assessment. The mediastinum contains the heart and great vessels, the trachea, oesophagus, thymus, lymph nodes, vagus and phrenic nerves, thoracic duct and a variable amount of fat. Cranially, it communicates with the deep fascial planes of the neck, and caudally with the retroperitoneal space via the aortic hiatus.

Abnormalities of the mediastinum

- pneumomediastinum
- mediastinal masses
- diffuse mediastinal widening
- mediastinal shift

Pneumomediastinum: The individual boundaries of the cranial mediastinal contents cannot normally be distinguished. The presence of free air within the

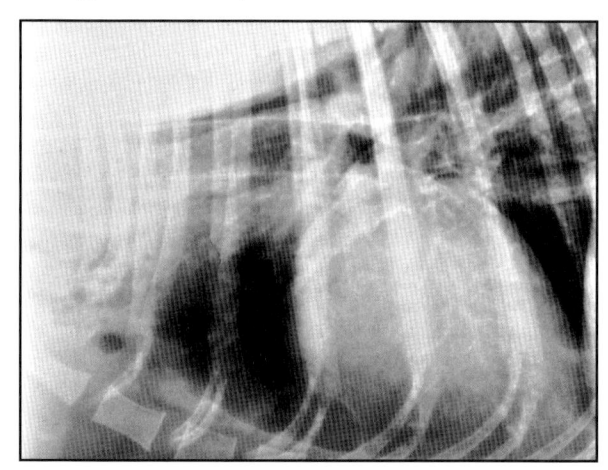

Figure 5.7*: Lateral left thoracic radiograph of a 2-year-old cross bred dog following a road traffic accident. Air in the mediastinum highlights the tracheal walls, great vessels cranial to the heart and the ventral border of the longus colli muscles.*

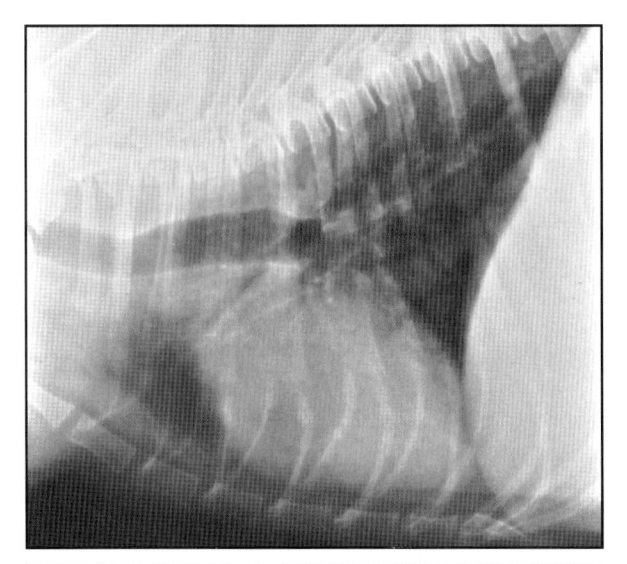

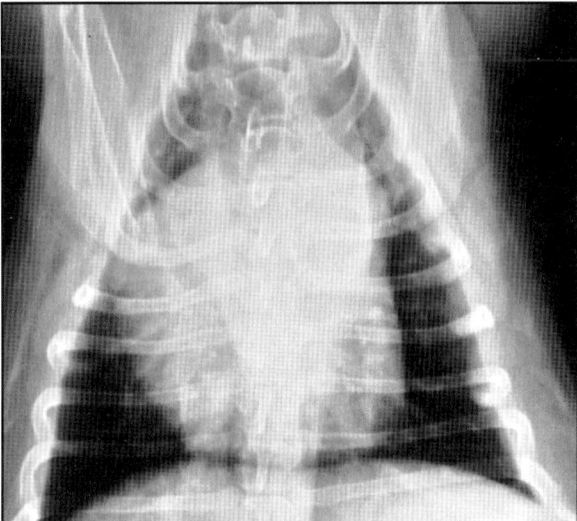

Figure 5.8: Normal thoracic radiographs of an obese 11-year-old Scottish Terrier. Fat within the mediastinum is seen dorsal to the sternebrae on the lateral view and causing mediastinal widening cranial to the heart on the DV view.

mediastinum (pneumomediastinum) provides contrast against which the outer wall of the trachea, the oesophagus, major branches of the aortic arch and cranial vena cava may be seen (Figure 5.7). Pneumomediastinum may arise due to leakage of air from a defect in the oesophagus, trachea or main stem bronchi, and deep puncture wounds in the neck may allow air to track into the mediastinum via the thoracic inlet. Air escaping from ruptured alveoli, e.g. secondary to blunt trauma, can dissect alongside pulmonary vessels to the hilus, causing pneumomediastinum. Whatever the cause of the pneumomediastinum, it may be accompanied by subcutaneous emphysema. If the air within the mediastinum accumulates very rapidly, the increase in pressure can occasionally be sufficient to rupture the mediastinal pleura and cause a pneumothorax.

Mediastinal masses: Mediastinal masses can be identified when they cause abnormalities in width or shape of the mediastinum, or displace the intrathoracic tra-

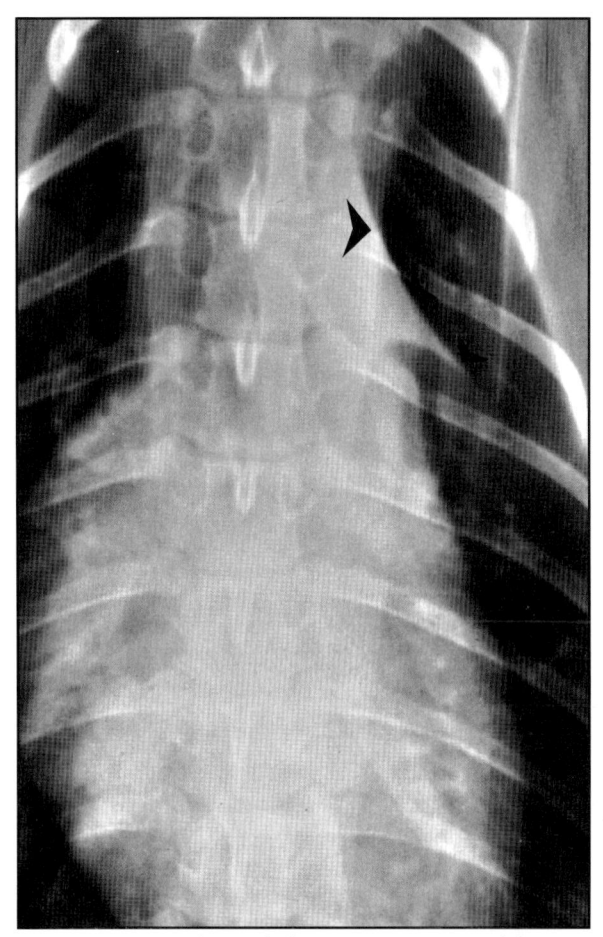

Figure 5.9: DV radiograph demonstrating a normal thymic 'sail' (arrowhead) in a young dog.

chea or cardiac shadow. The normal cranial mediastinum is no wider than the overlying vertebrae on the DV view in the cat. In older, small breed dogs *fat deposition* can cause marked widening of the cranial mediastinum and tracheal displacement (Figure 5.8). In young dogs the thymus can be identified to the left of the mid-line as a sail-shaped soft tissue mass (Figure 5.9). Mediastinal masses should be assessed on at least two views.

Localized soft tissue densities in the cranial mediastinum are most often neoplastic, but may also be due to an abscess or granuloma, and rarely, a haematoma or a cyst. *Cranial mediastinal masses* in young cats are most commonly due to *thymic lymphoma*, and may be large enough to displace the heart caudally.

Dilatation of the oesophagus may be generalized or localized. As a dilated oesophagus usually contains some air, it is nearly always distinguishable from a soft tissue mass on plain films. Where doubt exists, a barium meal will locate the oesophagus. Liquid barium should not be used alone because of the high risk of aspiration pneumonia in animals with compromised oesophageal function. Most caudal mediastinal masses are the result of oesophageal disease.

The *sternal lymph nodes* are located just dorsal to the sternum between the heart and thoracic inlet, and hilar lymph nodes are found adjacent to the tracheal

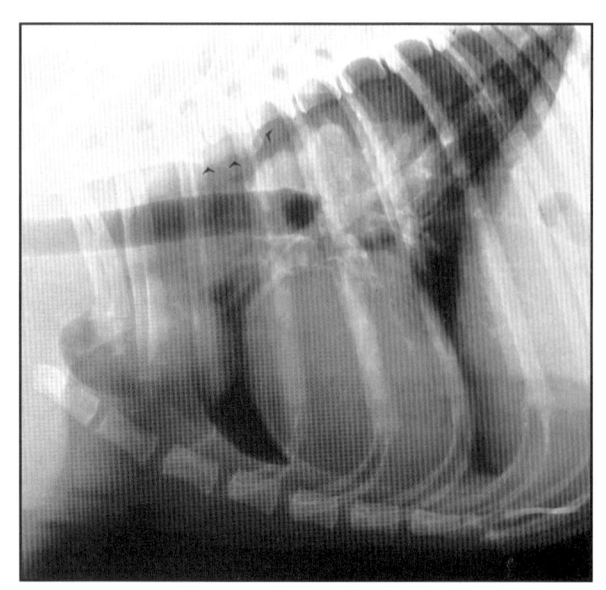

Figure 5.10: Sternal and hilar lymph node enlargement in a 4-year-old Airedale with lymphoma. The caudal border of the scapulae (arrowheads) should not be mistaken for a lesion.

bifurcation. Node enlargement is commonly due to lymphoma, and is a frequent finding in dogs with the multicentric form of the disease, but may be inflammatory, resulting from antigenic stimulation secondary to other intrathoracic disease (Figure 5.10).

Diffuse mediastinal widening: This is most often the result of mediastinal fat or fluid. It is difficult to appreciate on the lateral view. Mediastinal fluid is identified by the presence of *reverse fissure lines* on the DV projection. These appear as triangular or 'rose thorn' like soft tissue densities with the base toward the hilus at the division of the lung lobes.

Mediastinal fluid cannot be characterized by its radiographic appearance alone; however in most cases it is accompanied by at least a small volume of pleural fluid which can be analysed following thoracocentesis.

Mediastinal shift: Displacement of the mediastinum from the midline on the DV or VD view is referred to as *mediastinal shift*. It is most commonly seen as a physiological consequence of lateral recumbency, particularly in the anaesthetized animal, when the dependent lung collapses. This is recognized as displacement of the heart towards the side that was previously dependent, accompanied by an increase in the density of that hemithorax. It also occurs in diseases causing unequal lung expansion or in space occupying lesions including unilateral pleural effusion or pneumothorax.

The cardiac shadow

Despite the recent advances in echocardiography which have revolutionized cardiac imaging, thoracic radiography remains an important means of assessing cardiac disease. The modalities should be considered complementary to one another as each can provide different information.

The heart shadow is best assessed on the *DV* and *right lateral views*. In the dog, breed variation has a great effect on the appearance of the normal heart. Sternal contact is greatest in barrel-chested breeds, the heart appearing oval on the DV projection, whereas in deep-chested breeds the heart is more upright on the lateral view, and appears smaller and more circular on the DV radiograph.

Cardiac size

The *vertebral scale system* provides an objective measure of cardiac size (Figure 5.11). The maximal dimensions of the long and short axes of the heart are measured against the midthoracic vertebrae, starting with the cranial edge of T4. The sum of the long and short axes of the heart is 9.7 ± 0.5 vertebrae in normal adult dogs. In puppies the cardiac outline appears larger relative to the thoracic cavity than in the mature dog.

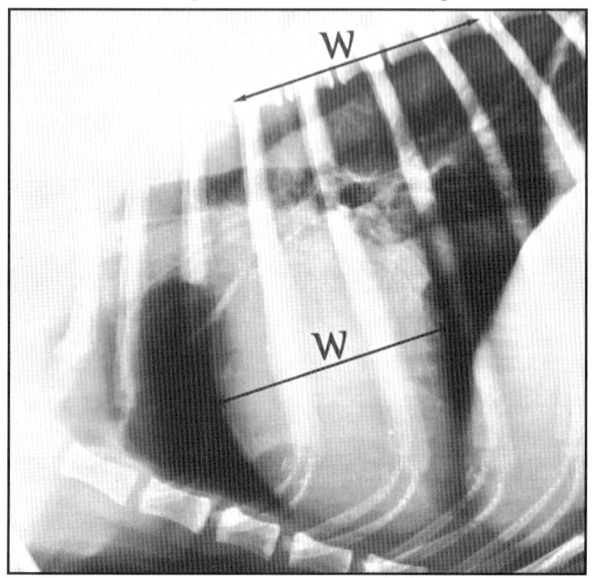

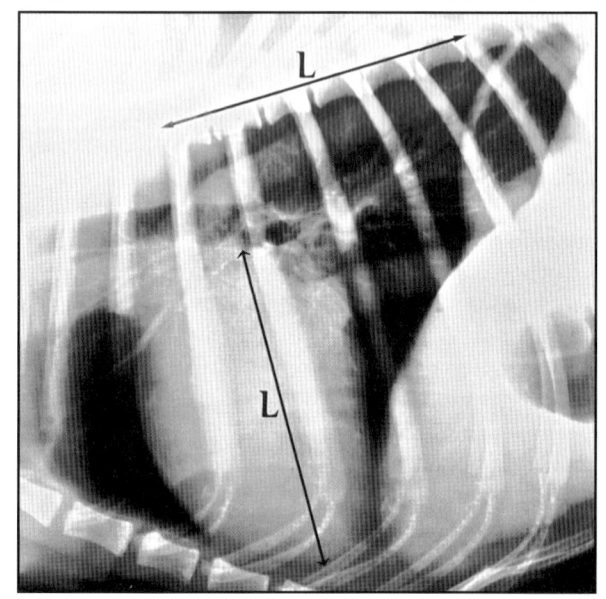

Figure 5.11: Vertebral scale system for assessment of cardiac size. The long axis (L) and short axis (W) of the cardiac silhouette are measured against the mid-thoracic vertebrae, starting with the cranial edge of T4. $L + W = 9.7 \pm 0.5$ vertebrae in normal adult dogs.

Recognition of abnormalities in cardiac shape may be of more value than assessment of size.

The appearance in the cat is more constant, the heart being angulated slightly in a craniodorsal to caudoventral direction. The width of the feline heart on the lateral view should not exceed two intercostal spaces (Figure 5.4).

In both species the height of the cardiac shadow on the lateral view should not exceed two-thirds the height of the thoracic cavity. The width on the DV view at the fifth intercostal space should be no greater than two-thirds the width of the thoracic cavity.

The cardiac shadow appears greater on expiration than inspiration. Valid comparisons of follow-up films can therefore only be made with films taken at the same phase of respiration, ideally at the point of maximum inflation of the lungs.

Microcardia

Overall reduction in cardiac size is a consequence of reduced venous return and is therefore seen in hypovolaemic states. The cardiac apex appears more pointed, and the pulmonary vessels and caudal vena cava are reduced in size. Microcardia in hypoadrenocorticism (Addison's disease) may be especially pronounced if the hypovolaemia is accompanied by a reduction in cardiac muscle mass.

Generalized cardiomegaly

Whilst moderate or marked cardiomegaly is a reliable indicator of heart disease, slight cardiomegaly must be interpreted with caution. It should also be remembered that significant heart disease can be present in a radiographically normal heart (e.g. arrhythmias, hypertrophic cardiomyopathy and subaortic stenosis).

With significant generalized cardiomegaly, the heart retains some of its contours which distinguishes true cardiomegaly from the globoid pattern of enlargement seen in pericardial effusions.

Diseases which cause generalized cardiac enlargement include dilated cardiomyopathy (Figure 5.12), concurrent tricuspid and mitral insufficiency, ventricular septal defects, and chronic anaemia.

Chamber enlargement

Whilst the signs given below are valuable indicators of chamber enlargement, it is unusual for any one chamber to be enlarged in isolation, and the overall shape of the heart and the appearance of the pulmonary circulation and great vessels should be considered in the assessment of cardiac enlargement.

Right atrium

Mild degrees of right atrial enlargement are not appreciable radiographically, but marked enlargement is recognized as:

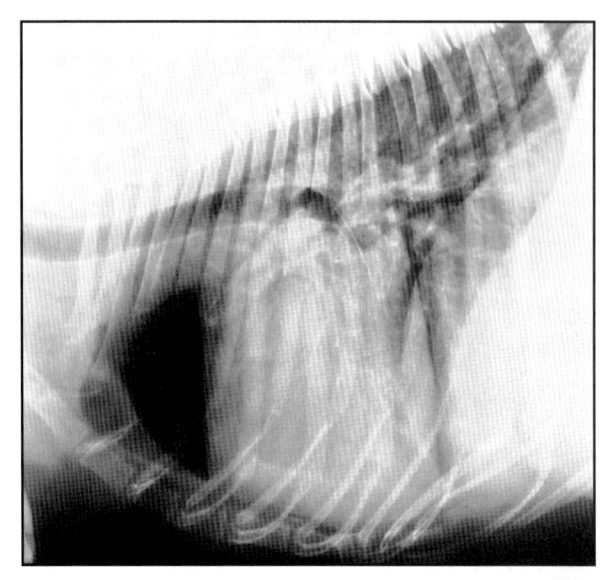

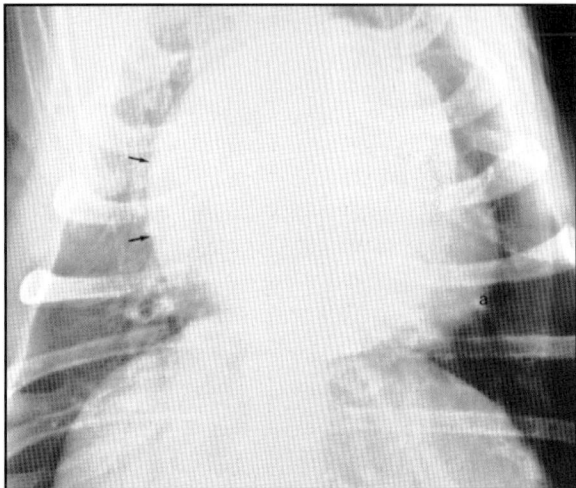

Figure 5.12: *Lateral and DV radiographs of a Dobermann with dilated cardiomyopathy and generalized cardiomegaly. Right sided enlargement is revealed by the apex of the heart being displaced to the left and the heart bulging towards the right body wall (arrows) on the DV view. The lateral view shows increased sternal contact and an intraventricular notch, the height of the heart revealing left sided involvement.*

- A distinct bulge in the DV projection at the 9–11 o'clock position
- Elevation of the trachea cranial to the carina on the lateral view
- A pronounced notch between right atrium and ventricle on the lateral view.

If, however, as is often the case, the right ventricle is also enlarged, then the cranial border will appear generally more rounded (Figure 5.13).

Right ventricle

Signs of right ventricular enlargement include:

DV view:

- a reverse D shape, the apex over to the left, and the right heart border bulging to the right chest wall.

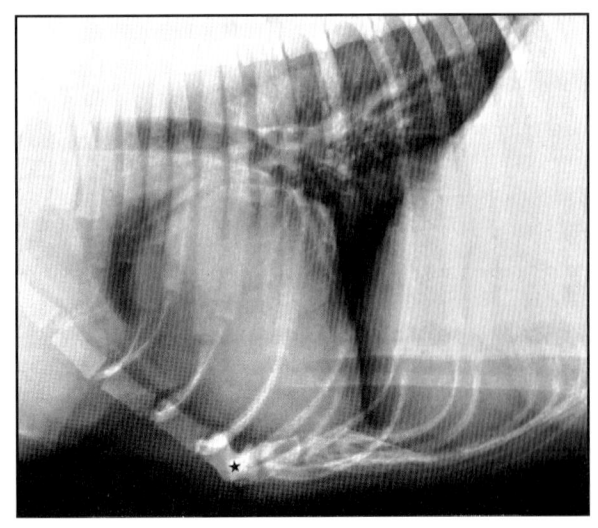

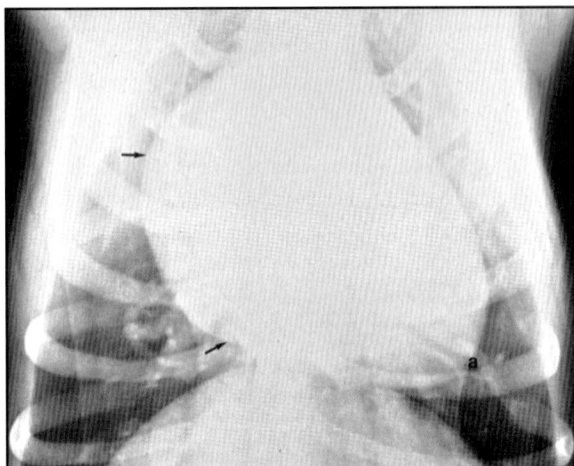

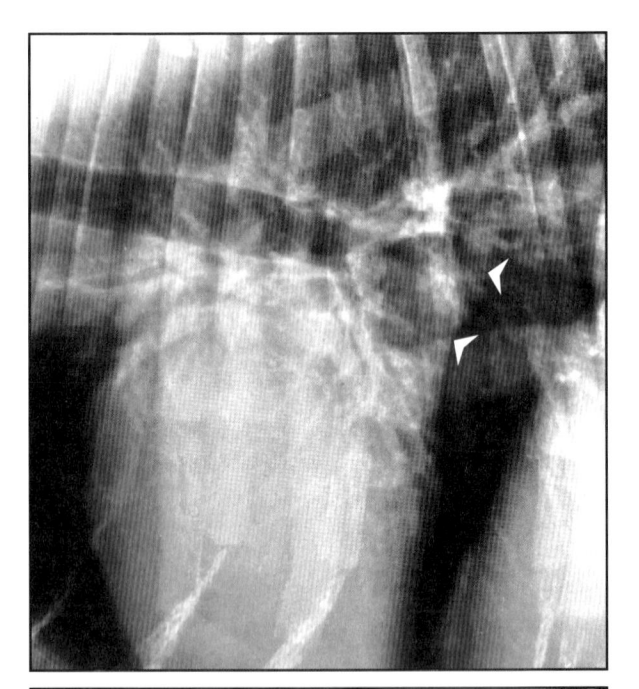

*Figure 5.13: Right atrial and ventricular enlargement secondary to tricuspid dysplasia. The trachea is elevated cranial to the carina on the lateral view. Note the congenital sternal deformity (★); abnormalities such as this may influence the position and appearance of the heart. The right border of the heart is rounded (arrows) on the DV view and the apex (**a**) is displaced to the left.*

Lateral view:

- Rounding of the cranial border
- Apex-tipping, the enlarged right ventricle elevating the apex off the sternum (especially with right ventricular hypertrophy)
- Elevation of the caudal vena cava as it runs towards the right atrium.

Left atrium
Signs of left atrial enlargement (Figure 5.14):

DV view:

- A dense soft tissue mass may be seen separating the left and right main stem bronchi, superimposed on the cardiac shadow
- The left auricular appendage may be seen as a bulge on the left cardiac border at the 2–3 o'clock position.

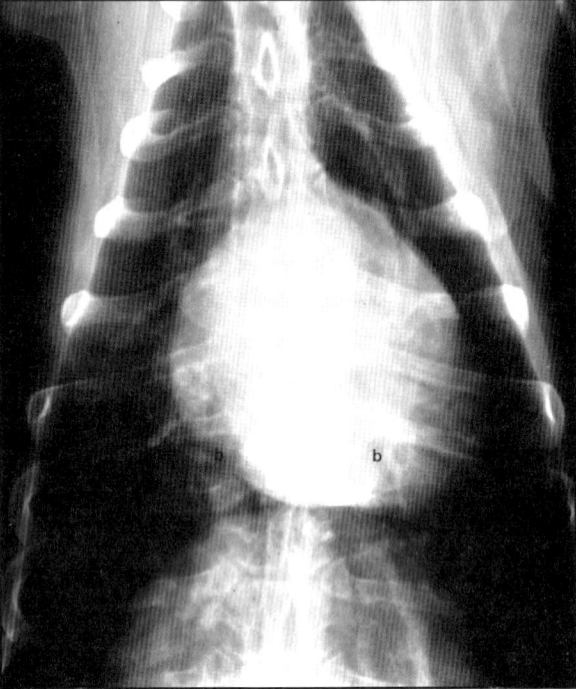

*Figure 5.14: Lateral and DV radiographs of a 7-year-old Dobermann with dilated cardiomyopathy demonstrating left sided enlargement. The caudal border of the left atrium is seen on the lateral view (arrowheads). Left atrial enlargement is less readily identified on the DV view, although an increase in soft tissue density between the mainstem bronchi to the caudal lobes (**b**) indicates its presence. There is no evidence of cardiogenic pulmonary oedema in this dog.*

Lateral view:

- More sensitive to left atrial enlargement
- A bulge in the caudodorsal cardiac shadow
- The left main stem bronchus is elevated, with the left atrium bulging up between right and left mainstem bronchi.

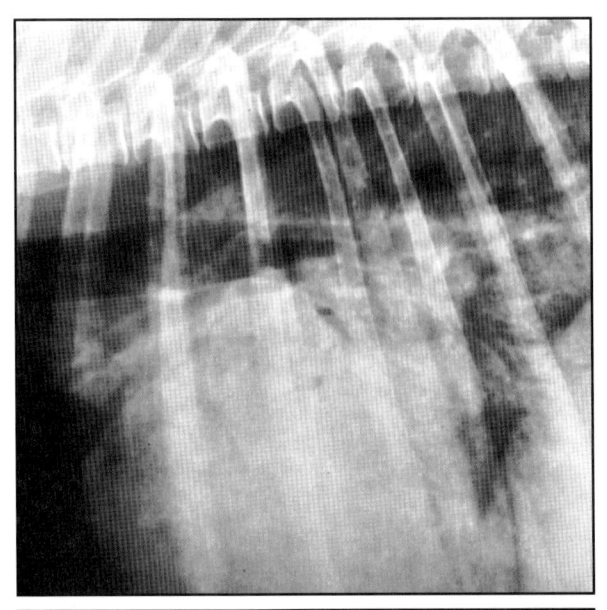

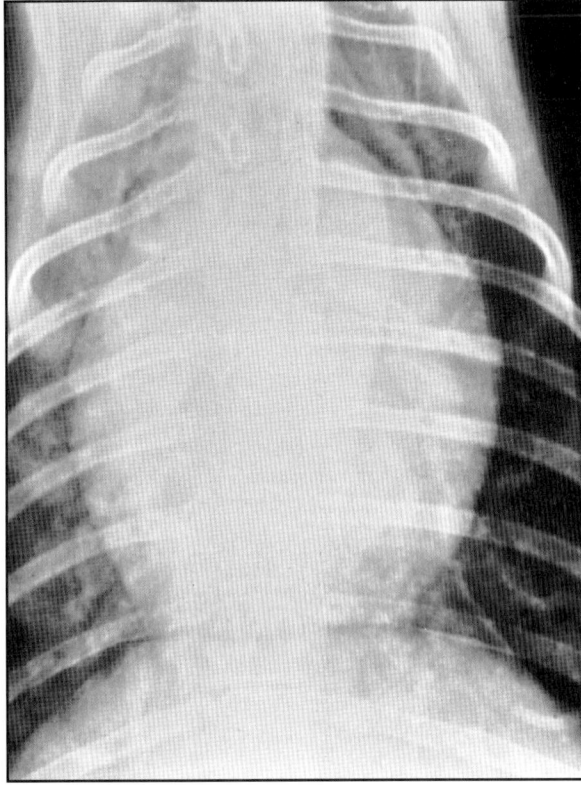

Figure 5.15: Lateral and DV radiographs of a cross bred dog with valvular endocardiosis. There is generalized cardiomegaly, with notable enlargement of the left ventricle. The caudal border of the heart is convex and the caudal trachea is elevated (lateral view). The DV view shows elongation of the cardiac silhouette. Opacification of the lung fields reflects left sided cardiac failure with interstitial oedema and patchy alveolar flooding.

Left ventricular enlargement

Signs of left ventricular enlargement (Figure 5.15):

DV view:

- Rounding of the cardiac apex
- Elongation of the cardiac shadow.

Lateral view:

- Increase in apicobasilar length of the heart, elevating caudal trachea and caudal vena cava
- Upright or convex caudal border.

The great vessels

Changes in the appearance of the great vessels can provide valuable clues as to abnormalities of cardiac function, and should be examined in conjunction with the cardiac shadow.

Caudal vena cava

The caudal vena cava may be elevated by enlargement of either ventricle. The maximal diameter of the caudal vena cava (not overlying heart or diaphragm) can be compared with that of the aorta at the same intercostal space on an inspiratory radiograph. A CVC/Ao ratio of >1.5 is strongly suggestive of right sided cardiac disease. Values between 1 and 1.5 do not, however, exclude a right sided abnormality. The diameter of the caudal vena cava may be increased in right sided congestive failure, and reduced in hypovolaemic states. Note that the normal appearance of the vessel alters with respiration.

Aorta

The ascending aorta is contained within the cranial mediastinum. Post-stenotic dilatation of the vessel may sometimes be seen in subaortic stenosis as an increase in soft tissue density of the dorsocranial heart shadow with cranial mediastinal widening on the lateral view. However, a normal appearance of the aorta on plain films does not rule out subaortic stenosis.

A localized dilatation may occasionally be recognized on the DV view in patent ductus arteriosus where the ductus leaves the descending aorta. This is referred to as a 'ductus bump'.

The aortic arch can be pronounced in cats with a sloping cardiac shadow on the lateral view, and the intrathoracic aorta may also occasionally appear somewhat undulant due to excessive length (so-called 'redundant aorta').

Pulmonary artery

The main pulmonary artery is located in the 1–2 o'clock position on the DV view in the dog, and a bulge here is generally the result of a post-stenotic dilatation or pulmonary hypertension. In the cat the vessel is closer to the mid-line and harder to identify.

On the lateral radiograph, gross enlargement of the pulmonary trunk (as a result of post-stenotic dilatation, patent ductus arteriosus or pulmonary hypertension), may be identified as a bulge highlighted by the caudal trachea.

The pulmonary circulation

Normal appearance

Pulmonary arteries are located dorsal and lateral to their accompanying bronchi and veins. On the lateral view, the vessels of the right cranial lobe are most readily assessed. The artery and vein should be similar in size, their diameter at the fourth intercostal space should not exceed the smallest diameter of the proximal part of the fourth rib. The vessels of the cranial part of the left cranial lobe are less apparent as they are usually superimposed on the craniodorsal mediastinum. The vessels of the caudal part of the left cranial lobe and the right middle lobe are superimposed on the heart shadow and are rarely seen clearly. The vessels of the caudal lobes are best seen on the DV view. They should not exceed the diameter of the ninth rib at the point where they cross it.

Overcirculation

Distension of the pulmonary vessels is seen in:

- Left to right shunts (e.g. PDA, VSD) (Figure 5.16)
- Overhydration.

Distension of pulmonary veins

Dilation of pulmonary veins is indicative of pulmonary venous congestion and is an important early sign of left sided congestive failure. The cranial veins on the lateral view appear larger than their accompanying arteries, and may sag ventrally.

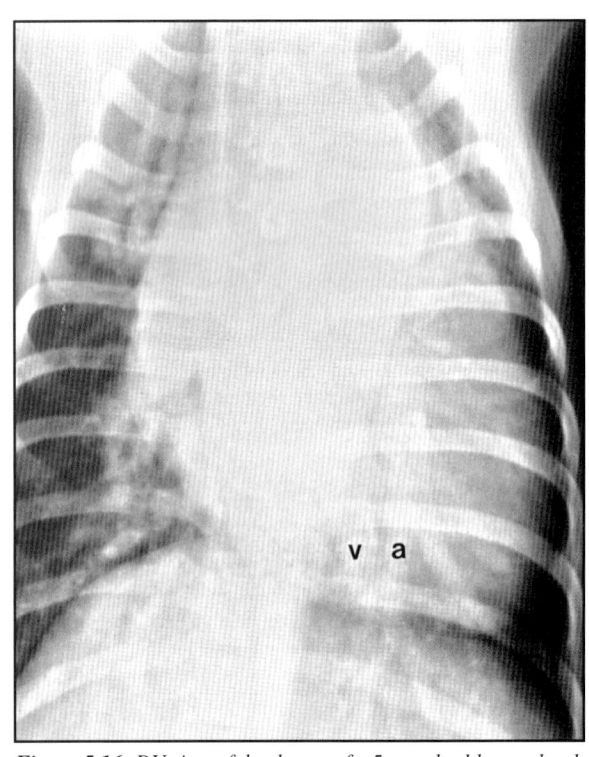

*Figure 5.16: DV view of the thorax of a 5-month-old cross bred dog with a patent ductus arteriosus. There is cardiomegaly, with distension of the pulmonary vessels. The pulmonary artery (**a**) and vein (**v**) of the left caudal lobe are labelled.*

Distension of pulmonary arteries

This is rarely seen in the UK. It arises as a consequence of pulmonary hypertension, or acute pulmonary thromboembolism.

It is a common finding in *heartworm disease* due to *Dirofilaria immitis*, which may rarely occur in imported dogs. Diffuse or patchy interstitial infiltrates frequently accompany the vascular changes. *Angiostrongylus vasorum* can cause similar features and has been reported in dogs in the south-west of England.

Undercirculation

Thin and thready looking pulmonary vessels are seen in:

- Hypovolaemia
- Right sided cardiac failure with reduced cardiac output
- Right to left shunts e.g. tetralogy of Fallot.

This appearance can be mimicked by overinflation of the lungs or overexposure.

Table 5.1 is intended only as a guide. Congenital cardiac defects vary in severity, and therefore the same type of defect can produce quite different radiographic appearances in different individuals. The changes associated with subaortic stenosis and small VSDs can be very subtle, the heart appearing normal in some cases.

A definitive diagnosis can rarely be reached on plain radiography alone, and usually requires echocardiography and/or cardiac catheterization and angiography.

Acquired cardiac disease

Echocardiography is also required for a definitive diagnosis in acquired cardiac disease. However, radiography remains the only practicable means of assessing the degree of left sided congestive failure and is important in determining therapeutic management.

Valvular endocardiosis and *dilated cardiomyopathy* are the most common acquired conditions in dogs, and both often cause a generalized cardiomegaly, which may be accompanied by signs of left or right congestive failure (Figure 5.15). A notable exception is dilated cardiomyopathy in the Dobermann, when the left atrium is commonly the only chamber to be enlarged (Figure 5.14).

Bacterial endocarditis is rare in the dog and cat, and radiographic findings are of limited value in diagnosing the condition. The cardiac silhouette may be normal, or show left atrial enlargement with pulmonary oedema.

Idiopathic hypertrophic cardiomyopathy is the most common acquired cardiac disease in the cat. Left atrial enlargement may be massive. This may confer a 'valentine' shape to the cardiac silhouette on the DV view. Left ventricular enlargement is sometimes apparent, but equally the cardiac shadow can appear normal.

Condition	LA	LV	RA	RV	Ao	PA	cVC	Lungfield
PDA	++	++	–	–	+	+	–	Overperfused
SAS	(+)	(+)	–	–	(+)	–	–	Normal
PS	–	–	(+)	++	–	++	(+)	Normal
VSD	+	++	–	++	–	–	–	Overperfused
MD	++	++	–	–	–	–	–	Veins dilated
TD	–	–	++	++	–	–	++	Normal
T of F	–	–	–	(+)	–	–	–	Underperfused

Table 5.1: *Patterns of enlargement seen in congenital cardiac disease.*
Key: + enlargement, ++ marked enlargement, (+) sometimes enlarged, – normal.
LA: left atrium, LV: left ventricle, RA: right atrium, RV: right ventricle, Ao: aorta, PA: pulmonary artery, cVC: caudal vena cava, PDA: patent ductus arteriosus,
SAS: subaortic stenosis, PS: pulmonic stenosis, VSD: ventricular septal defect, MD: mitral dysplasia, TD: tricuspid dysplasia, T of F: tetralogy of Fallot

Signs of left and/or right sided congestive failure are frequently seen. The radiographic appearance of *restrictive cardiomyopathy* is similar.

Dilated cardiomyopathy is now uncommon in cats, but the radiographic features are of generalized cardiomegaly with rounding of the cardiac apex. Pleural effusion is common, obscuring the cardiac shadow and masking any pulmonary oedema that may also be present.

Radiographic signs of left sided congestive failure
Radiography remains the only readily available means of assessing the degree of left sided heart failure (Figure 5.15). As described earlier, distension of pulmonary veins is the earliest radiographic sign, although this is not always seen. As pulmonary venous pressure builds up, oedema fluid is first formed in the interstitium, seen as a reticular pattern over the pulmonary parenchyma, blurring the outlines of the pulmonary vessels. The vessels remain visible however, until alveolar oedema develops. Cardiogenic pulmonary oedema in the dog typically has a perihilar distribution. This is not the case in the cat, where it is frequently patchy.

Radiographic signs of right sided congestive failure
Right sided congestive failure typically causes some or all of the following:

• Dilatation of the caudal vena cava
• Hepatic enlargement
• Ascites
• Pleural effusion
• Pericardial and mediastinal effusions (these often go undetected).

Pericardial disease
Generalized enlargement of the cardiac silhouette may be caused by pericardial abnormalities or true cardiac chamber enlargement.

Pericardial effusions result in the cardiac shadow assuming a globoid, football shaped appearance, with loss of the contours which are usually seen to delineate the cardiac chambers. It can usually be distinguished from true cardiac enlargement, although gross enlargement of the right atrium and ventricle as in tricuspid dysplasia can look similar. Non-selective angiocardiography (or echocardiography) can be used to confirm the diagnosis in equivocal cases.

Pericardioperitoneal diaphragmatic hernia is a congenital defect of the cat and dog where the pericardial sac is in direct communication with the peritoneal cavity. The diagnosis can often be made on plain films as gas in small intestinal loops is visible within the globoid cardiac shadow. The dorsal border of the hernia (the dorsal pericardioperitoneal mesothelial remnant) may be identified ventral to or superimposed over the caudal vena cava on the lateral view, connecting the pericardium to the diaphragm. When this is not clear, an upper gastrointestinal contrast examination with barium can be used to demonstrate herniated intestinal loops.

Non-selective angiocardiography
This technique can be performed in the practice situation. A bolus of warmed water soluble iodinated contrast (e.g. 440 mg/kg iodine) is injected rapidly through a catheter into the jugular vein. The passage of contrast may be demonstrated by rapid sequential radiography as it passes along the cranial vena cava, into the right atrium, right ventricle and pulmonary circulation. Because of dilutional effects in the pulmonary circulation, by the time the contrast material has returned to the left heart the bolus quality has deteriorated. The technique is therefore most useful for demonstration of abnormalities of the cranial vena cava and right heart (including right to left shunts). If rapid film changing equipment or a cassette tunnel is not available, useful information may still be obtained from an appropriately timed single radiograph. This is usually 3–5 seconds after the start of the injection, although timing of the exposure depends on the area of interest, speed of injection, length of catheter and circulation time of the patient, and is therefore subject to inaccuracies.

The lungfields

Normal radiographic appearance

The *right lung* is divided into cranial, middle, accessory and caudal lobes. The tip of the right cranial lobe crosses into the left hemithorax cranial to the cardiac shadow. The accessory lobe also crosses some distance into the left hemithorax, and its boundary may be identified on the VD and DV projection as a fold of mediastinum crossing obliquely from the cardiac apex to the left hemidiaphragm.

The *left lung* has two lobes, cranial and caudal. The cranial lobe is divided into a cranial and caudal part. The cranial part is the most cranially located lobe, overlapping the right cranial lobe at the thoracic inlet. A soft tissue line demarcating the division of right and left cranial lobes is frequently identified on the lateral view.

The *pulmonary arteries* are located dorsal and medial to the accompanying bronchus and pulmonary vein. The vessels taper towards the hilus, giving off many branches. A branch viewed end-on may appear very radiodense, and can be confused with a soft tissue nodule. Close inspection will show it to be the same diameter as the parent vessel with which it is in direct contact.

The *bronchial walls* may be seen in the normal animal close to the hilus as fine parallel white lines ventral to the pulmonary artery and dorsal to the vein. They are separated by a lucent stripe representing air within their lumen. Seen end-on they appear as ring shadows. They disappear towards the periphery.

The *pulmonary interstitium* is a fine lacy network of soft tissue density which represents the alveolar walls and connective tissue of the pulmonary parenchyma. It is seen throughout the lungfields, but is most obvious in the dorsocaudal area where lung tissue is thickest and the effects of superimposition are greatest. The interstitium becomes more apparent in ageing dogs.

Radiographic abnormalities

For assessment of the lungfield to be meaningful, the lungs must be adequately inflated. Soft tissue structures within the pulmonary parenchyma can only be identified if they are surrounded by alveolar air. Attempts to interpret changes in pulmonary parenchyma in poorly inflated lungs will lead to misdiagnoses. Every effort should therefore be made to obtain inspiratory radiographs. In the anaesthetized animal collapsed lungs should be reinflated with positive pressure ventilation prior to, and if necessary during, radiography. Pleural effusions and pneumothorax should be drained.

Radiographic abnormalities of the lungfield are most frequently described in terms of anatomical pattern recognition. No one pattern is diagnostic for a particular disease and a differential list should be considered in view of the distribution of the lungfield changes, other radiographic evidence of intrathoracic disease, and the clinical signs exhibited.

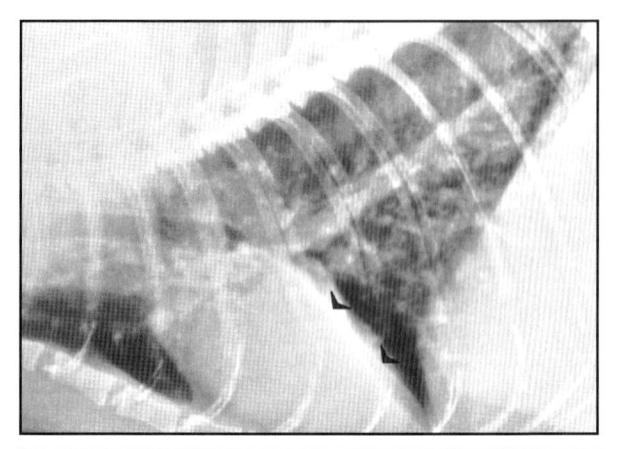

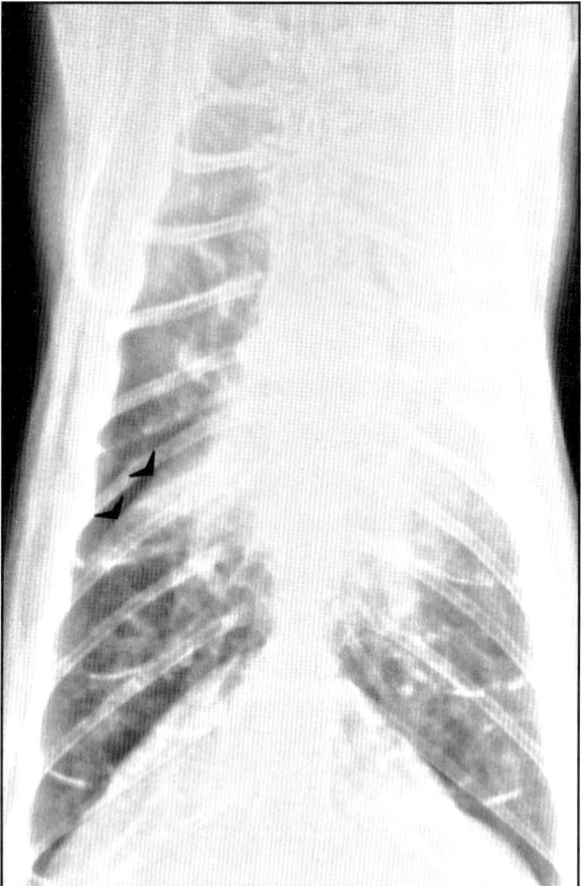

Figure 5.17: Severe bronchial disease in a cat. There is collapse of the right middle lobe (arrowheads). A mixed lung pattern, with bronchial, interstitial and patchy alveolar components, is seen throughout the lungfields.

Lungfield patterns

Abnormalities of the following patterns are described in pulmonary disease:

- Vascular (described earlier)
- Bronchial
- Alveolar
- Interstitial (nodular or diffuse).

It is most common, however, to see a mixed pattern with two or more of the above present (Figure 5.17).

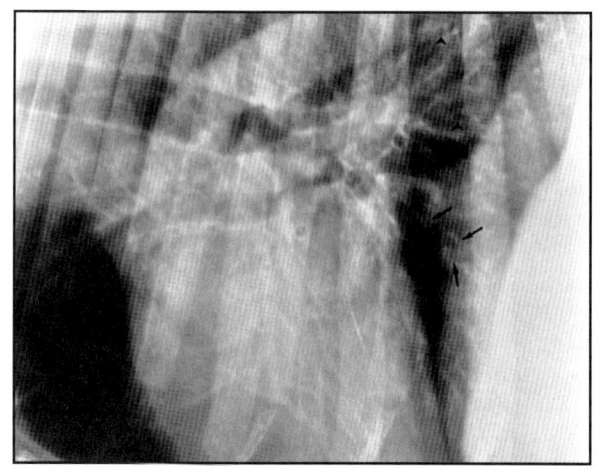

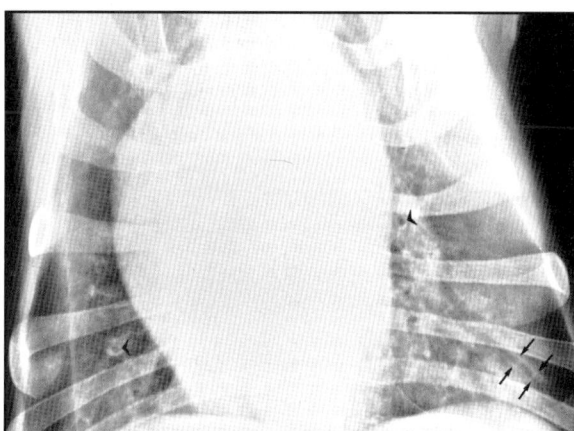

***Figure 5.18**: Bronchial pattern in an aged cross bred dog. The hallmark features of the bronchial markings, identified in cross section as 'ring shadows' (arrowheads) and 'tramlines' (arrows) are clearly seen.*

Bronchial patterns: The normal bronchial pattern may become exaggerated so that the bronchial markings become more obvious and are visible further into the lungfield periphery (Figure 5.18).

Calcification of bronchial walls: This may be an innocuous ageing change, especially in chrondrodystrophic breeds, but may also be seen in hyperadrenocorticism. The bronchial walls stand out very sharply, remaining narrow and clearly defined.

Thickening of bronchial walls: This results from a combination of the following:

* Exudate or mucus within the lumen, lining the mucosa
* Mucosal swelling with inflammatory infiltrates
* Hypertrophy of the muscularis
* Hyperplasia of the epithelium
* Peribronchial cuffing with inflammatory cells.

Thickened bronchial walls seen end on are graphically referred to as '*doughnuts*', and when struck at right angles to the primary beam, '*tramlines*'. The bronchial lumen is still visible as a lucency between the walls.

Bronchial patterns may be caused by the following conditions in the dog and cat:

* Chronic bronchitis
* Allergic bronchitis
* *Aelurostrongylus abstrusus* infection in the cat
* Bronchopneumonia.

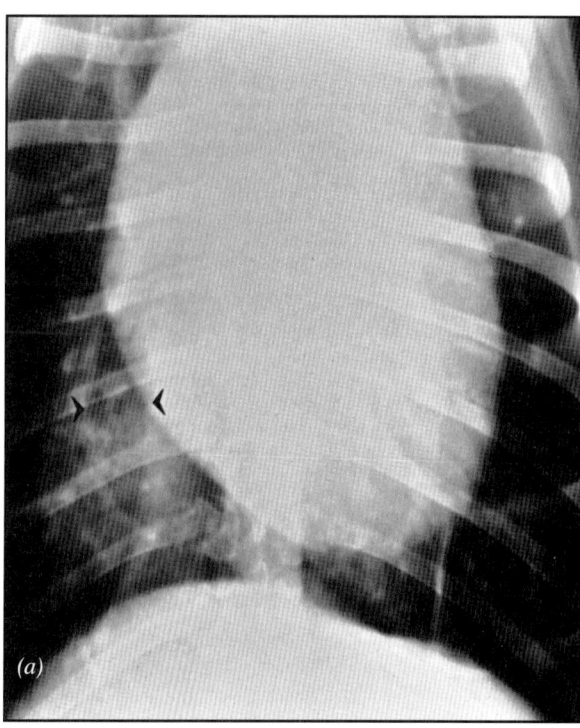

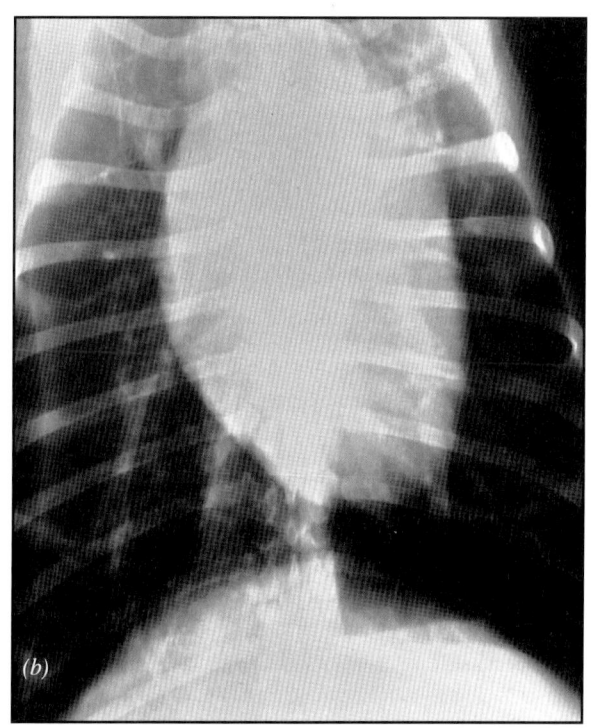

***Figure 5.19**: Sequential DV thoracic radiographs of a 3-year-old Springer Spaniel. (a) The bronchus to the right caudal lobe is widely dilated (arrowheads) with overlapping soft tissue opacification. (b) After retrieval of a bronchial foreign body, the bronchus remained grossly dilated.*

Bronchiectasis may occur in chronic bronchial disease, when the walls may become irreversibly damaged, with permanent dilatation and fibrosis (Figure 5.19). This is identified as saccular or cylindrical nontapering bronchial markings.

Alveolar patterns

Alveolar patterns arise when air within the alveoli is replaced by flooding with fluid or cells, or lost due to alveolar collapse. They are never visible in healthy, normally inflated lungs.

Alveolar patterns are most easily identified when *air bronchograms* are visible. These are formed when alveoli surrounding a bronchus are no longer air-filled and acquire a soft tissue density. The only structure to stand out in the affected tissue is the bronchial lumen, provided that it still contains air. The airway walls and the pulmonary vessels cannot be seen, and are 'lost' in the soft tissue density of affected alveoli (Figure 5.20).

When smaller areas of lung are affected, air bronchograms may not be apparent, but the affected lung tissue appears as fluffy, poorly marginated soft tissue densities within the lungfield. The vascular markings become invisible as they cross these areas. Affected areas show a tendency to coalesce.

Distribution of the alveolar filling pattern can be useful in determining the underlying cause.

Cardiogenic pulmonary oedema is one of the most commonly seen alveolar patterns. It has a perihilar distribution in the dog, but is patchy in the cat. Alveolar flooding is nearly always preceded by pulmonary venous congestion and interstitial oedema, so the pattern is most frequently mixed (Figure 5.15).

Aspiration pneumonia and bacterial bronchopneumonia are typically worse in the *ventral lungfield*, and the right middle lobe is most commonly affected (Figure 5.20).

Inhaled foreign bodies such as grass awns most often affect the *right caudal lobe*, producing a localized inflammatory response (Figure 5.19).

Neoplasms, abscesses and *granulomas* also produce local alveolar patterns.

Pulmonary contusion is a common cause of an alveolar pattern following trauma. Any area may be affected.

Interstitial patterns

The interstitium is composed mainly of the alveolar walls and interlobar septa, and provides a supporting framework for the lymphatics, vessels and bronchi. The interstitium is recognized as a *fine, lacy pattern* in the lungfield. It becomes more visible with the fibrosis which occurs as part of the normal ageing process.

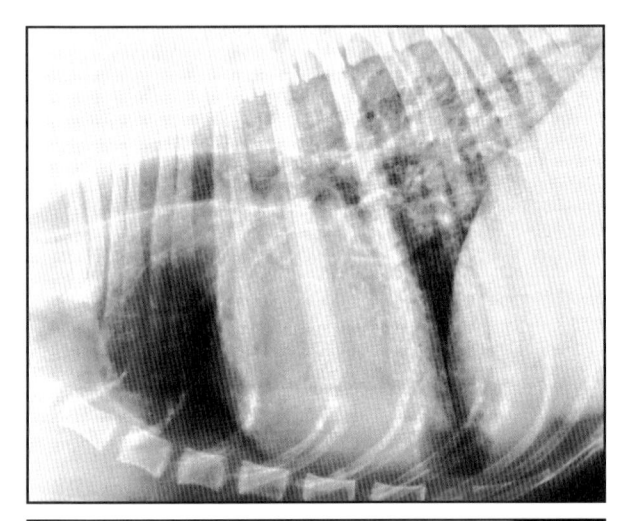

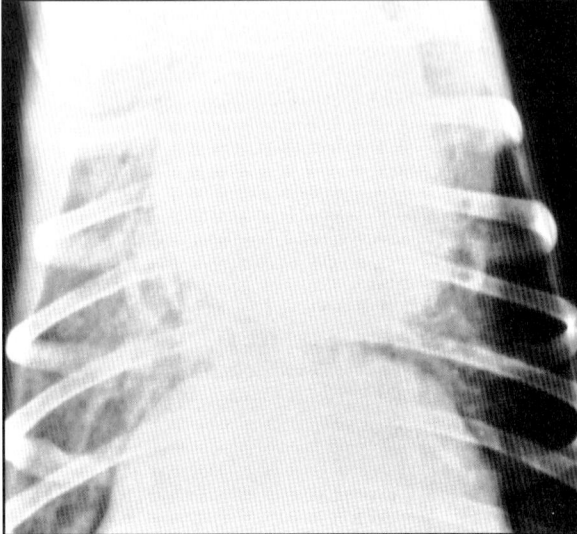

Figure 5.21*: Interstitial pattern in a Collie that had fallen into sheep dip. There is a generalized increase in lungfield density, which appears to be most marked in the lateral view in the dorsocaudal lungfield. The major pulmonary vessels may still be identified, but their margins are somewhat indistinct.*

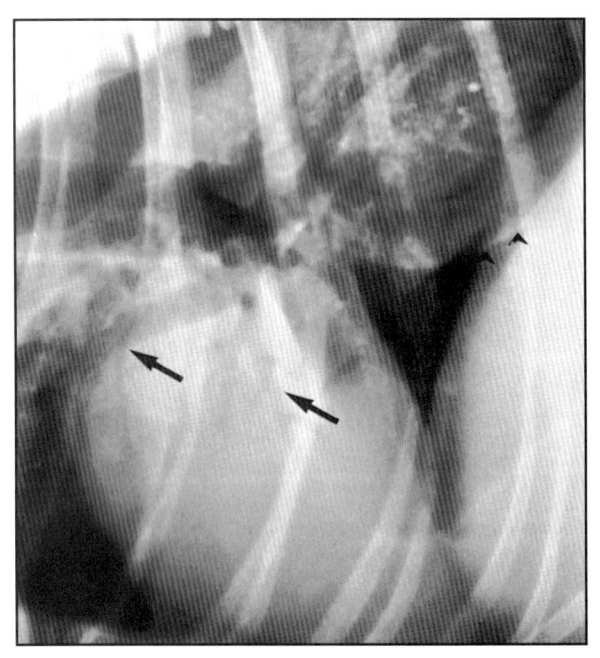

Figure 5.20*: Aspiration pneumonia in a Dachshund with megaoesophagus. The ventral wall of the oesophagus is identified (arrowheads). Mineralized ingesta is faintly visible within the caudal thoracic oesophagus. Air bronchograms are visible within the right cranial and middle lung lobes (arrows).*

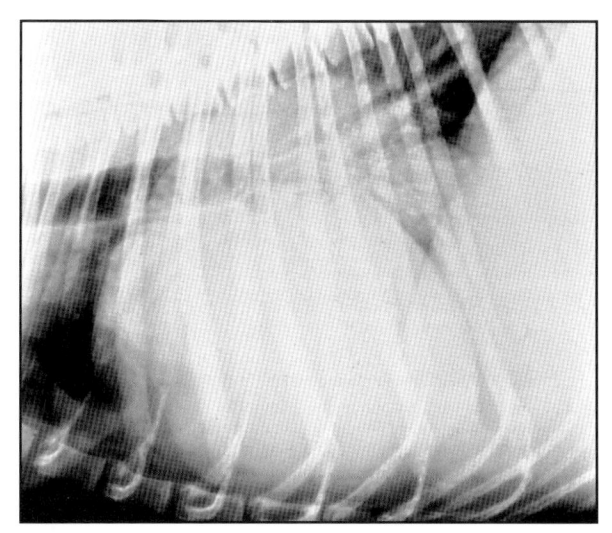

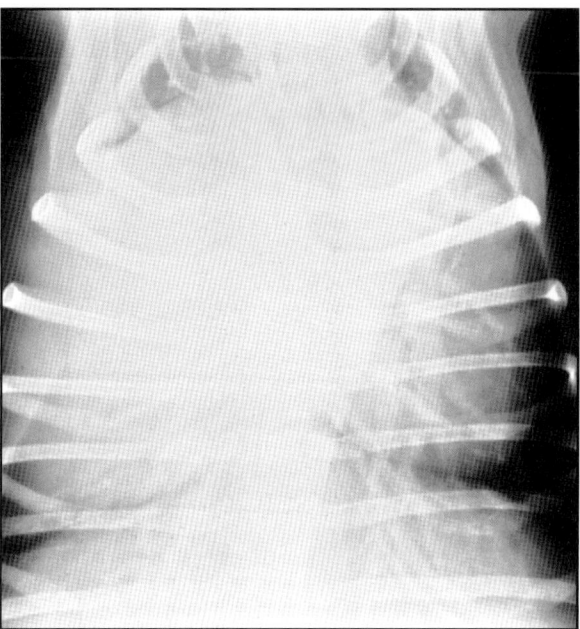

Figure 5.22: *Lateral and DV views of a 9-year-old Springer Spaniel with a massive primary lung tumour. The lung tumour originated from the right middle lobe, is displacing the heart, trachea and descending aorta to the left.*

A generalized unstructured increase in the interstitial pattern can be caused by oedema, inflammatory cells, haemorrhage or neoplasia (e.g. canine lymphoma) of the pulmonary interstitium. Vessels running through affected lung can still be detected (which distinguishes interstitial from alveolar patterns) but with some blurring of their margins (Figure 5.21). More structured *reticular or nodular patterns* of interstitial disease are less common, but are most often caused by miliary neoplastic infiltration.

Pulmonary mass lesions

Pulmonary mass lesions may be represented by solitary or multiple nodular densities. Most frequently these are *neoplastic*, but other causes such as *abscesses, cysts, granulomas* and *haematomas* should be considered. Fungal granulomas and Paragonimiasis may occur in dogs imported from endemic areas.

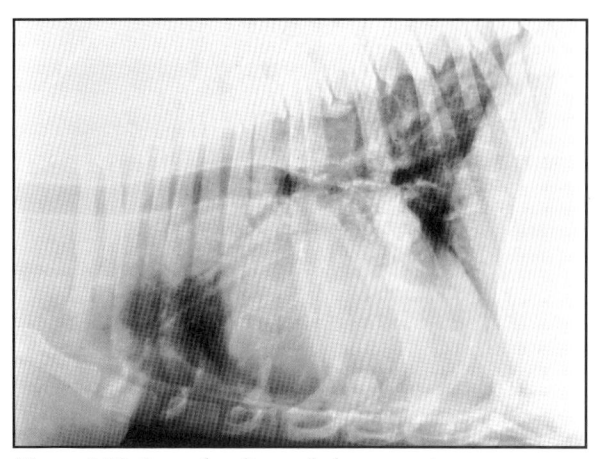

Figure 5.23: *Lateral radiograph demonstrating 'cannonball' metastases in a 10-year-old Rottweiler with a primary mammary tumour.*

Focal hyperlucencies may be due to cysts, bullae and blebs which are often, though not invariably, of limited clinical significance.

Cavitary pulmonary lesions are represented by a focus of increased radiodensity within which air has accumulated. This most frequently occurs within abscesses or primary pulmonary neoplasms.

Pulmonary neoplasia

Primary lung tumours: Large solitary nodules in the dog and cat are most frequently caused by primary lung tumours (Figure 5.22), although pulmonary granulomas should be considered. Bronchiolar carcinomas are usually found in the periphery of the caudal lobes. In the cat, they are often calcified. Bronchogenic carcinomas are found closer to the hilus.

Secondary neoplasia: Pulmonary metastatic disease classically appears as multiple well-defined nodules of varying sizes (Figure 5.23). Solitary nodules or interstitial patterns may also be due to secondary tumours. Although radiography is not particularly sensitive at detecting metastases, affected animals are often asymptomatic, and radiography plays an important role in their detection.

FURTHER READING

Berry CR, Koblik PD and Ticer JW (1990) Dorsal peritoneopericardial mesothelial remnant as an aid to the diagnosis of feline congenital peritoneopericardial diaphragmatic hernia. *Veterinary Radiology* **31**, 239

Buchanan JW and Bucheler J (1995) Vertebral scale system to measure canine heart size in radiographs. *Journal of the American Veterinary Medical Association* **206**, 194

Dennis R and Herrtage M (1995) In: *Manual of Small Animal Diagnostic Imaging* 2nd edn, ed. R Lee, pp. 43–67. British Small Animal Veterinary Association, Cheltenham, UK

Lehmkuhl LB *et al.* (1997) Radiographic evaluation of the caudal vena cava size in dogs. *Veterinary Radiology and Ultrasound* **38**, 94

Suter PF and Lord PF (1984) *Thoracic Radiology, a Text Atlas of Thoracic Diseases of the Dog and Cat.* Peter F. Suter, Wettswil, Switzerland

Thrall DE (1986) The mediastinum and the pleural space. In: *Textbook of Veterinary Diagnostic Radiology*, ed. DE Thrall, pp. 277–303. W.B. Saunders, Philadelphia, USA

(ii) Laboratory Tests

Christopher J.L. Little

INTRODUCTION

Laboratory investigations such as biochemistry and haematology seldom represent first line investigations in a small animal presented with a cardiorespiratory complaint. On the contrary, animals with cardiac or respiratory disorders often will exhibit no obvious haematological or biochemical abnormalities. Nevertheless, where practical, these investigations should form an integral part of the assessment of such patients principally to evaluate distant organ function, identify metabolic compromise and seek out occult disease which may impinge upon therapy or management of the patient. Moreover, in a substantial minority of cases, biochemistry and haematology investigations can help characterise cardiovascular and pulmonary diseases.

HAEMATOLOGY

Rapid basic haematology such as a packed red cell volume (PCV) estimation and examination of a stained blood smear will aid the evaluation of any patient presented in an emergency with signs such as pallor, pyrexia, epistaxis, tachycardia or tachypnoea. Haematology is essential where respiratory conditions such as pneumonia, pulmonary infiltrate of eosinophils, and lung tumours are suspected and where endocarditis is included in the differential diagnosis. Arrhythmias are not uncommon in the absence of obvious organic cardiac disease and a complete blood count should form a part of the further investigation of such cases.

Interpretation of haematology data should take into account absolute and relative leucocyte counts, red cell parameters, platelet size and numbers and cell morphology. Wherever possible, these should be evaluated alongside plasma protein and, arguably, fibrinogen or C-reactive protein levels as well as clinical findings. A working understanding of erythrocyte and leucocyte dynamics will aid the interpretation. These issues have been addressed in much greater detail elsewhere (Duncan and Prasse, 1986; Jain, 1993).

Anaemia

Anaemia is a frequent cause for animals to be presented with suspected cardiorespiratory disease. Tachypnoea, tachycardia, pallor and weakness are among the most common presenting signs particularly if the anaemia is of acute onset. If the PCV is less than 20%, a low grade early systolic murmur will usually be evident on the left hemithorax, typically over the heart base. Evaluation of a patient with anaemia must first establish whether the condition has arisen due to haemorrhage, haemolysis or bone marrow dysfunction. Anamnesis and careful clinical examination are vital, but further investigation will require full haematology; investigations such as clinical chemistry, urinalysis and bone marrow biopsy will usually be required (Squires, 1993). Dogs and cats with chronic inflammation or neoplasia frequently exhibit a mild normocytic normochromic anaemia. The aetiology of this condition is complex; therapy should be directed to the primary disease (Jain, 1993).

Polycythaemia

Polycythaemia, an elevated red cell mass, is found in some patients with suspected cardiorespiratory disorders. Relative polycythaemia, in which PCV rises but total body red cell mass is not increased, accompanies haemoconcentration in severely dehydrated animals and is not uncommon. In these patients, pallor and cardiovascular collapse are usually accompanied by microcardia, high urine specific gravity, prerenal azotaemia and other abnormalities related to the primary disease. A true polycythaemia caused by long-standing tissue hypoxia is not common but can sometimes be found secondary to chronic lung conditions such as chronic obstructive pulmonary disease (COPD). Congenital heart lesions associated with right-to-left shunting of blood (such as tetralogy of Fallot, or ventricular septal defects with Eisenmenger's physiology) may induce polycythaemia (Drazner, 1989). The affected animal may be cyanotic. In these cases, PCV can reach 65% or more; blood viscosity is dramatically increased, resistance to flow rises and cardiac output decreases.

Leucocyte abnormalities

Abnormalities of the leucocytes are sometimes present in animals presented for the investigation of cardiorespiratory signs. Acute and chronic bacterial pneumonias, which are more common in dogs, may be associated with leucocytosis due to neutrophilia and monocytosis (Thayer and Robinson, 1984; Tams, 1989). The extent of the elevation in white cell count will depend on the type, severity and duration of the bacterial infection. In acute conditions, toxic neutrophils and a high proportion of immature forms such as band cells, metamyelocytes and myelocytes may be seen. Where the mature forms outnumber the immature cells (a 'regenerative left shift'), this implies an appropriate bone marrow response to the inflammatory challenge and may be viewed as a favourable prognostic finding. If the neutrophil count is hardly elevated, or is depressed, and immature cells predominate (a 'degenerative left shift'), this can be an ambiguous finding, particularly early in the course of an acute infection. In this event, the outlook is potentially unfavourable. Vigorous antibiotic treatment must be undertaken and the investigation repeated regularly until either a regenerative neutrophilia or further deterioration ensues. In some animals with bacterial pneumonias the haematology will be normal or a stress leucogram will be present.

A similar leucocyte pattern to that seen in pneumonias may be found in dogs or cats with other cardiorespiratory complaints. Dogs with endocarditis usually exhibit an inflammatory leucogram although this is not always present (Anderson and Dubielzig, 1984; Bennett and Taylor, 1987; Elwood *et al.*, 1993). Pyothorax, pulmonary abscesses, bronchopulmonary disease and primary or metastatic thoracic neoplasia may be associated with the same haematological pattern (Chinn *et al.*, 1985; Dye *et al.*, 1996). Haemangiosarcoma, which may be located in the lungs and right atrium, or elsewhere in the body, can present with a catalogue of haematological disturbances. These vary but may include anaemia, anisocytosis, schistocytosis, neutrophilic leucocytosis, and alterations to the platelet count (Ng and Mills, 1985).

Eosinophilia

Eosinophilia ($>1.5 \times 10^9$/l) is not uncommon accompanying respiratory disorders of both cats and dogs. The associated conditions are believed to be of allergic origin and include feline asthma, allergic bronchitis and pulmonary infiltrate of eosinophils (PIE) (Bauer, 1989; Centre *et al.*, 1990). These terms are often used interchangeably. Parasitic infections and other pathology affecting the lungs are also sometimes accompanied by elevated eosinophil counts (Dye *et al.*, 1996). Radiography, faecal examination for parasites, bronchoscopy and/or bronchoalveolar lavage will be useful in differentiating these conditions (Martin *et al.*, 1993).

PLASMA BIOCHEMISTRY AND URINALYSIS

Plasma biochemistry facilitates more exact diagnosis and successful management of cardiorespiratory disorders in small animal patients. A variety of analytes may be measured but those which are most often helpful are listed in Table 5.2. Blood gas analysis, where available, will be of particular value and is dealt with elsewhere (see Chapter 6i). Biochemistry tests of plasma are enhanced when accompanied by urine tests, including specific gravity; because urinalysis is rapid, simple and inexpensive there is no excuse to avoid this investigation.

Prerenal azotaemia

In heart failure, the limited cardiac output is preferentially distributed to the coronary, cerebral and skeletal muscle vascular beds. A disproportionate drop in renal blood flow and glomerular filtration rate occurs. These effects contribute to renal retention of salt and water (see Chapter 3). Total body water and total body sodium increase, but the rise in sodium is often proportionately less than that of water so that a mild dilutional hyponatraemia can develop. In spite of the huge functional reserve of the normal kidney the reduction in glomerular filtration rate frequently leads to modest increases in plasma concentrations of *urea* and *creatinine*. In prerenal azotaemia, urea concentration rarely exceeds 50 mmol/l, creatinine concentrations are usually less than 500 mmol/l. This prerenal azotaemia must be differentiated from other prerenal causes such as dehydration or blood loss, and from renal and postrenal causes of azotaemia. Differentiation will largely be based on anamnesis and physical examination but can usually be facilitated by urinalysis and plasma protein assays, preferably before instituting diuretic therapy. In dehydrated patients, urine specific gravity and plasma protein levels will be high. Cats and dogs with clinically significant renal disease will exhibit urine specific gravity in the low or isosthenuric range. Ratios between urea and creatinine concentrations in the plasma are of no value in differentiating prerenal, renal and postrenal causes of azotaemia in the dog (Finco and Duncan, 1976).

Plasma creatinine concentration can be a crude but moderately accurate estimate of glomerular filtration rate in dogs, particularly where renal function is impaired (Finco *et al.*, 1995). An alternative but more complicated measurement of glomerular filtration rate is based on endogenous creatinine clearance. The patient's bladder is emptied. All urine produced over a set time (usually 8–24 hours) is collected and pooled. This urine volume, the creatinine concentration and plasma creatinine concentration midway through the test are measured.

Analyte	Principle reasons for measurement
Urea	Prerenal azotaemia may accompany severe heart failure and/or follow aggressive diuresis Renal failure affects drug excretion (digoxin, enalapril, etc.)
Creatinine	As for urea
Total protein	To assess hydration status and monitor diuresis To differentiate causes of ascites, hydrothorax and peripheral oedema
Albumin	To assess hydration and diuresis Albumin is a carrier protein for hormones, drugs and calcium
Globulin	To assess hydration status A non-specific indicator of immune challenge (pneumonias, abscesses, neoplasia, chronic infections etc.)
Alanine aminotransferase (ALT)	Evaluate hepatocellular disease in congestive heart failure
Alkaline phosphatase (ALKP)	Hepatocyte swelling and intrahepatic cholestasis may accompany congestive heart failure
Fibrinogen	Inflammation (insensitive marker in small animals) Disseminated intravascular coagulation (DIC)
Potassium	Hypokalaemia commonly accompanies diuresis Anorexic cats become hypokalaemic Hyperkalaemia can accompany widespread tissue damage and acute renal failure Hypoadrenocorticism (Addison's disease) Hypo- and hyperkalaemia promote arrhythmias
Sodium	Mild hyponatraemia can accompany congestive heart failure, especially where diuresis and salt restriction are used in management
Magnesium	Hypomagnesaemia quickly develops when diuresis is employed*
Thyroid hormone (T4)	Feline hyperthyroidism is frequently accompanied by hypertrophic cardiomyopathy

Table 5.2: *Clinical biochemistry tests of plasma in dogs and cats with cardiorespiratory disease.*
Alkalosis, an increase in plasma bicarbonate levels, and hypochloraemia may also occur.

Glomerular filtration rate (ml/min/kg) = Urine creatinine concentration (mmol/l) x Urine volume/plasma creatinine concentration (mmol/l) x Time (minutes) x Body weight (kg).

Normal dogs exhibit GFR around 2.5–4.4 ml/min/kg (Finco *et al.*, 1981, 1995; Gleadhill and Michell, 1996; Tennant, 1997). Alternative tests for assessment of azotaemia include urine creatinine to plasma creatinine ratio (>20:1 in prerenal azotaemia), urine sodium concentration (<10–20 mmol/l in prerenal azotaemia) and fractional excretion of sodium (<1% in prerenal azotaemia) (Graurer and Lane, 1995).

Many drugs, including digoxin, used in small animals with cardiac disease are excreted primarily by the kidneys. Where glomerular filtration rate is depressed, standard dose rates are inappropriate and the clinician should adjust doses downwards.

Liver enzymes

In congestive heart failure, venous congestion of the liver often leads to hepatomegaly, hepatocellular swelling and intrahepatic cholestasis. The plasma levels of hepatic enzymes, particularly *alanine aminotransferase* (ALT) and *alkaline phosphatase* (ALKP) can consequently rise. In cats, changes to ALKP activity are frequently subtle so that any change should be regarded as significant until proven otherwise. Hepatic venous congestion rarely causes liver failure, so plasma albumin concentration is unaffected by this pathology.

Electrolytes

Plasma electrolyte disturbances can have life-threatening effects on cardiac function. Electrolyte abnormalities most frequently arise from the treatment of cardiac failure in small animals. Diuretics, particularly thiazides, frusemide and bumetanide, can cause *hypokalaemia* and *hypomagnesaemia* as well as depletion of body sodium and chloride (Cobb and Michell, 1992). These derangements adversely affect cardiac rhythm. Other electrolyte disturbances such as hyperkalaemia and hyper or hypocalcaemia are more likely to arise from systemic disease but can also have detrimental effects on cardiac function.

Endocrine disturbances

Hyperthyroidism has become so frequent as a disease in elderly cats that T4 assays should be routinely performed in all elderly cats presenting with a medical abnormality. Conversely where feline hypertrophic cardiomyopathy or hypertension is diagnosed both thyroid and renal disease should be searched for (Dukes, 1992; Luis Fuentes, 1992).

Markers of myocardial damage

Measurements of plasma levels of aspartate aminotransferase (AST), an isoenzyme of creatinine kinase (CK–MB) and isoenzymes of lactate dehydrogenase (LDH–LD1 and LD2) are used in human medicine to diagnose and monitor the progress of myocardial infarction. Recently, more specific markers of myocardial damage such as the circulating levels of the myofibrillar proteins, troponin-T and troponin-I, have come to be used in human and experimental medicine (Bachmaier *et al.*, 1995; Voss *et al.*, 1995; Alonsozana and Christenson, 1996). Serum troponin-T has been found to be of particular value in the investigation of poultry with cardiac disease (Maxwell *et al.*, 1994). These tests certainly offer excellent prospects for the diagnosis of myocardial infarction and other acute cardiac insults in small animals, but they have yet to be fully evaluated in the clinical domain. Because acute myocardial insults such as infarction are believed to be relatively uncommon in small animal patients, the future role such tests may have in veterinary practice is difficult to judge.

Biochemical measurements of heart failure

Activation of the renin–angiotensin–aldosterone system plays a crucial role in the development and progression of heart failure. These and other mediators (for instance, noradrenalin, atrial naturetic peptide and endothelin) can be found in increased amounts in blood samples from small animals and people with heart failure (Watkins *et al.*, 1976; Knowlen *et al.*, 1983; Cohn *et al.*, 1984; Pellacani *et al.*, 1994). As yet, measurement of these substances is impractical and costly in most clinical circumstances. The levels of these analytes are affected by many variables such as the salt content of the patient's diet, body posture, level of arousal and previous medication. It seems likely that it will be some years before veterinary clinicians will find such data are of real value in the routine management of patients.

Laboratory tests in arrhythmias

Unexplained arrhythmias may arise for a wide variety of reasons. Where a primary cardiac cause is not found a profile of biochemical tests should form part of the investigation. These will sometimes indicate a cause of the arrhythmia such as renal or hepatic disease, endocrinopathies, electrolyte disturbances, neoplasia or pancreatitis (Fox and Nichols, 1988).

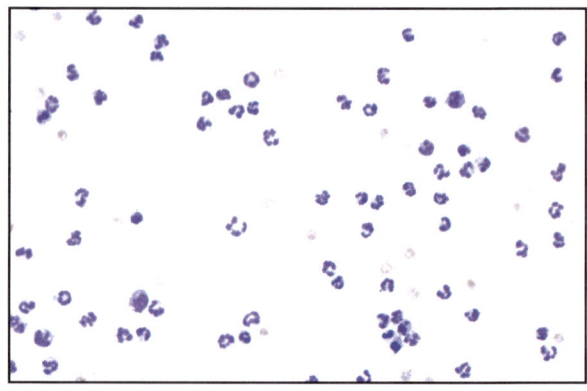

Figure 5.24: High-power view of a pleural effusion from a 2-year-old male Labrador with an intractable cough. Numerous mature neutrophils are present. Pyothorax was diagnosed.

Courtesy of A. May, R. Barron and Dr S. Toth.

EFFUSIONS AND TRANSUDATES IN BODY CAVITIES

Any accumulation of fluid within a body cavity should be sampled and inspected for diagnostic purposes. Sampling techniques for thoracic fluid are covered elsewhere in this manual (Chapter 29).

Samples for cytology and cell counts should be collected into EDTA. Smears are prepared in a similar manner to a blood film and should be submitted to a competent cytologist for evaluation. Pyothorax (empyema) is easily diagnosed in this manner (Figure 5.24). Where the effusion arises from a tumour the fluid will sometimes contain neoplastic cells (Figure 5.25), but their absence does not exclude this diagnosis. Where the fluid appears to be bloody its PCV should be measured and compared with that of a venous blood sample. Similarly the protein content of the fluid should be measured and compared with the plasma. True transudates have a low protein content (<25 g/l) and few cells. Exudates, such as pus or the

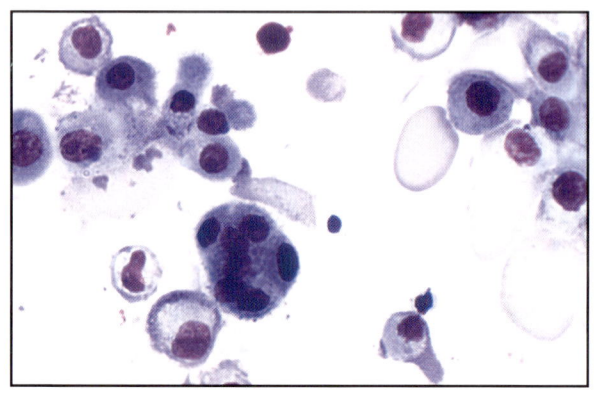

Figure 5.25: Cytology smear from a thoracic effusion in a male Labrador aged 14 years, viewed under oil immersion. Clinical signs were of weight loss and hyperpnoea. Clumps of pleomorphic cells of various sizes are present. The nuclear:cytoplasmic ratio is inconsistent. Nuclei show prominent nucleoli and are frequently located eccentrically. An adenocarcinoma was diagnosed.

Courtesy of A. May, R. Barron and Dr S. Toth.

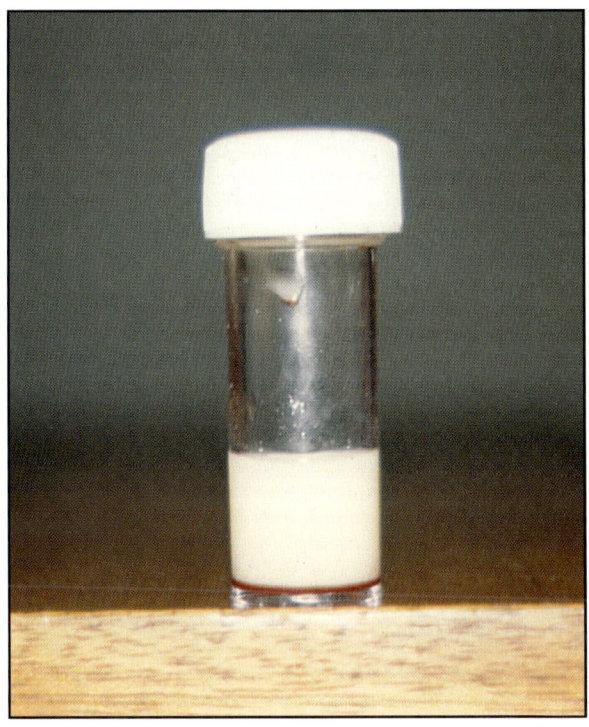

Figure 5.26: *Chylous pleural effusion withdrawn from the chest of a 4-year-old male Domestic Shorthair cat which had a restrictive cardiomyopathy.*

Courtesy of A. May.

effusion of feline infectious peritonitis (FIP) have a high protein content (>30 g/l), a high cell count, and will clot in the absence of an anticoagulant. Most frequently, the fluid is a modified transudate such as that associated with heart failure, and has accumulated over a number of days. Total protein content usually exceeds 25 g/l, the cell count is generally low but varies depending on the cause.

Chylothorax (Figure 5.26), a milky or pink opaque fluid, is not uncommon and presents an enigma. The opacity is due to the presence of triglyceride-rich chylomicrons so that when chyle is centrifuged it remains opaque. Accurate diagnosis of chylothorax is best achieved by measuring the triglyceride content of the fluid and comparing this with the plasma. If the effusion is chyle its triglyceride concentration will be higher than the plasma concentration and usually exceeds 1.0 mmol/l (Waddle and Giger, 1990). It should be noted that the ether clearance test for chylous effusions is unreliable. Contrary to accepted wisdom traumatic rupture of the thoracic duct seems to be an uncommon cause of chylothorax especially in cats where cardiac disease is a much more common cause (Fossum *et al.*, 1986, 1994; Waddle and Giger, 1990).

Diagnosis of the aetiology of pericardial effusions can be particularly challenging even to the most experienced clinicians and often cytology is of little help in this regard (Berg and Wingfield, 1984). Recently, it has been shown that measurement of the pH of pericardial effusions can facilitate the discrimination between non-inflammatory and inflammatory causes in a sub-

stantial proportion of cases. Pericardiocentesis samples were collected into plain plastic syringes and centrifuged. A single drop of supernatant was applied to the pH section of a urinalysis strip and the pH was assessed after 30 seconds. Where the effusion was of an inflammatory origin most samples gave a pH reading of 6.5, whereas where the samples were of non-inflammatory origin (usually neoplastic) the overwhelming majority exhibited a slightly alkaline reading (pH 7.5) (Edwards, 1996).

MICROBIOLOGY

Culture and antibiotic sensitivity tests are useful in dogs or cats with suspected pneumonia, pulmonary abscesses, pyothorax and similar conditions. Both aerobes and anaerobes should be sought.

Blood culture is the gold standard procedure for diagnosis of bacterial endocarditis. Antibiotic therapy should of course be withdrawn at least 24 hours before the investigation. Ideally, a series of two to five blood samples for culture, each of about 10ml, should be obtained over a period of 24–48 hours. Skin preparation must be thorough and the technique should be aseptic. The organisms most commonly isolated are the aerobes *Staphylococcus intermedius*, beta-haemolytic streptococci and *Escherichia coli*; however, anaerobic culture may be useful. Contaminants from the skin or elsewhere can hamper interpretation, consequently to make a confident diagnosis the same organism should be isolated from at least two cultures. The bacteria are often present in quite small numbers in the blood but various techniques have been developed to improve the yield of viable organisms. Close liaison between microbiologist and clinician will increase the success rate of this investigation (Bennett and Taylor, 1987; Calvert, 1988).

REFERENCES

Alonsozana GL and Christenson RH (1996) The case for cardiac troponin T: marker for effective risk stratification of patients with acute cardiac ischaemia. *Clinical Chemistry* **42**, 803–808

Anderson CA and Dubielzig RR (1984) Vegetative endocarditis in dogs. *Journal of the American Animal Hospital Association* **20**, 149

Bachmaier K, Mair J, Offner F *et al.* (1995) Serum cardiac troponin T and creatine kinase -MB elevations in murine autoimmune myocarditis. *Circulation* **92**, 1927–1932

Bauer T (1989) Pulmonary hypersensitivity disorders. In: *Current Veterinary Therapy X. Small Animal Practice*, ed. RW Kirk and JD Bonagura. W.B. Saunders, Philadelphia.

Bennett D and Taylor DJ (1987) Bacterial endocarditis and inflammatory joint disease in the dog. *Journal of Small Animal Practice* **29**, 347

Berg RJ and Wingfield W (1984) Pericardial effusion in the dog: a review of 42 cases. *Journal of the American Animal Hospital Association* **20**, 721–730

Calvert CA (1988) Endocarditis and bacteraemia. In: *Canine and Feline Cardiology*, ed. PR Fox. Churchill Livingstone, New York

Centre SA, Randolph JF, Erb HN and Reiter S (1990) Eosinophilia in the cat: a retrospective study of 312 cases (1975 to 1986). *Journal of the American Animal Hospital Association* **26**, 349

Chinn DR, Myers RK and Matthews JA (1985) Neutrophilic leukocytosis associated with metastatic fibrosarcoma in a dog. *Journal of the American Veterinary Medical Association* **186**, 806

Cobb M and Michell AR (1992) Plasma electrolyte concentrations in dogs receiving diuretic therapy for cardiac failure. *Journal of Small Animal Practice* **33**, 526

Cohn JN, Levine TB, Olivari MT *et al.* (1984) Plasma norepinephrine as a guide to the prognosis in patients with chronic congestive cardiac failure. *New England Journal of Medicine* **311**, 819-823

Drazner FH (1989) Polycythaemia. In: *Textbook of Veterinary Internal Medicine*, ed. SJ Ettinger. W.B. Saunders, Philadelphia.

Dukes J (1992) Hypertension: a review of the mechanisms, manifestations and management. *Journal of Small Animal Practice* **33**, 119

Duncan JR and Prasse KW (1986) *Veterinary Laboratory Medicine*, 2nd Edition. Iowa State University Press, Ames, Iowa

Dye JA, McKeirnan BC, Rozanski EA *et al.* (1996) Bronchopulmonary disease in the cat: historic, physical, radiographic, clinicopathologic and pulmonary function evaluation of 24 affected and 15 healthy cats. *Journal of Veterinary Internal Medicine* **10**, 385-400

Edwards J (1996) The diagnostic value of pericardial fluid pH determination. *Journal of the American Animal Hospital Association* **32**, 63-67.

Elwood CM, Cobb MA and Stepien RL (1993) Clinical and echocardiographic findings in 10 dogs with vegetative bacterial endocarditis. *Journal of Small Animal Practice* **34**, 420-427

Finco DR and Duncan JR (1976) Evaluation of blood urea nitrogen and serum creatinine concentrations as indicators of renal dysfunction: a study of 111 cases and a review of related literature. *Journal of the American Veterinary Medical Association* **168**, 593.

Finco DR, Coulter DB and Carsanti JA (1981) Simple accurate method for clinical estimation of glomerular filtration rate in the dog. *American Journal of Veterinary Research* **42**, 1874-1877

Finco DR, Brown SR, Vaden SL *et al.* (1995) Relationship between plasma creatinine concentration and glomerular filtration rate in dogs. *Journal of Veterinary Pharmacology and Therapeutics* **18**, 418-421

Fossum TW, Birchard SJ and Jacobs RM (1986) Chylothorax in 34 dogs. *Journal of the American Veterinary Medical Association* **188**, 1315

Fossum TW, Miller MW, Rogers KS and Bonagura JD (1994) Chylothorax associated with right-sided heart failure in five cats. *Journal of the American Veterinary Medical Association* **204**, 84

Fox PR and Nichols CER (1988) Cardiac involvement in systemic disease. In: *Canine and Feline Cardiology*, ed. PR Fox. Churchill Livingstone, New York

Grauer GF and Lane IF (1995) Acute renal failure. In : *Textbook of Veterinary Internal Medicine 4th Edn*, ed. EC Feldman and SJ Ettinger, pp 1720-1733. W.B. Saunders Co., Philadelphia.

Jain NC (1993) *Essentials of Veterinary Haematology*. Lea and Febiger. Philadelphia.

Knowlen GG, Kittleson MD, Nachreiner RF *et al.* (1983) Comparison of plasma aldosterone concentrations among the clinical status groups of dogs with chronic heart failure. *Journal of the American Veterinary Medical Association* **183**, 991-996

Luis Fuentes V (1992) Feline heart disease: an update. *Journal of Small Animal Practice* **33**, 130

Martin MWS, Ashton G, Simpson VR and Neal C (1993) Angiostrongylosis in Cornwall: clinical presentations of eight cases. *Journal of Small Animal Practice* **34**, 20

Maxwell MH, Robertson GW and Moseley D (1994) Potential role of serum troponin-T in cradiomyocyte injury in broiler ascites syndrome. *British Poultry Science* **35**, 663-667

Ng CY and Mills JN (1985) Clinical and haematological features of haemangiosarcomas in dogs. *Australian Veterinary Journal* **62**, 1

Pellacani A, Brunner HR and Nussberger J (1994) Plasma kinins increase after angiotensin-converting enzyme inhibition in human subjects. *Clinical Science* **87**, 567-574

Squires R (1993) Differential diagnosis of anaemia in dogs. *In Practice* **15**, 29

Tams TR (1989) Pneumonia. In: *Current Veterinary Therapy X. Small Animal Practice*, ed. RW Kirk and JD Bonagura. W.B. Saunders, Philadelphia

Tennant B (1997) *Small Animal Formulary, 2nd Edition*. BSAVA, Cheltenham.

Thayer GW and Robinson SK (1984) Bacterial bronchopneumonia in the dog: a review of 42 cases. *Journal of the American Animal Hospital Association* **20**, 731

Voss EM, Sharkey SW, Gernert AE *et al.* (1995) Human and canine troponin-T and creatine kinase-MB distribution in normal and diseased myocardium. Infarct sizing using serum profiles. *Archives of Pathology and Laboratory Medicine* **119**, 799-806

Waddle JR and Giger U (1990) Lipoprotein electrophoresis differentiation of chylous and nonchylous pleural effusions in dogs and cats and its correlation with pleural effusion triglyceride concentration. *Veterinary Clinical Pathology* **19**, 80

Watkins L, Burton JA, Haber E *et al.* (1976) The renin-angiotensin-aldosterone system in congestive heart failure in conscious dogs. *Journal of Clinical Investigation* **57**, 1606-1617

(iii) Electrocardiography

Serena E. Brownlie

USES OF ELECTROCARDIOGRAPHY

Electrocardiography is a technique for recording the electrical impulses associated with cardiac contraction on the surface of the body.

The uses of electrocardiography were summarized by Edwards (1987). He defined six main categories of use, as follows:

- Evaluation and prognosis of cardiac anatomical changes and arrhythmias, pericardial and pleural diseases and evaluation of cardiac therapy
- Differentiation of diseases which cause weakness, fatigue, lethargy, collapse or seizures
- Monitoring during anaesthesia and surgery
- Routine health checks, pre-anaesthetic examinations and evaluation of trauma cases
- Documentation of data from repeated examinations in the same animal
- Sharing information with colleagues.

These are all important indications for electrocardiograph (ECG) examination. However, it must be borne in mind that ECG examination should be carried out only after a careful clinical examination, and the results should be assessed along with findings from other diagnostic procedures if possible, such as chest radiographs, echocardiography and blood sample reports.

Recording the ECG

Interpretation of an ECG is easier if the recording is always made with the animal in the same position. The conventional position used is right lateral recumbency, with the fore and hind limbs as nearly perpendicular to the long axis of the body as possible (Figure 5.27). If the animal is uncomfortable in this position, or difficult to restrain, sternal recumbency may be used, but it is usually best to avoid the standing position because artefacts associated with movement and muscle tremor often make the trace unreadable. Movement is the enemy of a good ECG. In animals reluctant to lie still, gentle but firm handling is successful in the majority of animals. When this is unsuccessful, the electrodes may be attached and the animal left to settle into a comfortable position without restraint. A cat may be quieter in

its basket (Figure 5.28). Chemical restraint may cause changes in rhythm, but may be used as a last resort if the alternative is an uninterpretable ECG. The patient should be observed during recording so that movements may be marked on the trace and the normal rhythm changes associated with respiration identified.

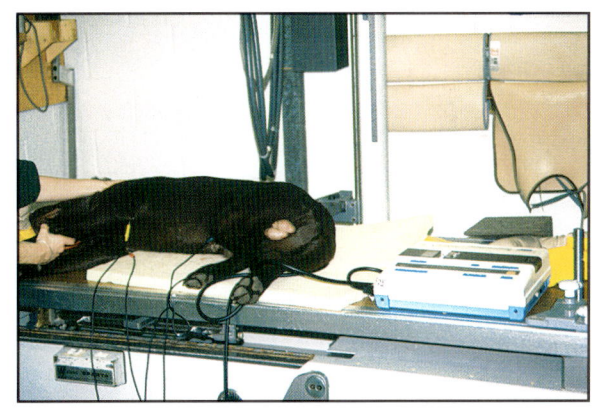

Figure 5.27: *Dog correctly positioned for ECG recording.*

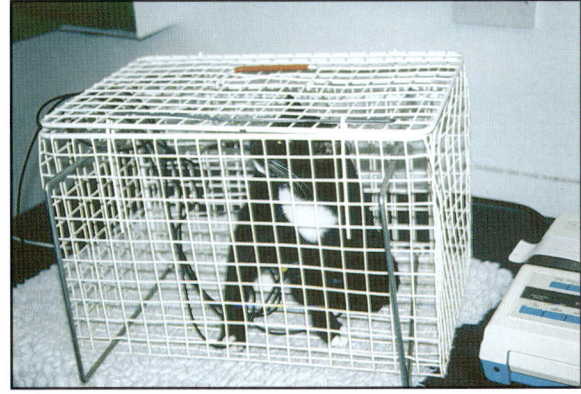

Figure 5.28: *Cat in a basket for ECG recording.*

For routine short ECGs, the electrodes are usually attached to the animal by crocodile clips, or occasionally by fine needles through the skin. An animal which is uncomfortable will be less willing to lie still and therefore it is wise to ensure that clips do not grip too tightly. Attaching them to the operator's hand soon identifies clips which are painful! For long-term ECG monitoring, sticky electrodes are best, but they do not adhere well to animal skin unless the coat is clipped and the skin cleaned. Even then, it is advisable to apply

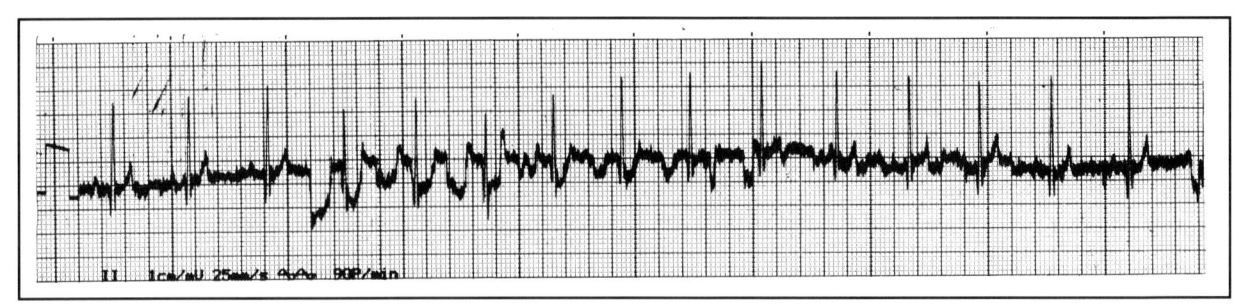

Figure 5.29: ECG showing interference caused by poor electrical contact.

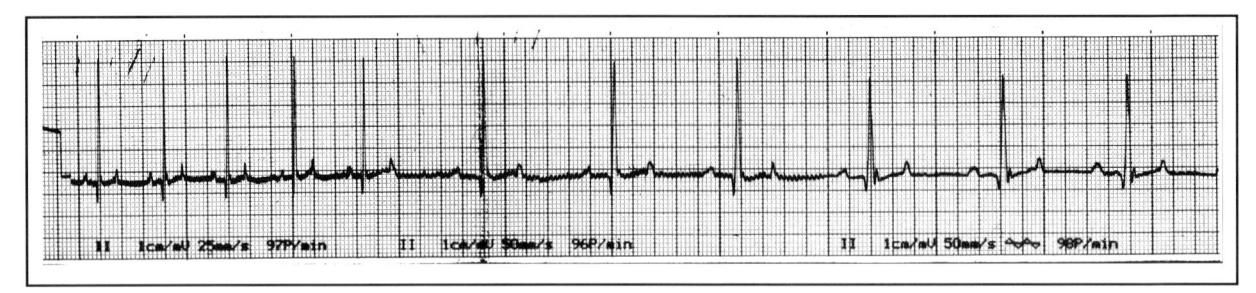

Figure 5.30: AC interference.

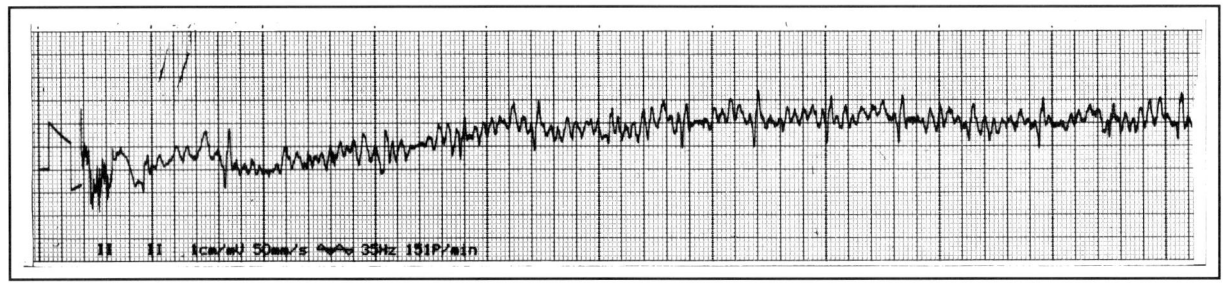

Figure 5.31: Movement artefact, caused by muscle tremor.

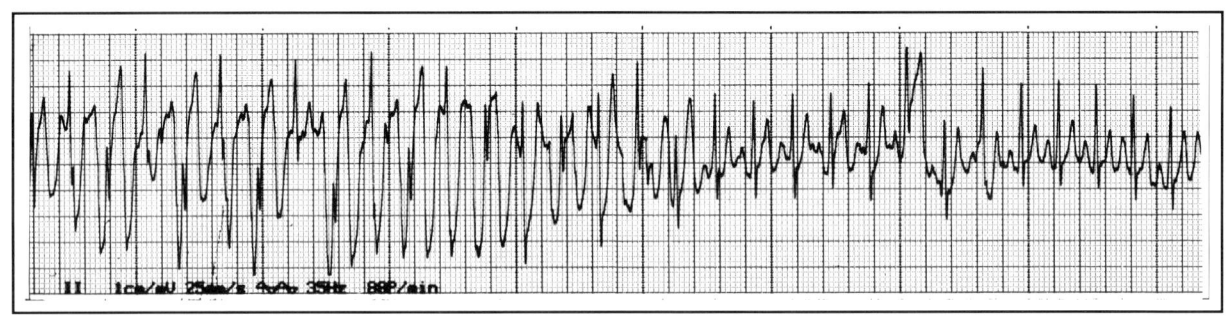

Figure 5.32: Movement artefact caused by panting.

adhesive tape so that they do not become dislodged. Good electrical contact is achieved by using electrode gel or cream, or even surgical spirit. The latter will evaporate quickly but has the advantage that it does not cause metal clips to corrode.

Important causes of interference artefacts

- Dirty or corroded clips causing poor electrical contact. Clean or replace clips (Figure 5.29)
- AC interference, i.e. small regular saw-tooth deflections on the whole trace (Figure 5.30). If this is severe enough to interfere with interpretation, switch off as many other electrical appliances as possible, insulate the animal on a rubber mat or move to another room
- Movement artefacts: twitching, trembling, tail-wagging, panting, purring (Figures 5.31 and 5.32).

ECG leads

Limb electrodes are usually positioned fairly near to the body to reduce movement, using the relatively hairless areas of skin just behind both elbows and in front of the left stifle. A neutral electrode may be placed anywhere but is usually placed in front of the right stifle. The hind limb electrodes may also be attached to the skin overlying the gastrocnemius tendon. The standard bipolar limb leads usually used in dogs and cats are as follows:

- Lead I – Right fore (-ve) compared with left fore (+ve)
- Lead II – Right fore (-ve) compared with left hind (+ve)
- Lead III – Left fore (-ve) compared with left hind (+ve)

The augmented leads (aVR, aVL and aVF) represent one limb compared with the other two.

The electrodes may be colour-coded and marked as for human use, e.g. the lead for attaching to the right fore is often red and marked RA (right arm), the left fore yellow, marked LA, the left hind green and marked LL or F (foot) and the neutral (N) lead is usually black.

Chest electrodes are rarely used in veterinary practice but, if needed, they are usually placed at the sixth left intercostal space near the sternum (CV6LL or V2), and at the costochondral junction (CV6LU or V4), at the fifth right intercostal space near the sternum (CV5RL or rV2) and in the dorsal midline between the scapulae (V10). Orthogonal leads are placed so that recording takes place in three planes across the chest, from right to left, craniocaudally and ventrodorsally. This system is often used in the horse but rarely in small animals.

ECG machine controls
Although ECG machines vary in design, they all operate in a similar way.

The sensitivity control
This allows the operator to vary the number of centimetres on the paper which are equivalent to 1 mV on the ECG. Most traces are recorded at 1 cm/mV, but if the complexes are so tall that they cannot be accommodated on the paper, decreasing the sensitivity will give a readable trace. It is important that the sensitivity is marked on the paper with a calibration mark so that it is immediately obvious, if the machine does not do this automatically.

Paper speed control
This allows the operator to choose how fast the trace is run. Basic single channel machines usually give a choice of only two speeds, 25 and 50 mm/s. More expensive and versatile machines give a choice of slower and faster speeds. Slow running may be useful to save paper in a long recording if one is looking for intermittent arrhythmias. Three channel machines use wider paper and record three lead tracings simultaneously, which allows artefacts to be identified more easily, e.g. a twitch of the left hind leg may be confused with an abnormal QRS on a single channel recording, but on a three channel recording it will only be present in leads II and III and not in lead I, demonstrating that it is an artefact. Of course the operator should have observed this anyway by watching the patient while recording.

Filter
This allows artefacts to be suppressed, evening out the trace. Its use often causes a marked decrease in the height of the QRS complexes, and this should be taken into account when the trace is interpreted.

Lead selector
Many modern ECG machines have an automatic programme of lead selection, but this may not always be suitable for the veterinary patient, therefore most operators prefer manual lead selection.

INTERPRETATION OF WAVEFORMS

The heart contains specialized pacemaker cells which are capable of spontaneous depolarization, and a system of rapidly conducting tissue which transmits the electrical impulse from the pacemaker cells in an organized and co-ordinated manner throughout the heart. Under normal circumstances, the impulse is initiated by the pacemaker with the fastest intrinsic rate, which is the sinoatrial node, located in the right atrium. It then spreads across the atria to the atrioventricular node, through the right and left branches of the bundle of His, down each side of the interventricular septum towards the apex of the heart, and then across the ventricular walls through the Purkinje fibres. The deflections on the ECG trace represent the sum of all the electrical forces involved in the cardiac cycle. Wavefronts moving towards an electrode will produce a positive deflection and those away from an electrode will produce a negative deflection. Those moving in opposite directions will cancel each other out, and those moving at right angles to an electrode will not produce a deflection either way by that electrode.

The first deflection of each cycle is known as the P wave, and this represents atrial depolarization. The right atrium begins to depolarize slightly before the left. There is then a brief delay as the impulse passes through the atrioventricular node, allowing blood from the atria to enter the ventricles, and this period is recorded as a short line which is neither positive nor negative (isoelectric). This is called the PR interval.

There are three main phases of ventricular depolarization in the dog and cat, which produce the Q, R and S deflections on the ECG. The Q wave is produced by the depolarization of the middle and apical parts of the septum, the R wave by the spread of the impulse towards the surface of both ventricles and the S wave by the activation of the myocardium at the base of the ventricles. There is then a short isoelectric period (the ST segment) before the ventricles repolarize and produce the T wave on the ECG (Figure 5.33). The pattern of ventricular depolarization in the dog and cat is fairly constant and although the height of the QRS complex may vary from animal to animal, its shape does not vary a great deal. The R wave is the main

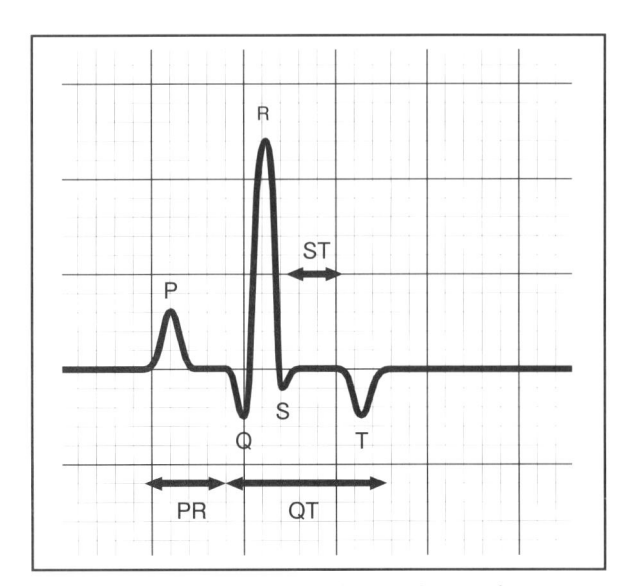

Figure 5.33: Normal canine lead II PQRST complex.

deflection and it is usually positive on lead II. However, the T wave in small animals is highly variable in size and polarity.

Waveform measurements

Normal ECG criteria have been defined and are quoted by many authors, such as Tilley (1992) (Table 5.3).

	Duration (s)		Voltage (mV)	
	Dog	Cat	Dog	Cat
P wave	0.04	0.04	0.4	0.2
PR interval	0.06-0.13	0.05-0.09		
QRS	< 0.06	< 0.04	≤ 3.0	< 0.9
QT interval	0.15-0.25	0.12-0.18		

Table 5.3: Normal ECG criteria.

P wave

The P wave in small animals is usually positive. In the dog, it may vary in height and even polarity in a cyclical manner associated with respiration. This is known as wandering pacemaker, and it is due to vagal inhibition of the sinoatrial node causing a temporary shifting of the pacemaker site to another part of the atrium. Prolongation of the P wave is known as *P mitrale* and it is often an indication of severe left atrial enlargement, because the impulse takes longer to cross it. Notching of the P wave is not necessarily abnormal unless it is also prolonged. P waves of 0.05 seconds are often seen in giant breed dogs with no evidence of left atrial enlargement. (Miller and Tilley, 1988). An increase in the height of the P wave is usually associated with right atrial enlargement, because the right and left voltages are summated instead of occurring at slightly different times. This is called *P pulmonale*.

PR interval

See Table 5.3. Prolongation of the PR interval is most often associated with digoxin therapy. A short PR interval may indicate ventricular pre-excitation.

QRS complex

The QRS complex height measurement in Table 5.3 may not apply to young deep-chested large breed dogs which may have taller R waves. In small breed dogs, 0.05 second duration is usual. Tall and/or wide QRS complexes may indicate left ventricular enlargement. Fat animals tend to have smaller R waves than thin animals of the same breed. However, if the R waves are much smaller than expected for a particular breed, it may suggest the presence of fluid in the pleural cavity or pericardial sac.

Right bundle branch block is a delay or block in conduction in the right branch of the bundle of His. It is characterized on ECG by wide, deep S waves, especially in leads I, II and aVF, and right axis deviation. It is often an incidental finding in animals with no signs of illness, although it may suggest that myocardial disease is present (Figure 5.34).

Left bundle branch block is a delay or block in conduction in the main left branch of the bundle of His, or in both anterior and posterior fascicles. It is characterized on ECG by prolongation of the QRS complexes to 0.08 seconds or greater. It is usually wide and

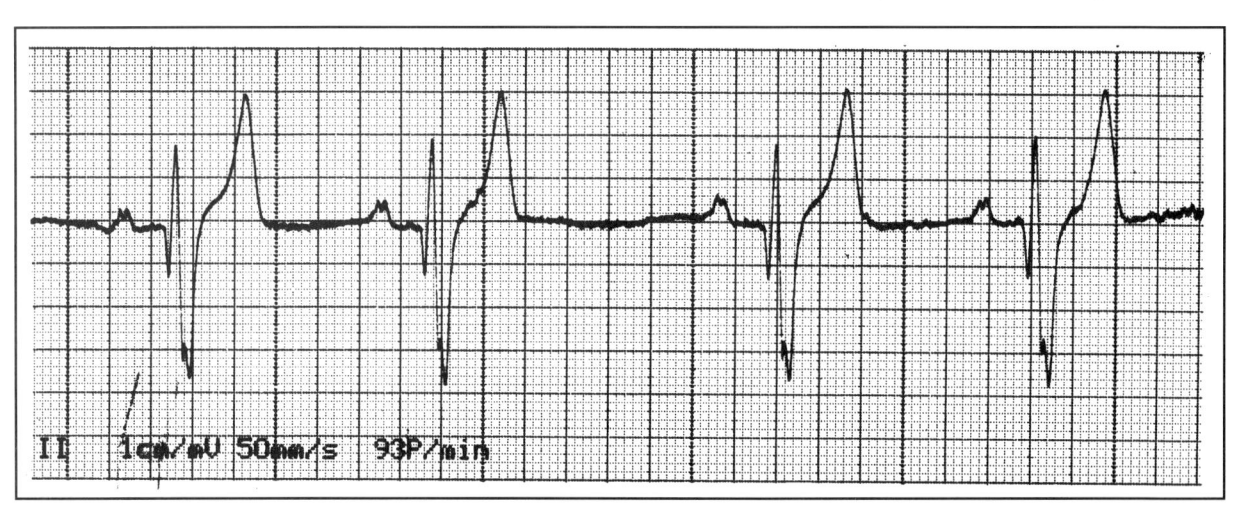

Figure 5.34: Right bundle branch block in a giant breed dog.

findings suggest myocardial hypoxia or ischaemia, e.g. due to myocardial infarction, and are particularly worrying if they develop during the course of an illness or during anaesthesia. Slurring of the ST segment into the T wave (coving) is often seen in heart failure.

QT interval

See Table 5.3. Alteration in the QT interval has also been associated with abnormalities in electrolyte and calcium levels.

T wave

The T wave in the dog should not measure more than 25% of the R wave. This should be interpreted with care as the T wave may be normal with a small QRS. The Chihuahua is reported to be unusual in having a positive T wave in lead V10. The maximum height quoted for cats is 0.3 mV. The author has never found any abnormality consistently associated with T wave changes. However, they are classically associated with plasma electrolyte abnormalities, particularly potassium, and if the T wave alters during the progression of an illness, careful patient monitoring is probably indicated.

Mean electrical axis

Even if the QRS complex is normal in overall height and duration, it is still possible that ventricular enlargement exists and the pattern of the QRS complexes in

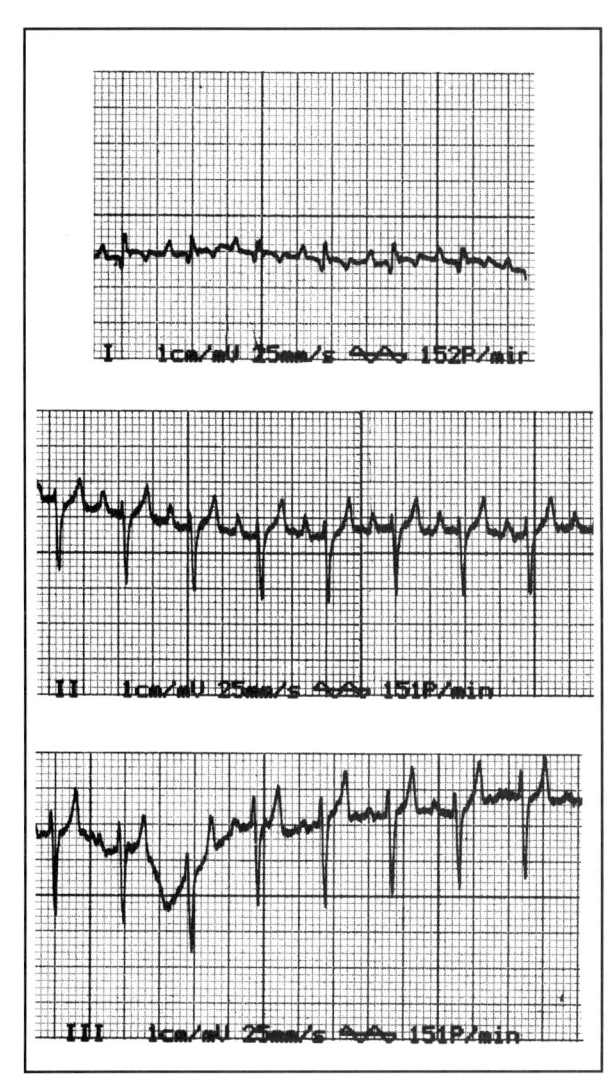

Figure 5.35: *Left anterior fascicular block in a giant breed dog.*

positive in leads I, II, III and aVF. It is considered to be an indication of severe myocardial disease, because the left bundle branch is a large structure which is not readily damaged, unlike the right branch. Only the anterior part of the left bundle may be damaged, (anterior fascicular block) and this is seen in animals with or without clinical signs (Figure 5.35). Posterior fascicular block is rare.

ST segment

The ST segment should have no depression greater than 0.2 mV or elevation greater than 0.15 mV. These

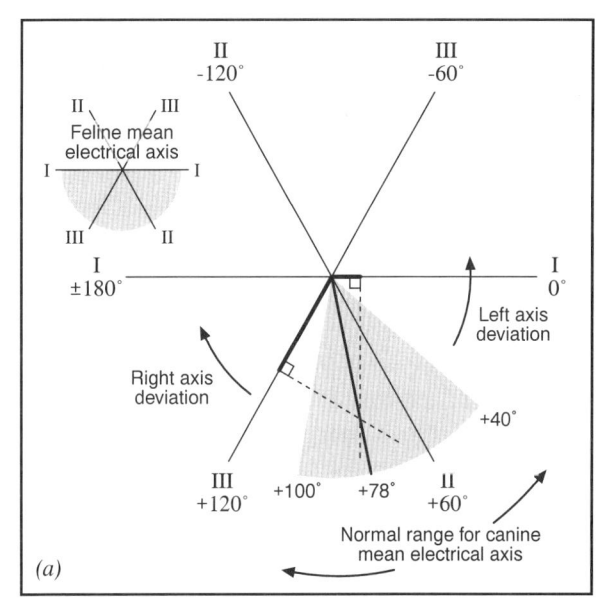

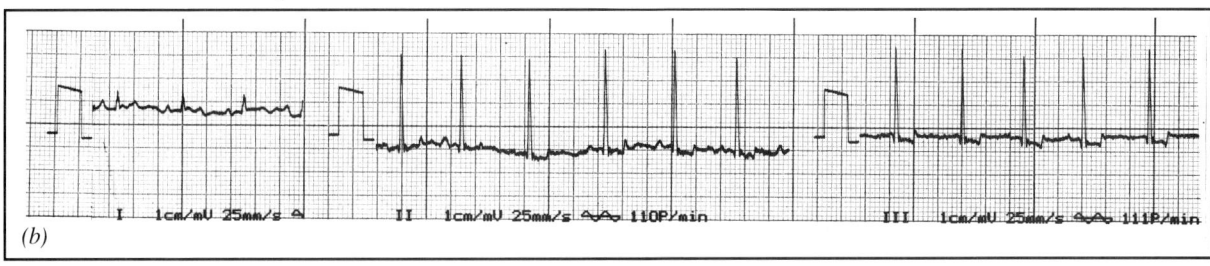

Figure 5.36: *(a) Use of the hexaxial reference diagram to calculate the mean electrical axis in the frontal plane in a normal dog. (b) Normal canine ECG from which the axis in (a) was calculated.*

different leads may be used to calculate the likelihood of this. The method usually used in small animals is calculation of the mean electrical axis in the frontal plane, which is in fact the average of all the vectors of electrical activity produced by ventricular depolarization. In order to determine the mean electrical axis it is necessary to construct a diagram (Figure 5.36). This is known as a *triaxial reference system*, or *hexaxial* if the augmented leads are included, which was originally based on Einthoven's triangle, i.e. lines joining the three limb electrodes on right and left arms and the left leg, with the heart in the centre. Using Figures 5.36, the axis is obtained as follows:

- Measure the algebraic sum of the positive and negative deflections of the QRS complexes in two leads (normally leads I and III)
- Plot these vectors in relation to the centre to scale along the lines on the diagram
- Draw lines perpendicular to these points
- Where the lines intersect, draw a line to the centre
- The angle which this line makes with the zero line is the *mean electrical axis*.

The accepted normal range in the dog is between +40 and +100 degrees. In the cat, the range is wider, between 0 and +180 degrees. An axis from +100 to -90 degrees in the dog is a fairly reliable indication of right ventricular enlargement, whereas an axis between +40 and -90 degrees in the opposite direction is associated with left ventricular enlargement.

There is a much simpler, though not so accurate method of axis calculation, which is to choose the lead which is nearest to isoelectric. The axis will be approximately at right angles to the position of this lead on the hexaxial diagram (Figure 5.36).

Normal rates and rhythms

Heart rate
It is a simple matter to calculate heart rate from an ECG trace, provided one knows the paper speed, and, although the rate should have been counted during the clinical examination, there are circumstances when auscultation is difficult, e.g. when the heart sounds are muffled by fluid or neoplasia, or when there is marked respiratory noise. Many modern ECG machines mark the paper each second or the paper itself may be printed with a mark after each 25 mm. To obtain the number of beats per minute, all that is required is to count the number in 6 seconds and multiply by 10, or some other preferred arithmetical combination.

Heart rate in the adult dog varies widely, usually between 70 and 180 beats per minute, depending on the animal's state of excitement, and values outside this range have been recorded in normal dogs. In the cat, the normal range quoted by Miller and Tilley (1988) is

160–240 beats per minute, with a mean of 197 per minute. In the author's experience, if a pet cat is handled gently during ECG recording, it is usually possible to achieve heart rates lower than this mean figure. The lower end of the range is much higher than that quoted by Edwards (1987), whose range is 90–240.

Heart rhythm
In the dog, the normal rhythms are *regular sinus rhythm* (Figure 5.37), sinus tachycardia associated with excitement, and sinus arrhythmia often with wandering pacemaker (Figure 5.38).

Sinus arrhythmia is a regularly irregular rhythm originating in the sinoatrial node in which the R-R intervals vary by more than 0.12 seconds or 10%. In brachycephalic breeds in which most individuals have a degree of airway obstruction, this sinus arrhythmia, which causes an increase in heart rate with inspiration and a decrease with expiration, may become so marked that the sinus pauses approach the definition of *sinoatrial block* or *sinus arrest*. Whether this is described as an abnormality or not has to be decided by the clinician in charge of the case and depends on whether the animal is showing any signs of illness. Sinus arrhythmia of all degrees is abolished by vagolytic drugs.

Normal sinus rhythm (Figure 5.39) and sinus tachycardia with excitement are the only rhythms accepted as normal in the cat.

Intermittent ECG abnormalities
One normal ECG does not rule out heart disease! Further diagnostic tests may be required, especially in cases having collapsing episodes. Intermittent arrhythmias may only be detected by 24 hour ECG monitoring, ambulatory monitoring or event recording.

ECG monitors are available for human hospitalized patients which detect rhythm disturbances and sound an alarm or print out the abnormality when it occurs. However these are programmed to detect human arrhythmias and may not be able to cope with normal canine sinus arrhythmia, artefacts such as panting or the movements of an animal in a hospital cage. Ambulatory (Holter) monitoring is a technique which allows an ECG to be continuously recorded for long periods of time. If an ECG can be recorded, without too many artefacts, from an animal which is going about its normal daily activities, there is a much greater chance that intermittent problems will be identified. Modern recorders are small and light enough for all but the smallest dogs to carry around, usually attached to a harness, and the tape, or recorded information in a microcomputer, is analysed later by high speed scanning devices.

Small event recorders are available for human patients which are applied by the patient when they feel

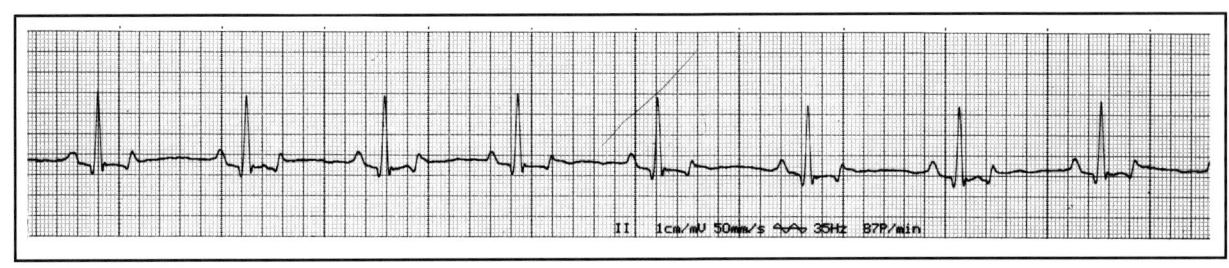

Figure 5.37: *Normal regular sinus rhythm in a dog.*

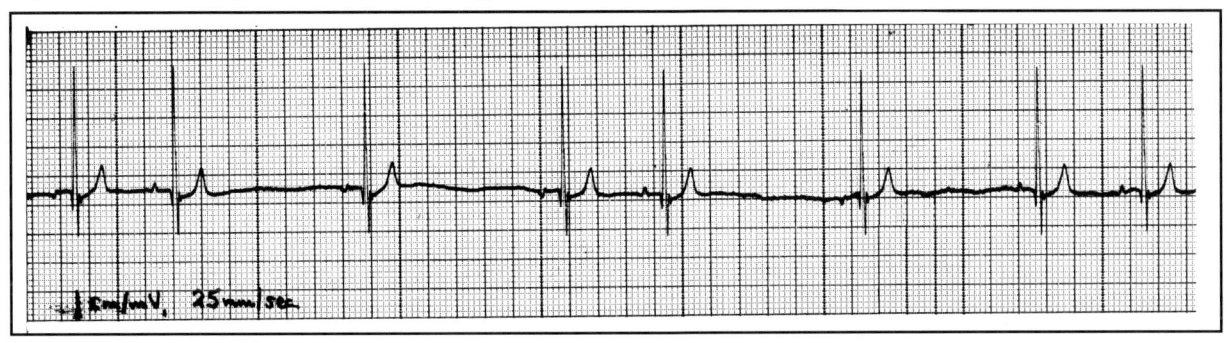

Figure 5.38: *Sinus arrhythmia with wandering pacemaker in a dog. Note the variation in appearance of the P wave.*

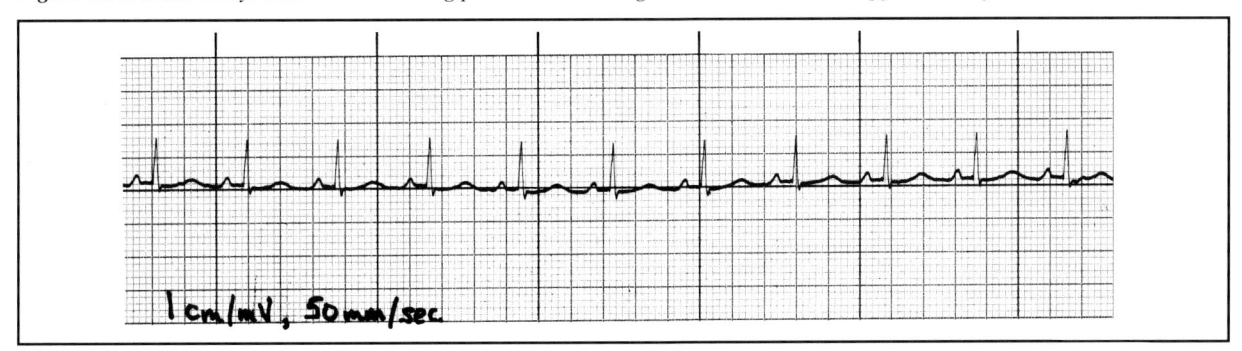

Figure 5.39: *Normal sinus rhythm in a cat.*

unwell or by someone else if the patient collapses. The ECG is recorded on tape and may be transmitted by telephone. These devices can be used in animals, although the event may be missed by the time the owner realizes that there is a problem and applies the electrodes.

REFERENCES

Edwards NJ (1987) *Bolton's Handbook of Canine and Feline Electrocardiography*, 2nd edn. WB Saunders, Philadelphia

Miller MS and Tilley LP (1988) In: *Electrocardiography In Canine and Feline Cardiology*, ed. PR Fox. Churchill Livingstone, New York

Tilley LP (1992) *Essentials of Canine and Feline Electrocardiography*, 3rd edn Lea & Febiger, Philadelphia

(iv) Bronchoscopy

Brendan C. McKiernan

INTRODUCTION

Bronchoscopy has been an integral part of respiratory speciality practices in veterinary medicine since at least the early 1970s, providing the clinician with valuable information about a patient's respiratory system. Performed by experienced veterinarians, bronchoscopy is invaluable in the diagnosis of many lower airway disorders.

Equipment

Both rigid and flexible endoscopes have been used for bronchoscopy.

Rigid bronchoscopes have been used in human medicine since the turn of the century, but after Ikeda introduced the flexible fibrescope in 1967, the use of flexible endoscopes increased significantly and they are now the most commonly used instruments for both veterinary and human bronchoscopy.

Flexible endoscopes have many advantages over rigid endoscopes, including versatility, improved manoeuvrability and an increased viewing area within the tracheobronchial tree. There are also disadvantages when compared with rigid endoscopes, including increased initial purchase cost, more expensive repair costs, a decreased quality of image transmission (noted primarily during endoscopic photography), decreased durability (the greater flexibility may lead to more optical bundle breakage), and less suction and instrumentation capability (the biopsy channel size is generally smaller). Despite these limitations, the versatility, manoeuvrability and increased viewing area make flexible endoscopes the preferred endoscopic instrument.

Species differences (for example, in the length and diameter of an animal's airways) result in certain limitations in the use and application of flexible human endoscopes, and often necessitate the selection of other endoscopes (e.g. the flexible paediatric gastroscope) for use as a 'veterinary bronchoscope'. The use of a paediatric gastroscope and two sizes of bronchoscope allows for excellent bronchoscopic evaluation in patients weighing from 2 kg to over 75 kg. Yet these have enough versatility to be used in other endoscopic procedures, such as rhinoscopy, cystoscopy, oesophagoscopy and gastroduodenoscopy. Endoscopes may be made specifically for human or veterinary use; a partial list of manufacturers is given in Table 5.4. Veterinarians have often obtained good quality second-hand endoscopes from a local hospital or endoscope salesperson.

Manufacturer and model	Working length/diameter	Channel size	Other uses
Olympus[1] BF3C30	55 cm/3.5 mm	1.2 mm	R, C
Olympus, BFP-30	55 cm/5.0 mm	2.2 mm	R, C
Olympus, XP-20	103 cm/7.9 mm	2.0 mm	GI; 4-way tip deflection
Olympus, Vet-XP10	140 cm/7.9 mm	2.0 mm	GI; 4-way tip deflection
Storz[2], 60001VB	55 cm/5.0 mm	2.0 mm	R, C
Storz, 60001VL	85 cm/5.0 mm	2.0 mm	R, C
Storz, 60002VB	54 cm/3.7 mm	1.2 mm	R, C
Storz, 60003VB	100 cm/2.9 mm	1.2 mm	R, C
Storz, 60511VG	150 cm/8.0 mm	2.5 mm	GI; 4-way tip deflection

Table 5.4: Examples of selected flexible endoscopes and sizes which would be suitable for bronchoscopy in dogs (larger diameter scopes) and cats (smaller diameter scopes). The overall length, diameter and relative flexibility of the endoscope will determine the scope's versatility and potential use in other endoscopic procedures such as rhinoscopy (R), gastroduodenoscopy (GI) and cystoscopy (C).

1 Olympus Endoscopes: Key Med Ltd, Southend-on-Sea; 2 Storz Instruments: Rimmer Brothers Ltd, London

Indications	**Diagnostic for visual assessment and sample collection**
	Chronic cough
	Chronic parenchymal (alveolar, interstitial) diseases
	Evaluation of suspected airway calibre disorders, including: dynamic changes (tracheobronchial collapse, tracheobronchial malacia); fixed changes (compression, bronchiectasis)
	Persistent halitosis, not of upper airway origin
	Haemoptysis
	Suspected tracheobronchial fistula
	Suspected large airway laceration
	Suspected lung lobe torsion
	Presurgical (lobectomy) staging
	Therapeutic
	Removal of a foreign body – main use
	Removal of copious/retained secretions or mucous plugs
	An aid in difficult intubations
Contraindications	**Relative**
	Resting expiratory effort – risk of exertional airway collapse (and severe hypoxaemia) during procedure and especially during the anaesthesia recovery period
	Uraemia – increased risk of haemorrhage
	Pulmonary hypertension – anaesthetic risk
	Poor cardiopulmonary reserve – increased risk of arrhythmias
	Absolute
	Uncorrected bleeding diathesis
	Nonreversible hypoxaemia (PaO_2 <65 mmHg while on oxygen) – increased risk of arrhythmias
	Unstable cardiac arrhythmias
	Cardiac failure
Complications	*Induced airway irritation* (laryngospasm, bronchospasm, paroxysmal coughing)
	Hypoxaemia
	Cardiac arrhythmias
	Fever
	New radiographic infiltrates
	Barotrauma – O_2 insufflation with significant air trapping
	Haemorrhage – friable tissue; post brushing/biopsy

Table 5.5: Indications, contraindications and potential complications of bronchoscopy in small animals. (Modified from Roudebush, 1990)

Care and cleaning

Flexible endoscopes are delicate, expensive instruments and should be handled, used, and cleaned with the utmost care. Improper handling (e.g. forceful insertion or bending) or cleaning (e.g. some instruments can be totally immersed, others should be gas sterilized) may result in instrument damage and expensive repair costs. Equipment sterility is often hampered by humidity. *Pseudomonas*, which favours damp environments, is a common contaminant of respiratory equipment, including endoscopic equipment. Flexible endoscopes should be hung up for storage, as leaving them in their cases will prevent them from completely drying out inside. Ethylene oxide, steam, and cold soaking techniques have been successfully used to sterilize endoscopes and biopsy equipment. Manufacturers outline the use, care and cleaning instructions with their instruments; this information should be clearly understood by anyone who will handle the endoscope.

BASIC BRONCHOSCOPIC TECHNIQUE

Indications and contraindications

Bronchoscopy may be used for diagnostic, therapeutic and prognostic purposes (McKiernan, 1989; Ford, 1990; Roudebush, 1990). Diagnostic bronchoscopy is used to obtain visual information concerning the airways (e.g. compression, dynamic collapse, and dilation) as well as to obtain samples (cytology, culture and occasionally biopsy) to help establish a specific diagnosis. Bronchoscopy is useful therapeutically, especially in the removal of airway foreign bodies (Lotti and Niebauer, 1992). It is also very helpful in determining prognosis when non-reversible anatomical or mucosal changes are recognized in lower airways. Other than the risks associated with the anaesthesia required for the procedure, this author does not feel that there are any absolute contraindications to bronchoscopy in veterinary medicine.

The clinician must weigh up any risks presented by the patient (e.g. anaesthesia, bleeding, hypoxaemia, arrhythmias) against the benefit which might be obtained from the procedure. Roudebush (1990) summarized the clinical indications and the potential contraindications for bronchoscopy, a modification of which is outlined in Table 5.5.

Anaesthesia for bronchoscopy is covered in Chapter 5(vii).

Monitoring and positioning the patient for bronchoscopy

Routine electrocardiographic monitoring is recommended during anaesthetic induction, the bronchoscopic procedure and for a period of time while the patient recovers. In humans, significant decreases in PaO_2 have been reported during bronchoscopy (Zavala, 1978; Roudebush, 1990). The frequency of this problem has not been assessed in veterinary medicine. If a similar decrease does occur, the potential exists for significant hypoxaemia and possibly cardiac arrhythmias to develop.

Two positions have commonly been used for bronchoscopy in small animals. Selection of either sternal or dorsal recumbency is based on preference and training. The author prefers that animals be in *sternal recumbency* because that position is more familiar to veterinarians, it avoids any possible gravitational influences on the airways and on cardiorespiratory function, and it is easier to maintain.

Bronchoscopic training

One of the biggest problems in bronchoscopy is learning how to manipulate the flexible endoscope. It is mandatory that the bronchoscopist be able to direct the instrument (e.g. for biopsy and collection of cytology specimens) without undue risk to the patient (prolonged anaesthetic time, excessive mucosal trauma) or damage to the endoscope, and be able to manoeuvre to specific lobar sites without difficulty.

Methods have been proposed for making tracheobronchial casts (inflated air-dried lung specimens) which serve as excellent training models (McKiernan and Kneller, 1983). These hollow bronchial casts allow beginners the opportunity to develop safely the manual dexterity and anatomical recognition skills that are absolutely necessary to become a competent bronchoscopist. The clinician should pursue some form of specialized training prior to using bronchoscopy as a routine diagnostic tool.

Bronchoscopists must have a good understanding of normal endoscopic lung anatomy if they are to recognize abnormalities and diseases. The differentiation (recognition) of normal from what is abnormal is a subjective one. Experience and practice greatly improve the clinician's ability to detect lesions at an early stage. Amis and McKiernan (1986) have proposed 'bronchoscopic terminology' for the identification of canine endobronchial anatomy (Figure 5.40). This reference and the dried lung models are helpful in correlating radiographic lesions to endoscopic findings (and vice versa), localizing lesions and for recording the location (in writing) of lesions, biopsies, or photographs for future comparison and reference. Bronchoscopic findings and colour changes in the respiratory mucosa are difficult to describe or depict through line drawings or black and white photography. The reader is strongly encouraged to review normal canine endobronchial anatomy (Amis and McKiernan, 1986) and consult colour photographs of endoscopic findings from healthy and diseased animals when beginning to learn bronchoscopy (Stradling, 1976; Venker-van Haagen, 1979; Venker-van Haagen *et al.*, 1985; Ford, 1990; Roudebush,

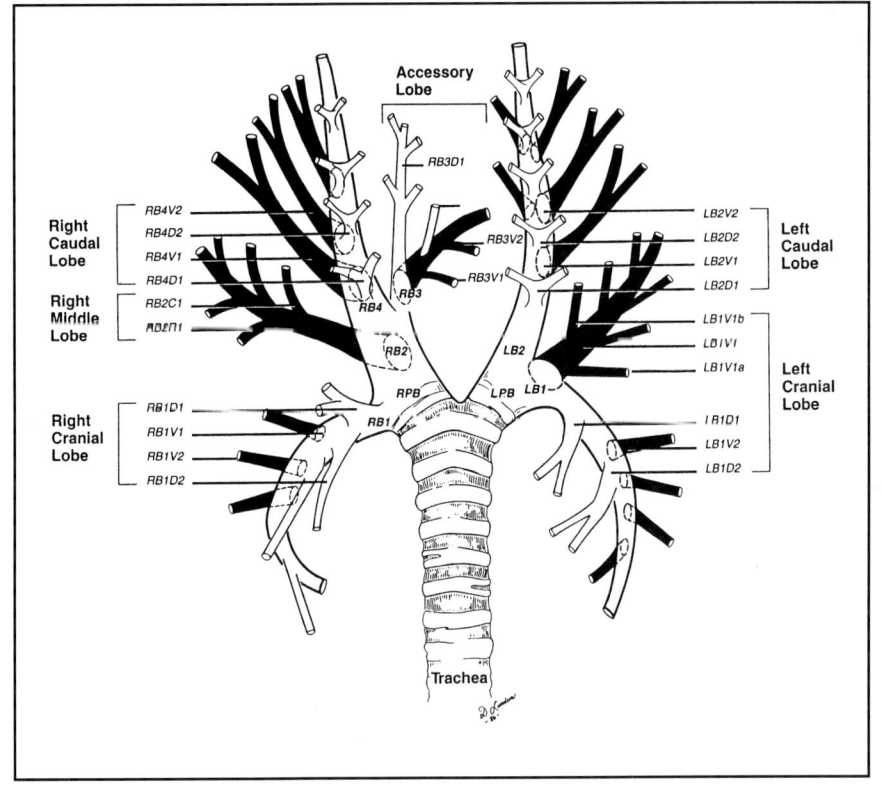

Figure 5.40: *Artist's representation of the canine bronchial tree using a proposed nomenclature system. This system uses letters and numbers to identify the principal, lobar, segmental bronchi by their bronchoscopic order of origination and their dorsal and ventral anatomic orientation. Key: R, right; L, left; B, bronchus; P, principal; V, ventral; D, dorsal; C, caudal; R, rostral. Numbers indicate origination order, and lower case letters indicate origination order of subsegmental bronchi (without anatomical orientation).*

From Amis and McKiernan (1986) with permission.

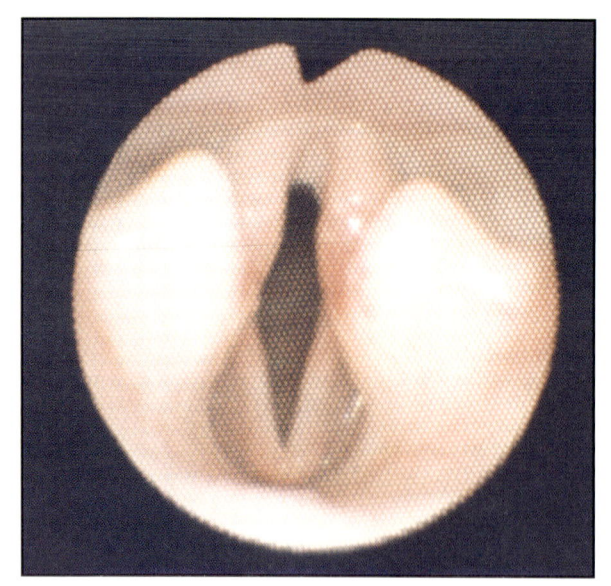

Figure 5.41: Endoscopic photograph of a normal canine larynx (slight hyperaemia noted on the dog's left arytenoid cartilage). The epiglottis is being held down ventrally, the cuneiform processes of the arytenoid cartilages are visible on the left and right side of the rima glottidis, the vocal folds (forming a 'V' at the bottom of the picture) and saccular crypts are visible at the ventral aspect of the rima glottidis.

1990; and Brearley *et al.,* 1991).

It is valuable for the bronchoscopist to be thorough and perform all endoscopies using a standard protocol, so as to not overlook any part of the examination. My preference is to examine the larynx, trachea, carina, the right side, and finally the left side of the tracheobronchial tree. Changes in gross anatomy, fixed and dynamic lumen size, abnormalities in airway shape, mucosal/submucosal characteristics, and the presence of secretions should be noted and recorded upon completing the procedure.

Bronchoscopic procedure

All supplies and equipment for bronchoscopy must be ready before starting the procedure so as to minimize anaesthetic time. Once an animal is sedated, connected to the monitoring equipment and positioned, it is ready to be anaesthetized. Following induction, dental mouth gags should be placed to protect the endoscope throughout the duration of the procedure. Supplemental oxygen should be administered.

Normal and abnormal bronchoscopic findings

Endobronchial anatomy is best described sequentially, as the bronchoscope is passed into the tracheobronchial tree. The author routinely examines the larynx (anatomy and intrinsic function/motion if possible; Figure 5.41), the cervical and intrathoracic trachea and then the carina before sequentially evaluating all the lobar and finally as many segmental and/or subsegmental bronchi as possible (the latter varies with patient and endoscope size).

As the endoscope is passed through the larynx, C-shaped cartilaginous rings are normally visible beneath the tracheal mucosa. The shape of the trachea should be noted, with healthy dogs and cats of most breeds having a nearly circular shaped cervical and intrathoracic trachea. The dorsal tracheal membrane is normally viewed as a longitudinal strip of muscle joining the ends of the 'C'-shaped rings. The tracheal membrane should be stretched relatively tightly so that there is little if any redundancy (visible protrusion or collapse into the airway) in the normal animal (Figure 5.42). Changes in fixed (static) as well as dynamic airway calibre and collapse of tracheal and/or bronchial lumens should be noted if present. During respiration a small dynamic calibre change may be noted but the airways will not completely collapse in the healthy animal, even during forceful respiration (e.g.

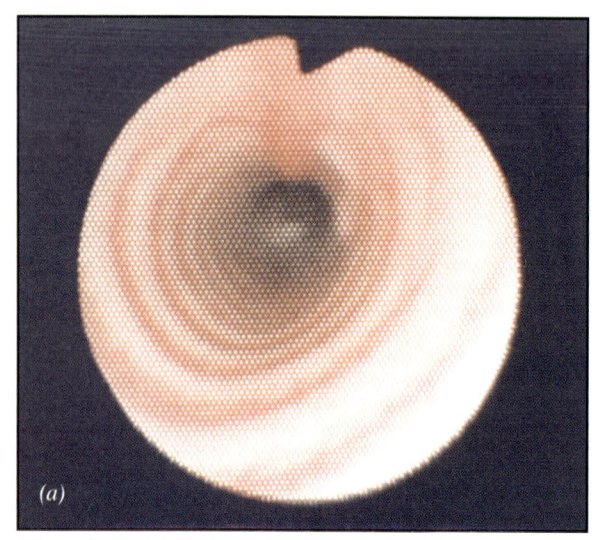

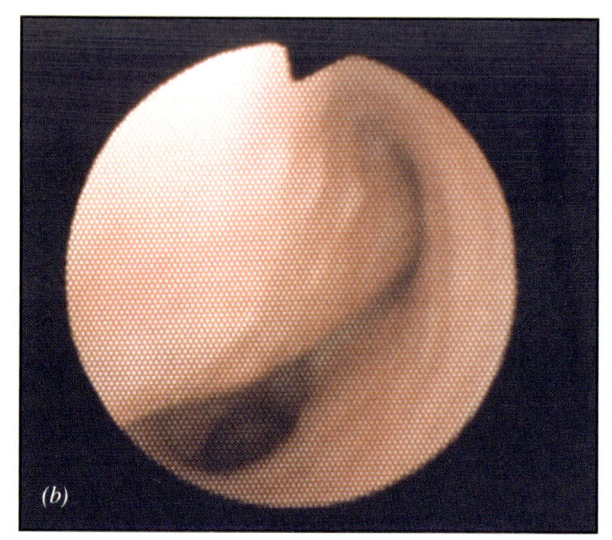

Figure 5.42: (a) Endoscopic photograph of the cervical trachea of a normal dog. Note the white 'C'-shaped tracheal rings, the tracheal membrane (visible under the notch at the top of the photo) and the fine submucosal vascularity (the reddened area between rings) which are typically seen. (b) Photograph of the caudal intrathoracic trachea and carina from a dog with chronic bronchitis and tracheal collapse. Note the redundant dorsal tracheal membrane which hangs down into the lumen of the trachea and nearly completely obstructs the left principal bronchus at rest. Upon exertion as the dog became lighter under the anaesthesia and with coughing all intrathoracic airways were observed to collapse completely.

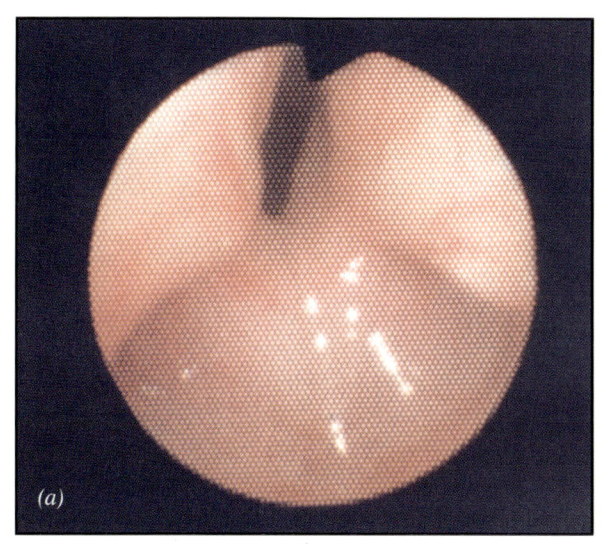 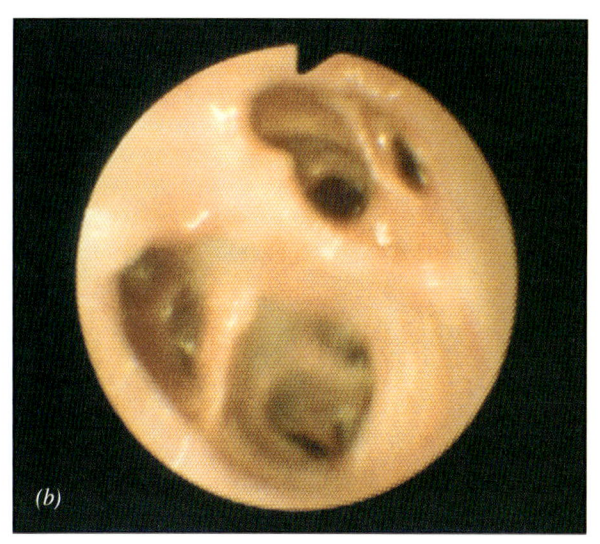

Figure 5.43: (a) Oedematous tissues within the respiratory tract are well demonstrated by this photograph of oedematous, everted laryngeal saccules. The entire ventral portion of the larynx is obstructed by gelatinous, glistening tissue (the everted saccules) which obstructed an estimated 40–50% of the entire rima glottidis of this dog. (b) Mucosal oedema in the lower airways is similar in appearance, as demonstrated by this photograph from the right caudal lobe of a dog with bronchiectasis (dilated bronchi of varying shape) and ongoing mucosal irritation.

coughing). Collapse is commonly observed in animals with tracheal collapse, bronchiectasis and tracheo-bronchial malacia, conditions where the structural integrity of the cartilaginous support of the airways has been altered.

Mucosal colour of the normal tracheobronchial tree should be light pink, although its appearance will vary depending on the intensity and proximity of the endoscopic lighting which is being used. A rich supply of submucosal vessels (mucosal capillaries) is usually visible within the submucosa and is especially notice-able between the cartilaginous rings of the trachea (Figure 5.42a). A slight glistening appearance of the normal mucosa is due to the presence of a thin periciliary fluid layer (the 'sol').

Oedema (excessive fluid accumulation in the mucosa) is readily apparent due to the gelatinous appearance it imparts to the epithelial surface (Figure 5.43). Mucosal oedema may be accompanied by blunting the bronchial bifurcations or 'spurs' (the carina is the only spur which is specifically named) and some degree of loss of detail of the submucosal vascular pattern. Generalized reddening of the mucosa (due to inflammatory changes, increased vascularity, and hyperaemia) is a common finding in chronic respiratory diseases. Because only diseased animals typically undergo bronchoscopy, care must be exercised in interpreting the appearance of the tracheobronchial mucosa so as not to accept the reddened mucosa as normal.

Mucus may be observed in healthy animals as small accumulations on the mucosa, stranding across the lumen, or pushed up in front of the bronchoscope during bronchoscopy (usually clear to white and slightly opaque). Larger accumulations and secretions of un-usual colour are associated with chronic irritation, infec-tion (bacterial, parasitic or fungal), allergies and trauma.

Stradling (1976) states that secretions are excessive if there is need to suction them from the airways during bronchoscopy, regardless of the gross appearance of the mucus. Larger accumulations of secretions are abnor-mal and should be sampled for analysis.

Haemorrhage from friable mucosal surfaces may be easily induced during endoscopy due to forceful or rough endoscope insertion, suction, brushings or bi-opsy procedures. When haemorrhage is present on initial examination (Figure 5.44) it may be associated with thoracic trauma (lung contusion, bite wounds), parasitic infection (e.g. *Paragonimus*), airway foreign body, mucosal trauma (e.g. from chronic coughing) or airway narrowing due to external compression such as hilar lymphadenopathy. In the author's experience, haemorrhage is rarely caused by primary lung tumours

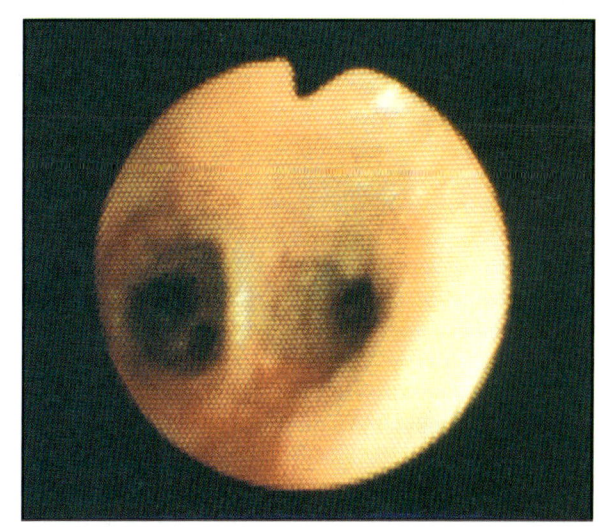

Figure 5.44: Endoscopic photograph taken at the carina of a dog diagnosed with chronic bronchitis of undetermined aetiology. Note the severe mucosal oedema, haemorrhage and submucosal nodules.

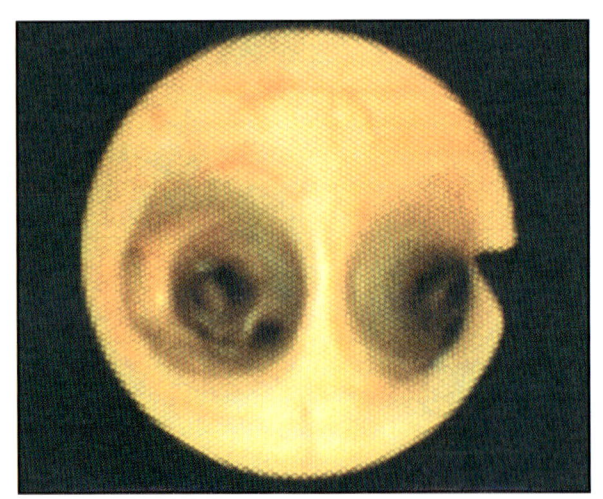

Figure 5.45: Endoscopic photograph of the carina from a normal dog. Looking down the right principal bronchus (on the left in the photo) the right cranial, caudal and accessory bronchi are visible, while in the left principal bronchus (on the right in the photo) the left caudal lobar bronchus is seen. (As noted from left to right in the photo, respectively).

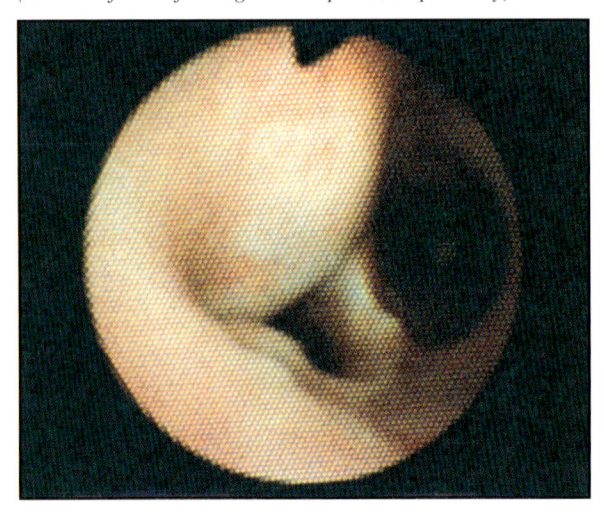

Figure 5.46: Tracheobronchial lymphadenopathy obstructs the right cranial lobar bronchus in a dog with systemic blastomycosis. The carina is commonly widened as the result of hilar lymphadenopathy in systemic fungal diseases as well as lymphosarcoma and primary lung tumours; no widening is noted in this case and the carina is seen as a narrow band of tissue dividing the trachea with the left principal bronchus extending into the distance.

in dogs, as they typically develop in the periphery and impinge on the airway without the mucosal invasion that is typical of many human lung cancer cases.

The *carina* is the name given to the bifurcation of the trachea into the left and right mainstem or principal bronchi (Figure 5.45). In the healthy animal, this bifurcation is relatively sharp with no evidence of mainstem bronchial compression secondary to hilar lymphadenopathy. Various systemic fungal diseases (histoplasmosis, blastomycosis, coccidiodomycosis) and tumours (lymphosarcoma, primary lung tumours) may involve these lymph nodes and lead to mainstem bronchial compression and coughing, especially following exertion (Figure 5.46).

Focal or generalized changes may be observed in the *tracheobronchial tree* of a diseased animal, including those involving:

- *lumen size* (intraluminal obstruction, stricture, external compression, or bronchiectasis - see Figure 5.44)
- *lumen shape* (dynamic collapse - see Figure 5.42(b))
- *mucosal abnormalities* (oedema, accumulations of secretions, irregularity or erosions, mucosal hyperplasia, and thickening or folding)
- *submucosal changes* (increased vascularity or hyperaemia, haemorrhages, or nodule formation - see Figures 5.43(b) and 5.44.

Sample procurement and handling

The recognition of normal from abnormal involves a subjective interpretation in many instances. Experience and practice will improve an endoscopist's ability to detect early lesions. The lung (bronchial epithelium) appears to respond to irritation in limited ways, and therefore the abnormalities seen (even by an experienced bronchoscopist) may not be pathognomonic for any specific disease (Haschek, 1986). Samples obtained (cytology, culture and biopsy) are therefore relied upon to establish a specific diagnosis.

Whether or not abnormalities are noted, samples should be obtained for tests such as cytological evaluation (via brush, curette, washing pipe, or most commonly the bronchoalveolar lavage - BAL), for culture (from washings, lavage or tissue biopsy), and on occasion for histopathological evaluation (via cup biopsy forceps). Collection of samples for cytological examination is covered in Chapter 5(v). The normal BAL results from cats and dogs are summarized in Table 5.6.

Complications

Bronchoscopy is generally a safe procedure and lacks any serious complications. There are a number of potential complications which have been associated with bronchoscopy in human medicine but these have rarely been encountered during canine and feline bronchoscopy. Complications that have been mentioned in veterinary medicine are few in number and can easily be anticipated by reviewing these items and the contraindications listed in Table 5.5. Despite the potential for complications, few serious complications have been documented in animals. The most serious complications that I have encountered were in dogs with severe chronic obstructive pulmonary disease (usually those with diffuse malacic changes and severe airway collapse). These animals may develop exercise or stress-related cyanosis following bronchoscopy, i.e. during recovery from anaesthesia. Dogs which present with a chronic history of coughing (often with cyanosis) and/ or severe expiratory effort (an abdominal push) while

Reference	Scott *et al.,*[1]	Rebar *et al.,*[2]	Padrid *et al.,*[3]	King *et al.,*[3]
Year	1993	1980	1991	1988
Species	canine	canine	feline	feline
(*n*)	46	9	24	11
Total cell count/μl	NR	516 (240–630)	301(±126)	241(±101)
% Macrophages	75 (27–92)	83	64 (±22)	70.6 (±9.8)
% PMN	3 (0–30)	5	5 (±3)	6.7 (±4.0)
% Lymphocytes	10 (1–43)	5.7	4 (±3)	4.6 (±3.2)
% Eosinophils	3 (0–28)	4.2	25 (±21)	16.1 (±6.8)
% Mast cells	1 (0–5)	2.3	<1 (±<1)	NR
% Epithelial cells	NR	NR	2 (±2)	NR
% Goblet cells	NR	NR	<1 (±<1)	NR

Table 5.6: *BAL results from clinically healthy dogs and cats. NR = not reported*

[1] *Results are median values and (range) obtained from second lavage performed;* [2] *Results are mean values and (range) from six lung lobes from all dogs;* [3] *Results are mean values (±SD) obtained from all cats*

breathing at rest should be considered at risk for developing this problem. In these cases, care must be taken in choosing an anaesthetic protocol which allows for a non-excitable, slow anaesthetic recovery.

Topical 1% lignocaine sprayed at the carina at the completion of the bronchoscopic procedure may minimize coughing and therefore airway collapse during the post-bronchoscopy period. Close patient monitoring is imperative during the recovery period as well.

Practical applications of bronchoscopy

There is no question that bronchoscopy (including cytology and culture) is the gold standard for the diagnosis of lower respiratory tract diseases in small animals. The direct visualization of lesions and selected collection of airway samples, the appreciation of dynamic airway calibre changes and the possibility for therapeutic intervention (foreign body removal) are a few of the reasons why this diagnostic technique is clearly superior to others such at transtracheal aspiration biopsy or fine needle lung aspiration. The primary limitations which might be considered relative to bronchoscopy are financial (it is more expensive to perform a complete bronchoscopic examination), and concerns about the anaesthesia required for the procedure. Despite these concerns, bronchoscopy should be considered the diagnostic test of choice in any case with significant (and especially chronic) lower respiratory tract disease in the dog and cat.

REFERENCES AND FURTHER READING

Amis TC and McKiernan BC (1986) Systemic identification of endobronchial anatomy during bronchoscopy in the dog. *American Journal of Veterinary Research* **47**, 2649

Brearley M J, Cooper JE and Sullivan M (1991) *Color Atlas of Small Animal Endoscopy.* Mosby-Year Book, St Louis, MO

Ford RB (1990) Endoscopy of the lower respiratory tract of the dog and cat. In: *Small Animal Endoscopy,* ed. TR Tams. CV Mosby, St Louis, MO

Haschek WM (1986) Response of the lung to injury. In: *Current Veterinary Therapy* 9th edn, ed. RW Kirk. WB Saunders, Philadelphia

Hawkins EC, Denicola DB and Kuehn NF (1990) Bronchoalveolar lavage in the evaluation of pulmonary disease in the dog and cat. *Journal of Veterinary Internal Medicine* **4**, 267

Hoffmann W E and Wellman ML (1986) Tracheobronchial cytology. In: *Current Veterinary Therapy* 9th edn, ed. RW Kirk. WB Saunders, Philadelphia

King RR, Zeng QY, Brown DJ, Kunkle GA and Courtney CH (1988) Bronchoalveolar lavage cell populations in dogs and cats with eosinophilic pneumonitis. *Proceedings of the 7th Veterinary Symposium, Comparative Respiratory Society*

Lotti U and Niebauer GW (1992) Tracheobronchial foreign bodies of plant origin in 153 hunting dogs. *Compendium of Continuing Education for the Practicing Veterinarian* **14**, 900

McKiernan BC (1989). Bronchoscopy in the small animal patient. In: *Current Veterinary Therapy* 10th edn, ed. RW Kirk. WB Saunders, Philadelphia.

McKiernan BC and Kneller SK (1983) A simple method for the preparation of inflated air-dried lung specimens. *Veterinary Radiology* **24**, 58

Padrid PA, Hornof WJ, Kurpershoek C J and Cross CE (1990) Canine chronic bronchitis. *Journal of Veterinary Internal Medicine* **4**, 172

Padrid PA, Feldman BF, Funk K, Samitz EM, Reil D and Cross CE (1991) Cytologic, microbiologic, and biochemical analysis of bronchoalveolar lavage fluid obtained from 24 healthy cats. *American Journal of Veterinary Research* **52**, 1300

Rebar AH, Denicola DD and Muggenburg BA (1980) Bronchopulmonary lavage cytology in the dog: normal findings. *Veterinary Pathology* **17**, 294

Rebar AH, Hawkins EC and Denicola DB (1992) Cytologic evaluation of the respiratory tract. *Veterinary Clinics of North America* **22**, 1065

Roudebush P (1990) Tracheobronchoscopy. *Veterinary Clinics of North America* **20**, 1297

Scott M, Dennis J, Watson G and Oliver N (1993). Bronchoalveolar lavage of histologically normal and diseased canine lung lobes. *Veterinary Pathology* **30**, 433

Stradling P (1976) *Diagnostic Bronchoscopy: An Introduction,* 3rd edn. Churchill Livingstone, New York

Venker-Van Haagen AJ (1979) Bronchoscopy of the normal and abnormal canine. *Journal of the American Animal Hospital Association* **15**, 397

Venker-Van Haagen AJ, Vroom WM, Heijn A and Van Ooijen PG (1985) Bronchoscopy in small animal clinics: an analysis of the results of 228 bronchoscopies. *Journal of the American Animal Hospital Association* 21, 521

Zavala DC (1978) *Flexible Fiberoptic Bronchoscopy.* Pepco Litho Press, Cedar Rapids, IA

(v) Cytological Collection Techniques

Brendan Corcoran

INTRODUCTION

Cytological evaluation of material collected from the airways and the lung is invaluable in the diagnosis of respiratory disease. While culturing of organisms in the respiratory tract is necessary for the accurate assessment of respiratory infections and selection of suitable antimicrobial agents, identification of the cellular reaction in the airways is more likely to result in a definitive diagnosis than any other single respiratory diagnostic technique.

Airway cytology is particularly useful in identifying pulmonary neoplasia and pulmonary infiltration with eosinophilia and can be used to support diagnoses of acute and chronic airway and pneumonic diseases.

BASIC TECHNIQUES AND EQUIPMENT REQUIREMENTS

Airway sampling should be carried out preferably with the aid of bronchoscopy, so as to allow accurate collection of material that is likely to aid diagnosis. However, good quality samples can be obtained using blind sampling techniques and are feasible techniques in general practice. Airway sampling should be attempted in all acute and chronic respiratory disease cases, with the exception of acute tracheobronchitis (kennel cough).

Sampling should not be carried out immediately prior to thoracic radiography, as the sampling fluid will be seen on radiographs. The basic equipment required for each technique includes a suitable sampling catheter, syringes containing the sampling fluid, a 20 ml syringe for suction, suitable containers and transport media (Figure 5.47).

Sampling catheters should be long enough to reach close to the lung periphery, semi-rigid to ease advancement into the airways, and have a narrow lumen to assist suction. Purpose-made endoscope catheters are preferable and are easy to use, but dog urinary catheters can also be adapted for airway sampling.

The preferred sampling solution is warmed sterile normal saline. Cytological preservatives should not be instilled into the airways. Arrangements should be made with the laboratory for suitable transport media

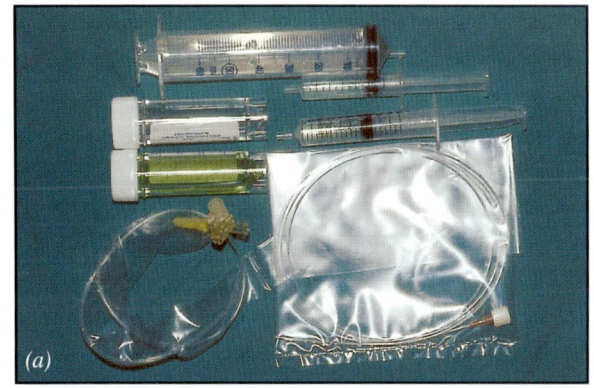

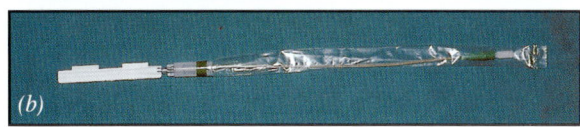

Figure 5.47: *The basic equipment required for airway sampling is readily available and inexpensive. (a) Examples of sampling equipment: Portex bronchoscope biopsy catheter, bitch urinary catheter, syringes, Bijou bottles and fixative material (Cytofix®, Shandon Ltd, UK). (b) Jugular through-the-needle catheter for transtracheal sampling.*

and fixatives. If material cannot be analysed on the day of collection, the author uses a 50:50 dilution of Cytofix® to preserve cellular elements during transport to the laboratory. Alternatively, centrifuge the sample and make air-dried smears. Specific transport media may also be required for identification of viruses, microaerophilic and anaerobic bacilli and chlamydial organisms, and your laboratory should be contacted for suitable advice.

Opinion on the volume of saline necessary to obtain sufficient diagnostic material varies. In general, sample volumes should be restricted to a minimum, with very large sample volumes being used if there is a constant suction facility. The author uses 2 ml aliquots in cats and between 2 and 15 ml per aliquot in dogs (three aliquots in total). Between 40 and 50% of the instilled saline can be retrieved. The use of large sample volumes will not necessarily improve the amount or quality of material retrieved, and may be mildly hazardous in cats.

Once the procedure is completed the samples are pooled and two aliquots are made for cytological and microbial analysis.

CYTOLOGICAL COLLECTION TECHNIQUES

Several techniques have been described for the collection of representative cell samples from the airways.

Visualized sampling

Sample collection with the aid of an endoscope with a biopsy channel will give the best results. For tracheal and bronchial sampling, identify material suitable for collection and aspirate with the biopsy catheter or collect with a biopsy brush. To carry out bronchoalveolar lavage (BAL), the endoscope, with the pre-loaded catheter in the biopsy channel, is lodged in the bronchus serving the lung area of interest. After approximately 10 seconds, the aliquot of saline is injected and immediately aspirated. Multiple samples can be collected from the same site, with three samples usually being sufficient. Up to 50% of the aliquot can be retrieved with the remainder being removed by normal lung transport mechanisms. The procedure can be repeated at different sites of interest. If a constant suction facility is available, the collection of larger numbers of samples, using large volumes of solution, can be carried out. However, in the author's experience three samples collected from selected sites are usually sufficient (either from the same site or three different sites) to give representative material, and more intensive sampling will not necessarily give any additional information.

Blind sampling

These techniques are used where an endoscope is not available or where general anaesthesia would be hazardous to the patient. The sampling catheter is advanced as far as possible into the respiratory tract, the solution is infused and immediately aspirated. Approximately 20–30% of the solution may be retrieved and high quality diagnostic material can be obtained by this method. In fact, blind sampling is the method commonly used in cats, unless a very small diameter endoscope is available. The distance that the catheter is advanced may determine the type of sample collected (tracheobronchial wash or bronchoalveolar lavage (BAL)), but in practice the sample is less likely to be a true BAL than if collected using endoscopy.

Per-oral sampling can be carried out in anaesthetized patients. The catheter is passed via an endotracheal tube into the respiratory tract and material is collected in the usual manner. On occasions, diagnostic material becomes trapped at the end of the endotracheal tube and can be harvested for analysis.

Transtracheal and translaryngeal sampling involve a similar procedure (Figure 5.48). The site where the catheter is to be introduced is clipped and aseptically prepared. The patient should be sedated and local anaesthetic injected through to the airway lumen. A 2–4 mm skin incision is made. With the patient restrained in the sternal position and the head elevated, the airway is held in place and a wide bore (12–14 G) hypodermic needle is inserted into the airway lumen, between tracheal rings in the case of the transtracheal technique, and through the cricothyroid ligament, rostral to the ridge of the cricoid cartilage, in the case of translaryngeal sampling. The sampling catheter is advanced through the needle a predetermined distance or as far into the airway as possible. The solution is instilled and then aspirated. This will usually cause paroxysmal coughing which may assist retrieval of material. After withdrawal of the needle digital pressure should be applied to the site for approximately 2 minutes.

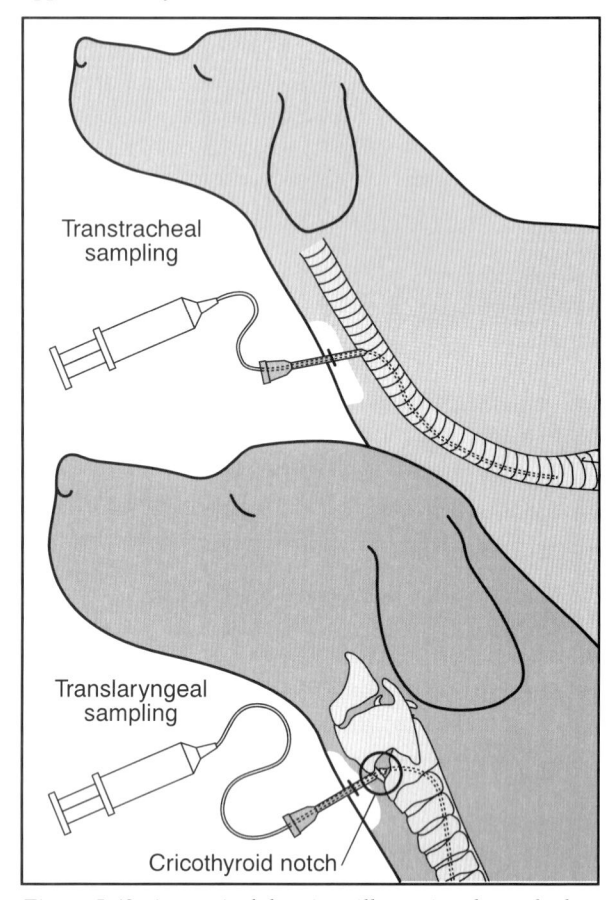

Transtracheal sampling

Translaryngeal sampling

Cricothyroid notch

Figure 5.48: *Anatomical drawings illustrating the methods for translaryngeal (cricothyroid ligament) and transtracheal airway sampling.*

INTERPRETATION OF AIRWAY CYTOLOGICAL RESULTS

The interpretation of airway cytology must be made in the context of the other clinical findings. In a large number of cases with obvious respiratory disease, the sample findings will be inconclusive, but in others they will be diagnostic. There are also differences in the cell types and differential percentages between tracheobronchial and bronchoalveolar lavage samples. BAL samples tend to have higher numbers of macrophages compared with tracheal samples, illustrating the lower airway and alveolar source of the material.

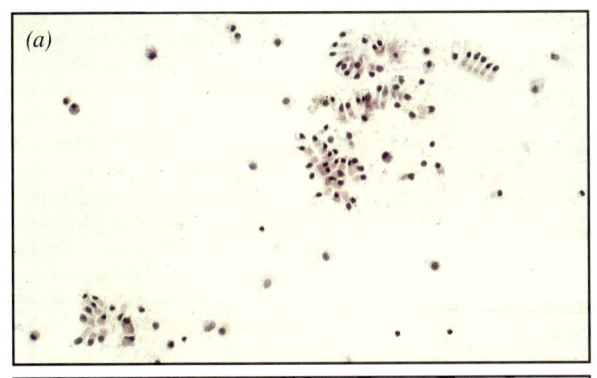

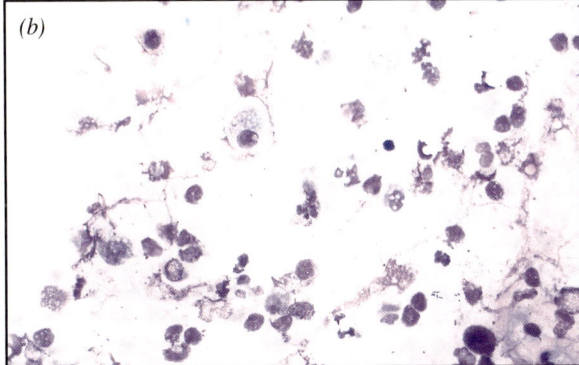

Figure 5.49: *(a) Normal airway cytology sample with small numbers of mononuclear cells and mucin background staining. The majority of cellular elements are epithelial cells. (b) Example of an abnormal sample from a cat with asthma. There are large numbers of cells and debris including monocytes, plasma cells and eosinophils.*

In normal animals, some cellular material is usually found. Small numbers of ciliated epithelial cells, neutrophils, macrophages and plasma cells are consistent with a normal or non-diagnostic sample (Figure 5.49). Macrophages tend to be the most common cell type in normal samples. In situations where the normal cell numbers are large or atypical cells are detected, such as eosinophils or neoplastic cells, the sample is diagnostic.

Neoplastic cells may be found in airway samples where the disease is sufficiently advanced to erode the airway walls and shed cells into the airway lumen. Cells can be found with both primary and secondary neoplasms, and the cell type can allow differentiation of the tumour type.

The presence of large numbers of neutrophils and macrophages suggests a non-specific inflammatory reaction. Neutrophils are often seen with acute and chronic airway inflammation. Macrophages are mononuclear cells that appear in response to alveolar and lower airway inflammation and may be supportive of a diagnosis of bronchopneumonia. Diseases restricted to the pulmonary interstitium rarely produce an airway cellular reaction that can assist diagnosis.

The quantity of mucus in the sample should be assessed, although the degree of mucus accumulation in the airways is better assessed by bronchoscopy. Excessive quantities of mucus are associated with chronic bronchitis and are due to mucous hypersecre-tion by increased numbers of mucous glands and goblet cells in the airways.

The presence of even small numbers of eosinophils, in the author's experience, is significant and is suggestive of parasitic or airway hypersensitivity diseases such as *Oslerus (Filaroides) osleri* infection and pulmonary infiltration with eosinophilia. In normal cats eosinophils are reported to be found in airway samples. This is a contentious and unresolved issue. In the author's opinion, eosinophils in airway samples collected from cats with overt signs of respiratory disease should be regarded as significant. Nevertheless, airway eosinophilia is not a consistent finding with feline asthma syndrome.

COLLECTION OF LUNG PARENCHYMAL SAMPLES

The collection of samples from the lung parenchyma usually involves transthoracic needle biopsy techniques, although samples can also be retrieved during thoracotomy. Transbronchial sampling can also be attempted using an endoscope and suitable spring-loaded endoscope biopsy needle. However, endoscopy tends to be used to obtain samples of airway mucosa.

Successful collection of samples is best achieved where the lesion is well delineated, consolidated, close to the chest wall and away from vital structures (heart and major blood vessels). The best results are achieved with primary pulmonary neoplasms. Sampling from lung where the pathological changes are minimal is usually unsuccessful.

Percutaneous collection techniques involve using either a 1.5–3.0″, 21–23 gauge needle attached to a large syringe, or purpose-made biopsy needles designed to collect a core of tissue. With both techniques, the site should be clipped and scrubbed and standard aseptic procedures should be followed. The site for optimum sampling is identified from thoracic radiographs. Lung puncture is painful, and sedation and local anaesthesia should be considered.

With needle biopsy, the needle and syringe are directed straight into the sample area, and suction is applied. Suction should be stopped before the needle is withdrawn. To process the collected material, disconnect the needle from the syringe, fill the syringe with air, re-attach it to the needle and empty the contents of the needle onto microscope slides, make a smear and air-dry.

When using a commercial biopsy needle, a small skin incision is made one or two rib spaces from the needle insertion site. Place the needle in the incision and slide towards the site, inserting the needle into the sample site. Collect the material and remove the needle applying digital pressure to the area. The collected plug of tissue should be mounted on a piece of card and immersed in 10% formalin.

There are potential hazards with transthoracic biopsy techniques. Simple needle biopsy is the least hazardous, but also the least productive. Complications can result from pneumothorax and damage to pulmonary vessels. While pneumothorax can be avoided by the operator using care during the procedure, puncture of a large vessel, particularly by a cutting biopsy needle, cannot always be guarded against and can be fatal.

COLLECTION OF MATERIAL FROM THE PLEURAL SPACE

Collection of material from the pleural space is attempted if a pleural effusion has been identified on radiographs. A simple needle technique similar to that for lung needle biopsy will suffice. Collected material is submitted for routine analysis and aerobic and anaerobic culture.

FURTHER READING

Creighton SR and Wilkins RJ (1974) Transtracheal aspiration biopsy: technique and cytologic evaluation. *Journal of the American Animal Hospital Association* **10**, 219–226

Rebar AH and DeNicola DB (1988) The cytologic examination of the respiratory tract. *Seminars in Veterinary Medicine and Surgery (Small Animal)* **3**, 109–121.

Teske E, Stokhof AA, van den Ingh TSGAM, Wolvekamp WThC, Slappendel RJ and DeVries HW (1991) Transthoracic needle aspiration biopsy of the lung in dogs with pulmonic diseases. *Journal of the American Animal Hospital Association* **27**, 289–294

(vi) Diagnostic Ultrasonography

Michael E. Herrtage

Diagnostic ultrasonography has proved to be of great value in veterinary medicine as a complementary imaging technique to radiology. This chapter will deal primarily with the use of diagnostic ultrasound in the examination of the heart, usually referred to as *echocardiography*. Echocardiography has revolutionized veterinary cardiology by providing a non-invasive means for the accurate qualitative and quantitative assessment of cardiac function that is required for the diagnosis and management of congenital and acquired heart disease. Its use has supplanted invasive techniques such as cardiac catheterization and angiocardiography, and because echocardiography can be repeated without causing undue stress to the patient, the technique can also be used to monitor the effects of treatment.

Diagnostic ultrasound can also be used successfully in the examination of non-cardiac thoracic disease and can provide useful diagnostic information in selected patients. The indications and limitations of this technique are dealt with in the section at the end of this chapter.

PRINCIPLES OF ULTRASOUND IMAGING

The principle of ultrasonography is similar to that of sonar devices used by bats and submarines. Ultrasound is high frequency sound above the audible range of the human ear, i.e. greater than 20 000 Hz. Diagnostic ultrasound usually employs sound waves of frequencies between 2.25 and 10 MHz.

Transducer

Diagnostic ultrasound is produced by a transducer which consists of one or more crystals with piezo-electric properties. These crystals are able to convert mechanical signals (such as sound waves) into electrical signals, and *vice versa*. Ultrasound waves are generated by a piezo-electric crystal, when it vibrates at high frequency after the application of a short burst of an alternating current.

If the transducer is placed in contact with the surface of the patient, the sound waves travel through the tissues. These pressure waves are propagated through the tissue by transfer of energy to adjacent molecules. As the wave front advances, small quantities of sound energy are reflected back from successive tissue interfaces. The returning echoes interact with the transducer, causing slight deformation of the piezo-electric crystal. This generates an electric current that can be amplified and analysed according to the strength and depth of the reflected echoes. The transducer thus acts as both an emitter and receiver of sound energy.

Sound reflection

Most of the transmitted sound energy is scattered or absorbed; however, a little is reflected back at interfaces between tissues of differing *acoustic impedance*, for example, between the pericardium and the myocardium. If there is a large difference in acoustic impedance, most of the sound beam is reflected back, as with the interface between soft tissue and bone or soft tissue and gas.

Two types of reflected ultrasound occur at an acoustic interface: *specular echoes* and *scattered echoes* (Figure 5.50). Specular echoes are produced by

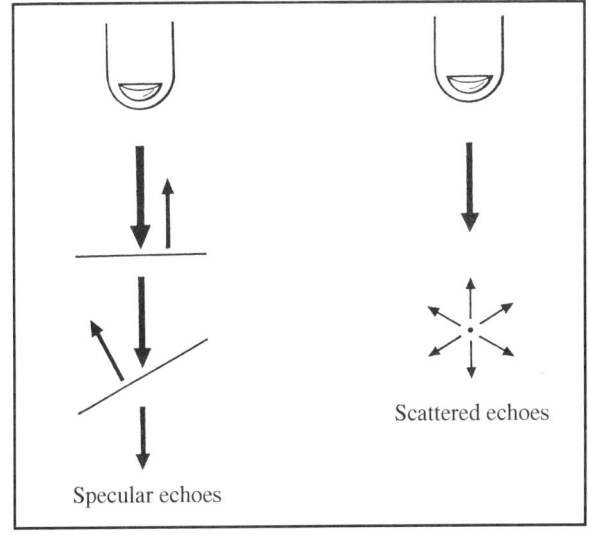

Scattered echoes

Specular echoes

Figure 5.50: Specular and scattered echo production. Specular echoes originate from relatively large acoustic interfaces that reflect a proportion of the beam with the remainder passing on undeviated into tissue beyond the interface. Specular echoes are angle dependent. Scattered or non-specular echoes originate from small, weakly reflective objects and are less angle dependent.

objects that are fairly large with respect to the wavelength and that present a relatively smooth surface to the ultrasound beam. These objects regularly reflect the ultrasound beam and are angle dependent. The object is best seen when the beam hits the interface at an angle of 90 degrees. Scattered echoes are ultrasound waves reflected back from small irregular objects, similar to or smaller in size than the wavelength of the beam, and the reflection is not angle dependent. The scattered or non-specular echoes give organs their characteristic echo texture.

Depth determination

Since the speed of sound in soft tissue structures is relatively constant, by measuring the time delay between when a pulse is emitted and when the reflected sound is detected, the depth of the interface can be calculated.

Resolution

Resolution is the ability of the image to represent individual structures and is *dependent on wavelength*. High-frequency transducers are useful to image superficial structures and can take advantage of high resolution. In order to image deeper structures, however, lower-frequency transducers must be used with a resultant compromise in resolution. The ideal frequency for transducers used in veterinary ultrasonography is shown in Table 5.7.

DISPLAY FORMATS

The reflected ultrasound can be displayed in a number of different ways. The most important forms of display are:

Transducer frequency	Veterinary applications
2.25 MHz	Equine hearts
3 MHz	Large breeds of dog
5 MHz	Small–medium sized dogs
7.5 MHz	Cats
	Equine tendons
10 MHz	Eyes (all species)

Table 5.7: *The ideal transducer frequency for veterinary ultrasonography.*

B-mode (brightness mode)

In B-mode, the amplitude of the reflected signal is displayed on the cathode ray screen as a spot of variable brightness. A large signal produces a bright spot and a small signal a dim spot. By collecting information from successive scan lines as the transducer is moved to different positions, a two-dimensional (2D) image of the slice or plane is built up. To form a typical sector scan, pulses of ultrasound are transmitted along about 120 scan lines over a 90° arc. In 'real time' screening the image produced is continuously updated at a rate of 30–60 pictures per second to allow movement to be appreciated (Figure 5.51).

Real time scanning is the most commonly used technique in veterinary diagnostic ultrasound. It is the simplest display to interpret because it provides an anatomical cross-sectional image.

There are three types of transducer capable of producing 2D images, mechanical and electronic sector scanners and linear array scanners:

Mechanical sector scanners use either a small number of crystals on a rotating wheel or a single crystal which oscillates back and forth to produce a fan-shaped field.

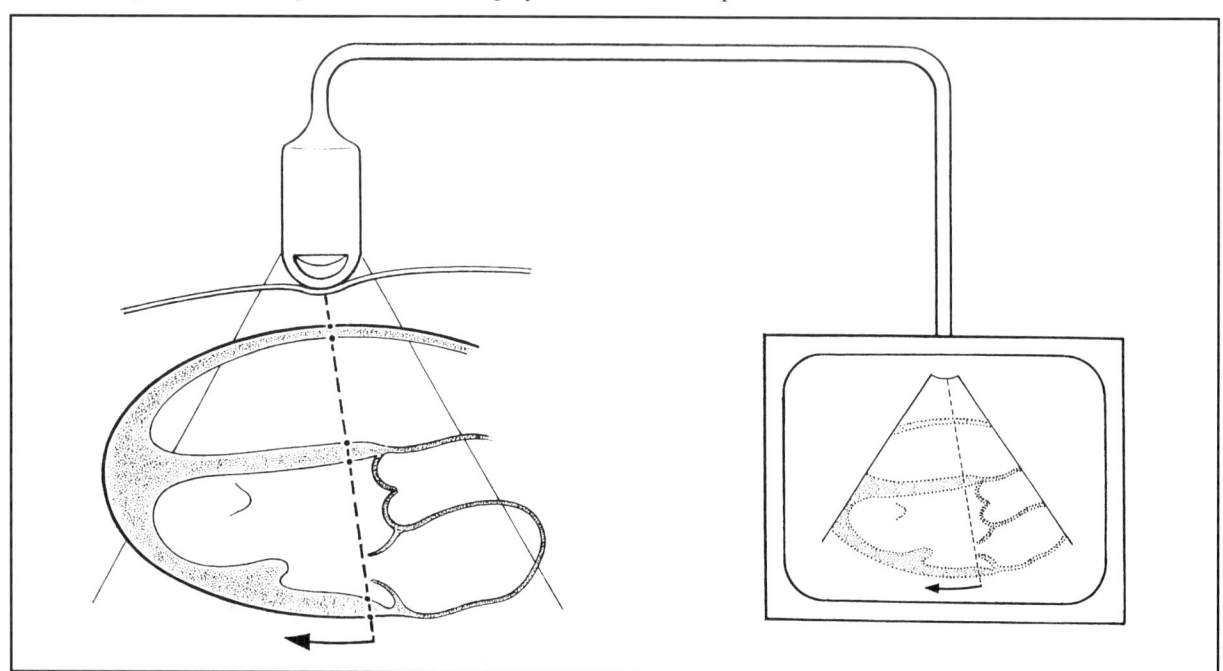

Figure 5.51: *Diagram showing the production of a sector scan image of the heart. The B-mode echoes received from each successive scan line are used to build up an image of the heart on the oscilloscope.*

Phased array sectors or electronic sector scanners use an array of small static crystals which are electronically triggered to sweep through a fan-shaped field.

Linear array scanners use small crystals (60–250) arranged in a line. The crystals are electronically triggered in groups. These transducers produce a rectangular image and require good contact with the skin over a large area.

A transducer with a small contact area (footprint) is essential to allow access between the ribs for echocardiography and non-cardiac thoracic ultrasonography; only mechanical and electronic sector scanners are suitable for this purpose.

M-mode (motion mode)

M-mode is an adaptation of B-mode, which uses a single crystal to produce a pencil beam of ultrasound. The beam is used to examine a small area of the heart. Ultrasound is reflected back from the tissue interfaces to the transducer when it is placed at right angles to moving structures. The single vertical line composed of dots of varying brightness is continuously updated and plotted against time, thus displaying the motion of the structures during the cardiac cycle. M-mode has a high sampling rate (pulse repetition rate of 1000–2000 per second) which facilitates the accurate resolution and definition of rapidly moving structures, such as the cardiac wall or valves, for evaluation (Figure 5.52). It is particularly useful for cardiac measurements.

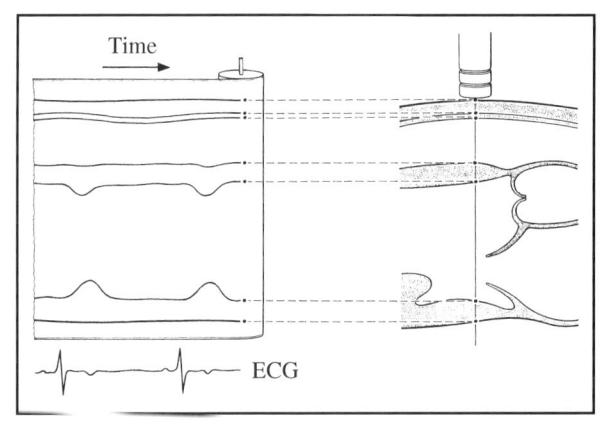

Figure 5.52: *Diagram showing the production of an M-mode recording of the heart. The reflected B-mode echoes received from a single scan line through the heart are plotted against time.*

Mechanical and electronic 2D sector scanners are available with integrated M-mode capability. The direction of the M-mode beam can be controlled and is represented as a cursor on the 2D image. With duplex imaging, it is possible to steer the M-mode in order to gain traces from precise anatomical locations.

Doppler ultrasound

Ultrasound waves are transmitted from a transducer at a specific frequency. When the sound waves strike red blood cells which are moving relative to the ultrasound beam, the frequency of the returning echoes differs slightly from that of the transmitted waves as a consequence of the Doppler effect. The frequency shift is directly proportional to the velocity of the blood. Maximum velocities can be measured when the Doppler beam is parallel to blood flow.

There are two basic Doppler techniques: continuous wave and pulsed wave Doppler. Continuous wave Doppler is very sensitive and allows the measurement of high maximum velocities. However, an important drawback is that all velocities along the length and width of the ultrasound beam are recorded and the regions of abnormal flow cannot be localized accurately.

This problem is circumvented by using pulsed wave Doppler, which records reflected signals from a particular depth, so that localization within a 2D image is possible. However the pulsed wave system is unable to detect high frequency Doppler shifts (i.e. high velocities) due to a phenomenon known as *aliasing*. This disadvantage is greatly reduced by colour flow Doppler, a two dimensional version of pulsed wave Doppler.

Doppler uses low-frequency transducers (1.5–2.0 MHz) to reduce the problem of aliasing.

Terminology

It is conventional to display the ultrasound image as white on a black background. There are a number of terms that may be used to describe the image (Table 5.8).

Term	Description
Anechoic Echolucent Sonolucent	Appears black on conventional scans, due to the absence of reflected ultrasound. Represents complete transmission of sound (e.g. fluid)
Hyperechoic Echogenic	Reflected ultrasound appears as bright white echoes on a conventional scan. Represents a highly reflective tissue interface (e.g. bone or gas)
Hypoechoic Relatively echolucent	Reflected ultrasound appears dark grey on conventional scans. Represents minimal reflection of ultrasound from tissue interface (e.g. most soft tissue structures)

Table 5.8: *Terminology used in echocardiography.*

Artefacts

A number of artefacts can occur during routine ultrasound examinations. It is important to recognize the most common artefacts to avoid misinterpretation.

Acoustic shadowing. Acoustic shadows are seen deep to a highly reflective acoustic interface, for example gas or bone. An intensely bright white outline is seen at the border of the tissue, but as most of the ultrasound beam has been reflected, no information can be gained from beyond the interface and it therefore appears dark on the scan. Both ribs and lung tissue can cause acoustic shadowing.

Distant enhancement. If the ultrasound beam passes through a relatively homogeneous echolucent medium, for example a gallbladder or a cyst, less attenuation occurs than if the beam passes through the surrounding echogenic tissues. When the sound beam strikes the far wall of this cystic structure, the echoes appear to be brighter than the surrounding structures.

Reverberation. Strongly reflected echoes can cause an echo to form at the transducer face. This will re-enter the patient and cause a second echo to be displayed twice as deep as the original acoustic interface. Reverberations are usually caused at highly reflective air-fluid interfaces and appear as highly echoic parallel lines recurring at regular intervals.

Mirror-image artefact. This artefact is also produced at highly reflective tissue interfaces and is caused by multiple internal reverberations between an organ and the reflective surface. Mirror-image artefacts are often seen at the pericardium–lung interface with a 'second heart' beating deep to the original.

ECHOCARDIOGRAPHY

Echocardiographic technique

In order to obtain the maximum amount of information from an echocardiographic examination, it is important to adopt a systematic approach to ensure that nothing is overlooked. For a complete examination, the heart should be imaged from the right and left parasternal positions. Occasionally, suprasternal and subcostal views are also required.

Patient preparation

To ensure good contact between the transducer and the skin, the hair should be clipped from a small area extending for several intercostal spaces over the apex beat of the heart on each side of the thorax. In most dogs this is usually from the third to the sixth intercostal space at the level of the costochondral cartilages. The skin should be clean and any scale, dirt or grease should be removed with spirit.

Most animals do not require chemical restraint, although this may facilitate studies in uncooperative patients, particularly young puppies and cats. Sedation may affect the cardiac indices, including heart rate, chamber dimensions and contractility. Firm but reassuring physical restraint from a trained veterinary nurse in quiet subdued surroundings will be sufficient to examine the majority of patients.

Patient positioning

The patient should be restrained in right and left lateral recumbent positions for the standard right and left parasternal views. It is helpful to have a working surface with a notch or hole cut out of it, so that the operator can scan from the dependent side with the animal in lateral recumbency. This reduces the interference caused by air-filled lung and increases the size of the acoustic window (the area where the heart is in contact with the thoracic wall).

Alternatively, patients can be scanned from above in lateral recumbency or in the upright (standing, sitting or sternal) position with the foreleg pulled forward. The latter position is particularly useful in cats and dyspnoeic patients.

Equipment

A full echocardiographic examination takes time to complete. It is therefore important that the operator adopts a comfortable working position within easy reach of both the patient and the ultrasound machine. The most appropriate transducer is then chosen according to the patient's size, 3.0–5.0 MHz for dogs and 5.0–7.5 MHz for cats. A simultaneous ECG is recorded, and is essential for determining accurate timings within the cardiac cycle.

A generous quantity of water-soluble coupling gel is applied to the thorax to eliminate air and improve sound transmission between the transducer and the skin. Two dimensional, M-mode and Doppler studies may then be undertaken after adjusting the depth and gain settings to produce an optimal image.

Time–gain compensation (TGC)

The overall brightness of the image can be altered by changing the power output of the transducer. Too little power results in loss of fine detail, while too much power obliterates detail due to too many echoes. Therefore select the lowest power that provides good differentiation of the structures.

Attenuation occurs at approximately 1 dB/cm/MHz. Without TGC or depth-compensation, when examining a homogeneous organ, distant echoes would be reduced by attenuation producing a false effect of a hypoechoic pattern in the deeper tissues.

TGC controls allow the operator to suppress the echoes from close to the transducer and to increase selectively echoes returning from distant regions to compensate for attenuation. The aim is to adjust the gain until there is an even image density throughout the field.

Contrast echocardiography

Contrast echocardiography can be performed by injecting a bolus of fluid containing microbubbles into a peripheral vein while imaging the heart. The microbubbles are harmless to the patient, but will be highly reflective to the ultrasound beam and thus appear hyperechoic. Saline, blood and colloid infusion fluids have been used immediately after agitation through a three-way tap from one syringe to another to produce microbubbles. The contrast can be seen entering and leaving the right side of the heart. The left cardiac chambers are not normally opacified, as the microbubbles do not pass through the pulmonary circulation. The appearance of hyperechoic bubbles on the left side of the heart suggests a right to left shunt.

2D assessment

The 2D assessment of the heart provides anatomical and functional information. A systematic approach is essential to ensure that all structures have been assessed. In dogs and cats the left side of the heart is better imaged than the right owing to the proximity of the right to the transducer and difficulty in adjusting the near-field echoes.

Three parasternal (parallel and adjacent to the sternum) transducer positions are commonly used and provide consistent imaging planes: the right parasternal location, the left caudal (apical) parasternal location and the left cranial parasternal location. A long axis view transects the heart from base to apex, while a short axis view is perpendicular to the long axis. The optimum transducer locations vary from patient to patient and must be determined during the examination. The subcostal (just caudal to the xiphoid cartilage) and suprasternal (thoracic inlet) positions do not provide ideal or consistent images of the heart, but may be useful especially for Doppler studies in some animals.

It is important to display the image in a consistent manner, so that the operator becomes familiar with the standard views and can quickly detect changes from normal. The transducer has an index mark that indicates the plane of the scan. The structures close to the index mark are displayed to the right side of the screen, although most ultrasound machines have a left–right reversal capability so that proper orientation can be maintained regardless of the position of the index mark. The image should be displayed with the transducer at the top and the deeper structures to the bottom of the display. As a general rule, *the heart should be displayed with the heart base or cranial aspect of the heart to the right of the screen.* The only exception is the left cranial (apical) four chamber view, where the heart is displayed vertically from apex to base with the left chambers to the right of the screen.

Image planes

Recommendations for standards in transthoracic 2D echocardiography in the dog and cat have been published (Thomas *et al.*, 1993) and these should be followed. A summary of the standard planes and views is given in Table 5.9. Note that when describing positioning of the transducer, the terms *clockwise* and *anticlockwise* refer to rotation of the transducer as if looking along its axis towards the thoracic wall, and not the rotation of the hand which will depend on whether the patient is being scanned from above or below. Each view should be optimized to show the

anatomical structures listed for each view. Apart from the assessment of anatomy and function, the views can be helpful for alignment of M-mode and Doppler cursors.

Some of the more common echocardiographic findings seen with certain cardiac disorders during a 2-D examination are listed in Table 5.10.

M-mode measurements

M-mode echocardiography allows measurement of chamber size and wall thickness and provides characterization and timing of motion, relative to the ECG, during the cardiac cycle. Guidelines for recording and measurement of the echocardiogram have been published by the American Society of Echocardiography (Sahn *et al.*, 1978) and are recommended for use in the dog and cat.

Measurements from the M-mode tracing are made from leading edge to leading edge. End-diastole is taken as the onset of the first rapid deflection of the QRS complex of the ECG. End-systole is taken at the nadir of septal motion in patients whose septal motion is normal, alternatively measurements can be taken at the peak of left ventricular free wall motion. The peak downward motion of the septum occurs slightly before the maximum upward excursion of the left ventricular free wall (Figure 5.59).

Left ventricular indices

Correct alignment of the M-mode cursor is required in both the right parasternal long and short axis planes for accurate and reproducible measurements to be made. The left ventricular dimensions should be obtained when the ultrasonic beam is directed between the papillary muscles in the right parasternal short axis view at the level of the chordae tendineae. M-mode measurements are listed in Table 5.11.

Mitral valve measurements

These measurements are taken after aligning the M-mode cursor across the tips of the mitral valve leaflets in the right parasternal long axis view (Figure 5.60).

Systolic time intervals

These measurements are taken after alignment of the M-mode cursor across the aorta in the right parasternal long axis view. In the M-mode tracing, only one aortic cusp is usually seen (Figure 5.61).

Interpretation of the M-mode measurements must take into account body weight, breed, heart rate, age and physical training (Morrison *et al.*, 1992). Normal values for the cat are listed in Table 5.12.

Doppler echocardiography

Doppler echocardiography provides information about the flow of blood within the heart chambers, across the valves and in the great vessels. It is complementary to 2D and M-mode echocardiography and provides a more

Right parasternal long axis views (Figure 5.53)

Position	• 3rd–6th intercostal space at the level of the costochondral junction
	• Transducer index mark pointing towards the heart base
	• Rotate index mark cranially (clockwise) for view 2
View 1	• Left ventricle and mitral valve
	• Left atrium and pulmonary veins
	• Right ventricle, tricuspid valve and right atrium
View 2	• Left ventricle, outflow tract, aortic valve and proximal ascending aorta
	• Left auricular appendage, usually referred to as the left atrium
	• Right pulmonary artery
Display	• Cardiac apex to the left and the base (atria or aorta) to the right
Additional uses	• M-mode alignment for the mitral valve (view 1) and for the aortic valve (view 2)

Right parasternal short axis views (Figure 5.54)

Position	• 3rd–6th intercostal space at the level of the costochondral junction
	• Transducer index mark pointing cranioventrally, perpendicular to the long axis view
	• Optimize for symmetry of the left ventricle and papillary muscles
	• Angle beam dorsally from the apex to the base to obtain each view
View 1	• Left ventricular apex
	• Right ventricle
View 2	• Left ventricle, high papillary muscle level
	• Right ventricle
View 3	• Chordae tendineae of the left ventricle
	• Right ventricle
View 4	• Mitral valve
	• Right ventricle
View 5	• Aortic root and valve
	• Left atrium and left auricular appendage
	• Right ventricle, tricuspid valve, right ventricular outflow tract and pulmonary valve
Display	• Cranial part of the image (right ventricular outflow) to the right with the right heart encircling the left ventricle and aorta clockwise
Additional uses	• M-mode alignment for left ventricular indices (view 3) and for the aorta (view 5)
	• Doppler alignment for pulmonary valve flow

Left parasternal caudal (apical) long axis view

Position	• 5th–7th intercostal space at the level of the costochondral junction
	• Transducer index mark pointing dorsally towards the heart base for the two chamber views, but pointing caudally and to the left for the four chamber views
	• May help to place transducer vertically over the gallbladder and angle cranially

Left apical two chamber views (Figure 5.55)

View 1	• Left ventricle, mitral valve and left atrium
View 2	• With slight anticlockwise rotation the left ventricular outflow and ascending aorta can be seen
Display	• Left ventricular apex to the left and left atrium or aorta to the right

Left apical four chamber views (Figure 5.56)

View 1	• Left ventricle, left atrium, right ventricle and right atrium (four chamber view)
View 2	• With slight cranial angulation, the left ventricular outflow tract and aorta comes into view (five chamber view)
Display	• Left heart to the right and right heart to the left
Additional uses	• Doppler alignment for mitral, tricuspid and aortic valve flow

Left cranial parasternal long axis views (Figure 5.57)

Position	• 3rd–4th intercostal space at the level of the costochondral junction
	• Transducer index mark pointing cranially
View 1	• Left ventricular outflow tract, aortic valve and ascending aorta
View 2	• Angling the beam ventrally reveals an oblique view of the left ventricle with a long axis view of the right ventricle, tricuspid valve and right atrium
View 3	• Angling the beam dorsally reveals the right ventricular outflow tract, pulmonary valve and main pulmonary artery
	• In most animals, the main pulmonary artery can be followed dorsally to the division into the left and right pulmonary artery
Display	• Left ventricular apex to the left and aorta or right ventricle to the right
Additional uses	• Doppler alignment for tricuspid and pulmonic valve flow

Left cranial parasternal short axis view (Figure 5.58)

Position	• 3rd–4th intercostal space at the level of the costochondral junction
	• Transducer index mark pointing dorsally approximately perpendicular to the long axis plane
View	• Right ventricular inflow and outflow with short axis view of aorta
Display	• Right heart encircling the aorta clockwise (right ventricular inflow to the left, right ventricular outflow and pulmonary artery to the right)

Table 5.9: Standard echocardiographic views.

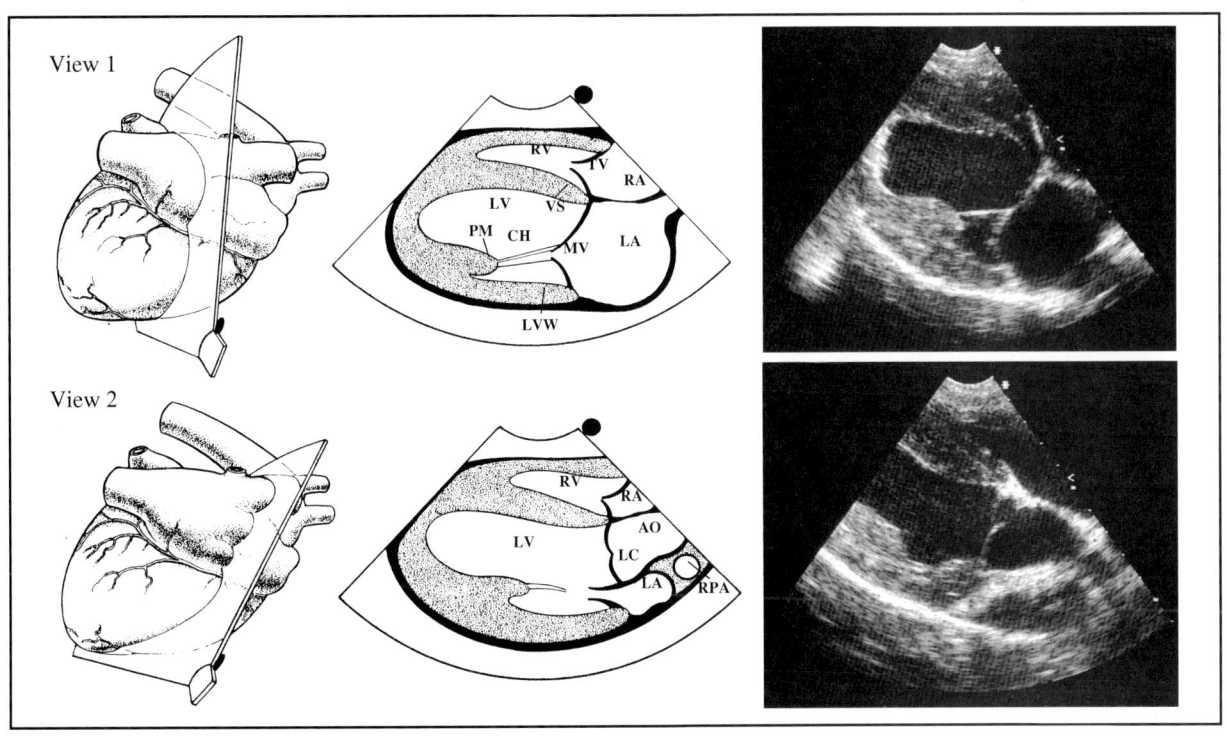

Figure 5.53: *Right parasternal long axis views (adapted from Thomas et al., 1993).*

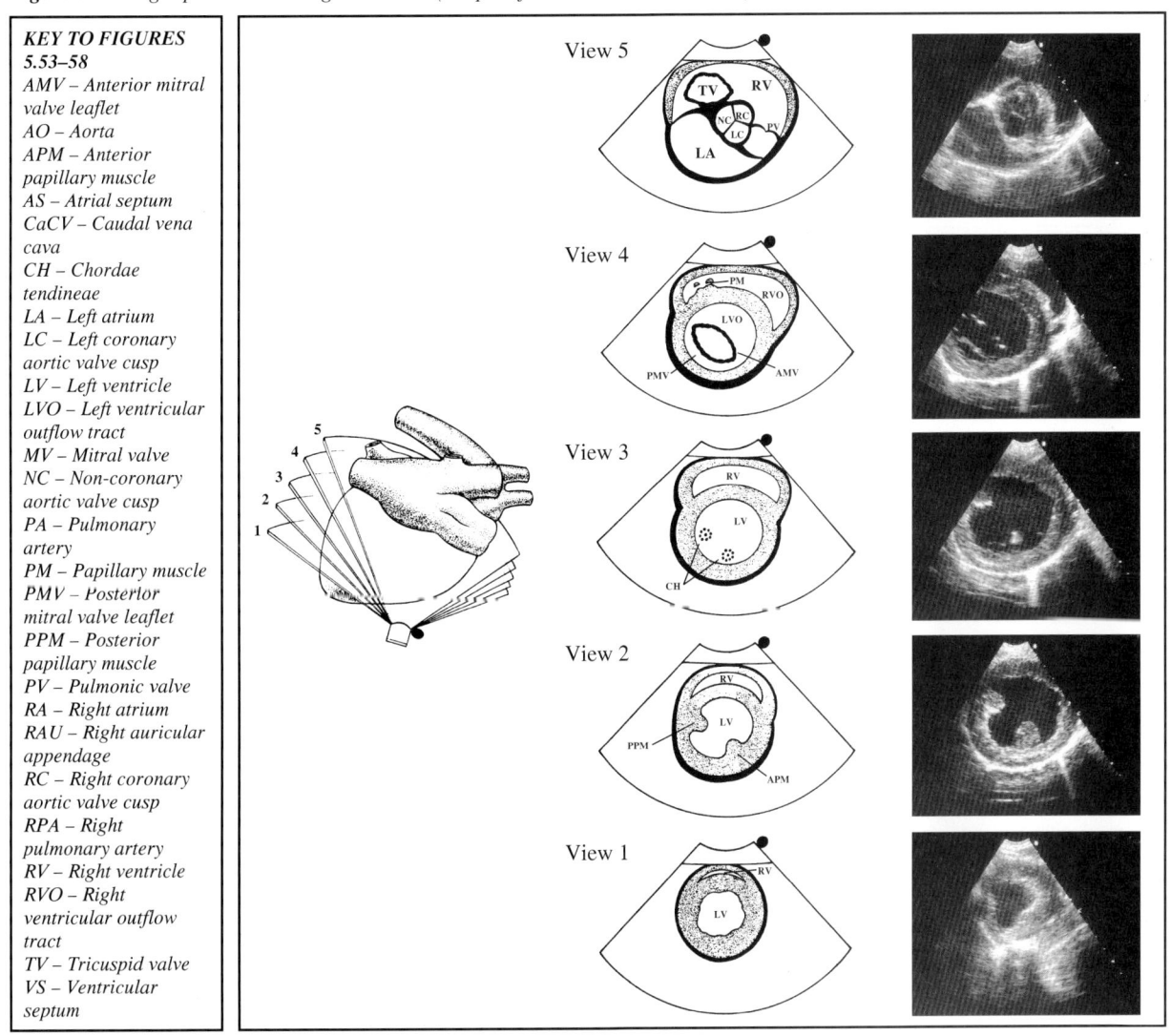

KEY TO FIGURES 5.53–58
AMV – Anterior mitral valve leaflet
AO – Aorta
APM – Anterior papillary muscle
AS – Atrial septum
CaCV – Caudal vena cava
CH – Chordae tendineae
LA – Left atrium
LC – Left coronary aortic valve cusp
LV – Left ventricle
LVO – Left ventricular outflow tract
MV – Mitral valve
NC – Non-coronary aortic valve cusp
PA – Pulmonary artery
PM – Papillary muscle
PMV – Posterior mitral valve leaflet
PPM – Posterior papillary muscle
PV – Pulmonic valve
RA – Right atrium
RAU – Right auricular appendage
RC – Right coronary aortic valve cusp
RPA – Right pulmonary artery
RV – Right ventricle
RVO – Right ventricular outflow tract
TV – Tricuspid valve
VS – Ventricular septum

Figure 5.54: *Right parasternal short axis views (adapted from Thomas et al., 1993).*

complete, non-invasive evaluation of cardiac function. The technique is discussed further in Chapter 6(ii).

NON-CARDIAC THORACIC ULTRASONOGRAPHY

Echocardiography is a well established technique in veterinary medicine for the assessment of cardiac disease. However, the use of diagnostic ultrasound for the examination of non-cardiac thoracic disease is often overlooked. Certainly, the inability of ultrasound to penetrate air-filled structures precludes its use for the examination of normal lungs, but in disease states where the normally air-filled lung is collapsed, consolidated or replaced by fluid or mass lesions, ultra-

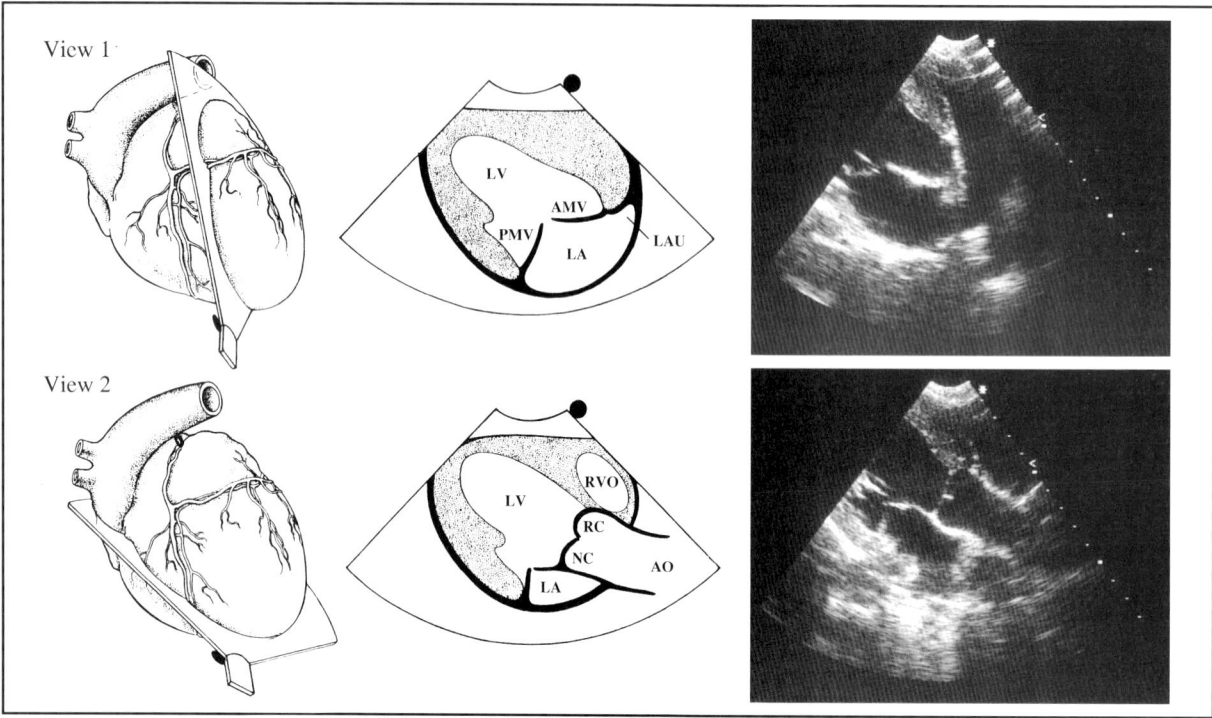

Figure 5.55: Left apical two-chamber views (adapted from Thomas et al., 1993).

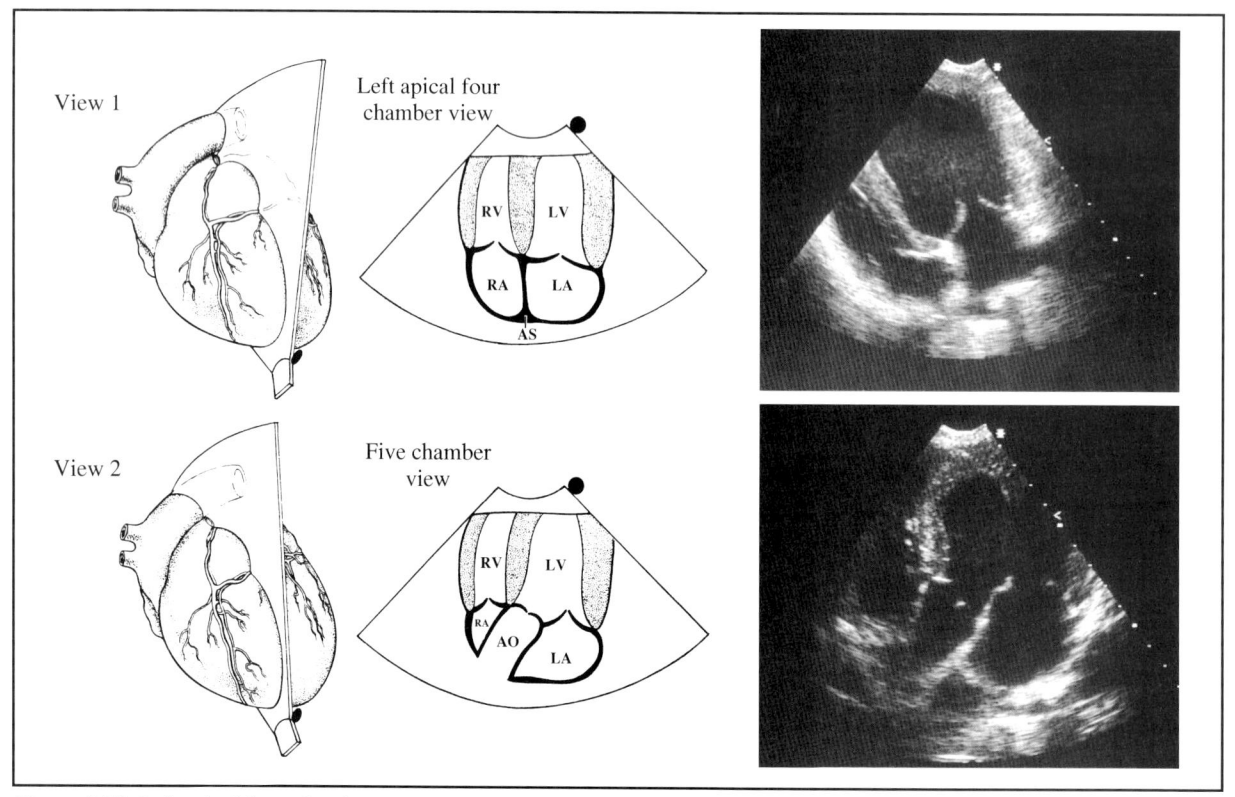

Figure 5.56: Left apical four-chamber views (adapted from Thomas et al., 1993).

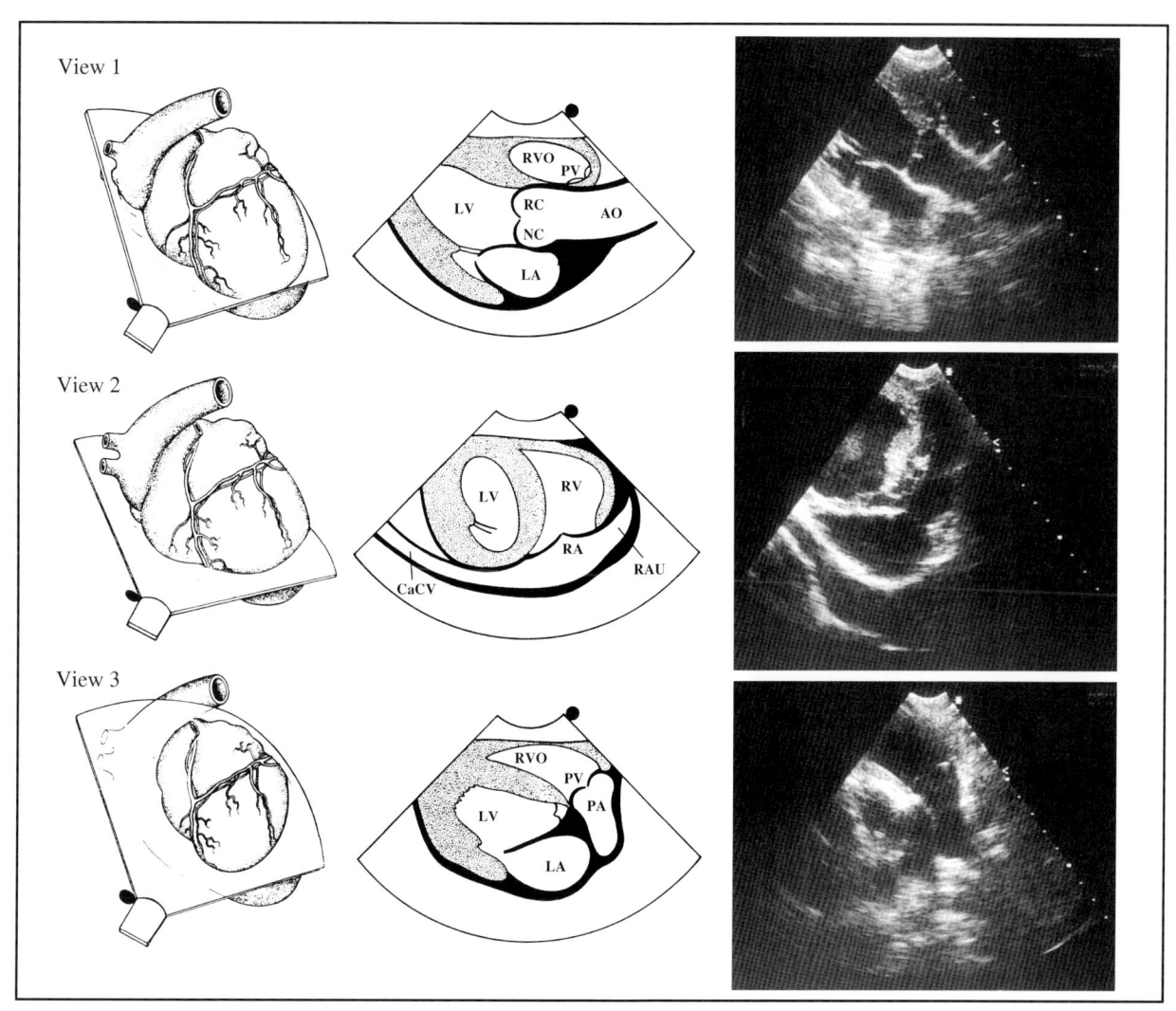

Figure 5.57: *Left cranial parasternal long axis views (adapted from Thomas et al., 1993).*

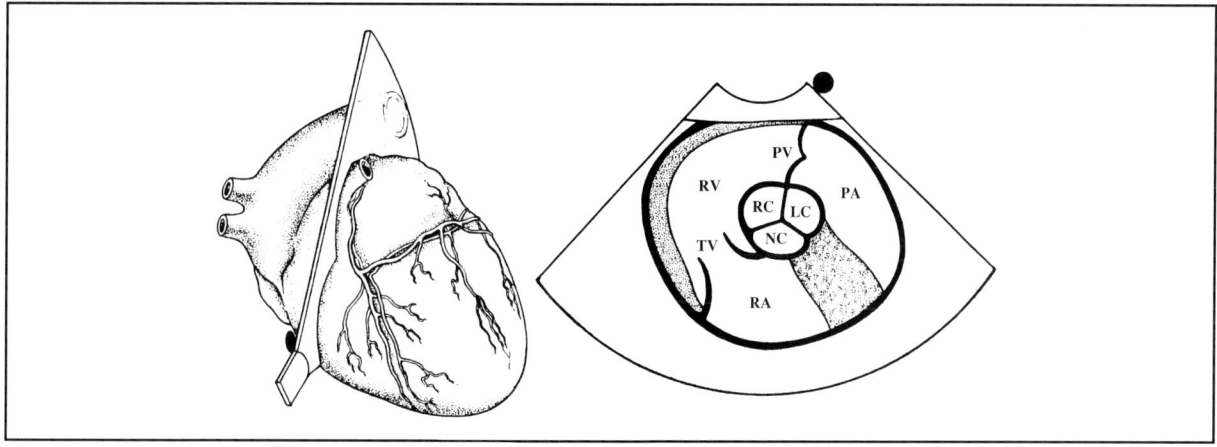

Figure 5.58*: Left cranial parasternal short axis view (adapted from Thomas et al., 1993).*

sound waves can penetrate the thorax and the examination may provide valuable information to complement the radiographic findings.

In addition to pulmonary lesions, ultrasonography may also provide useful information about thoracic wall lesions, pleural effusions, mediastinal pathology and diaphragmatic rupture. Ultrasound-guided thoracocentesis or biopsy of pleural, mediastinal or pulmo-

nary lesions can help in diagnosis of the underlying pathology.

Technique

The thorax may be examined, using the standard intercostal windows described for echocardiography or using any other intercostal, subcostal or suprasternal approach. The area where the pathology may come

Echocardiographic findings in pericardial effusion
- Echolucent space between the epicardium and pericardium
- There may be abnormal cardiac motion
- Fluid space is greatest at the cardiac apex
- Fluid may contain echodense material – fibrin, clots or tumour

Echocardiographic findings in dilated cardiomyopathy
- Marked dilation of left side or all four chambers
- Hypokinetic left ventricle
- Reduced fractional shortening
- Reduced aortic root excursion
- Late aortic valve opening and early closure

Echocardiographic findings in hypertrophic cardiomyopathy
- Normal to decreased left ventricular systolic and diastolic internal dimensions
- Increased septal and left ventricular free wall systolic and diastolic thickness
- Hypertrophy of left ventricular papillary muscles
- Normal to increased indices of left ventricular function

Echocardiographic findings in mitral insufficiency
- Thickened mitral valve leaflets
- Left atrial and left ventricular dilation
- Increased fractional shortening unless myocardial failure
- Prolapse of mitral valve into left atrium
- Chaotic fluttering of mitral valve if chordae tendineae have ruptured

Echocardiographic findings in patent ductus arteriosus
- Difficult to image ductus
- Changes reflect fluid overload – dilated left heart
- Left ventricular contractility may be reduced in advanced cases

Echocardiographic findings in ventricular septal defect
- Defect usually high in septum
- Defect should be visible in several imaging planes
- Left atrial and left ventricular dilation
- Hyperkinetic left ventricle if shunt is large
- Right ventricle is usually normal or slightly dilated in left to right shunt
- Right ventricular hypertrophy and flattened septum if pulmonary hypertension present

Echocardiographic findings in aortic stenosis
- Sub-aortic fibrous ring
- Thickening or doming of aortic valve leaflets if valvular stenosis
- Left ventricular hypertrophy
- Papillary muscles may appear hyperechoic
- Premature aortic closure
- Systolic fluttering of the aortic valve
- Systolic anterior motion of the mitral valve
- Post-stenotic dilation of the aorta

Echocardiographic findings in pulmonic stenosis
- Abnormal thickening or doming of pulmonic valve
- Post-stenotic dilation of main pulmonary artery
- Right ventricular hypertrophy
- Flattened or paradoxical septal motion

Echocardiographic findings in tetralogy of Fallot
- High septal defect
- Right ventricular hypertrophy
- Pulmonic stenosis
- Over-riding aorta
- Flattened or paradoxical septal motion
- Left heart may be smaller than normal
- Contrast study shows right to left shunt

Table 5.10: Common echocardiographic findings in heart disease.

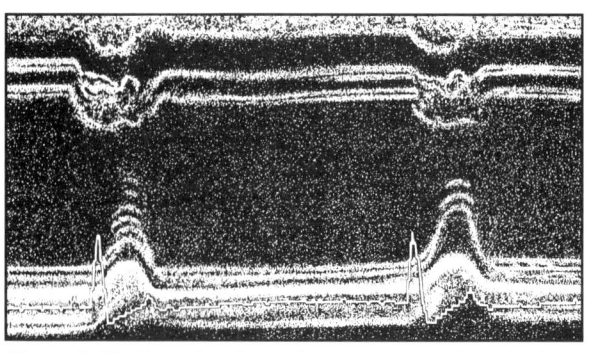

Figure 5.59: M-mode echocardiogram of the left ventricle used for measurement of the left ventricular indices.

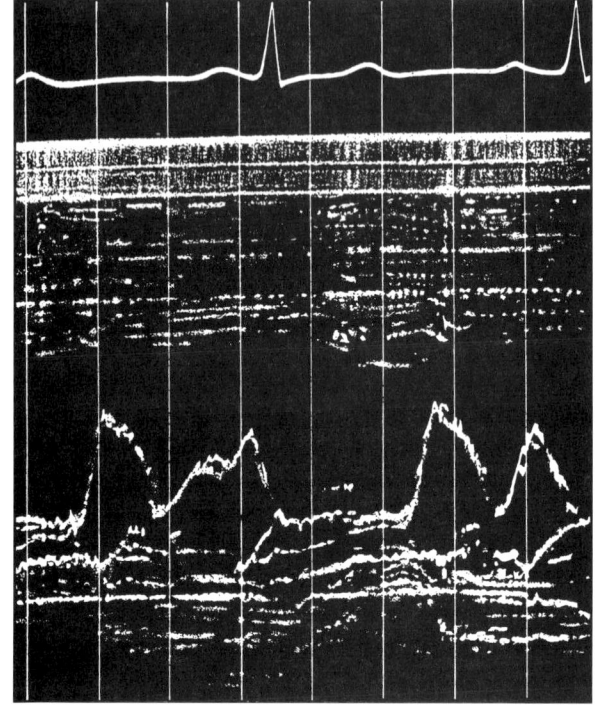

Figure 5.60: M-mode echocardiogram of the mitral valve.

into direct contact with the thoracic wall is often best assessed from radiographs.

Thoughtful positioning of the patient to improve the image may be required. For example, it may be beneficial to place the animal in lateral recumbency with the affected side down and scan from underneath the patient in order to increase the size of the acoustic window.

Fine needle aspiration or needle biopsy techniques can be used accurately and safely following identification and localization of the lesions, with a much greater chance of gaining representative tissue and with less risk of damaging vital structures.

Normal appearance
If the transducer is moved away from the heart and diaphragm in the normal animal, only interference from air-filled lung is seen beyond the chest wall.

Thoracic wall lesions
Thoracic wall masses are easy to identify clinically, if

Chordae tendineae level
- LVID-S   left ventricular internal dimension in systole
- LVID-D   left ventricular internal dimension in diastole
- FS%   fractional shortening

$$FS\% = \frac{LVID\text{-}D - LVID\text{-}S}{LVID\text{-}D} \times 100$$

- LVFW-S   left ventricular free wall in systole
- LVFW-D   left ventricular free wall in diastole
- IVS-S   interventricular septum in systole
- IVS-D   interventricular septum in diastole

Mitral valve level
- EPSS   E-point (of AMV) to septal separation

Aortic valve level
- Aortic root dimension measured at end-diastole
- LA dimension or more accurately the left auricle dimension measured at end-systole
- LV pre-injection period is the time taken from the first deflection of the QRS to the opening of the aortic cusp
- LV ejection time is measured from the opening to the closure of the aortic valve

Table 5.11: M-mode measurements.

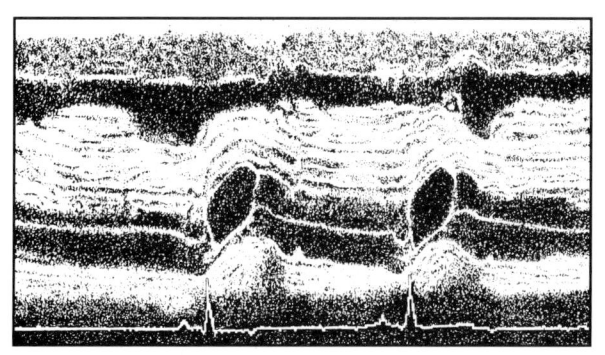

Figure 5.61: M-mode echocardiogram of the aorta and left atrium used for measurement of the systolic time intervals.

they grow externally. However, ultrasound is useful to determine their echo pattern and structure, and can define the full extent of masses which grow into the thoracic cavity. The displacement and involvement of intrathoracic structures can be assessed.

Pleural fluid

Pleural effusion is readily identified ultrasonographically as a hypoechoic or anechoic space between the thoracic wall or diaphragm and the lung. The volume and location of the fluid will dictate the degree of lung displacement. Fluid collects between the lung and thoracic wall and between the lung lobes, causing the lung lobes to retract towards the pulmonary hilus.

Transudates appear as anechoic space. Pyothorax or haemothorax may contain internal echoes and sometimes appear complex or septated. Occasionally, however, anechoic fluid may be infected.

Mediastinal lesions

Cranial mediastinal masses are usually easy to image.

As the transducer is moved cranial to the heart, the echo pattern of solid tissue is seen rather than normal lung interference.

Cranial mediastinal masses have a variable ultrasonographic appearance. Lymphomas are often, but not invariably, homogeneous, hypoechoic and avascular. Masses of other histological types vary in echogenicity, architecture and vascularity. Irregular anechoic areas represent areas of fluid, haemorrhage or necrosis, while bright echogenic areas represent fibrosis or calcification. A fine needle aspirate or biopsy is required for a histological diagnosis.

Mediastinal fluid may also be recognized on ultrasonography as an anechoic space between the moving echogenic confines of the mediastinum. Appreciation of this finding will allow fine needle aspiration to be performed in order to make a diagnosis.

Pulmonary lesions

Pulmonary masses and pulmonary consolidation may be imaged if a suitable ultrasonographic window can be obtained. This depends on the affected structure contacting the thoracic wall or diaphragm without interposed air-filled lung. Once imaged, ultrasound-guided aspiration or biopsy can be performed to provide samples for diagnosis.

Lung tumours and abscesses have variable echogenicity and irregular borders. They displace the air-filled lung and may be distinguished from pulmonary consolidation by the lack of vascular and bronchial structures.

Pulmonary consolidation will result in a parenchyma-like appearance similar to liver. Small pockets of air produce focal hyperechoic areas. Fluid filled

Measurement	Cardiac timing	Mean ± SD
Interventricular septum	diastole	3.1 ± 0.4 mm
	systole	5.8 ± 0.6 mm
Left ventricular internal diameter	diastole	15.9 ± 1.9 mm
	systole	8.0 ± 1.4 mm
Left ventricular free wall	diastole	3.3 ± 0.6 mm
	systole	6.8 ± 0.7 mm
Fractional shortening		49.8 ± 5.3 %
E point to septal separation	diastole	0.2 ± 0.9 mm
Aorta	diastole	9.5 ± 1.1 mm
Left atrium	systole	12.3 ± 1.4 mm
Heart rate		194 ± 23 /min
Body weight		4.1 ± 1.1 kg

Table 5.12: Normal M-mode echocardiographic values in the cat.

blood vessels or bronchi appear as anechoic branching tubular structures.

Diaphragmatic rupture

Ultrasonography may aid diagnosis of diaphragmatic rupture particularly in patients with equivocal radiographic findings. A small rupture resulting in entrapment of a liver lobe will cause a marked pleural effusion and is an ideal candidate for ultrasonography.

Abdominal viscera such as omentum, spleen, stomach and intestine may be imaged in the pleural space after more severe damage to the diaphragm. However it is important to recognize a mirror-image artefact of the liver (see above) to avoid a false positive diagnosis.

CONCLUSION

Diagnostic ultrasound has made a major contribution to the improved diagnosis and management of cases in veterinary medicine. However the technique does require considerable operator skill and experience to gain the best results. The learning curve is steep, but some conditions, for example dilated cardiomyopathy or pericardial effusion are relatively easy to diagnose and this should give the novice confidence to continue to work and improve their technique.

REFERENCES AND FURTHER READING

General
Barr F. (1990) *Diagnostic Ultrasound in the Dog and Cat.* Blackwell Scientific Publications, Oxford
Nyland TG and Mattoon JS (1995) *Veterinary Diagnostic Ultrasound.* WB Saunders, Philadelphia

Cardiac
Atkins CE and Synder PS (1992) Systolic time intervals and their derivatives for evaluation of cardiac function. *Journal of Veterinary Internal Medicine* **6**, 55-63
Jacobs G and Knight DH (1985) M-mode measurements in nonanaesthetized healthy cats: effects of body weight, heart rate, and other variables. *American Journal of Veterinary Research* **46**, 1705-1711
Moise NS (1988) Echocardiography. In: *Canine and Feline Cardiology,* ed. PR Fox. Churchill Livingstone, New York
Morrison SA, Moise NS, Scarlett J, Mohammed H and Yeager AE (1992) Effect of breed and body weight on echocardiographic values in four breeds of dogs of differing somatotype. *Journal of Veterinary Internal Medicine* **6**, 220-224
Sahn DJ, Demaria A, Kisslo J and Weyman A (1978) Recommendations regarding quantitation in M-mode echocardiography: results of a survey of echocardiographic measurements. *Circulation* **58**, 1072-1083
Thomas WP, Gaber CE, Jacobs GJ, Kaplan PM, Lombard CW, Moise NS and Moses BL (1993) Recommendations for standards in transthoracic two-dimensional echocardiography in the dog and cat. *Journal of Veterinary Internal Medicine* **7**, 247-252

Thoracic (non-cardiac)
Konde LJ and Spaulding K (1991) Sonographic evaluation of the cranial mediastinum in small animals. *Veterinary Radiology* **32**, 178-184
Stowater JL and Lamb CR (1989) Ultrasonography of noncardiac thoracic diseases in small animals. *Journal of the American Veterinary Medical Association* **195**, 514-519

(vii) Sedation and Anaesthesia for Special Investigations

R. Eddie Clutton

In human beings with cardiopulmonary disease, a range of non-invasive tests can be performed and a diagnosis established without recourse to invasive and stressful procedures that require sedation or anaesthesia. This is not the case with animals and the veterinary clinician is in an Escherian dilemma; the risk of anaesthesia is increased when an accurate diagnosis is missing but frequently, the latter cannot be established without anaesthesia. Anaesthetics may precipitate a haemodynamic and/or hypoxic crisis in animals with advanced cardiopulmonary disease, yet severe stress caused by examination in conscious animals may have the same effect.

GENERAL PROBLEMS WITH ANAESTHESIA AND CARDIOPULMONARY DISEASE

- Some 'sedatives' and most anaesthetics depress cardiopulmonary function; animals with pre-existing cardiopulmonary disease will be at a greater risk of cardiopulmonary failure than 'normal' animals
- Cardiac failure alters drug pharmacokinetics, so responses to normal drug doses may be unpredictable, or predictably different, e.g. the rate of induction with volatile agents may be more rapid, or the effects of normal injectable agent doses may be more profound
- Drugs used in the treatment of heart disease may interact adversely with anaesthetics.

Preoperative examination will allow formulation of an appropriate plan for anaesthesia and the measures needed to optimize cardiopulmonary function. Ideally, formulation of the anaesthetic plan should be influenced by the way in which the disease process affects oxygen delivery to the brain and myocardium. The way in which the disease influences the pharmacokinetics and pharmacodynamics of anaesthetics and adjunct drugs is also important. It is desirable to know or predict how anaesthesia and surgery will affect the function of diseased organs. Proper assessment is based on an accurate diagnosis.

GENERAL APPROACH

Preliminary investigation

A complete physical examination is important in risk assessment. Exercise tolerance is particularly informative of an animal's suitability for anaesthesia.

A tentative diagnosis can often be established with tests performed using restraint alone. These will indicate which additional tests may be required and establishes 'potential' anaesthetic risk. Physical examination, haematology, electrocardiography, echocardiography and blood gas analysis are included here.

Haematology (including haemoglobin concentration) and *biochemistry* may be helpful in pre-anaesthetic assessment. Under specific circumstances, serum protein, potassium and glucose levels should be established and liver and renal function tests performed, as all may influence anaesthesia. Blood samples should be taken from a suitable vein without fuss, otherwise a 'stress haemogram' with associated artefacts results.

Electrocardiography should be used to identify arrhythmias before anaesthesia, and can be taken from the standing or resting animal should enforced recumbency prove stressful. In animals that resist, electrocardiography can be dispensed with unless physical examination indicates pulse deficits or perturbation of rhythm; in these cases, sedation will be required. Unfortunately most drugs used for this purpose will affect test results (see below).

Arterial blood gas analysis provides useful information on the lungs' ability to oxygenate blood, eliminate carbon dioxide (CO_2) and influence acid–base status. While venous samples are easily obtained, taking samples from the femoral artery requires physical restraint. In obese or restless animals, accurate arterial puncture is difficult and may require multiple, stressful attempts. 'Stress' will affect arterial blood gas results usually by lowering CO_2 through hyperventilation or decreasing O_2 tension. Depending on the drugs used, lowering 'stress' with sedatives will increase $PaCO_2$ by respiratory depression, and lower O_2 tension by a number of mechanisms.

A tentative diagnosis indicates the need for further investigations and allows preliminary therapeutic measures to be taken prior to anaesthesia.

Patient preparation

Preparation aims to lower the risk of anaesthesia and the investigation itself by limiting the effects of pre-existing disease and securing functional reserve. Some conditions found on preliminary examination require treatment. The extent of preparation depends on the degree of pathology present.

Given that the broad goal of cardiopulmonary function is to oxygenate blood and pump it to peripheral tissue, optimizing preoperative function can be assisted by analysis of the equation for oxygen flux, which indicates the volume of oxygen being distributed by the heart per minute:

$$\text{Oxygen flux } (DO_2) = \text{oxygen content of arterial blood } (CaO_2) \text{ x cardiac output } (Qt)$$

The oxygen content of arterial blood, CaO_2, is influenced by haemoglobin saturation, the partial pressure of O_2 in arterial blood and the haemoglobin concentration. Therefore, optimizing cardiopulmonary function involves optimizing blood oxygenation, cardiac output and haemoglobin concentration and function.

Blood oxygenation

This has three components:

- Ventilation
- Gas distribution within the lung
- Gas exchange across the alveolar–capillary membrane.

Ventilation is improved by removing abnormal accumulations of fluid or gas. Pleural and/or abdominal effusions should be drained.

Adequate distribution of inspired gas can be achieved with a dry, 'clean', low-resistance airway, but this may not be possible without specific therapy (and therefore a diagnosis).

Gas diffusion within the alveolus may improve if pulmonary oedema is treated.

Cardiac output

Cardiac output is optimized through control of *heart rate* and *stroke volume*.

Therapy to improve stroke volume will vary according to the underlying cardiac disease. Conservative management of congestive heart failure (such as cage rest) is entirely compatible with anaesthesia. However, many cardiac drugs are associated with untoward effects and potentially severe interactions with anaesthetics (see Table 5.13). Nevertheless, withholding 'cardiac' medications immediately before anaesthesia in order to avoid intraoperative complications may precipitate acute decompensation and is not recommended.

Arrhythmias are a common feature of cardiopulmonary disease, and may be associated with significant haemodynamic effects (e.g. hypotension) which are aggravated by anaesthetics. Arrhythmias may 'worsen' after sedatives or anaesthetics are given, i.e. deteriorate into lethal forms like ventricular fibrillation or pulseless electrical activity (PEA). In contrast, some may resolve under anaesthesia. The effects of anaesthetics on arrhythmias are, however, probably less than the effects of poorly managed anaesthesia. Some anti-arrhythmic drugs (e.g. propranolol) may interact with anaesthesia (see Table 5.13).

As a rule, arrhythmias should be treated if:

- They are haemodynamically significant
- They are likely to deteriorate under anaesthesia.

If there is no way of knowing the latter, it is wiser to treat preoperatively. Alternatively, therapy can be made available and only given if the rhythm deteriorates.

Drug	Complications
Digoxin	Arrhythmias
Frusemide	Hypovolaemia, hypokalaemia, hypochloraemia
Non-selective β_1 or β_2 blocking agents*	Hypotension, bradycardia, bronchospasm, obtunded sympathetic responses to hypovolaemia, hypercapnia, hypoxaemia, acute aggravation of congestive failure
Ca^{2+} channel blocking agents†	Bradycardia, other arrhythmias, hypotension, acute aggravation of congestive failure
Nitroglycerine	Hypotension, tachycardia
Nitroprusside	Hypotension, tachycardia
Hydralazine	Acute: hypotension, tachycardia Chronic: hypernatraemia, hypokalaemia
α_1 antagonists§	Hypotension, tachycardia
ACE inhibitors‡	Hypovolaemia, hypotension, tachycardia

*e.g. propranolol †e.g. verapamil, diltiazem §e.g. prazosin ‡e.g. captopril, enalapril, benazepril

Table 5.13: *Cardiac preparation drugs potentially affecting anaesthesia.*

This is less preferable because some antiarrhythmics produce adverse effects, especially when injected rapidly, e.g. procainamide causes hypotension.

Some arrhythmias are unpredictable in terms of response to anaesthetics and anti-arrhythmic drugs, e.g. canine sick-sinus syndrome. Before these patients are anaesthetized, it is prudent to establish which treatment is likely to be effective should problems arise after induction. In this example, atropine, glycopyrrolate, dobutamine or isoprenaline should be evaluated if a transvenous pacing unit is unavailable.

Haemoglobin concentration

Polycythaemia (haematocrit more than 0.55) is an occasional feature of cardiopulmonary disease and is important in anaesthesia. First, it elevates blood viscosity and mimics an elevation in systemic vascular resistance. Second, the presence of polycythaemia may signal right to left shunts of intrapulmonary (neoplasm, bronchitis) or extrapulmonary (ventricular septal defect) origin. Polycythaemia, which exerts an adverse haemodynamic effect, should be treated using normovolaemic haemodilution.

Anaemia increases risk from anaesthesia. Adequate plasma haemoglobin concentrations are especially important for maintaining DO_2 during anaesthesia in animals with cardiopulmonary disease; however, the rate of development of anaemia and the severity of cardiopulmonary disease are also factors. Chronic anaemia influences risk less than acute haemorrhagic anaemia.

The risks of tests must be appreciated, not all are benign and the cost–benefit ratio must be established before starting.

ANAESTHETIC TECHNIQUE SELECTION

Any technique under consideration must be safe, and remain safe irrespective of what pathology the investigation reveals. It must also provide conditions that allow the investigation to be performed effectively. Ease of administration is important. More specific determinants of technique and drug selection are:

Species

Drugs may, according to species, be predictably ineffective (acepromazine in cats), unpredictable (benzodiazepines in dogs and cats), produce undesirable effects (ketamine in dogs), or be hazardous (alphaxalone in dogs). Drug pharmacokinetics may depend on species, e.g. propofol in dogs and cats. Drugs may not be licensed for use in the species under investigation.

Individual

Techniques and drugs should suit the individual in terms of temperament, breed, age and health status.

Recalcitrant, boisterous animals usually, though not always, tolerate less safe techniques than animals incapacitated by sickness. Some breeds respond differently to certain drugs, e.g. Sight Hounds and thiobarbiturates. Breed-related conditions complicating anaesthesia may be present, e.g. airway obstructive syndrome in brachycephalic breeds.

Nature of the test

The anaesthetic must suit the investigation in terms of duration and degree of invasion. Greater risk is associated with invasive, prolonged investigations and so anaesthesia is likely to be more complicated. Ideally, the technique should have minimum effects on the variables under scrutiny, otherwise the effects must be predictable and quantifiable, so that the results can be interpreted accurately.

Experience

In higher risk cases, it is wiser for anaesthetists to use techniques and drugs with which they are acquainted, rather than attempt new, unfamiliar methods that are theoretically more appropriate. This does not, however, justify the use of a totally inappropriate technique because 'it's the only one ever used'.

With cardiopulmonary disease, the technique should possess the following features:

- Have minimal adverse or preferably, beneficial effects on underlying pathophysiological processes, e.g. alteration of heart rate; alteration of afterload
- Avoid harmful interactions with therapeutics given perioperatively
- Take account of the altered pharmacokinetic state produced by disease.

Sedatives versus general anaesthesia

That sedation is safer than general anaesthesia seems intuitive: protective reflexes are preserved to some extent and 'less' central nervous depression is imposed. Furthermore, sedative techniques are more convenient. Frequently, these represent very minor advantages that are far outweighed by the *overall* convenience and safety of general anaesthesia produced with inhaled anaesthetics.

Disadvantages of sedation

Unpredictability: The efficacy of sedative techniques depends on several factors: time must be allowed for drugs to exert peak effect, during which stimulation must be kept to a minimum. The animal's temperament is also important; aggressive or very anxious dogs may be difficult to sedate effectively without recourse to high doses that may also produce adverse effects. However, some sedative techniques do not always produce conditions that allow the anticipated investigation. When this occurs, the investigator will either have to postpone the current test, repeating it later under more effective sedation, or increase the 'level' of sedation by giving additional drug. This may produce depression, which is physiologically more disturbing than a light level of general anaesthesia, as well as being longer lasting. An alternative is to give a general anaesthetic. Most anaesthetics are compatible with sedative techniques; the latter come to represent pre-anaesthetic medication. However, embarking on this option from the onset would have avoided the wastage of time and drugs.

Predictable effects are particularly desirous in sedative techniques for cats, which are poorly tolerant of interference like the imposition of abnormal positioning for radiography.

Inadequate duration of effects: It is often difficult to predict how much time an investigation will require. Unless short-acting, titratable drugs showing non-cumulative effects are used from the onset, sedative top-ups must be used and their aforementioned disadvantages endured. Apart from those drugs whose effects can be antagonized, central nervous depression with sedative techniques can only be increased, not lessened; recovery form the effects of these depends on the cardiac, renal or hepatic function.

Adverse effects: Some sedatives, e.g. α_2 agonists like xylazine and medetomidine, are potent cardiopulmonary depressants and have arrhythmogenic effects at low doses.

Consciousness and 'stress': Sedated animals remain aware of unpleasant stimuli and may respond with potentially hazardous catecholamine release.

'Standard of care': Because sedation is generally, though erroneously, regarded as safer than anaesthesia, fewer preparations are made for adverse events. Sedation is not normally associated with the routine pre-placement of a venous catheter; fluids are not given; vital signs beyond the level of consciousness are not periodically assessed. Indeed, the important haemodynamic variables at risk of deterioration, e.g. blood pressure, ECG cannot easily be monitored because the patient may not tolerate instrumentation. Usually, an anaesthetic record is deemed unnecessary. Endotracheal intubation is impossible, and means of positive pressure ventilation and O_2 support may be unavailable.

Individuals involved with sedated rather than anaesthetized animals are usually less alert to the animal's needs, presumably because they feel the animal is capable of looking after itself. This is not true; for example, a sedated animal is more likely to fall off a radiography table than an anaesthetized one. After the investigation, the sedated animal is less likely to be nursed and monitored even though the risk of problems, for example arrhythmias and hypothermia, remains high.

Advantages of general anaesthesia
The airway is protected, so positive pressure ventilation (PPV) can be rapidly imposed if necessary and inspired gas enriched with oxygen. Intravenous access is present for fluids and emergency drug administration. Intensive monitoring is possible. The level of anaesthesia can be adjusted to suit the need of the investigation at any moment. Importantly, general anaesthesia with volatile agents can be safely extended yet still provide rapid recoveries after prolonged investigations providing some agents (e.g. methoxyflurane) and hypothermia are avoided.

Drug choice
The major determinants of drug choice are species, breed, size, age, temperament, disease state and the proposed investigation. In general, anaesthesia should attempt to create the haemodynamic conditions that would be the desired aims of medical therapy, for example, a reduction in heart rate and an increase in stroke volume, or bronchodilation. However, the use of 'general information' on the haemodynamic effects of anaesthetics (popularly tabulated; see Table 5.14) is misleading, as they tend to oversimplify drug effects. Data on the haemodynamic effects of anaesthetics are applicable only when the precise experimental conditions in which they were obtained are replicated in the clinic. Most are derived from healthy animals; the effect of disease on drug behaviour often escapes evaluation. For example, the adverse versus desirable effects of halothane on cardiac output depends on whether the myocardium is normal or hypertrophic.

It is also inappropriate to recommend the use of a given agent without reference to indirect physiological effects which may be more perturbing in a physiological sense than the drug's direct effects. For example, isoflurane would seem to be preferable to halothane in an animal with ventricular premature complexes (VPCs) because the latter render the propagation of arrhythmias more likely in the presence of catecholamines. However,

Drug	Cardiac output	Mean arterial blood pressure	Systemic vascular resistance
Halothane	↓	↓	↔
Isoflurane	↑ ↔	↓	↓ ↓
Methoxyflurane	↓	↓	↓

Table 5.14: Haemodynamic effects of anaesthetics. ↔ = no change.

isoflurane depresses ventilation more than halothane and is associated with greater CO_2 retention; hypercapnia is itself arrhythmogenic. Under these circumstances, isoflurane is the preferred drug only if normocapnia is ensured by positive pressure ventilation.

Similarly, an understanding of underlying pathophysiological processes is necessary for rational drug selection. Ketamine would appear to be a useful drug in animals in which myocardial depression is poorly tolerated, because it maintains cardiac output. However, this effect is mediated through the autonomic nervous system. In animals in which autonomic activity is already high, e.g. those in congestive heart failure, ketamine can induce little, if any, incremental inotropic or chronotropic effect. Indeed, a depressant effect becomes apparent making the use of ketamine inadvisable.

When underlying pathophysiological processes are poorly understood, selecting drugs on the basis of 'common knowledge' may prove hazardous. In animals with ventricular ectopic activity, it would seem fair to choose isoflurane over halothane, providing normocapnia is maintained. However, when ectopic activity arises from hypoxic foci within the ventricle, the result of the choice may be disappointing. Isoflurane maintains ventricular contractility, and is therefore more likely to maintain damaged myocardium near the threshold of negative oxygen balance and thus assist in exacerbating arrhythmias.

The selection of the most appropriate drugs does not guarantee success. Safe anaesthesia only results when drugs are used within the context of good anaesthetic management. Patient position, ventilation, fluid administration and temperature management must be considered along with the drugs producing unconsciousness. For example, the fact that halothane lowers the 'fibrillation threshold' to catecholamines, would indicate that the appropriate response to the appearance of intraoperative VPCs would be the reduction of inspired halothane concentration. In most cases, the reverse is true; the arrhythmia is occurring because of inadequate levels of anaesthesia and responds to increasing halothane concentrations.

In conclusion, drug choice in animals with cardiopulmonary disease is influenced by several factors. The one usually deemed most important, i.e. pharmacodynamic effect, often transpires to be of minor importance; familiarity with a given technique often proves to be the most appropriate determinant. Nevertheless, broad guidelines may be given:

- A well managed anaesthetic is usually more effective and safer than sedation
- Short-acting, titratable drugs are preferred to long-acting agents
- Any apparent advantage in using drugs that may be antagonized (medetomidine, etorphine) is usually outweighed by the undesirable effects of the drugs themselves. While medetomidine may be less hazardous than xylazine, it nevertheless causes mucous membranes to appear cyanotic, leaving the anaesthetist wondering whether this represents normal drug action or imminent death. Pharmacological antagonism *is* useful with drugs like acepromazine, whose adverse effect (hypotension) responds to alpha$_1$ agonists like methoxamine (0.05–0.1 mg/kg i.v.)
- Pharmacological preparation should be made for the widest possible range of adverse effects; antiarrhythmic drugs, positive and negative chronotropes and inotropes should be available as well as the means of oxygen administration and positive pressure ventilation. *Monitoring should be as extensive as the animal will tolerate.*

PROBLEMS WITH SPECIFIC TESTS

Bronchoscopy

Bronchoscopy is poorly tolerated in sedated people and requires general anaesthesia in dogs and cats. The major problem with bronchoscopic examination is that varying degrees of upper airway occlusion are inevitable, ranging from partial to absolute, depending on the relative diameters of the endoscope and trachea. The problem is most significant in cats and toy breeds. In addition, bronchoscopy often elicits marked laryngospinal reflex activity (e.g. coughing, gagging, 'bucking') which promotes lung collapse and predisposes to hypoxia as well as inducing trauma and precluding straightforward evaluation. This activity is eliminated at 'deeper' levels of anaesthesia that ideally should be produced with short-acting drugs (e.g. halothane, propofol, 'Saffan'), otherwise slow recoveries will result. A common underlying problem in animals undergoing bronchoscopy is chronic bronchitis. Anaesthetics, medical gases and endotracheal intubation inhibit mucociliary escalator function for a considerable time postoperatively, and some safeguards against this may be required.

Problems with upper airway obstruction are in large part dependent on the design of bronchoscope and the 'dwell-time' it is left *in situ*. If the bronchoscope is to be left *in situ* for hazardous periods (which depends on the time it takes for the animal to become hypoxic), a means for providing positive pressure ventilation (PPV) must be found. The use of pulse oximetry is very useful for defining the time when PPV must be imposed or bronchoscopy discontinued. With modern rigid endoscopes, PPV can be provided by a Venturi system that injects oxygen down the device's lumen which entrains air through the open end. Earlier methods, for example apnoeic diffusion oxygenation or simple oxygen insufflation down the bronchoscope, inevitably result in either hypoxia or hypercapnia.

With fibreoptic bronchoscopes, the trachea may be intubated as normal and the bronchoscope passed through an air-tight gasket positioned on a commercially available elbow connector that joins the endotracheal tube to the anaesthetic breathing system. Ventilation is then maintained by manual compression of the rebreathing bag. If there are no means by which the lungs may be rhythmically inflated with oxygen – an inevitability in cats using older pattern bronchoscopes without a Venturi – the endoscope must be removed at 20–30 second intervals (or whenever the mucous membrane colour, ECG or pulse oximeter indicates critical blood gas derangement) and the lungs inflated three to four times using oxygen. Repeated removal and re-introduction of the bronchoscope is likely to produce some degree of traumatic laryngotracheitis, although the temptation to keep it *in situ* for as long as possible must be overcome. Lubricating the endoscope with gels should be avoided, as animals may be incapable of effective postoperative expectoration. Residual gel may produce distal airway collapse and in a small diameter airway, create a disproportionately greater reduction of airway dimensions. If a biopsy is taken, animals should be positioned so that any blood drains away from the 'good' lung and down the trachea.

Anaesthesia for bronchoscopy should allow a rapid recovery of consciousness and the return of protective reflexes. Consequently, long-acting drugs should be avoided. A venous catheter should be placed to allow aliquots of anaesthetic to be given should an animal 'lighten' during a time when volatile agent administration is interrupted. Pre-anaesthetic medication should be given to smooth induction and recovery, and to provide a 'background' against 'swings' in anaesthesia that may follow the periodic interruption of volatile agent administration. Acepromazine (12.5–100 µg/kg) is appropriate in both cats and dogs. In cats, low doses of ketamine at 2.5 mg/kg may be used to augment the sedative effect, while in dogs, butorphanol (100–300 µg/kg) provides a useful anti-tussive effect. Induction to anaesthesia involves no special considerations beyond the usual requirements, e.g. species. Endotracheal intubation should be performed in most cases to allow PPV between bronchoscopic sessions. Anaesthesia may be maintained either with short-acting injectable anaesthetics (methohexitone, alphaxalone–alphadolone, propofol) or insoluble volatile agents (halothane, enflurane or isoflurane). Nitrous oxide (N_2O), however, should not be used if continuous oxygenation is impossible; diffusion hypoxia may occur and augment the effects of upper airway obstruction. 'Deep levels' of anaesthesia become unnecessary if the upper airway is desensitized with 1.0–2.0 ml of 1% lignocaine solution. This is introduced through the rima glottidis before tracheal intubation. Periodic monitoring is required but during bronchoscopy should be continuous; especial interest should be taken of signs indicating hypoxia: ECG; heart rate; mucous membrane colour; SpO_2.

Laryngeal examination

Examining reflex laryngeal activity in dogs and cats involves maintaining the animal within a narrow 'band' of unconsciousness for (usually) very short periods of time. Anaesthesia must be 'deep' enough to suppress struggling and allow mouth opening yet 'light' enough that reflex activity is retained. This is most easily achieved using short-acting injectable drugs like methohexitone, propofol (dogs) or alphaxalone (cats).

Occasionally, animals with laryngeal paralysis are cyanotic and present *in extremis.* In this situation, an airway must be established rapidly and oxygen provided; this may require general anaesthesia.

Anaesthesia for laryngeal examination should allow a rapid recovery and return of protective reflexes. A venous catheter should be placed to allow aliquots of anaesthetic to be given should an animal 'lighten' during examination (indicated by 'bucking' or head-shaking). Pre-anaesthetic medication may be given to smooth induction and recovery, although it will prolong the effects of incremental injections of intravenous anaesthetic so that if an overdose is given and laryngeal activity is obliterated, the laryngoscopist must wait a little longer before reflexes return and allow the examination to continue. In dogs, anaesthesia may be induced with methohexitone (1–10 mg/kg i.v.), propofol (2–5 mg/kg i.v.), or thiopentone (2–20 mg/kg i.v.), with the absolute dose influenced by several factors, particularly the effects of pre-anaesthetic medication. Slight under-dosage is desirable (in contrast with the normal goals of intravenous induction to anaesthesia). In cats, increments of alphaxalone-alphadolone (6–12 mg/kg i.v.) may be used although induction by halothane in a chamber (after pre-anaesthetic medication with acepromazine) is useful when venous access is difficult to achieve. Induction by mask is another option in cats, although pre-anaesthetic medication must produce relatively greater sedation in order to reduce the risk of vigorous resistance. Acepromazine at 12.5 (µg/kg i.m. combined with ketamine at 2.5 mg/kg i.m. and midazolam at 0.25 mg/kg i.m. is a useful combination for this. When profound sedation is present, anaesthesia is induced by mask delivery of halothane or isoflurane in oxygen (and N_2O). Laryngoscopy is attempted as soon as consciousness is lost. If laryngeal reflexes are absent, the investigator waits until drugs redistribute or are expired and reflexes return. The onset of laryngeal activity indicates the beginning of a short period during which evaluation will be most fruitful. In a short while, reflexes become stronger and eventually the animal begins to struggle. If the examination is incomplete a further aliquot of injectable (or exposure to volatile) anaesthetic becomes necessary.

Radiography

The disadvantages of sedation compared with general anaesthesia are even greater during radiological examination of animals with cardiopulmonary disease. General anaesthesia almost guarantees adequate immobility and so diminishes the need for repeated exposures, reducing exposure to ionizing radiation, and cost. Endotracheal intubation under general anaesthesia in combination with an anaesthetic breathing system allows lung inflation during exposure, which improves radiographic contrast of thoracic structures. Anaesthetic breathing systems with long hoses in which the expiratory valve is positioned at the proximal (machine) rather than the distal (patient) end, e.g. Lack or Bain systems, are ideal; they permit the anaesthetist to inflate the lungs while positioned behind radiation screens some distance from the animal. This feature is especially important during fluoroscopic examination. The risk of pulmonary barotrauma during lung inflation is low (see Chapter 23), although holding the lungs in the inspiratory position for unnecessarily long periods (beyond those needed to produce satisfactory radiographs) may reduce venous return and invoke compensatory tachycardia.

There are few particular anaesthetic requirements for dogs and cats undergoing radiographic examination beyond those mentioned above; the use of short-acting drugs that allow rapid recoveries should be favoured. The 'level' of anaesthesia required in most investigations is that which just ensures the absence of reflex responses to the endotracheal tube. One frequently overlooked problem during radiography in unconscious animals is related to patient positioning. Stabilizing position or improving contrast by the injudicious placement of sand-bags or restrictive use of 'ties' may limit ventilation or reduce functional residual capacity; animals must be positioned in a way that does not impair physiological function.

Echocardiography

From the anaesthetist's perspective, the ultrasonic examination of the heart (using high frequency sound waves) is a 'benign' test. It is not associated with exposure to hazardous radiation and the image produced is itself a useful way to monitor the effects of anaesthetics. Doppler echocardiography allows mechanical activity, valve action and blood flow to be observed on a beat-for-beat basis.

Sympathetic physical restraint alone may suffice for echocardiography, although sedation is required when restraint is vigorously resisted or for prolonged investigations (in which animals appear to become 'bored'). Occasionally, general anaesthesia may be required.

The selection of suitable 'sedative combinations' is based more on pre-existing disease and personal preference than the examination itself (see Table 5.15) In comparison with general anaesthetics, the effect of sedatives on ultrasound variables has not been extensively examined in companion animals.

Cardiac catheterization

Some diagnostic procedures like selective angiography, manometry (pressure determinations) and oximetry (oxygen content measurement) involve catheterization of the heart and so usually require general anaesthesia. In the diseased heart, catheters and contrast material can precipitate arrhythmias, including ventricular ectopic beats or ventricular tachycardia. Many arrhythmias result from tactile stimulation of the endocardium by the catheter tip (the region of the right atrioventricular annulus seems to be particularly sensitive), and so repositioning the catheter is often remedial. However, many iatrogenic arrhythmias appear to be well tolerated; this is usually the case if disease is not advanced and ventilation is supported vigorously. Arrhythmias can occur after injection of contrast media, although a modest, transient and inconsequential increase in heart rate is the usual response. Irrespective of cause, severe ventricular arrhythmias often respond to lung ventilation with 100% oxygen imposed every 20-30 seconds. If the animal appears to be 'light', the inspired concentration

---

Dogs

Acepromazine (12.5-50 μg/kg) given with one of the following:

Morphine	0.1-1.0 mg/kg i.m. or s.c.
Pethidine	2.0-5.0 mg/kg i.m. or s.c.
Butorphanol	50-200 μg/kg i.m. or s.c.
Buprenorphine	5-10 μg/kg i.v., i.m. or s.c.

Medetomidine (5-10 μg/kg) with Pethidine (2-5 mg/kg i.m.)

Cats

Acepromazine (12.5-50 μg/kg) with Ketamine (2.5-7.5 mg/kg i.m.)

Acepromazine (12.5-50 μg/kg) and Ketamine (2.5-7.5 mg/kg i.m.) with Midazolam (0.25 mg/kg i.m.)

Table 5.15: Sedative combinations suitable for echocardiographic examination in companion animals.

of volatile anaesthetic should be increased. If, after 30–60 seconds or so, ventricular ectopic activity persists, intravenous aliquots of lignocaine (2–4 mg/kg i.v.) should be given. If the examination cannot be suspended but arrhythmias persist, a lignocaine infusion (25–75 µg/kg per minute), with continued ventilatory support is advised.

Anaesthesia for cardiac catheterization should allow a rapid recovery. A venous catheter should be positioned to allow anti-arrhythmic drug administration. Pre-anaesthetic medication incorporating acepromazine (12.5–100 µg/kg) is usually appropriate in both cats and dogs as this drug exerts a useful anti-arrhythmic effect. Induction involves no special considerations. Endotracheal intubation should be performed in most cases to allow PPV. Anaesthesia may be maintained with insoluble volatile agents (halothane or isoflurane) delivered in nitrous oxide. The ECG and pulse characteristics should be continuously monitored during catheterization, at which time, ventilation should be supported using an appropriate anaesthetic breathing system.

Specialist Techniques

(i) Blood Gas Analysis

R. Eddie Clutton

INTRODUCTION AND OVERVIEW

Blood gas analysis provides useful information in the evaluation of pulmonary, cardiovascular and renal function and gives critical information in cases where several organ systems are affected by disease (e.g. congestive heart failure), injury, drugs (e.g. anaesthesia) or toxins.

These days, the most difficult part of blood gas analysis is sample collection. Once obtained, blood is presented to the 'probe' of the blood gas analyser. A sample of 35–70 µl is aspirated and passed through three sampling chambers:

- An oxygen electrode measuring O_2 tension (PO_2)
- A CO_2 electrode measuring CO_2 tension (PCO_2)
- A glass pH meter measuring pH.

In response to prompts, the technician 'inputs' the patient's temperature, the barometric pressure (P_b) and haemoglobin concentration [Hb]. An integral computer takes pH and PCO_2 measurements and with input data, derives further variables like bicarbonate concentration $[HCO_3^-]$, base excess (BE), total CO_2 (tCO_2) and percentage haemoglobin saturation (SO_2).

Sample results are displayed and a printout provided, usually within 60 seconds. This allows rapid diagnosis and treatment; for example, the moment-to-moment adjustment of ventilator patterns in the intensive care unit or operating room. Modern devices are self-calibrating. The small blood volume required means samples can be taken from very small animals. Modern analysers have a sample cycle time, including automatic rinsing, that allows up to 55 tests per hour.

Blood gas analysis equipment costs in excess of £7500 per unit and service contracts on second hand ex-laboratory equipment are similarly expensive. Such costs are difficult to justify, even in the most progressive practices. However, any general hospital which has an intensive care unit or performs surgery will possess blood gas analysis equipment and usually, will analyse veterinary samples providing blood has been adequately heparinized.

Sampling

In conscious dogs, arterial blood is most easily taken from the femoral artery. In anaesthetized animals, the dorsal metatarsal or lingual arteries may be used. Venous blood may be used in special circumstances.

When necessary, the skin overlying the intended puncture site is clipped and surgically prepared. In contrast to venepuncture, in which the needle tip is advanced by sight into the lumen of a raised vein, arteriopuncture relies more on palpation. In the right-handed sampler, a needle and pre-heparinized (1 or 2 ml) syringe is advanced beneath that point where fingers of the left hand feel the maximum arterial pulsation; very mild negative pressure is applied to the syringe plunger. If puncture is unsuccessful, the needle tip is withdrawn and re-directed. When enough blood is collected, a sterile swab is applied with pressure over the puncture site and the needle is withdrawn. Firm pressure must be applied for at least 5 minutes, or until there is no evidence of haemorrhage.

Samples are drawn into glass or plastic syringes whose dead space only is filled with heparin (excessive anticoagulant is undesirable; its low pH influences results). Air bubbles must be eliminated rapidly from the sample and the syringe capped, otherwise atmospheric gas contamination occurs. If a delay between collection and analysis is likely, samples should be collected in glass syringes and placed on ice slush. This retards metabolism and minimizes time-related changes in PO_2 and PCO_2. Delay between collection and analysis of samples should be kept to a minimum, ideally less than 30 minutes.

Information provided by blood gases and pH

Blood gas analysis provides primary information on ventilation and acid–base status. Some elements of cardiac and metabolic function may be inferred from these data. Ventilation and acid–base homeostasis are related. CO_2 rapidly influences the concentration of bicarbonate $[HCO_3^-]$, which is the principal pH buffer. Renal control of $[HCO_3^-]$ is a slower process. Through CO_2 levels, ventilation rapidly influences arterial pH:

$$CO_2 + H_2O \rightleftharpoons H_2CO_3 \rightleftharpoons H^+ + HCO_3^-$$

Arterial blood values

PaO_2 — arterial partial pressure of oxygen
$PaCO_2$ — arterial partial pressure of carbon dioxide
pHa — arterial pH

Arterial blood values indicate:

- The lungs' ability to oxygenate blood (PaO_2)
- The lungs' ability to eliminate CO_2 ($PaCO_2$)
- Pulmonary influence on acid–base status (pHa and $PaCO_2$).

This information is useful when ventilatory disease is present, during controlled ventilation or anaesthesia. (Note: arterial blood variables are indicated by the suffix 'a', venous samples with a 'v' and alveolar samples with 'A').

Venous blood values

PvO_2 — venous partial pressure of oxygen
$PvCO_2$ — venous partial pressure of carbon dioxide
pHv — venous pH

Venous blood values indicate:

- Metabolism-related variables such as tissue O_2 consumption
- CO_2 production
- Acid (H^+) generation.

Although venous blood values may be of value in diseases associated with primary acid–base abnormalities, they do not indicate the compensatory effects of ventilation on pHa. Consequently, arterial and venous blood gas values are not interchangeable (see Table 6.1). However, during anaesthesia, cutaneous vasodilation and hyperaemia cause peripheral venous blood gas values to approach arterial levels and allow $PvCO_2$ and pHv values to become valid estimates for ventilation and acid–base status. Peripheral venous PO_2 does not accurately indicate PaO_2, although if PvO_2 values are greater than 7.98 kPa (60 mmHg), it can be assumed that arterial hypoxaemia is absent.

ASSESSING VENTILATION

Arterial oxygen tension (PaO_2)

Hypoxaemia = PaO_2 < 7.98 kPa (60 mmHg)

Oxygen tension in arterial blood (PaO_2) indicates the ability of the lungs to oxygenate blood. However, PaO_2 values will vary according to the fractional inspired concentration of oxygen (FiO_2).

An animal breathing 100% O_2 may have high PaO_2 levels in the presence of significant lung pathology. Breathing room air (21% O_2) with healthy lungs could produce a theoretical maximum PaO_2 value of 13.3 kPa (100 mmHg), according to the alveolar gas equation:

$$\text{Alveolar } O_2 \text{ tension } (PAO_2) = FiO_2\,(P_b - P_{H_2O}) - \frac{PaCO_2}{0.8}$$

P_b is the barometric pressure
P_{H_2O} is the saturated vapour pressure of water
$PaCO_2$ is the arterial partial pressure of carbon dioxide
0.8 is the respiratory quotient (the ratio of volumes of CO_2 produced: O_2 produced)
When 100% oxygen is breathed (FiO_2: 1.0), the theoretical maximum PAO_2 is 85.1 kPa (640 mmHg).

When investigating lung function, PAO_2 is calculated using the alveolar gas equation and compared with PaO_2; the difference between the two values, the alveolar–arterial oxygen tension gradient ($P(A-a)O_2$) may be used to assess the extent of pulmonary dysfunction (see Chapter 2).

When breathing room air, $P(A-a)O_2$ ranges from 0.66 to 3.3 kPa (5–25 mmHg). The difference arises because of mixing of blood from lung units with differing degrees of oxygenation. Greater differences in $P(A-a)O_2$ result from:

- Reduced oxygen tension in mixed venous blood (increased O_2 extraction by tissues)
- venous admixture ('shunt' or low ventilation-perfusion ratios) indicates lung pathology.

	Room air (20% O_2)				Oxygen (100% O_2)			
	Arterial		Venous		Arterial		Venous	
pH	7.40		7.376		7.40		7.376	
	kPa*	mmHg	kPa	mmHg	kPa	mmHg	kPa	mmHg
PO_2	13.3	100	5.33	40	85.1	640	7.11	53.5
PCO_2	5.32	40	6.11	46	5.32	40	6.11	46

Table 6.1: Arterial and venous blood gas values breathing room air and oxygen.
The kilopascal (kPa) is the accepted SI unit of gas tension and replaces mmHg; 1 kPa = 7.52 mmHg.

'Shunt' describes the passage of blood from right (pulmonary) to left (systemic) circulations without exposure to alveolar gas. Hypoxaemia from right to left shunting represents dilution of oxygenated arterial blood with shunted, desaturated venous blood. A shunt may be *intrapulmonary* (neoplasm, bronchitis, pneumonia, atelectasis) or *intracardiac* (e.g. ventricular septal defects). The presence of 'shunt' is demonstrated by PaO_2 values which do not improve when 100% oxygen is breathed.

Low ventilation/perfusion (V/Q) lung zones are overperfused and/or underventilated; blood receives some O_2 but is not saturated. Inspiring pure O_2 eliminates N_2 from poorly ventilated alveoli and raises O_2 tensions in pulmonary capillaries, elevating PaO_2.

Arterial carbon dioxide tension ($PaCO_2$)

Hypercapnia = $PaCO_2$ > 5.85 kPa (44 mmHg)

Arterial CO_2 tension is a sensitive index of the efficiency of alveolar ventilation (*V*a) in removing CO_2 from the body.

The level of CO_2 in the blood is directly proportional to the rate of CO_2 production (VCO_2 or metabolic production), and inversely proportional to the rate of CO_2 elimination (*V*a, or minute alveolar ventilation).

Hypercapnia results from either decreased alveolar ventilation (anaesthesia, head injury) or increased CO_2 production (e.g. pyrexia, malignant hyperthermia). In anaesthetic practice another cause is rebreathing, which occurs when gas flow in non-rebreathing systems is insufficient to elute CO_2 from the circuit, or when soda-lime is exhausted in rebreathing systems.

A $PaCO_2$ less than 4.78 kPa (36 mmHg) indicates hyperventilation. This occurs in response to pain or may be iatrogenic, when ventilation is controlled excessively. When severe hypoxia is present (e.g. major shunt) PaO_2 replaces $PaCO_2$ as the principal respiratory stimulant, and ventilation may become excessive with respect to CO_2.

ASSESSING CARDIAC OUTPUT/OXYGEN CONSUMPTION

Arterio–venous oxygen content differences

An estimate of the adequacy of cardiac output relative to whole body oxygen consumption (VO_2) is provided by calculating the difference between arterial and mixed venous oxygen content ($C(a-v)O_2$). This requires taking arterial and mixed venous blood samples simultaneously. The traditional units of $C(a-v)O_2$ are ml/dl.

Normal $C(a-v)O_2$ is 4–6 ml/dl. Decreased cardiac output, prolonged circulation time or sluggish perfusion increases the $C(a-v)O_2$ value. If cardiac output is stable, increased $C(a-v)O_2$ indicates increased metabolic O_2 consumption, i.e. a hypermetabolic state.

Pulse oximetry

Pulse oximetry uses the relative absorption of red light by oxyhaemoglobin and haemoglobin to determine the percentage saturation of haemoglobin with oxygen (SaO_2). This is linked to the PaO_2 by the oxyhaemoglobin dissociation curve and so PaO_2 and SaO_2 measurements are complementary.

Technique

A probe is attached to a perfused and light-proofed mucous membrane. Despite its ease of application, SaO_2 is a 'cliff-edge' variable; the arterial PaO_2 value of 8 kPa (60 mmHg) represents the 'shoulder' of the oxyhaemoglobin dissociation curve and corresponds to an SaO_2 of 0.9. Between SaO_2 values from 1.0 to 0.9, PaO_2 remains in excess of 8 kPa (60 mmHg) and haemoglobin remains saturated with oxygen. However, SaO_2 values less than 0.9 lie on the steep slope of the dissociation curve, and indicate large falls in haemoglobin saturation will occur with small reductions in PaO_2. In short, the pulse oximeter does not show the animal's proximity to a hypoxaemic cliff edge, but indicates when it has fallen off.

ACID–BASE BALANCE

Blood gas analysis permits examination of acid–base status through measurement of pH and $PaCO_2$. From these, [HCO_3^-] is calculated by analyser software applying the Henderson–Hasselbalch equation. This indicates that normal pHa depends on the maintenance of a HCO_3^-:CO_2 ratio of 20. The normal range of arterial pH (pHa) is 7.44–7.36.

$$pH = pK + \frac{\log [HCO_3^-]}{0.225 \times PaCO_2}$$

Interpretation (see Table 6.2)

Increased [H⁺]

Processes in which [H⁺] rises include metabolic and respiratory acidosis. If changes are severe and compensation incomplete, acidaemia (pH < 7.36) results.
Causes include:

- Acid accumulation (e.g. diabetic ketoacidosis)
- Base [HCO_3^-] loss (e.g. renal failure)
- Carbon dioxide retention (hypercapnia; hypoventilation).

Acute metabolic acidosis: pH falls as HCO_3^- is lowered by reaction with accumulating H⁺. Irrespective of added acid strength, the resulting pH fall is less than

Condition	pH	$PaCO_2$	HCO_3^-	*BE*
Acute metabolic acidosis	↓ ↓	↓	↓ ↓	↓ ↓
Chronic metabolic acidosis	↓	↓ ↓	↓	↓
Acute metabolic alkalosis	↑ ↑	↑	↑ ↑	↑ ↑
Chronic metabolic alkalosis	↑	↑ ↑	↑	↑
Acute respiratory acidosis	↓ ↓	↑	↑	↑
Chronic respiratory acidosis	↓	↑ ↑	↑ ↑	↑ ↑
Acute respiratory alkalosis	↑ ↑	↓ ↓	↓	↓
Chronic respiratory alkalosis	↑	↓	↓ ↓	↓ ↓

Table 6.2: *Altered acid–base states.*

expected because HCO_3^- (and other buffer systems) react with H^+ to form only weak acids (e.g. H_2CO_3) in reaction with H^+. Within minutes of this immediate buffering response, hyperventilation begins, lowering $PaCO_2$ and partly raising pHa.

Chronic metabolic acidosis: Several hours later, renal compensation involving HCO_3^- retention and enhanced H^+ excretion begins in order to restore normal pH.

Metabolic acidosis is, therefore, characterized by reduced pH, reduced HCO_3^-, reduced $PaCO_2$ and base deficit, or negative base excess (*BE* < 0).

Acute respiratory acidosis: pH falls because CO_2 is retained, with $PaCO_2$ rising above 5.85 kPa (44 mm Hg). Concurrently, $[HCO_3^-]$ rises about 1 mmol/l per 1.33 kPa (10 mmHg) rise in $PaCO_2$ because accumulating CO_2 is hydrated in plasma ($H_2O + CO_2 \rightleftharpoons H_2CO_3 \rightleftharpoons H^+ + HCO_3^-$).

Chronic respiratory acidosis: In time, renal retention of HCO_3^- raises $[HCO_3^-]$ by about 3 mmol/l per 1.33 kPa rise in $PaCO_2$ which restores normal pH.

Features of chronic respiratory acidosis include reduced pH, raised $PaCO_2$ and raised $[HCO_3^-]$.

Decreased [H⁺]

Alkalosis describes pathological metabolic and respiratory processes lowering $[H^+]$. Severe alkalosis or incomplete compensation causes alkalaemia (pH > 7.44).

Acute metabolic alkalosis: Buffering is the immediate response to pH increases. Within minutes, hypoventilation begins, raising $PaCO_2$ and lowering pH.

Chronic metabolic alkalosis: Hours later, renal compensation involving HCO_3^- excretion and H^+ retention restores normal pH. The result is an increased pH, increased HCO_3^-, increased $PaCO_2$ and positive base excess (*BE* > 0).

Acute respiratory alkalosis: pH rises because CO_2 is

'blown off' ($PaCO_2$ < 4.78 kPa, 36 mmHg). Initially, $[HCO_3^-]$ falls by about 2 mmol/l per 1.33 kPa (10 mmHg) fall in $PaCO_2$.

Chronic respiratory alkalosis: Renal excretion of HCO_3^- reduces $[HCO_3^-]$ levels by about 5 mmol/l per 1.33 kPa fall in $PaCO_2$ restoring normal pH. Features include increased pH, decreased $PaCO_2$, and decreased HCO_3^-.

OVERALL APPROACH TO BLOOD GAS ANALYSIS

Clinical history

Clinicians should predict the blood gas 'picture' on the basis of history. Examination must appraise specifically renal, gastrointestinal, cardiovascular disease, fluid disturbances and the ventilatory rate pattern and depth. This 'prediction' is entirely permissible because it simplifies the process of distinguishing primary from compensatory changes and forms the basis of rational treatment.

Sample site

The site of blood collection depends on the type of information sought. Lung function evaluation requires an arterial sample, while metabolic processes are best interpreted by analysis of mixed venous blood. Samples should be submitted for additional pertinent tests such as [Hb] and haematocrit.

Interpretation (see Table 6.3)

pH	< 7.36 = acidaemia >7.44 = alkalaemia
$PaCO_2$	< 4.78 kPa (36 mm Hg) = respiratory alkalosis > 5.85 kPa (44 mm Hg) = respiratory acidosis
$[HCO_3^-]$	> 27 mmol/l = metabolic alkalosis < 23 mmol/l = metabolic acidosis

Table 6.3: *Variables generated by blood gas analysis.*

- Examination of pH should determine the presence of acidaemia or alkalaemia
- Low $PaCO_2$ levels indicate respiratory alkalosis; high $PaCO_2$ levels indicate respiratory acidosis
- High bicarbonate concentrations indicate metabolic alkalosis, low bicarbonate concentrations indicate metabolic acidosis.

The primary problem is then identified by matching $PaCO_2$, $[HCO_3^-]$, or both with pHa. The extent of compensation is determined by adjusting $[HCO_3^-]$ for acute or chronic elevations/reductions in CO_2 (see Table 6.4).

Assessment of PaO_2

- Is hypoxaemia (PaO_2 < 7.98 kPa, 60 mmHg) present?
- If so, does low FiO_2 explain this?
- If not, can hypoxaemia be linked to pH and, or $PaCO_2$ changes?

$PaCO_2$ change	Change in $[HCO_3^-]$ per 1.33 kPa change in $PaCO_2$
Acute ↑	1 mmol/l
Chronic ↑	3 mmol/l
Acute ↓	2 mmol/l
Chronic ↓	5 mmol/l

***Table 6.4**: Compensatory changes in $[HCO_3^-]$ with $PaCO_2$.*

- Hypoxaemia with low or normal $PaCO_2$ = shunt, or V/Q mismatching
- Hypoxaemia with elevated $PaCO_2$ = hypoventilation.

REFERENCES AND FURTHER READING

Adams AP and Hahn CEW (1982) *Principles and Practice of Blood Gas Analysis*. 2nd edn. Churchill-Livingstone, Edinburgh

(ii) Doppler Echocardiography

Peter G.G. Darke

INTRODUCTION

With ultrasound, cardiologists can examine intracardiac structures in detail: echocardiography is used to evaluate cardiac dimensions, and congenital and acquired lesions of the valves, myocardium and pericardium (Moise, 1988; Weyman, 1994; Kienle and Thomas, 1995). The ultrasound image is formed from signals reflected by cardiac structures.

Physical principles of Doppler

Ultrasound is emitted by the transducer at a known frequency. By the Doppler principle, when this signal is reflected by moving tissues, it will be received by the transducer at a changed frequency (Figure 6.1). This frequency shift is directly proportional to the velocity and direction of the moving tissue. As the bulk of moving tissues in the heart and great vessels are blood cells, Doppler analysis of the reflected signal demonstrates the velocity and direction of blood flow (Goldberg *et al.*, 1988; Hagan and De Maria, 1989; Weyman, 1994). A skilled operator can then measure

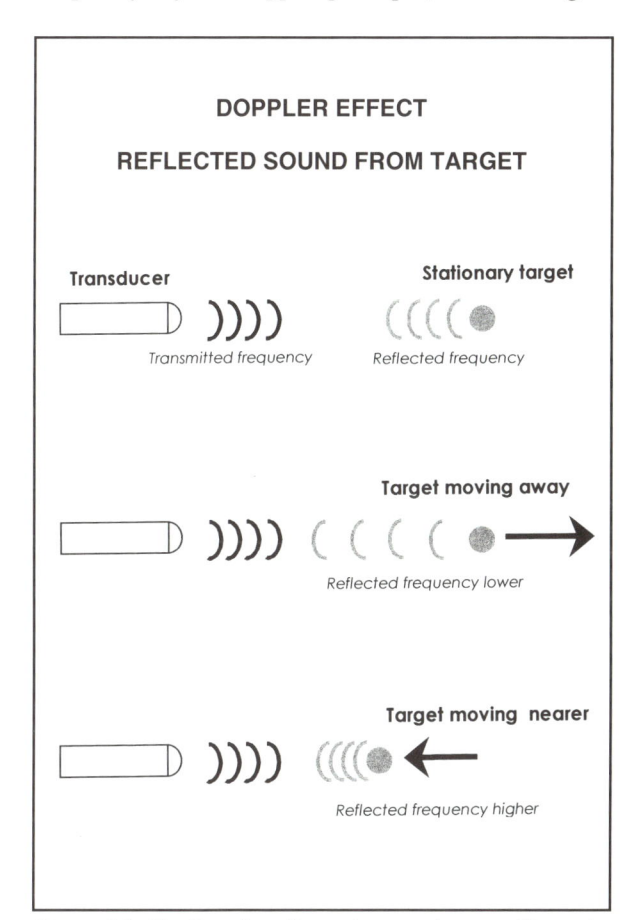

Figure 6.1: The Doppler effect: when an ultrasound beam is reflected by moving tissues, it will be reflected at a changed frequency. This shift in frequency will be directly related to the velocity and direction of the moving tissue.

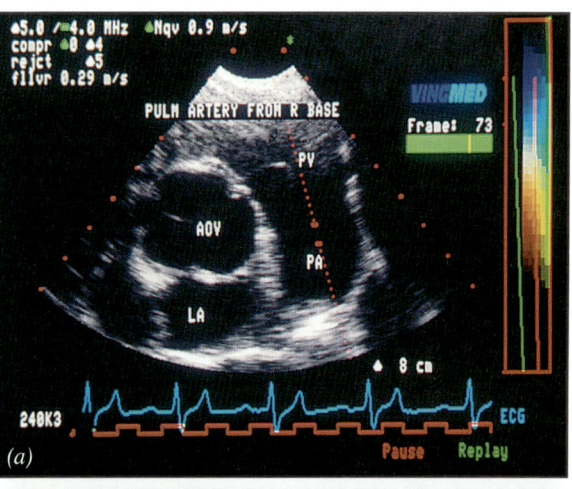

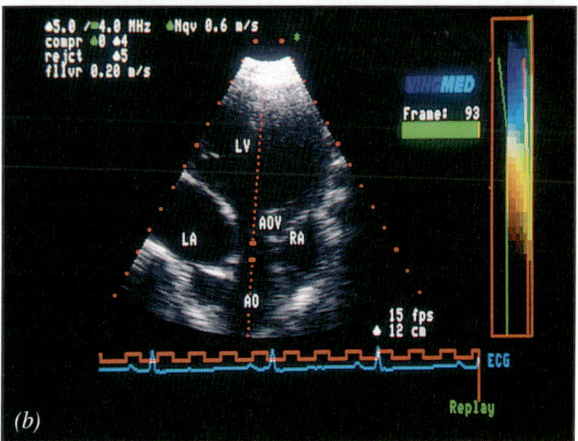

Figure 6.2: Precise alignment of the Doppler beam with blood flow, and accurate placement of the sample volume (indicated by a pair of red dots) at a point just beyond semilunar valves: (a) in the pulmonary artery of a Greyhound, from a left cranial short-axis view; (b) in the ascending aorta of a West Highland White Terrier from the subcostal site, imaging through the liver.

flow at almost any site in the heart and great vessels of dogs and cats (Brown *et al.*, 1991; Darke *et al.*, 1993, 1996) and this facility can be further enhanced by transoesophageal echocardiography (Loyer and Thomas, 1995) (Figure 6.2).

Types of Doppler and signal portrayal

The data are portrayed as a velocity-time graph of blood flow (spectral Doppler), usually synchronous with an ECG (Figure 6.3). If the ultrasound signal is transmitted in pulses (pulsed-wave Doppler), the echocardiograph can determine the depth from which the Doppler signal is being recorded. However, there are physical limits to the maximum velocity that can be measured by this technique without 'aliasing'. Aliasing occurs at velocities higher than can be handled by pulsed-wave Doppler, and the spectral Doppler recording shows the flow as 'wrapped round' the

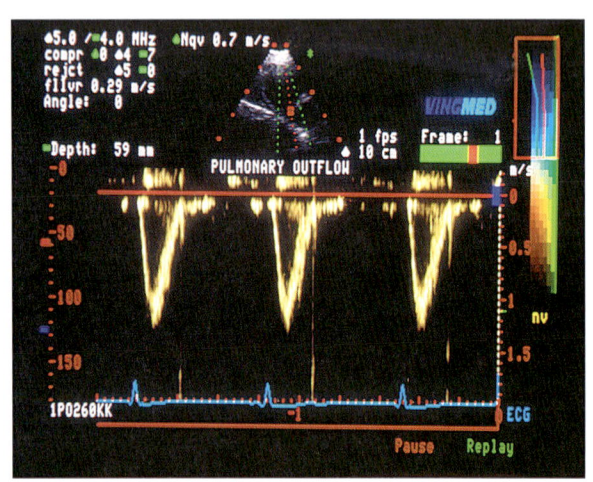

Figure 6.3: *Pulsed-wave 'spectral' Doppler recording of flow in the pulmonary artery of a normal Boxer, synchronously with an ECG. Note the ejection immediately after QRS complex, to a maximum velocity that just exceeds 1.2 m/s.*

display (Figure 6.4a). Higher velocities require the use of continuous-wave Doppler, which cannot discriminate the depth at which blood flow is being evaluated, or high pulsed repetition Doppler (HPRF), which is a compromise between the two techniques (Figure 6.4b).

Evaluation of blood flow at each heart valve by spectral Doppler can be used to demonstrate abnormal flow (e.g. valve regurgitation) (Figure 6.8). Furthermore, the velocity of flow will be elevated through any narrow orifice during systole (e.g. with ventricular septal defect, aortic valve stenosis or atrioventricular regurgitation). Doppler demonstrates whether flow is laminar (Figure 6.3) or disturbed (Figure 6.5), and the presence of turbulence often helps to indicate the source of cardiac murmurs.

Use of Doppler in clinical diagnosis

Many haemodynamic phenomena can be evaluated objectively and non-invasively by Doppler echocardiography (Goldberg *et al.*, 1988; Weyman, 1994). These include:

- *Abnormal flow* with valve regurgitation or through congenital shunts (e.g. patent ductus arteriosus or septal defect)
- *Pressure gradients* across stenotic or regurgitant valves, or shunts such as septal defects
- *Ventricular diastolic function*: the pattern of ventricular inflow through the atrioventricular valves may be disturbed
- *Ventricular systolic function*: a number of parameters may be affected by ventricular performance
- *Volume of flow* through the valves and great vessels can be derived from the velocity–time integral (VTI or 'stroke distance').

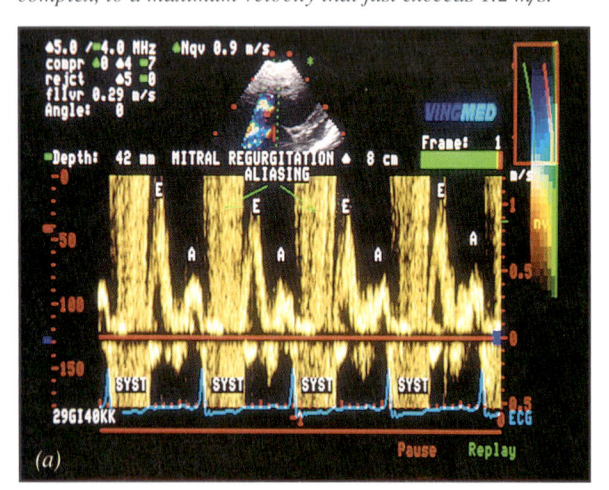

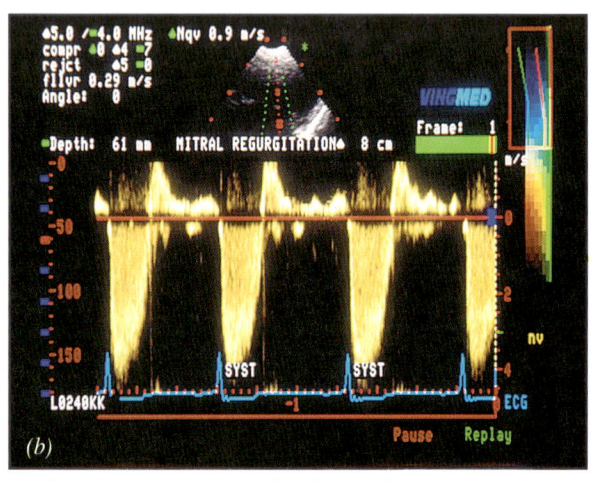

Figure 6.4: *Pulsed-wave spectral Doppler recording from the mitral valve of a Springer Spaniel with mitral regurgitation secondary to dilated cardiomyopathy. (a) An aliased signal, with which the regurgitant flow (away from the transducer – below the baseline) is of too high a velocity to be accommodated by the pulsed-wave Doppler; passive (E) and active (A) ventricular filling waves are seen (above the baseline, towards the transducer), but the signal is overlaid by the regurgitant flow that is wrapped round the trace in systole. (b) The systolic regurgitation can now be accommodated when high pulse repetition frequency Doppler (HPRF) is used, to a maximum velocity that just exceeds 4 m/s. Similar recordings can be made by continuous-wave Doppler, with which there are no practical limits.*

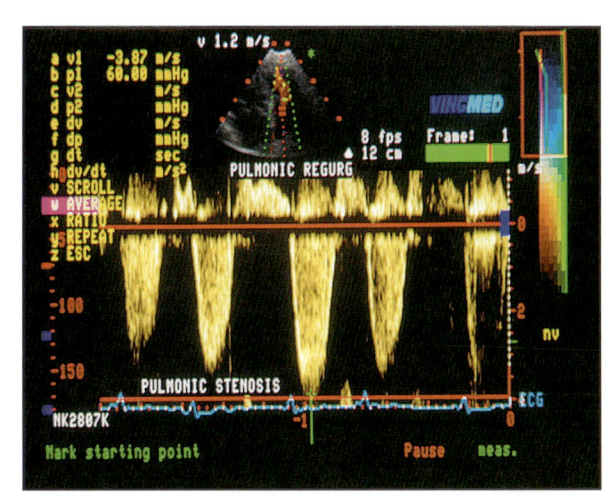

Figure 6.5: *Disturbed flow in the pulmonary artery of a Boxer with pulmonic stenosis, recorded with HPRF Doppler. Compare with normal flow in Figure 6.3, and note that the 'envelope' of the trace is no longer clearly outlined, due to variations in velocity recorded from disturbed flow, and note also that the maximum velocity of flow is higher (3.87 m/s), owing to the stenosis. By the modified Bernoulli equation, this equates to a pressure gradient over the valve of about 60 mmHg.*

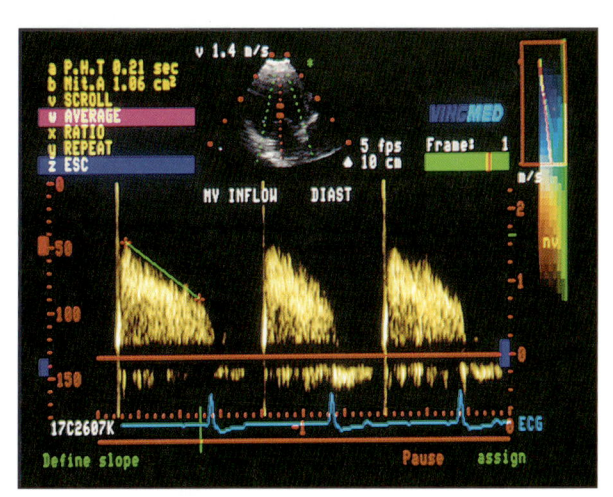

Figure 6.6: *Pulsed-wave Doppler recording from the mitral valve of a Springer Spaniel with mild mitral stenosis. Compare with Figure 6.9a, and note that there are no longer two clear envelopes, of passive and active filling of the ventricle, in diastole, but a prolonged filling wave of higher-than-normal velocity (approximately 1.5 m/s) and some disturbance to the laminar flow.*

Doppler echocardiography can confirm the diagnosis and severity of disease in most congenital cardiac disorders (Moise, 1989) and in acquired valvular diseases (Darke *et al.*, 1996).

Pressure gradients

A pressure gradient exists between two cardiac chambers, or across a heart valve if the flow of blood is constricted. For example, if the flow pathway is narrow through a stenotic valve (e.g. pulmonic stenosis), with valve regurgitation (as in mitral insufficiency), or across a restrictive shunt (e.g. ventricular septal defect), the velocity of flow will be increased (Figure

6.5). The maximum pressure gradient is closely related to the maximum velocity of flow detected beyond a constriction. By a modification of the Bernoulli equation, $p = 4V_2^2$, where V_2 is the maximum velocity of flow recorded beyond the lesion (in m/s), and p is the pressure gradient in mmHg.

Pressure gradients derived by Doppler echocardiography have been validated against instantaneous pressure gradients measured by cardiac catheterisation (Currie *et al.*, 1986; Thomas, 1990; Weyman, 1994). For recording high velocities, continuous-wave Doppler is essential. Doppler has proved to be a reliable and rapid, non-invasive technique when used by a skilled technician. With a valvular stenosis (mitral, aortic, pulmonic), generally the higher the velocity and pressure gradient, the more severe the lesion. As a rule of thumb, velocities less than 2.2 m/s, representing pressure gradients less than 50 mmHg across the aortic or pulmonic valves, indicate mild stenosis; gradients of 50–100 mmHg indicate moderate stenosis; and velocities over 5 m/s, representing gradients greater than 100 mmHg, are found with severe stenosis, and these carry a poor prognosis. With mitral stenosis, as seen frequently in English Bull Terriers, not only do relatively high velocity of flow (>2 m/s) and turbulence indicate severe stenosis, but a shallow descending slope, representing prolongation of the flow curve of passive ventricular filling, is also found with severe disease (Fox *et al.*, 1992; Weyman, 1994; Kienle and Thomas, 1995; Darke *et al.*, 1996) (Figure 6.6).

However, relatively high flow velocity with valve regurgitation (e.g. mitral or tricuspid insufficiency) indicates that a high pressure gradient is being maintained between the ventricles and atria, and that the regurgitation may therefore be relatively mild. Similarly, with shunts such as ventricular septal defects or

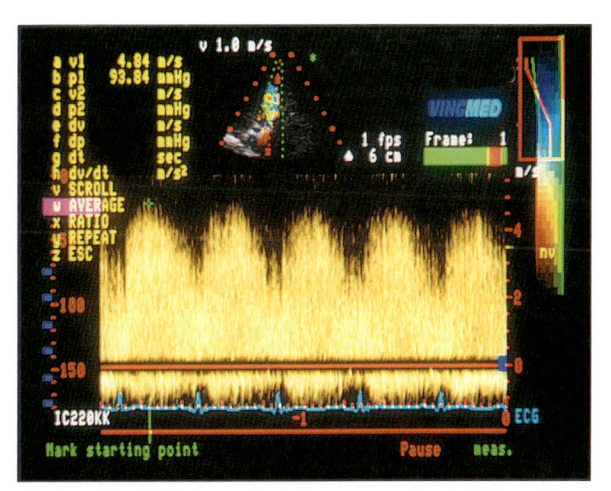

Figure 6.7: *HPRF recording from a crossbred Collie with patent ductus arteriosus. Note the continuous disturbed flow that varies throughout systole and diastole, with a maximum velocity of 4.84 m/s. By the modified Bernoulli equation, this represents a pressure gradient between the aorta and the pulmonary artery of about 94 mmHg, demonstrating that pulmonary hypertension is almost certainly not present in this case.*

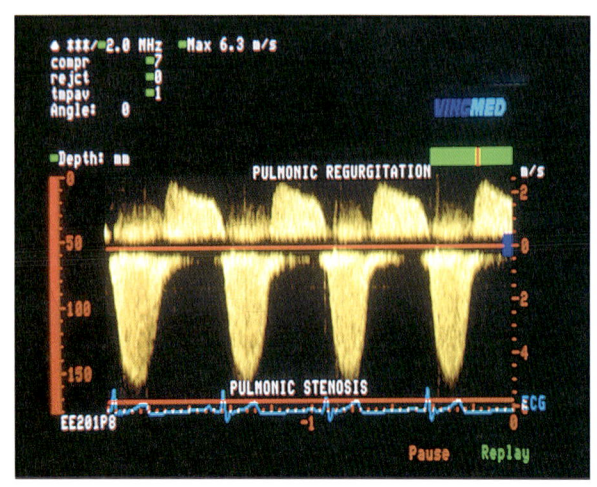

Figure 6.8: *Pulmonary regurgitation (above the baseline in diastole – towards the transducer) recorded by continuous-wave Doppler in a Labrador with pulmonic stenosis. Note that there is no great reduction in velocity of regurgitation until systole commences, indicating a mild regurgitation with minimal loss of pressure gradient across the valve.*

patent ductus arteriosus, high velocity flow implies mild to moderate disease, with a good (normal) pressure gradient being maintained between left and right sides of the circulation (Figure 6.7).

Furthermore, in aortic or pulmonic insufficiency, a shallow slope in the fall of the regurgitant velocity curve suggests a slow decline in diastolic pressure (Figure 6.8), while a rapid fall-off suggests severe disease (Weyman, 1994; Kienle and Thomas, 1995).

Ventricular diastolic function

Non-invasive evaluation of ventricular diastolic dysfunction (e.g. abnormal relaxation, or lack of ventricular compliance) is very difficult without Doppler. Even with this technique, the results are rather variable. However, one of the most common indications of diastolic dysfunction is reversal of the E wave to A wave ratio in atrioventricular valve inflow. Normally, most ventricular filling is passive, giving a larger inflow in early diastole, followed by a smaller atrial 'kick' (Figure 6.9a). However, in many cases of abnormal ventricular relaxation, the atrial contraction contributes a higher velocity of flow (A wave) than the passive filling (E wave) (Figure 6.9b).

Ventricular systolic function

Dilated cardiomyopathy is one of the most common causes of cardiac failure in large dogs. Investigations have shown a reduction not only in the fractional shortening measured by echocardiography, but also in the maximum velocity and acceleration (dv/dt) of flow in the aorta (Figure 6.10) and pulmonary artery. Furthermore, the pre-ejection period tends to be prolonged, and the ejection time reduced, in this disease. Although these phenomena are influenced by preload and afterload, they can be helpful in the evaluation of myocardial function.

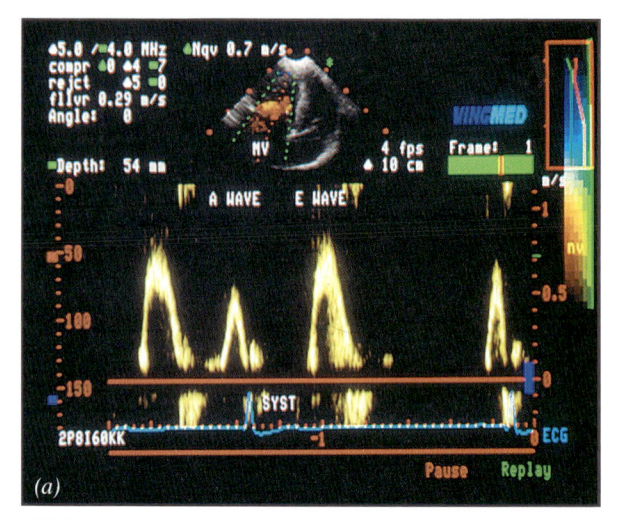

(a)

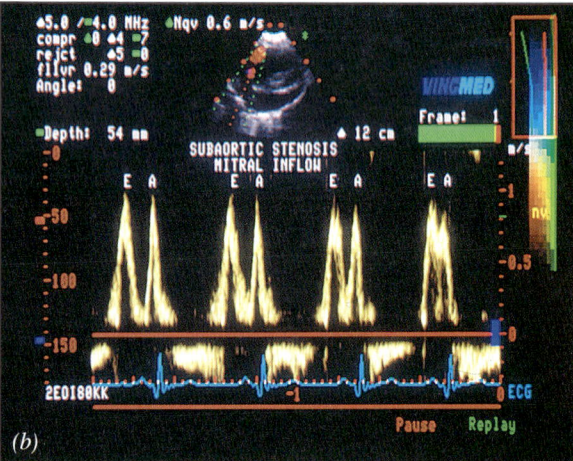

(b)

Figure 6.9: *Pulsed-wave Doppler recordings from the mitral valve of two dogs: (a) a normal Boxer, showing the two inflow waves, the larger flow being in early diastole (E wave – to about 0.8 m/s) and the smaller being associated with the atrial contraction (A wave – to about 0.6 m/s); (b) a Labrador with aortic stenosis and evidence of impaired ventricular relaxation: the active filling (A) wave is of higher velocity than normal, to be almost the equal of the passive filling (E) wave.*

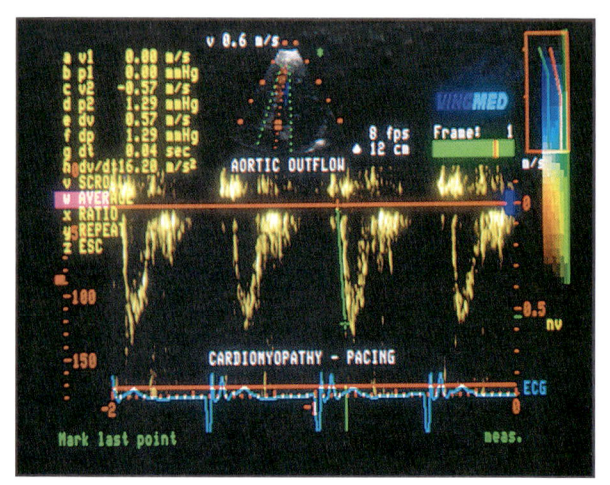

Figure 6.10: *Pulsed-wave Doppler recording from the ascending aorta of a dog with cardiac pacing and chronic left ventricular failure (a form of 'dilated cardiomyopathy'). Note the low maximum velocity (0.5 m/s), the weak signal and the poor acceleration of flow (dv/dt) in the aorta (16.2 m/s²).*

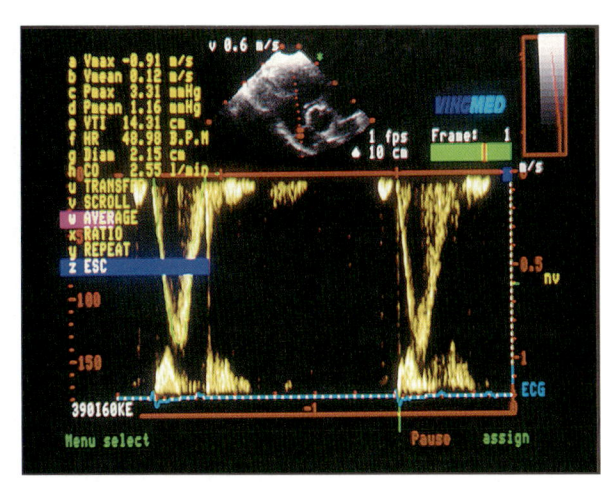

Figure 6.11: Measurement of cardiac output from a pulsed-wave Doppler recording from the pulmonary artery of a Border Collie. The spectral 'envelope' has been traced (in green) by use of a tracker-ball, giving the velocity–time integral (VTI: 14.31 cm). The diameter of the pulmonary artery has been previously carefully measured (2.15 cm), and this value entered on the screen. From this the machine will calculate πr^2, and multiply this by the VTI and the heart rate (48.98/min) to produce the cardiac output (2.55 l/min).

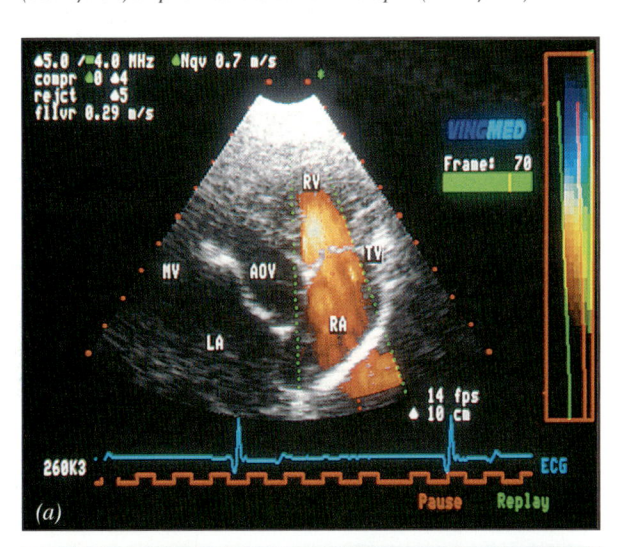

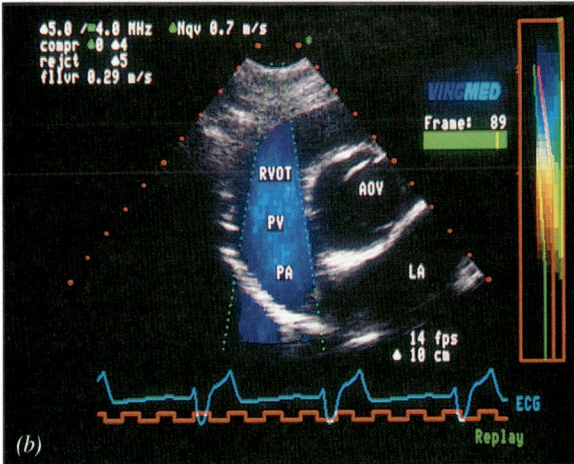

Figure 6.12: Colour-flow Doppler recordings from normal dogs. (a) Tricuspid valve inflow in a German Shepherd Dog. Flow is towards the transducer near the cardiac apex, coded in red. (b) Pulmonic valve outflow in a Greyhound. The flow is away from the transducer, coded in blue.

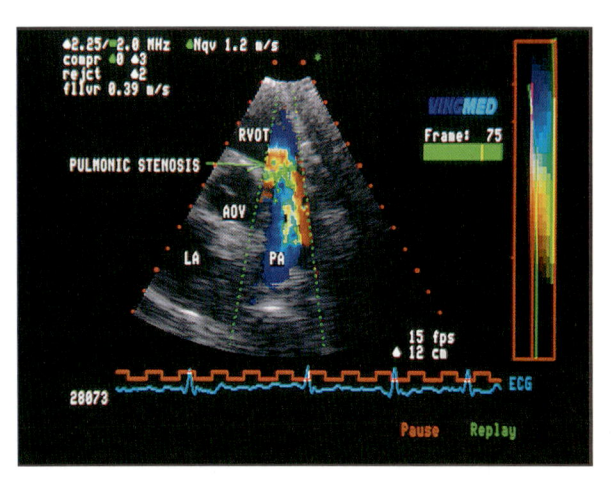

Figure 6.13: Colour-flow Doppler recording from a Boxer with pulmonic stenosis. Although some of the flow is still coded in blue, there are green and yellow patches, indicating disturbed flow, and red areas suggesting aliasing associated with high-velocity flow.

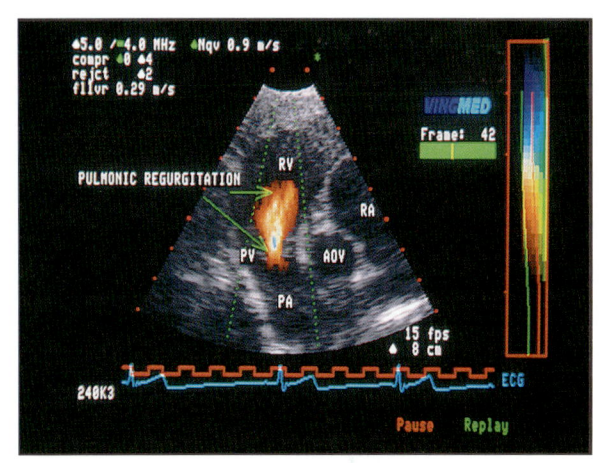

Figure 6.14: Colour-flow Doppler recording from a Labrador with pulmonic stenosis, showing pulmonic regurgitation as a red jet (towards the transducer, into the right ventricle from the valve) during diastole. Valve stenosis is often accompanied by regurgitation, detected by Doppler even in the absence of an audible diastolic murmur.

Flow volume

The velocity–time integral is derived from the area under the spectral Doppler curve (which is a velocity–time graph). If this VTI is multiplied by the cross-sectional area of the vessel or valve from which the Doppler signal is being recorded, stroke volume is estimated, and from which cardiac output can readily be calculated (Bonagura *et al.*, 1990) (Figure 6.11).

Cardiac output tends to fall late in severe cardiac failure, but it can be evaluated by Doppler echocardiography. Careful use of this technique produces results comparable to those gained by thermo-dilution with cardiac catheterization. As the greatest source of error is in the measurement of the cross-sectional area of the vessel from which flow is measured, evaluation of flow can be most useful in non-invasive monitoring of haemodynamic changes due to therapy in an individual animal in which the cross-sectional area should remain relatively constant.

The cardiac output can be assessed from both the ascending aorta and the pulmonic valve, which should normally be equal. In congenital shunts, however, the flow through the two sides of the circulation will not be balanced, and the degree of shunting (shunt ratio) can be derived by comparing pulmonary flow to systemic flow (Qp:Qs). This has proved to be of value in assessing haemodynamic overload in patent ductus arteriosus in dogs (Darke, 1991). In this disease, the flow through the aortic valve is equivalent to pulmonary flow, and flow at the pulmonic valve represents systemic flow.

Colour-flow Doppler is a form of angiogram in which the flow of blood is superimposed on a two-dimensional echocardiographic image. This colour coding of blood flow is composed by the Doppler echocardiograph from pulsed-wave Doppler signals (Weyman, 1994). Flow away from the transducer is usually shown in blue, and flow towards the probe is coded red (Figure 6.12). Velocities are graded by intensity, with the brightest signal demonstrating the highest velocities. Disturbed (turbulent) flow is often portrayed as another colour, typically green or yellow (Figure 6.13). Colour-flow Doppler helps to speed the cardiac examination, as abnormal flow (e.g. valve regurgitation (Figure 6.14) or septal defects) is readily demonstrated, and the visual indication of disturbed flow is invaluable in detecting the origin of cardiac murmurs (Kisslo *et al.*, 1988; Miller and Bonagura, 1989; Darke, 1992; Darke *et al.*, 1996).

REFERENCES

Bonagura JD, Darke PGG, Long K and Haigh AL (1990) Doppler echocardiographic estimation of heart function: comparison with invasive measurements in closed-chest dogs. *Proc 8th ACVIM Forum*, American College of Veterinary Internal Medicine, Blacksburg, Virginia, pp 863–866

Brown DJ, Knight DH and King RR (1991) Use of pulsed-wave Doppler echocardiography to determine aortic and pulmonary velocity and flow variables in clinically normal dogs. *American Journal of Veterinary Research* **52**, 543–550

Currie PJ, Hagler DJ, Seward JB, Reeder GS, Fyfe DA, Bove AA & Tajik AJ (1986) Instantaneous pressure gradient: a simultaneous Doppler and dual catheter correlation study. *Journal of the American College of Cardiology*, **7**, 800–806

Darke PGG (1992) Doppler echocardiography. *Journal of Small Animal Practice* **33**, 104–112

Darke PGG, Bonagura JD and Kelly DF (1996) *Color Atlas of Veterinary Cardiology*. Mosby-Wolfe, London

Darke PGG, Bonagura JD and Miller M (1993) Transducer orientation for Doppler echocardiography in dogs. *Journal of Small Animal Practice* **34**, 2–8

Darke PGG and Luis Fuentes V (1991) Estimation of congenital shunt ratios by Doppler. *Proc 9th Annual ACVIM Forum*, American College of Veterinary Internal Medicine, Blacksburg, Virginia, pp 699–701

Fox PR, Miller MW and Liu S-K (1992) Clinical, echocardiographic and Doppler inaging characteristics of mitral valve stenosis in two dogs. *Journal of the American Veterinary Medical Association* **201**, 1575–1579

Goldberg SJ, Allen HD, Marx GR and Donnerstein RL (1988) *Doppler Echocardiography*, 2nd edn, Lea & Febiger, Philadelphia

Hagan AD and De Maria AN (1989) *Clinical Applications of Two-Dimensional Echocardiography and Cardiac Doppler*, 2nd edn. Little Brown, Boston

Kienle RD and Thomas, WP (1995) Echocardiography. In: *Veterinary Diagnostic Ultrasound*, ed. TG Nyland and JS Mattoon. Saunders, Philadelphia

Kisslo J, Adams DB and Belkin RN (1988) *Doppler Color Flow Imaging*. Churchill Livingstone, New York

Loyer C and Thomas WP (1995) Biplane transesophageal echocardiography in the dog: technique, anatomy and imaging planes. *Veterinary Radiology and Ultrasound* **363**, 212–226

Miller MW and Bonagura JD (1989) Doppler colour-flow imaging. *Proc 7th Annual ACVIM Forum*. American College of Veterinary Internal Medicine, Blacksburg, Virginia, pp 823–829

Moise NS (1988) Echocardiography. In: *Canine and Feline Cardiology*, ed. PR Fox. Churchill Livingstone, New York

Moise NS (1989) Doppler echocardiographic evaluation of congenital heart disease. *Journal of Veterinary Internal Medicine* **3**, 195–207

Thomas, WP (1990) Doppler echocardiographic estimation of pressure gradients in dogs with congenital pulmonic and subaortic stenosis. *Proc 8th Annual ACVIM Forum*. American College of Veterinary Internal Medicine, Blacksburg, Virginia, pp 867–869

Weyman, AE (1994) *Principles and Practice of Echocardiography*, 2nd edn. Lea & Febiger, Philadelphia

(iii) Cardiac Catheterization

Linda Lew and J. David Fowler

Cardiac catheterization is indicated when less invasive methods of demonstrating or evaluating cardiac lesions either are unavailable or have been unsuccessful. Cardiac catheterization involves the placement of catheters into selective chambers and great vessels of the heart for the purposes of determining pressure (manometry), oxygen tension (oximetry) and cardiac output. Selective angiography is performed for anatomical identification and description of cardiac lesions. The goals of cardiac catheterization are to confirm a suspect diagnosis, to evaluate the characteristics and severity of cardiac lesions, and to identify multiple or complicating abnormalities.

CATHETER SELECTION

Cardiac catheters are available with various material, size, shape and construction characteristics (see Figure 6.15). Catheters are generally constructed of polyethylene, polyurethane, Dacron (polyethylene terephthalate) or Teflon (polytetrafluoroethylene). The composition of the catheter affects its shape, stiffness and coefficient of friction. Stiffer catheters are more easily manipulated, but carry a greater risk of inducing trauma. Softer catheters are generally used for right-sided cardiac catheterization, whilst stiffer catheters are used for manipulation into the left ventricle. Cath-

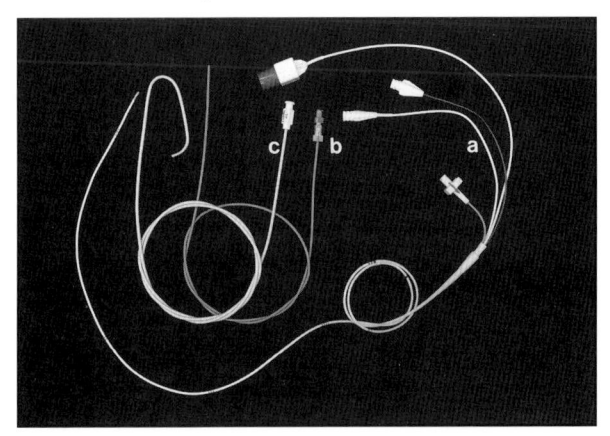

*Figure 6.15: Examples of catheters useful in cardiac catheterization include the Swan–Ganz multilumen catheter (**a**), multiple side-hole catheter (**b**), and moulded or 'gooseneck' end-hole catheter (**c**).*

eters tips may also be moulded into various shapes, varying from straight to curved to pig-tail. Moulded catheters are selected to assist manipulation into specific cardiac structures.

Catheters may be further classified by the position and number of the holes in the catheter. End-hole catheters are best suited for pressure measurements. High pressure injection of contrast material during selective angiography can cause end-hole catheters to recoil, resulting in catheter displacement or endocardial trauma. Side-hole catheters are therefore more appropriate for angiography. In order to obtain the most accurate measurements, the shortest and largest diameter catheter that can be accommodated should be used. Most dogs require 5–8 French catheters; cats and very small dogs may need narrower catheters.

Swan–Ganz catheters are multilumen catheters used primarily for right-sided cardiac catheterization. The catheter contains an inflatable balloon end which facilitates catheter flow-through from the right atrium into the pulmonary artery. Right atrial, right ventricular, pulmonary artery and pulmonary wedge pressures may be attained. Simultaneous blood sampling from multiple levels may be taken for determination of oxygen tensions. Swan–Ganz catheters may also be used for determination of cardiac output using a thermodilution method.

TECHNIQUE

Left-sided cardiac catheterization

Access to the left heart is gained via a peripheral artery, usually the carotid or femoral. Following exposure of the vessel, rubber stents or umbilical tapes are placed around the artery for ease of manipulation and to control haemorrhage. A small transverse arterotomy is performed. The catheter is placed into the arterial lumen with the aid of a catheter introducer and advanced retrograde to the level of the aortic root and left ventricle. Left ventricular systolic and end-diastolic, and aortic systolic, diastolic and mean pressures are recorded. Samples from the left ventricle, aortic root and descending aorta are obtained for blood gas analysis. Angiography may be performed from the level of the left ventricle or aortic root, depending on the specific suspected diagnosis. After completion of catheterization the femoral or carotid artery may be repaired, but is more often ligated with no adverse sequelae.

Right-sided cardiac catheterization

The technique for right-sided catheterization is similar to that for left-sided catheterization. The femoral or jugular vein is generally used for access and the catheter is advanced from the right atrium, through the right ventricle and into the pulmonary artery. Systolic and diastolic pressure determinations are made from the pulmonary artery and right ventricle. Pulmonary wedge pressures may be obtained as an indirect indication of left atrial pressure. Central venous pressure may be determined from the right atrium. Oxygen tensions are obtained from pulmonary artery, right ventricular, right atrial and vena caval blood samples. Right-sided angiography is generally performed from the level of the right ventricle.

GUIDELINES FOR INTERPRETATION

It is beyond the scope of this section to provide detailed interpretation of cardiac catheterization data pertinent to specific cardiac defects. The following principles are intended to assist the reader in understanding the methodology used to interpret cardiac catheterization results. Normal values are provided in Table 6.5.

Pressure measurements

Pressure measurements are used to diagnose and determine the severity of stenotic lesions. Normal values are presented in Table 6.5. Pressures across an opened cardiac valve should be equal. With valvular stenoses, pressures are greater proximal to the lesion than distal to it. An equivalent example would be placing a thumb partially over the end of a garden hose. This results in an increased pressure within the garden hose, and a 'jetting' of water from the hose. The magnitude of the pressure gradient across the

lesion is used to determine the severity of the stenosis. Atrioventricular valvular stenoses are associated with increased diastolic pressure gradients, whereas pulmonic and aortic stenoses are associated with increased peak systolic pressure gradients. Care must be taken in interpreting pressure data, since heart failure, anaesthetic agents and hypovolaemia can decrease transvalvular flow and falsely decrease pressure gradients. Combinations of lesions that reduce transvalvular flow across the stenotic lesion, such as tricuspid regurgitation with pulmonic stenosis, can also diminish pressure gradients. Large left-to-right shunting lesions, such as ventricular septal defects, may falsely increase pulmonic valve gradients because of the excessive blood flow across an otherwise normal valve.

Pulmonary or systemic hypertension is associated with increased systolic and mean pressures in the pulmonary artery or aorta, respectively. Mean pulmonary artery pressure greater than 15 mmHg and systolic pulmonary artery pressure greater than 25 mmHg indicate pulmonary hypertension. Mean aortic pressure greater than 120 mmHg and systolic aortic pressure greater than 150 mmHg occur with systemic hypertension.

Pulmonary wedge pressure is used as an indirect measure of left atrial pressure. Mean right atrial or pulmonary wedge pressure greater than 15 mmHg is seen with right-sided or left-sided heart failure, respectively.

Oximetry

The location and relative severity of shunting lesions are determined with oximetry. In left-to-right shunting lesions, oxygenated blood from the left side of the heart is shunted into the right side of the heart. This may occur at the level of the ventricle in the case of ventricular septal defect, the atrium in atrial septal defect or the great vessels in patent ductus arteriosus. Comparisons of the oxygen tensions in the right and left sides, and above and below the level of the shunt, are used to estimate the relative pulmonic to systemic flow ratio (an indication of the degree of shunting). The formula to determine

Location	Pressure (mmHg) (systolic/diastolic)	Oxygen saturation (%)
Left ventricle	120/0	98
Aorta	120/80	98
Pulmonary wedge pressure	12/6	NA
Pulmonary artery	20/10	75
Right ventricle	20/0	75
Right atrium	5/–1	75
Vena cava	5/–1	75

Table 6.5: Normal pressure and oximetry values from selected cardiac chambers and great vessels.

pulmonic to systemic flow ratio is derived from the Fick principle and is expressed as:

$$\frac{\text{Aorta } O_2 \text{ saturation } - \text{ Vena caval } O_2 \text{ saturation}}{\text{Aorta } O_2 \text{ saturation } - \text{ Pulmonic } O_2 \text{ saturation}}$$

Clinically significant left-to-right shunting lesions are associated with pulmonic to systemic flow ratios greater than 2.5:1.

Right-to-left shunts are associated with the shunting of poorly oxygenated blood from the right side into the oxygenated blood of the left heart. These shunts, therefore, produce a decrease in left-sided oxygen tension downstream from the shunt. Right-to-left shunts occur in the presence of severe pulmonary hypertension and are, therefore, always clinically significant.

Selective angiography

Selective angiography involves the rapid injection of iodinated contrast material into a specific chamber of the heart. Movement of the contrast material, and shape and size of the cardiac chambers and great vessels, is determined through rapid sequential radiographs or videotaping of fluoroscopic images (see Figures 6.16

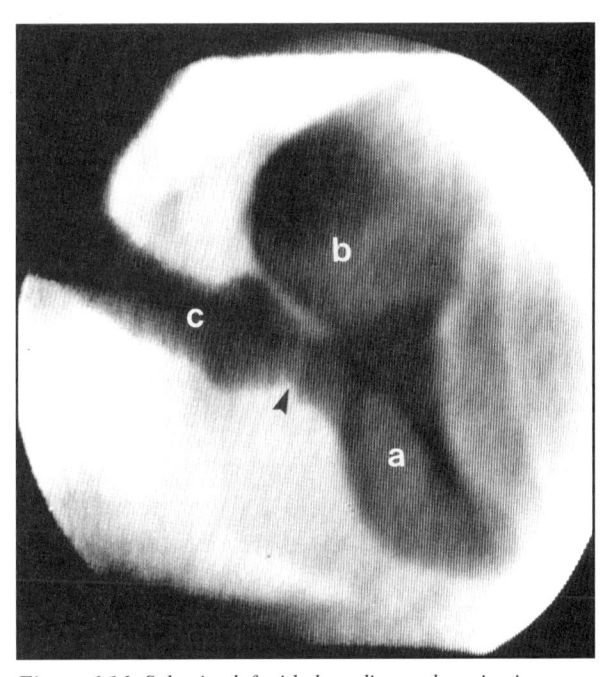

Figure 6.16: *Selective left-sided cardiac catheterization. Contrast material has been injected into the left ventricle. Ejection of contrast from the left ventricle into the aorta is apparent. Congenital mitral valve dysplasia in this dog resulted in retrograde flow of contrast from the left ventricle into the left atrium. Left ventricle (**a**), left atrium (**b**), aorta (**c**), aortic valve (arrow).*

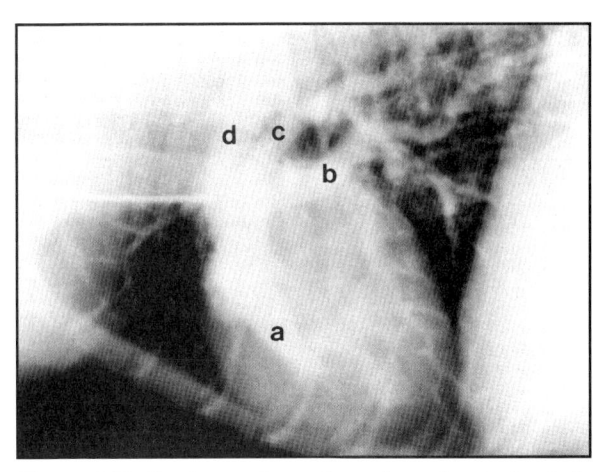

Figure 6.17: *Cardiac angiography performed at the level of the right atrium. Contrast material is being ejected from the right ventricle into the tortuous and dilated pulmonary arteries. Simultaneous filling of the aorta is consistent with a diagnosis of right-to-left shunting patent ductus arteriosus. Right ventricle (**a**), pulmonary arteries (**b,c**), aorta (**d**).*

and 6.17). Angiography provides localization and anatomical description of cardiac defects.

Cardiac output

Cardiac output may be obtained using an indicator dilution technique. The thermodilution technique is relatively safe, accurate and simple and allows repeated measurements over time. Right-sided catheterization is accomplished using a Swan–Ganz multilumen catheter with a thermistor mounted on the catheter tip. A known quantity of cold saline solution is rapidly infused through the catheter into the cranial vena cava or right atrium. The thermistor, positioned in the pulmonary artery, continuously records resultant blood temperature changes which are monitored by a dedicated cardiac output computer and expressed as cardiac output (litres/minute blood flow). Cardiac output may be further converted to a cardiac index (expressed as $l/min/m^2$ body surface area) to facilitate comparison between individuals.

FURTHER READING

Anderson LK (1993) Diagnostic method. In: *Textbook of Small Animal Surgery vol. 1. 2nd edn*, ed. D Slatter, pp.842–856. WBSaunders, Philadelphia

Bonagura JD (1989) Congenital heart disease. In: *Textbook of Veterinary Internal Medicine vol 1. 3rd edn*, ed. SJ Ettinger, pp. 976–1031. WBSaunders, Philadelphia

Fox PR and Bond BR (1983) Nonselective and selective angiocardiography. *Veterinary Clinics of North America: Small Animal Practice* **13**, 259–272

(iv) Pulmonary Function Testing

Brendan C. McKiernan

INTRODUCTION

Changes in respiratory function may be suggested from historical findings (e.g. exercise intolerance), an abnormal physical examination (e.g. increased effort or rate of breathing at rest), and certain radiographic results (e.g. dynamic airway collapse or diaphragmatic flattening). None of these, however, provides an actual functional assessment of the respiratory system. With the exception of arterial blood gas analyses, tests for the functional assessment of the respiratory system have not been clinically available. This chapter will introduce the recent developments towards pulmonary function testing in small animal medicine.

Physiology

The flow of air in and out of the lungs is the result of the difference between atmospheric and alveolar/pleural pressures (ΔPpl). In the healthy resting animal, inspiration is an active process, as muscular work expands the chest wall and diaphragm, creating the pressure difference. At rest, expiration is a passive process, occurring as tissues (lung, chest wall) stretched during inspiration recoil to their resting position at functional residual capacity (FCR). The entire tidal volume of a breath occurs during quiet breathing as the result of generation of ΔPpl of only a few cmH_2O. An increased amount of muscular effort (the 'work of breathing') is required to meet increased tissue demands during exercise or during certain disease conditions. The inspired tidal volume (V_T), the patient's lung compliance (C_L) and airway resistance (R_L), and the air flow rate (V) are all factors which determine the actual pressures (work) required to breathe (Robinson, 1992). The relationship between these parameters and the pressure required for air flow are shown in the following formula (Robinson, 1992):

$$\Delta P\text{pl} = V_T/C_L + R_L V$$

By taking the integral of flow, tidal volume may be obtained. With the aid of pulmonary function computers, and setting one of the two components on the right side of the above equation to 0 (i.e. measure at zero flow or isovolume points), the equation can then be solved for R_L or C_L, i.e.

$$C_L = \Delta V_T/\Delta P\text{pl}, \text{ when } \Delta V \text{ is } = 0$$
$$R_L = \Delta P\text{pl}/\Delta V, \text{ when } \Delta V_T \text{ is } = 0$$

The reader is referred to West (1990) and Robinson (1992) for a more detailed discussion of the physiology behind pulmonary function testing.

Respiratory diseases precipitate changes either in C_L (usually making the lung stiffer and less easily inflated; decreased C_L), or in R_L (by narrowing the airways; increased R_L). Changes in these parameters alter the strategy an animal uses to breathe (minimizing the energy cost of breathing), and results in the classical obstructive and restrictive breathing patterns which we recognize clinically. It is now possible to obtain measurements of pleural pressure (indirectly with an oesophageal balloon) and air flow (with a pneumotachograph) relatively easily, and derive the classical pulmonary mechanics measurements of R_L and C_L.

PULMONARY FUNCTION TESTS

Functional assessment of the respiratory system may involve measurements of gas exchange (blood gas analyses), of airway obstruction (tidal breathing flow–volume loops, lung resistance), and/or the elastic recoil or stiffness of the lung (lung compliance). Some of these tests may be performed in the awake patient, others require general anaesthesia.

Arterial blood gas analysis

The measurement of the partial pressure of oxygen and carbon dioxide in arterial blood was the first pulmonary function test used on a routine basis in clinical veterinary medicine. Although the equipment required for blood gas measurements is moderately expensive, samples may be kept on ice and analysed at a human hospital or reference laboratory hours after collection. Solid state, portable blood gas analysis machines have recently been developed which have enabled routine blood gas analysis to be performed at many veterinary hospitals. Arterial blood gas analysis provides a simple and easy method of quantifying the adequacy of alveolar ventilation (via $PaCO_2$), oxygenation (via PaO_2)

and the overall efficiency of gas exchange in the lung (via the difference between alveolar and arterial PO_2, DA-aO_2) (refer to Chapters 2 and 6(i) for a more thorough discussion).

Tidal breathing flow–volume loop analysis

Flow–volume curves (loops), and especially the maximal or forced flow–volume manoeuvre, have been an important component of human pulmonary function testing since the 1950s. Measurements of forced vital capacity (FVC), forced expiratory volume during the first second (FEV_1) and various flow rates during expiration (e.g. the average flow during the middle portion of expiration, $FEF_{25-75\%}$) are routinely measured and are good indicators of lung disease (West, 1990). Similar 'forced' manoeuvres are only possible in dogs and cats on a research basis, as general anaesthesia and externally generated airway pressures are required (negative pressure to the airway or positive pressure to the chest wall), techniques which preclude routine clinical cases (Robinson, 1992).

Following reports of tidal breathing flow volume loop (TBFVL) analysis in infants, the use of this technique was reported in conscious dogs in the detection of airway obstruction (Amis and Kurpershoek, 1986a). The technique has since been computerized for easy and rapid clinical application in dogs and cats (McKiernan and Jones, 1987; McKiernan and Johnson, 1992). Using the criteria established for normals in dogs and cats, TBFVLs are beginning to be used in university settings for the detection of obstructive airway diseases. The TBFVL technique is performed in the conscious animal with a face mask, pneumotachograph, and a differential pressure transducer (Figure 6.18). Signals sent to a pulmonary function computer are processed by respiratory loop analysis software for loop analysis and plotting. Normal values (Table 6.6) have been published for dogs and cats (Amis and Kurpershoek, 1986a; McKiernan *et al.*, 1993). Changes in TBFVL indices, as well as overall loop shape, are

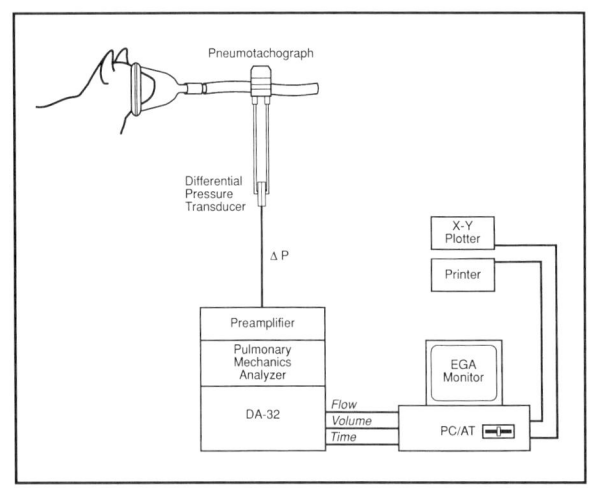

Figure 6.18: *Diagram of the laboratory set up used to obtain tidal breathing flow–volume loops in conscious cats.*

From McKiernan et al., 1993, with permission.

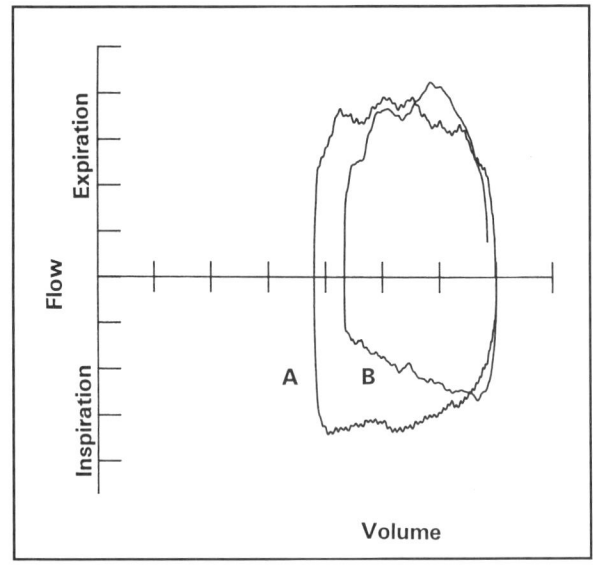

Figure 6.19: *Example of tidal breathing flow–volume loops (TBFVL) obtained from a healthy dog (A) and a dog with laryngeal paralysis (B). Note the reversal of inspiratory flow in the dog with laryngeal paralysis, when flow decreases as the arytenoid cartilages are abducted during a forceful inspiration.*

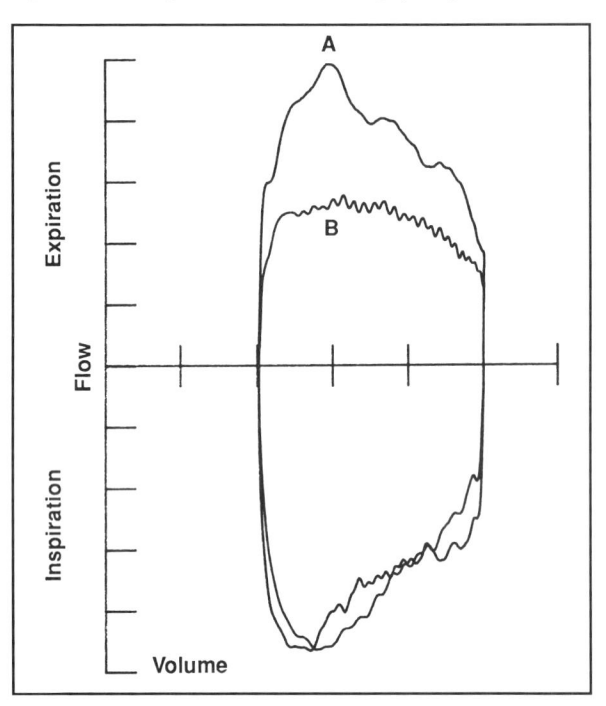

Figure 6.20: *Example of tidal breathing flow–volume loops obtained from a healthy cat (A) and a cat with chronic bronchitis (B). Note the decrease in the amplitude of the expiratory flow loop in the bronchitic cat. Expiratory time was also prolonged in the bronchitic cat but is not depicted on these axes.*

From McKiernan et al., 1993, with permission.

used to determine the type and location of obstructive lesions (Amis *et al.*, 1986b; Robinson, 1992; McKiernan *et al.*, 1993). TBFVL are capable of detecting functional changes in both upper and lower airways, and have been used clinically in the diagnosis and treatment of various obstructive airway diseases (Amis *et al.*, 1986b; Smith *et al.*, 1986; Padrid *et al.*, 1990; McKiernan *et al.*, 1993) (Figures 6.19 and 6.20).

Reference	Amis and Kurpershoek, 1986a	Amis et al., 1986b	Amis et al., 1986b	McKiernan et al., 1993	McKiernan et al., 1993
Species	Dog	Dog	Dog	Cat	Cat
Diagnosis	Clinically healthy	Type II paralysis, Non-fixed obstruction	Type III paralysis, fixed obstruction	Clinically healthy	Chronic bronchitis
(n)	33	17	10	19	7
Tidal volume V_T (ml)	460 ± 180	0.55 ± 0.16	480 ± 190	57.9 ± 15.4	46.0 ± 4.0
Peak expiratory flow PEF (ml/s)	780 ± 230	1000 ± 290 *	790 ± 350	113.7 ± 29.1	79.8 ± 19.8 *
Peak inspiratory flow PIF (ml/s)	740 ± 240	800 ± 280	830 ± 320	110.9 ± 26.6	103.4 ± 26.1
PEF/PIF	1.07 ± 0.13	1.33 ± 0.52	0.94 ± 0.17 *	1.04 ± 0.18	0.78 ± 0.10 *
Expiratory flow at 50% V_T EF_{50} (ml/s)	590 ± 210	810 ± 280 *	720 ± 360	104.4 ± 27.6	70.5 ± 19.4 *
Inspiratory flow at 50% V_T IF_{50} (ml/s)	680 ± 220	690 ± 240	760 ± 320	91.7 ± 22.3	85.3 ± 18.4
EF_{50}/IF_{50}	0.88 ± 0.16	1.25 ± 0.52	0.93 ± 0.22	1.16 ± 0.22	0.82 ± 0.10 *
Expiratory flow at 25% V_T EF_{25} (ml/s)	440 ± 180	600 ± 250 *	610 ± 320	86.3 ± 26.5	61.4 ± 21.7 *
Inspiratory flow at 25% V_T IF_{25} (ml/s)	590 ± 200	720 ± 280	700 ± 280	82.4 ± 19.8	75.4 ± 17.3
EF_{25}/IF_{25}	0.74 ± 0.18	870 ± 290	870 ± 300	1.06 ± 0.19	0.81 ± 0.17 *
Time in expiration T_E (ms)	1170 ± 480	1100 ± 470	960 ± 470	703.7 ± 133	800.1 ± 68.6
Time in inspiration T_I (ms)	920 ± 350	1060 ± 450	820 ± 270	716.6 ± 139.5	614.0 ± 71.1
T_E/T_I	1.26 ± 0.26	1.07 ± 0.33 *	1.14 ± 0.30	1.00 ± 0.15	1.31 ± 0.14 *
Respiratory rate RR (bpm)	32.2 ± 10.3	32.5 ± 14.2	39.2 ± 15.5	43.3 ± 7.1	42.1 ± 4
PEF/EF_{50}	1.35 ± 0.19	1.27 ± 0.17	1.14 ± 0.11 *	1.10 ± 0.06	1.14 ± 0.09
PEF/EF_{25}	1.89 ± 0.45	1.82 ± 0.45	1.37 ± 0.30 *	1.35 ± 0.17	1.35 ± 0.21
EF_{50}/EF_{25}	1.4 ± 0.26	1.41 ± 0.81	1.20 ± 0.16 *	1.23 ± 0.11	1.19 ± 0.17
PIF/IF_{50}	1.09 ± 0.05	1.16 ± 0.16	1.10 ± 0.08	NR	NR
PIF/IF_{25}	1.26 ± 0.14	1.14 ± 0.10 *	1.18 ± 0.08	1.38 ± 0.23	1.37 ± 0.16
IF_{50}/IF_{25}	1.16 ± 0.11	0.99 ± 0.12 *	1.08 ± 0.11	1.12 ± 0.08	1.14 ± 0.09
Expiratory volume at 0.1 s into expiration $TBEV_{0.1}$ (ml)	NR	NR	NR	6.3 ± 2.3	3.7 ± 1.5 *
Expiratory volume at 0.5 s into expiration $TBEV_{0.5}$ (ml)	NR	NR	NR	44.8 ± 12.2	29.5 ± 9.0 *

Table 6.6: *Selected tidal breathing flow–volume loop (TBFVL) indices from healthy dogs and cats; from dogs either with type II or type III laryngeal paralysis; and from cats with chronic bronchitis. NR - not reported. (n) - number of animals in study; * - significantly different (P ≤ 0.05) from values obtained for healthy dogs or cats, respectively.*

Airway mechanics

Measurements of R_L and C_L have been obtained from dogs and cats in the research laboratory for decades. Unfortunately the techniques employed relied upon surgical (e.g. tracheostomy, pleural space cannulation) and/or anaesthetic protocols which are not acceptable for use with clinical patients. In most instances, measurement of airway mechanics is done in the anaesthetized patient, because of the need to pass an oesophageal balloon to obtain a measurement of Ppl (McKiernan and Johnson, 1992). In intubated patients, measurements obtained are a reflection of the resistance and compliance of the lower respiratory tract (Robinson, 1992). By using a face mask and measuring the tracheal–atmospheric ΔPpl, the R_L of the upper airway has been determined in conscious dogs (Rozanski et al., 1994).

Airway resistance

Bronchitic cats are often briefly anaesthetized and intubated to obtain culture and cytology by transtracheal wash. We have utilized the same short-acting anaesthetic protocol to also collect data for pulmonary mechanics measurements. The protocol used involves light general anaesthesia, intubation with a sterile, standard diameter/length endotracheal tube, and passage of a paediatric oesophageal balloon into the caudal thoracic oesophagus. Following connection to differential pressure transducers, signals are processed by a pulmonary function computer and measurements of resistance and compliance calculated. Normal values (mean ± SE) for R_L (30.6 ± 0.56 cmH$_2$O/ml/s) and dynamic lung compliance (C_{dyn}) (16.8 ± 0.72 ml/cmH$_2$O) have been reported for cats using this technique (McKiernan et al., 1989). This procedure has enabled measurements of R_L and C_{dyn} in clinical cases of feline bronchitis which, for the first time, has allowed quantification of bronchodilator efficacy in clinical patients (Figure 6.21) (McKiernan and Johnson, 1992; Dye et al., 1996).

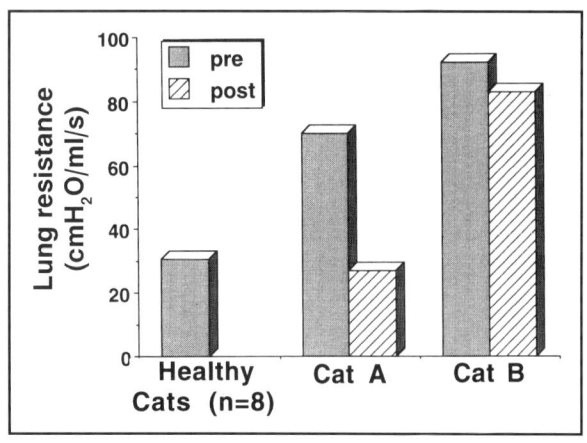

Figure 6.21: Demonstration of the immediate efficacy of intravenous terbutaline (0.01 mg/kg) as measured by lung resistance (R$_L$) in two cats diagnosed with chronic bronchial disease. Although there were no substantial differences between cat A and cat B (on history, physical or radiographic examination) there is a marked difference in their response to bronchodilator therapy. The mean R$_L$ obtained in healthy cats is shown for comparison. (From McKiernan and Johnson, 1992, with permission).

Compliance

Compliance may be measured either on a breath-to-breath basis (dynamic lung compliance, C_{dyn}) or under steady state (static) conditions which allow enough time for the volume in all lung regions to equilibrate (C_{stat}). If the inspiratory and/or expiratory breath time is inadequate for volume changes to occur fully (e.g. into and out of partially obstructed regions), the resulting measurement of C_L will be affected, and is why C_{dyn} is said to be frequency dependent. Changes in C_{dyn} reflect diseases of small airway as well as changes in tissue elasticity. C_{stat}, measured during periods of zero flow and after allowing sufficient time for equilibration to occur, is thought to be a more accurate reflection of changes in the actual elastic properties of the lung tissue (King *et al.*, 1991; Robinson, 1992). The technique has been reported to be of value in detecting changes in lung compliance of dogs in the critical care setting (King *et al.*, 1991). This technique can be easily performed in the clinical setting with only minimal equipment requirements. Differences in lung compliance are noted between dogs of varying sizes (King *et al.*, 1991; Robinson, 1992). King attempted to standardize the compliance measurement obtained by reporting a mean (±SD) body weight-adjusted thoracic compliance value for dogs of 1.85 ± 0.56 ml/cmH$_2$O per kg. Four of seven dogs with respiratory diseases had a mean compliance ≥2 SD below this value. In the clinical and research settings, dynamic lung compliance is the measurement most often obtained. The mean value (±SE) for C_{dyn} in healthy cats has been reported to be 16.8 ± 0.72 ml/cmH$_2$O (McKiernan *et al.*, 1989).

Clinical applications

Articles pertaining to pulmonary function tests in small animals are beginning to appear in the literature. Arterial blood gas analysis is a technique which is readily available to the practitioner. PaO_2, $PaCO_2$ and the $DA-aO_2$ are sensitive tests of overall lung function. Both TBFVL and pulmonary mechanics are being performed at selected speciality facilities on clinical patients. We have noted changes in either C_{dyn} or R_L (or both) in the clinical cases of feline chronic bronchitis on which we have performed these tests. The value of these tests is in the ability to quantify changes in lung function, hopefully with the objective of understanding the pathophysiology of disease processes and the efficacy of various medical and surgical treatments of respiratory tract diseases in dogs and cats. Like any new diagnostic modality, the future of these procedures in veterinary clinical practice remains to be determined.

REFERENCES

Amis TC and Kurpershoek C (1986a).Tidal breathing flow-volume loop analysis for clinical assessment of airway obstruction in conscious dogs. *American Journal of Veterinary Research*, **47**, 1002

Amis T C, Smith MM, Gaber CE and Kurpershoek C (1986b) Upper airway obstruction in canine laryngeal paralysis. *American Journal of Veterinary Research*, **47**, 1007

Dye JA, McKiernan BC, Rozanski EA, Hoffmann WE, Losonsky JM, Homco LD, Weisiger RM and Kakoma I (1996) Bronchopulmonary disease in the cat. Historical, physical, radiographic, clinicopathologic and pulmonary function evaluation of 24 diseased and 15 healthy cats. *Journal of Veterinary Internal Medicine*, **10**, 385–400

King LL, Drobatz KJ and Hendricks JA (1991) Static thoracic compliance as a measurement of pulmonary function in dogs. *American Journal of Veterinary Research*, **52**, 1597

McKiernan BC and Johnson LR (1992) Clinical pulmonary function testing in dogs and cats. *Veterinary Clinics of North America*, **22**, 1087–1099

McKiernan BC and Jones SD (1987) Computerized flow-volume loop acquisition in the dog. *Proceedings of the 6th Veterinary Respiratory Symposium*, p. 28. Chicago, IL

McKiernan BC, Dye JA, Rozanski EA, Jones SD and Hayes B (1989). Lung resistance and dynamic compliance in normal cats. *Proceedings of the 8th Veterinary Respiratory Symposium*, p. 24. Liège, Belgium

McKiernan BC, Dye JA and Rozanski EA (1993) Tidal breathing flow-volume loops in healthy and bronchitic cats. *Journal of Veterinary Internal Medicine*, 7, 388–393

Padrid PA, Hornof WJ, Kurpershoek CJ and Cross CE (1990) Canine chronic bronchitis. *Journal of Veterinary Internal Medicine*, **4**, 172

Robinson NE (1992) Airway physiology. *Veterinary Clinics of North America*, **22**, 1043

Rozanski EA, Greenfield CL, Alsup JC, McKiernan BC and Hungerford LL (1994) Measurement of upper airway resistance in awake untrained dolichocephalic and mesaticephalic dogs. *American Journal of Veterinary Research*, **55**, 1055

Smith MM, Gourley IA, Kurpershoek C and Amis TC (1986) Evaluation of a modified castellated laryngofissure for alleviation of upper airway obstruction in dogs with laryngeal paralysis. *Journal of the American Veterinary Medical Association*, **188**, 1279

West JB (1990) Tests of pulmonary function. In: *Respiratory Physiology*, 4th edn. Williams and Wilkins, Baltimore.

PART TWO

Clinical Problems

Differential Diagnosis of Dyspnoea

Virginia Luis Fuentes

INTRODUCTION

Respiratory patterns are frequently disturbed in cardiopulmonary disease. 'Breathing problems' may be the primary reason for presentation, although owners are often surprisingly unobservant of respiratory difficulties compared with more obvious clinical signs such as coughing, inappetence or exercise intolerance. Dyspnoea nearly always represents significant disease, and a dyspnoeic animal always merits closer inspection.

DEFINITIONS

Dyspnoea is a term derived from the Greek words *dys* (painful or difficult) and *pnoia* (breathing). In human medicine it is generally taken to mean the subjective sensation of 'shortness of breath' that may be experienced by patients with respiratory disease, or healthy individuals following exertion. In humans, dyspnoea is considered to be a symptom analogous to pain, and is therefore different from objective terms such as tachypnoea or cyanosis. Severity of dyspnoea in humans may correlate poorly with the degree of physiological impairment. This makes dyspnoea a difficult concept to apply to animals. Nevertheless, animals undoubtedly experience dyspnoea, just as they do pain. In the same way, we are faced with similar difficulties in assessing dyspnoea in animals as those found in the assessment of pain. We can overcome some of these problems by using objective measurements such as respiratory rate, arterial blood gas measurement or oxyhaemoglobin saturation.

Tachypnoea is another term frequently used in the description of breathing abnormalities, and means an increase in respiratory rate.

Hyperpnoea is often taken to mean increased depth of respiration, although it is sometimes used to describe any laboured breathing.

Orthopnoea is a state where the animal adopts an unusual posture to assist ventilation; dogs are often reluctant to lie down, and will stand with their elbows abducted to facilitate chest excursion.

MECHANISMS OF DYSPNOEA

The neurophysiological mechanisms underlying dyspnoea are poorly understood. In humans, an increase in ventilation will result in the sensation of dyspnoea in both normal subjects and patients with respiratory disease, although the onset of dyspnoea occurs with much lower levels of ventilation in the abnormal individuals. Chemoreceptor input is one of the factors influencing ventilatory drive, and dyspnoea has been recorded in paralysed human patients with fixed mechanical ventilation when levels of inspired CO_2 were increased (Banzett *et al.*, 1989). Increased respiratory muscle work and respiratory muscle fatigue will also result in a sensation of dyspnoea. This may be mediated by increased efferent traffic to respiratory muscles, or by afferent activity from respiratory muscle receptors. There is also a psychological component, and in humans the perception of the severity of dyspnoea may be influenced by fear, or experience.

The different causes of dyspnoea can be subdivided according to the type of stimulus, although there is usually some overlap.

Mechanical interference with ventilation can cause hypoxia. The interference to ventilation may be caused by airway obstruction (e.g. laryngeal paralysis), or 'restrictive' lung disease, where the lungs may be stiffer than normal (e.g. pulmonary oedema). Chest wall abnormalities may also limit chest expansion (e.g. pectus excavatum), restricting the magnitude of ventilation that can be achieved.

Weakness of the respiratory muscles may not cause dyspnoea at rest, but early onset of respiratory muscle fatigue may result in dyspnoea with minimal exertion (e.g. with neuromuscular disorders). The respiratory muscles may become inefficient with large pleural effusions if the chest is distended; the intercostal muscles will be positioned abnormally and will not be operating at optimum mechanical efficiency. This may be sufficient in itself to cause dyspnoea, even without any direct factors associated with the pleural effusion, such as hypoxia resulting from the restriction of ventilation.

Increased respiratory drive is often associated with metabolic disturbances, such as metabolic acidosis or anaemias.

Wasted ventilation such as with pulmonary thromboembolism mainly causes dyspnoea via the hypoxia that results.

APPROACH TO THE INVESTIGATION OF THE DYSPNOEIC ANIMAL

The dyspnoeic patient requires extremely gentle handling. Dyspnoeic cats and dogs may be critically hypoxaemic even at rest, and any restraint that results in struggling may be fatal. Nevertheless, with acutely dyspnoeic animals it is necessary to carry out a rapid but accurate assessment in order to institute corrective measures as quickly as possible. There are many causes of dyspnoea, and appropriate treatment usually requires an accurate diagnosis.

The first priority must be to ensure adequate oxygenation. Administering oxygen may be counterproductive if it results in undue stress to the patient. Non-stressful methods include oxygen cages, or administering oxygen via a transparent plastic bag over the animal's head (see Chapter 20). Sometimes a few minutes of cage rest without handling will help by reducing oxygen demand.

In some circumstances, oxygen administration will fail to relieve clinical signs unless the underlying cause is also addressed (e.g. draining a pleural effusion).

Obtaining a few details about the animal's history, assessing the animal's respiratory patterns, and palpating, auscultating and percussing the chest may allow recognition of the type of respiratory problem present and allow the condition to be specifically treated. In many situations, radiography will be necessary to narrow the list of differential diagnoses, but great care must be taken when carrying out this procedure in dyspnoeic animals. Sedation should be avoided if possible, as this may further reduce respiratory reserve, however psychological stress may be just as dangerous. In a proportion of animals, the cause of dyspnoea may remain unclear after these measures, and further investigations may still be required.

Potential causes of dyspnoea are listed in Table 7.1.

History

- Was the onset gradual or sudden?
  Chronic causes of dyspnoea may result in gradual or progressive signs (e.g. pulmonary fibrosis), a sudden onset (pneumothorax, pulmonary thromboembolism), or intermittent signs (feline asthma, excitement with laryngeal paralysis).
- Is coughing also present?
  Coughing and dyspnoea may be present with

Pathophysiological problem	Categories	Key features	Examples	Specific features
Mechanical interference with ventilation	Airway obstruction	↑ Respiratory noise	Brachycephalic obstruction syndrome Laryngeal paralysis Feline asthma Bronchitis	Characteristic breed Dysphonia ± Coughing ± Coughing
	Resistance to lung expansion	↑ Respiratory rate	Pulmonary oedema Interstitial fibrosis Pleural disease	± Crackles, cardiac signs Older WHW terriers Dullness on percussion
	Resistance to expansion of chest wall	↑ Respiratory rate	Obesity Abdominal masses Ascites	
Weakness of the respiratory pump	Absolute		Neuromuscular diseases	Concurrent neurological signs
	Relative – pleural disease (muscles at a relative disadvantage)	'Barrel'-shaped chest Heart sounds may be muffled	Pleural effusion Pneumothorax Hyperinflation	Dullness on percussion Hyper-resonance
Increased respiratory drive	Metabolic acidosis	Concurrent disease	Diabetic ketoacidosis	Ketones in urine
	↓ effective haemoglobin	Change in mucous membrane colour	Anaemia Right-to-left cardiac shunts Methaemaglobinaemia	Pale mucous membranes Cyanosis 'Chocolate'-coloured mucous membranes
Wasted ventilation			Pulmonary thromboembolism	Suggestive concurrent systemic disease
Psychological			Anxiety, pain	

Table 7.1: Causes of dyspnoea. WHW = West Highland White.

tracheal collapse, congestive heart failure, pneumonia, pulmonary infiltration with eosinophils (dogs), and with feline asthma and mediastinal masses.
- Is respiratory noise present?
Respiratory noise is often associated with airway obstruction. Inspiratory noise is usually caused by upper airway obstruction, whereas expiratory noise occurs with intra-thoracic airway obstruction.

The owner should be questioned to make sure any intermittent bouts of respiratory noise are not episodes of reverse sneezing, which may be seen in normal dogs as well as in dogs with pharyngeal problems. These episodes usually only last for a few minutes, and the animal is usually normal before and immediately following the 'attack'. The owner may describe choking or gasping noises, and the episode can often be terminated by distracting or comforting the animal. Reverse sneezing is not normally associated with cyanosis or syncope.

- Is the animal depressed or systemically ill?
Animals with bacterial pneumonia may be dull and inappetent. Dogs with abnormal respiration secondary to diabetic ketoacidosis may have a history of polydipsia with recent inappetence and vomiting.
- Is there a history of regurgitation?
Megaoesophagus and swallowing difficulties should alert the clinician to the possibility of aspiration pneumonia.

Physical examination
Observation of the animal's breathing patterns can provide invaluable information about the underlying cause.

Respiratory patterns

- Increased respiratory rate (tachypnoea) is often associated with resistance to lung expansion. This may be because the lungs are 'stiff' (pulmonary oedema, interstitial fibrosis), because of pleural disease (effusions, pneumothorax), or because of restriction of chest wall movement (obesity, ascites, abdominal masses)
- Increased respiratory effort and increased respiratory noise may be associated with airway obstruction. The timing of the noise may provide a clue as to the site of obstruction. These noises may be clearly audible without a stethoscope
- Inspiratory noise (stridor or stertor) tends to be associated with upper airway obstruction (stenotic nares, elongated soft palate, laryngeal paralysis)
- Expiratory noises (wheezes) are more likely with lower airway obstruction (feline asthma).

Palpation of the chest

- 'Barrel'-shaped chests may be suggestive of a large pleural effusion, pneumothorax or hyperinflation (feline asthma)
- An incompressible cranial chest may be found with mediastinal masses
- Displacement of the apex beat may occur with right ventricular enlargement, right lung lobe collapse, or pulmonary masses
- Precordial cardiac thrills or arrhythmias may be detected with cardiac disease.

Respiratory system
Auscultation should not just be restricted to the chest, but should include the upper airways. Upper airway noise is often referred to the chest. Respiratory sounds can be classified according to their character:

- Normal breath sounds are the sounds heard in normal animals (sometimes called 'bronchovesicular' sounds)
- Wheezes may be heard in association with narrowing of small airways. This may be a result of bronchoconstriction, or mucus occluding airways (feline asthma, chronic bronchitis)
- Crackles are inspiratory sounds heard with closure of small airways (interstitial fibrosis) or when air flows through secretions (severe pulmonary oedema)
- Rhonchi are loud, low pitched sounds emanating from large airways and are often associated with increased respiratory rate and effort. Stridor and stertor are the sounds generated in the larynx and nasal passages respectively.

Thoracic percussion

- Ventral dullness often indicates a pleural effusion
- Localized dullness suggests a mass lesion, or an area of consolidation.

Cardiovascular system

- Murmurs and gallop sounds may indicate a possible cardiac cause for dyspnoea; however, it is possible for compensated cardiac disease to coexist with respiratory disease (e.g. acquired mitral valve disease and chronic bronchitis).
- Heart rate and rhythm can help to identify signs of congestive heart failure. Generally cardiac disease causes dyspnoea as a result of congestive heart failure: this will usually be accompanied by tachycardia in dogs (although less reliably in cats). The presence of sinus arrhythmia in dogs may suggest a non-cardiac cause of dyspnoea.

Upper airway/tracheal obstruction (key features: *respiratory noise, increased respiratory effort*)

Condition	History	Physical examination	Radiography	Further tests
Brachycephalic syndrome	Characteristic breed: stertor, stridor, from early age. Acute exacerbations	± Stenotic nares, marked upper airway noise	± Elongated soft palate, hypoplastic trachea	Examination under GA
Pharyngeal masses	Stertor, halitosis, difficulty swallowing, gagging	Mass may be visible on inspection	Mass may be visible on radiographs	Examination under GA/ biopsy
Laryngeal paralysis	Labradors, Setters; dysphonia, progressive with acute exacerbations	Inspiratory stridor, worsens on constriction of larynx	Usually unhelpful	Examination under GA
Tracheal collapse	Toy breeds, ↑ respiratory noise history of 'goose-honk' cough	Flattened trachea on palpation	Narrowed OR widened trachea	Bronchoscopy, fluoroscopy
Tracheal foreign body	Sudden onset	↑ Respiratory effort and noise	FB may be visible if radiopaque	Bronchoscopy
Tracheal masses	↑ Respiratory noise young kennelled dog (*Oslerus osleri*)	↑ Inspiratory and expiratory noises audible over trachea	Mass(es) may be visible on plain radiography	Bronchoscopy, tracheal cytology/biopsy

Lower airway disease (key features: *wheezing, expiratory effort*)

Condition	History	Physical examination	Radiography	Further tests
Chronic bronchitis	Terrier breeds, coughing,	Wheezes/ crackles may be audible	↑ Bronchial markings, (interstitial pattern)	Bronchoscopy, bronchial cytology
Feline asthma	± Coughing, paroxysmal attacks	Wheezes/ crackles ± barrel-shaped chest (hyperinflation)	Increased bronchial markings ± air-trapping	Bronchial cytology
Smoke inhalation	History of exposure	External burns, tachypnoea and crackles/ wheezes	Generalized mixed bronchial/interstitial/ alveolar patterns	CoHb estimation

Pulmonary parenchymal disease (key feature: *increased respiratory rate*)

Condition	History	Physical examination	Radiography	Further tests
Chronic pulmonary interstitial disease	Terrier breeds (West Highland White), progressive course, ± coughing	Loud coarse crackles, ↑ respiratory effort	↑ Interstitial markings, ± bronchial pattern	Bronchoscopy, biopsy
Cardiogenic pulmonary oedema	± Coughing/exercise intolerance/syncope. May cough frothy oedema fluid if severe	Murmurs, arrhythmias, gallop sounds tachypnoea ± crackles	Cardiac enlargement, especially left atrium interstitial/alveolar pattern distended pulmonary veins	ECG, echocardiography
Non-cardiogenic pulmonary oedema	Sudden onset. May cough frothy oedema fluid. Concurrent systemic disease/ trauma (electrocution)	Tachypnoea ± crackles	Alveolar pattern, normal cardiac silhouette	Echocardiography, bronchial cytology to rule out other causes
Severe bacterial pneumonia	Dullness, inappetence; soft, productive cough ± History of regurgitation	Pyrexia, localized/ventral dullness on percussion	Alveolar pattern often in dependent lobes, ± ↑ bronchial markings ± megaoesophagus	Tracheal/bronchial cytology/culture
Pulmonary infiltrates with eosinophils	± Coughing	Tachypnoea, crackles may be present	Variable bronchial/ interstitial pattern	Bronchoscopy, cytology, routine haematology
Intra-pulmonary haemorrhage	Soft cough, ± haemoptysis ± history of trauma/ingestion of rodenticides	Tachypnoea, ± signs of bleeding elsewhere	Patchy alveolar distribution	Clotting tests
Pulmonary neoplasia	Dyspnoea less common – usually history of coughing, haemoptysis, progressive course ± weight loss	Localized dullness on percussion, ± end-expiratory 'snap' if dynamic airway compression	Localized consolidation, mediastinal shift	Bronchoscopy, ultrasound, cytology from wash/fine needle aspirate/biopsy
Pulmonary thromboembolism	Sudden onset concurrent predisposing illness (hyperadrenocorticism, AIHA, etc)	Tachypnoea	Variable, from no significant changes to localized alveolar patterns	Pulmonary angiography
Near-drowning	History of drowning	Tachypnoea, crackles	Alveolar pattern	

Table 7.2: Differential diagnosis of dyspnoea.

Pleural diseases (key features: *distended chest* if severe, *increased respiratory effort*)

Condition	History	Physical examination	Radiography	Further tests
Pneumothorax	± History of trauma sudden onset	Hyper-resonance dorsally on percussion decreased breath sounds, cardiac sounds	Retraction of lung lobes, increased lucency of periphery with absence of vascular markings	Thoracocentesis
Pleural effusions	Often relatively sudden onset	Loud breath sounds dorsally, muffled ventrally	Retraction of lung lobes with interlobar fissures	Fluid analysis, repeat radiography post-thoracocentesis, ultrasound
Ruptured diaphragm	± History of trauma	± Muffled heart sounds, empty abdomen	Loss of diaphragmatic line, displacement of abdominal viscera, gas-filled loops in thorax	Barium studies
Mediastinal masses	± Regurgitation, ± Horner's syndrome	Incompressible cranial chest, ventral dullness on percussion if pleural effusion	Displacement of trachea/heart, widening of mediastinum, ± pleural fluid	Ultrasound, cytology/fine needle aspirate/biopsy

Extra-thoracic causes (key features: *normal thoracic radiographs*)

Condition	History	Physical examination	Radiography	Further tests
Anaemia	Weakness, exercise intolerance	Pale mucous membranes, ± haemic murmur, bounding pulse	Not usually helpful	Haematology
Right-to-left shunts	Exercise intolerance	Cyanosis, ± murmur	Under-perfused lung fields ± cardiac enlargement	Echocardiography, haematology
Metabolic acidosis	Concurrent disease, e.g. ketoacidosis, renal failure	Tachypnoea/panting	Not helpful	Biochemistry, urinalysis, acid base status
Heatstroke	Previously in hot car/exertion in heat	Tachypnoea, rectal temperature >105°F	Not helpful	
Fear, pain	Suggestive history	Tachypnoea		

AIHA = autoimmune haemolytic anaemia, COHb = carboxyhaemoglobin, GA = general anaesthesia

Table 7.2 continued: Differential diagnosis of dyspnoea.

Ancillary tests

Radiography
As can be seen from Table 7.2, radiography is diagnostically useful with many causes of dyspnoea. This subject is covered more fully in Chapter 5(i).

Blood gas analysis
Blood gas analysis can help to characterize the type and severity of functional impairment caused by respiratory disease by measuring arterial oxygen tension (see Chapter 6i). It can also be useful in identifying metabolic causes of 'dyspnoea', where increased respiratory drive results from non-respiratory disease, e.g. metabolic acidosis.

Haematology
Significant right-to-left cardiac shunts are usually accompanied by polycythaemia; anaemias will also be confirmed by haematology. Dogs with infiltrates with eosinophils will sometimes also have a peripheral eosinophilia (see Chapter 5ii).

Biochemistry
Uncontrolled diabetes mellitus may progress to ketoacidosis, which may result in apparent breathing difficulties together with other causes of metabolic acidosis.

Bronchoscopy
Bronchoscopy may allow some respiratory tract abnormalities to be directly visualized, and is also one of the most effective ways to gain cytological material from the lower airways (see Chapter 5).

Electrocardiography
Whilst an ECG may be invaluable for the identification of arrhythmias, it is rarely of much use for identifying the cause of dyspnoea. If an arrhythmia is present, this will often be detected on physical examination. Arrhythmias rarely cause dyspnoea in the absence of congestive heart failure, which is more readily detected by radiography.

Echocardiography
Echocardiography is indicated where cardiac disease is suspected, in order to make a specific diagnosis. However, radiography may be preferable for identifying congestive heart failure as a cause of dyspnoea, and a specific diagnosis may not be required until the congestive cardiac signs have been treated.

Sometimes echocardiography is less stressful than radiography for a dyspnoeic animal, particularly when the animal is allowed to adopt its own favoured position. Left atrial enlargement and dilated pulmonary veins may suggest left-sided cardiac failure, although radiographs are better for demonstrating the actual pulmonary oedema. Pleural effusions are readily demonstrated by ultrasound (see Chapter 5vi).

Some of the more common conditions which may result in dyspnoea are listed in Table 7.2, together with their key features and suitable further tests.

REFERENCES

Banzett RB, Lansing RW, Reid MB, Adams L and Brown R (1989) 'Air hunger' arising from increased PCO_2 in mechanically ventilated quadriplegics. *Respiratory Physiology* **76**, 53-67

Differential Diagnosis of Coughing

Brendan Corcoran

THE COUGH MECHANISM

The reader is referred to Chapter 2 for more detailed discussion of the physiology of the cough reflex.

In cardiorespiratory diseases, it should be remembered that coughing can be caused by airway compression in addition to airway inflammation. This is particularly pertinent with tracheal collapse, primary pulmonary neoplasia and left atrial enlargement.

Assessing the character of the cough can be useful in assisting diagnosis, but over-emphasis or interpretation of this finding should be avoided. The presence of nocturnal coughing or an association with exercise are non-specific signs, and rarely assist diagnosis. Eliciting coughing by tracheal compression is equally difficult to interpret, although with specific tracheal disorders there is often a heightened tracheal cough reflex. A dry hacking cough is associated with large airway disease, particularly acute tracheobronchitis, and a 'seal-bark' or 'goose-honk' cough is typical of tracheal collapse. Soft ineffectual coughing occurs with lower airway and lung diseases such as bronchopneumonia, and is due to the paucity of cough receptors at this level of the respiratory tract. Deciding whether or not a cough is productive is difficult, as most dogs and cats swallow expectorated material. Expectoration of a thick mucoid material can occur with chronic bronchitis, but usually expectorated material consists of saliva that accumulates in the pharynx during paroxysms of coughing and retching.

CLINICAL HISTORY

Signalment

Age and breed predilections for various cardiorespiratory diseases are well recognized and can give initial valuable diagnostic information. Sex predisposition is not readily recognized. A variety of congenital and acquired breed-associated cardiac diseases are documented, and the reader should be familiar with the more commonly recognized types (see Chapter 14). Anatomical respiratory abnormalities are usually seen in the brachycephalic breeds, with tracheal collapse being particularly prevalent in toy breeds. Chronic bronchial disease and pulmonary neoplasia are usually seen in middle-aged to elderly dogs, while acute tracheobronchitis is more common in young dogs.

General historical features

Enquiries about vaccination and worming status, the possibility of exposure to infective agents (kennels etc.) and the presence of a dusty and polluted environment, particularly in the case of young animals with respiratory disease, should be made. Coughing in other affected individuals in the owner's house or known contacts is highly suggestive of infection. The history of the siblings and the parents should also be sought, particularly if there is evidence of congenital cardiac disease or lung worm infection.

The onset and progression of coughing can assist diagnosis, and more detail is given in the discussion of specific diseases in other chapters.

The additional presence of tachypnoea, dyspnoea and exercise intolerance should be noted, and these signs are usually indicative of advanced or severe cardiac and respiratory disease. Care should be taken where the owner confuses panting with tachypnoea. Non-cardiorespiratory causes of exercise intolerance also need to be considered. Similarly, collapsing and syncope may be reported, and these are usually associated with cardiovascular disease. The presence of cyanosis may be noted by the owner, particularly if exercise intolerance and collapsing are present. In the majority of instances cyanosis is associated with respiratory impairment. Cyanosis occurring at rest can be attributed to either cardiac or respiratory disease, and is a serious finding.

A history of current or previous diseases affecting other body systems including gastrointestinal diseases and endocrinopathies, can be significant as they can result in secondary respiratory diseases. A history of trauma (recent or long-term), recent major soft tissue surgery (pulmonary thromboembolism), surgical removal of malignant neoplasms within the previous 12 months, and consumption of toxins (e.g. paraquat, warfarin) can greatly assist in obtaining a diagnosis.

PHYSICAL EXAMINATION

The physical examination should allow differentiation of cardiac from respiratory causes of coughing in the majority of cases, and attention should be paid to both systems, as the subsequent diagnostic approaches will be markedly different.

General physical examination

Debility and cachexia are common findings with chronic respiratory diseases, such as pulmonary neoplasia and chronic bronchitis, and with long-standing congestive heart failure. Pyrexia in a coughing case is highly suggestive of acute pneumonia, and the presence of lymphadenopathy or other body-surface masses would alert the clinician to a possibility of metastatic pulmonary neoplasia. Lameness and long bone pain may be associated with a thoracic mass (hypertrophic pulmonary osteoarthropathy). Obesity often complicates respiratory diseases, and can have significant bearing on the clinical presentation of several chronic diseases, particularly tracheal collapse. Attention should be paid to physical signs of diseases that can have secondary effects on the respiratory system, such as hyperadrenocorticalism and hypothyroidism.

Examination of the cardiovascular system

Since coughing is usually due to left atrial enlargement and congestive heart failure, which can be caused by several cardiac conditions, the main aim of the cardiovascular examination in a coughing dog or cat is to exclude possible cardiac involvement, and so allow the clinician to concentrate on the respiratory system. It should be noted that cats rarely cough with cardiac diseases. The presence of a murmur, suggestive of mitral regurgitation, even if there are no signs of congestive heart failure, is sufficient to suspect a cardiac cough.

- The colour of the mucus membranes, capillary refill time, strength and character of the femoral pulse are assessed for evidence of left ventricular output problems
- The heart and pulse rates are counted and compared, and the rhythm of both noted and compared. The presence of jugular distension or pulsation should be noted, although right-sided failure alone is unlikely to cause coughing
- The chest is palpated to assess the strength of the apex beat, subjectively assess the size of the heart, and identify precordial thrills
- The presence of murmurs is noted, their point of maximal intensity, radiation, character, grading and position in the cardiac cycle
- Palpating the abdomen for ascites or percussing the chest to identify pleural effusions should also be carried out, but will only be relevant to coughing if biventricular failure has occurred.

Examination of the respiratory system

Physical examination of the respiratory system rarely allows a diagnosis to be made, but enables assessment of the severity of the respiratory disease, and in some instances, the possible location of the problem.

- The external nares and eyes should be examined for discharges, and it should be remembered that nasal material may be tracking from the airways
- The respiratory rate is counted and the respiratory pattern noted. The presence of dyspnoea can be appreciated if the respiratory rate is sufficiently slow and can be described as either inspiratory or expiratory. At fast respiratory rates (tachypnoea), the presence of dyspnoea can be difficult to observe. Inspiratory and expiratory dyspnoea are often best appreciated on auscultation. A combination of tachypnoea and dyspnoea is called hyperpnoea
- Chest percussion can allow detection of pleural effusions and consolidated lung areas. Coughing can often be elicited by percussing directly over the affected lung area
- Manually compressing the chest can give a rough assessment of thoracic compliance. This is particularly useful in cats with cranial mediastinal masses
- The respiratory system should be auscultated from the larynx to the periphery, and a decision made as to the contribution of upper airway noise to the sound heard in the chest. Auscultation during panting should be avoided, or at least taken into account
- Respiratory sounds are classified as rhonchi, wheezes and crackles. Rhonchi can be heard in normal individuals if they are excited/stressed or after exercise
- Rhonchi are loud, low pitched sounds emanating from large airways and are often associated with increased respiratory rate and effort. Stridor and stertor are the sounds generated in the larynx and nasal passages, respectively
- Wheezes are generated from small bronchi and are associated with airway narrowing, either due to bronchoconstriction or plugging with airway secretions
- Crackles are inspiratory sounds generated by the re-opening of airways that close during expiration. The intensity of the sound can be increased if there are concurrent airway secretions. Crackles are associated with conditions that reduce lung compliance, the best example of which is chronic pulmonary interstitial disease
- Mixed sounds are a combination of rhonchi, crackles and wheezes, but with close attention each sound should be identifiable. The terms rales and bronchovesicular sounds have minimal descriptive value and are gradually being omitted from the terminology.

DIAGNOSTIC TECHNIQUES

A wide range of diagnostic techniques is available for investigating the coughing case, but it is rare that a single test is diagnostic by itself, and the combined information from several tests is pooled to give the most likely diagnosis. However, some findings are very characteristic of certain diseases, and can be diagnostic in their own right. The reader is referred to other sections for detailed discussion of each technique.

Radiography

Radiography usually only allows a *radiographic* diagnosis to be made as several diseases can produce similar radiographic changes. The common radiographic changes include cardiomegaly, altered vascularity, increased bronchial markings, and increased interstitial and alveolar densities. The reader is referred to Chapter 5(i) for detail on assessment of cardiac changes. In many instances, a mixed bronchial, interstitial and alveolar pattern is present. The distribution of any changes can be of use in diagnosis. For example, with cardiogenic pulmonary oedema (interstitial/alveolar pattern) changes predominate in the hilar region, while with pneumonic lesions involvement of dependent lung areas and sites away from the central area occurs. Anatomical abnormalities of the trachea can be readily identified (e.g. tracheal collapse, hypoplastic trachea).

Bronchoscopy

Bronchoscopy allows: direct inspection of the airways; assessment of airway inflammation and the amount and source of purulent exudates (bronchopneumonia); confirmation of excess mucous secretion and chronic mucosal changes (chronic bronchitis); identification of foreign bodies; and visualization of dynamic airway collapse (pulmonary neoplasia; chronic pulmonary interstitial disease).

Bronchial cytology

Bronchial cytological analysis can deliver a definitive diagnosis in certain instances, such as pulmonary neoplasia, parasitic diseases and pulmonary infiltration with eosinophilia. For the remainder of cases, cytology will only allow assessment of the degree of airway inflammation, but will not necessarily enable a definitive diagnosis to be made. Bronchial samples can be cultured (aerobic, anaerobic and microaerophilic organisms), but it should be remembered that most organisms cultured are secondary pathogens.

Blood gas analysis

The presence of blood gas abnormalities will not allow identification of specific conditions, but can be used to separate ventilation–perfusion (V/Q) mismatching from alveolar hypoventilation, as the cause of the arterial blood gas changes, by calculating the alveolar–arterial oxygen difference (A–a). Typically, alveolar hypoventilation is associated with upper airway obstruction or severe pleural effusion, and V/Q mismatching with severe lung parenchymal disease. The major benefit of blood gas analysis is in assessing the degree of respiratory impairment and the need for oxygen supplementation.

Electrocardiography

The ECG is primarily used to identify arrhythmias and rarely allows definitive diagnosis of coughing. Increased complex height and width may suggest cardiomegaly and consequent compression of the mainstem bronchi, but such changes are better appreciated on radiography.

Echocardiography

Echocardiography will confirm cardiomegaly and the probable cause of congestive heart failure (e.g. dilated cardiomyopathy versus mitral valvular endocardiosis).

DIFFERENTIAL FEATURES OF DISEASES CAUSING COUGHING

The detailed clinical features of these diseases are presented in the relevant chapters, and in this section only the major or specific differential features of each disease are presented. Conditions causing coughing are presented in Table 8.1.

Oro-pharyngeal disorders

Oro-pharyngeal disorders usually cause gagging and choking, rather than coughing. Expectoration of frothy saliva often occurs.

Upper airway disorders

- *Laryngitis*: similar presentation to oro-pharyngeal disorders, with gagging rather than true coughing
- *Laryngeal paralysis*: inspiratory stridor and exercise intolerance in middle-aged to old, large and giant breed dogs. Coughing can occur, but is not a typical finding. Diagnosis by confirmation of paralysis under light general anaesthesia
- *Laryngeal neoplasia*: this is rare and more likely to cause dyspnoea
- *Tracheal collapse*: seal-bark or goose-honk cough in middle-aged toy breeds, particularly the Yorkshire Terrier, coupled with varying degrees of dyspnoea. The tracheal collapse can be confirmed on radiography, fluoroscopy or bronchoscopy
- *Tracheal stenosis, hypoplastic trachea, tracheal neoplasia, extra-mural compression of the trachea*: these conditions are rare and more likely to cause dyspnoea than coughing. Diagnosis by a combination of radiography and bronchoscopy.

| **Oro-pharyngeal disorders** |
| tonsillitis |
| pharyngitis |

| **Upper airway disorders** |
| larynx inflammation, neoplasia and paralysis |
| tracheal collapse |
| hypoplastic trachea |
| tracheal stenosis |
| tracheal neoplasia |
| extra-mural compression of trachea |

| **Lower airway disorders** |
| acute tracheobronchitis |
| chronic tracheobronchial syndrome |
| chronic bronchitis |
| bronchiectasis |
| bronchial neoplasia |
| *Oslerus (Filaroides) osleri* infection |
| airway foreign bodies |
| feline asthma syndrome |

| **Lung parenchymal diseases** |
| pneumonia |
| non-cardiogenic pulmonary oedema |
| chronic pulmonary interstitial disease |
| (idiopathic pulmonary fibrosis) |
| pulmonary abscess |
| intra-pulmonary haemorrhage |
| pulmonary neoplasia |
| pulmonary thromboembolism |

| **Cardiac disease** |
| left atrial enlargement |
| pulmonary oedema |
| interstitial |
| airway wall |
| alveolar |

| **Mediastinal disease** |
| neoplasia |
| infections |

Table 8.1: *Conditions causing coughing*

Lower airway disorders

- *Acute tracheobronchitis*: a dry harsh hacking cough in dogs that have been in suitable environments (e.g. dog kennels). The condition is self-limiting and signs resolve usually within 3 weeks. Diagnosis is made from the history and clinical presentation
- *Chronic tracheobronchial syndrome*: recurrent or chronic coughing in dogs that have had a history of kennel cough. An increased bronchial pattern may be present on radiographs, but there is no, or minimal, airway inflammation on bronchoscopy
- *Chronic bronchitis*: chronic paroxysmal coughing for two of the previous 12 months, with varying degrees of respiratory distress and exercise intolerance. Increased bronchial markings are seen on radiographs and excess mucus is found on bronchoscopy (confirmation of diagnosis). A roughened and nodular appearance to the mucosa might also be seen. Episodes of bronchopneumonia occur as the condition progresses and complicates the clinical picture
- *Bronchiectasis*: clinical signs similar to chronic bronchitis, with dilated airways seen on radiographs. Dilated bronchi, containing large quantities of muco-purulent material, visible on bronchoscopy confirms the diagnosis. More likely to be a complication of chronic bronchitis
- *Bronchial neoplasia*: neoplasms of the bronchial wall are rare (see Pulmonary neoplasia)
- Oslerus (Filaroides) osleri *infection:* chronic coughing, typically in dogs under 2 years of age, that may show temporary remission with glucocorticosteroids. Reactive nodules visible at the carina on bronchoscopy, which occasionally can be appreciated on radiography. Confirmation by demonstration of adult worms, larvae or embryonated eggs in tracheal samples
- Aelurostrongylus abstrusus *infection:* chronic coughing and/or respiratory distress in cats that are known to hunt. Some affected cats do not cough. Diagnosis is by demonstration of larvae in the faeces, although this can be difficult, supported by nodular or interstitial pattern on radiographs. An airway and circulating eosinophilia may be found
- *Airway foreign bodies*: acute onset of severe coughing, with or without respiratory distress depending on the location of the foreign body, associated with a typical event (e.g. running through a wheat field, playing with small objects etc.). The severity of coughing decreases within the first week and becomes chronic with halitosis developing over the following weeks or months. Confirmation of diagnosis by bronchoscopy, or on radiography if object is sufficiently radiodense
- *Feline asthma syndrome*: paroxysmal coughing and wheezing episodes in otherwise healthy cats, that are glucocorticosteroid responsive. Diagnosis is supported by radiographic changes, bronchial cytology (inflammatory reaction) and haematology, although these tests are not always diagnostic. Cutaneous reactivity to putative aeroallergens may be found.

Lung parenchymal disorders

- *Pneumonia*: soft and ineffectual coughing with or without pyrexia, lethargy, inappetence, leucocytosis with a neutrophilia and left shift, dyspnoea and exercise intolerance. Alveolar densities are noted on radiography and may be diffuse or localized. Mucopurulent material is visible on bronchoscopy, often exiting from single lobar bronchi, but the airway mucosa may appear normal. A polymorphonuclear-rich exudate is usually present, with moderate to large numbers of macrophages. The presence of airway eosinophilia gives a diagnosis of pulmonary infiltration with eosinophilia (eosinophilic pneumonia). Additional features of specific causes of bronchopneumonia may be present such as viral infections (e.g. canine distemper virus) and mega-oesophagus (aspiration pneumonia)
- *Non-cardiogenic pulmonary oedema*: dyspnoea is a more likely presentation than coughing. Typical features are a predisposition among brachycephalic dogs, and history of electrocution, strangulation (choke-chain injuries), severe hyperthermia and consumption of toxins (e.g. Paraquat). It can also be associated with systemic illness, septicaemia and toxaemia such as acute pancreatitis
- *Chronic pulmonary interstitial disease (idiopathic pulmonary fibrosis)*: chronic coughing and variable degrees of dyspnoea and exercise intolerance in small breeds, typically the West Highland White and Cairn Terriers. Widespread crackles on chest auscultation is practically diagnostic, but is supported by diffuse increased interstitial density on radiography and dynamic expiratory airway collapse on bronchoscopy
- *Pulmonary abscesses*: with respect to coughing, lung abscesses behave like primary neoplasms
- *Intrapulmonary haemorrhage*: pulmonary haemorrhage can be very similar to pneumonia. A history of trauma, consumption of anticoagulants, or other evidence of a coagulopathy with pneumonia lesions on radiography, and the presence of blood in the airways, is highly supportive of a diagnosis of intrapulmonary haemorrhage. Coagulopathy profiles will assist diagnosis
- *Pulmonary neoplasia*: chronic coughing in middle to old-aged dogs, with gradual development of cachexia, inappetence, dyspnoea and exercise intolerance. Lameness due to hypertrophic pulmonary osteoarthropathy may also be present in a minority of cases. Diagnosis is supported by radiography and the demonstration of airway collapse on bronchoscopy. The presence of blood-tinged mucus is also supportive, but a diagnosis is made by demonstrating neoplastic cells in airway washes or transthoracic biopsy material
- *Pulmonary thromboembolism*: acute onset of tachypnoea without radiographic evidence of severe lung disease. Coughing rarely occurs but may be present if the affected lung area becomes consolidated (pneumonic).

Cardiovascular disorders

Coughing in cardiac cases is a consequence of the development of left-sided congestive heart failure, for which there are a variety of possible underlying cardiac conditions (see Chapter 12).

- *Left atrial enlargement*: left atrial enlargement is usually appreciated on thoracic radiographs, supported by echocardiography. This is the most common cause of coughing in cardiac disease, and is particularly common in small breeds
- *Cardiogenic pulmonary oedema*: cardiogenic pulmonary oedema is diagnosed on radiography where there is evidence of cardiac abnormalities. The coughing is often soft and ineffectual, and similar to bronchopneumonia. Cardiomegaly, particularly left-sided changes, should be apparent and congested pulmonary venous circulation can be appreciated. The accumulation of oedema fluid in the interstitium and alveoli mainly occurs in the central hilar region, extending into the caudal lung field as the condition deteriorates.

Mediastinal disorders

- *Neoplasia* (e.g. *lymphosarcoma*): distension of the cranial mediastinum usually results in dyspnoea and swallowing problems, but can also cause coughing. Mediastinal widening is confirmed on radiography, although a specific diagnosis is often difficult to make without biopsy material. Diagnosis is most likely to be made on post mortem
- *Infections* (e.g. *Nocardiosis*): similar to neoplasia, widening of the mediastinum secondary to infectious processes; can be difficult to diagnose ante mortem.

Syncope, Collapse and Episodic Weakness

Anne French

Animals may be presented for evaluation of episodes of weakness, fainting, seizures, collapse or with a history of fatigue or exercise intolerance. Symptoms may be present at rest, on excitement, during feeding or with exercise. This is a challenging diagnostic area, as the differential diagnosis encompasses a long list of disease entities. Frequently the clinician does not witness one of the 'episodes', and is dependent on the client for a description . This chapter will describe the common presenting symptoms and causes. This will be followed be a more general discussion on aetiology and then a logical approach to the diagnostic work-up. A full discussion of pathophysiology and therapeutic modalities is beyond the scope of this chapter.

COMMON PRESENTING SYMPTOMS

Syncope

Typical features

*   Occurs at exercise
*   Flaccid collapse
*   Loss of consciousness
*   Rapid recovery.

Syncope refers to a sudden transient loss of consciousness due to deprivation of energy substrates that briefly impairs cerebral metabolism. The metabolism of the brain is entirely dependent on the perfusion of oxygen.

A syncopal episode is transient and recovery occurs within seconds to minutes. The first symptom is generalized muscle weakness, progressing to ataxia, which may be followed by collapse and a short period of loss of consciousness. In most cases, the animal is motionless with relaxation of the skeletal muscles, but in some cases this may progress to tonic spasms and incontinence. Vocalization may occur. Recovery is rapid, although a brief period of confusion may follow. Syncope usually occurs during exercise or upon excitement, but may occasionally occur at rest.

Presyncope

Presyncope is a transient episode of altered consciousness, and is a form of incomplete syncope. The animal may show a transient weakness progressing to ataxia, but there is no loss of consciousness.

The common causes of syncope are shown in Table 9.1. A summary of recent human studies has shown that non-cardiac syncope accounted for 46% of cases, obstructive cardiac disease 2.5%, arrhythmias 16%, and 36% were undetermined (Lewis *et al.*, 1994). No similar studies have been published for animals.

Seizures

Typical features

*   Usually at rest
*   Motor activity during collapse
*   Salivation/loss of sphincter control
*   Prodromal and post-ictal phases.

A seizure is an abnormal excessive paroxysmal synchronous discharge in a population of neurons. A seizure is a symptom of dysfunction in the grey matter of the brain which may be primary, or secondary to a metabolic abnormality.

Grand mal/tonic–clonic seizures are frequently preceded by a prodromal period of altered behaviour (an *aura*). The 'ictus' follows where the animal typically falls and becomes unconscious; the limbs are extended rigidly, opisthotonos is usually present and respiration stops. A brief tonic phase occurs which is rapidly followed by clonic limb movements in the form of running or paddling activity. Chewing movements of the mouth are common. Visceral activity may start in the tonic or clonic phase and may include pupillary dilatation, salivation, urination, defecation and piloerection. The ictus usually lasts 1–2 minutes. The post-ictal phase may include confusion, disorientation, restlessness, pacing and blindness lasting for minutes to hours. Seizures typically occur at rest. Seizures may occur singly, several close together (as *clusters*) or continuously (*status epilepticus*).

Absences or *petit mal seizures* are characterized by a brief loss of consciousness (lasting only seconds). There is no spontaneous motor activity, and a transient collapse may occur. These attacks are either uncommon in animals or uncommonly recognized.

Partial motor seizures are restricted to one part of

Cardiac disease	Obstruction to outflow		Aortic stenosis/subaortic stenosis Pulmonic stenosis Mitral stenosis HOCM Atrial tumours Ball valve thrombi Valvular endocarditis
	Arrhythmias	Bradyarrhythmias	Atrioventricular (AV) block Sinus bradycardia Atrial standstill Sick-sinus syndrome 'Brady–tachy' syndrome
		Tachyarrhythmias	Atrial fibrillation Supraventricular tachycardias Ventricular tachycardias
	Myocardial disease		Dilated cardiomyopathy Hypertrophic cardiomyopathy Restrictive cardiomyopathy Myocardial failure
	Pericardial disease		Pericardial effusion Constrictive pericarditis
	Cyanotic congenital heart disease		Tetralogy of Fallot Shunts with pulmonary hypertension
	Severe atrioventricular valvular incompetence		Endocardiosis Congenital AV valve disease
Respiratory tract disease	Hypoxia		Upper respiratory tract obstruction Severe lower respiratory tract disease Severe pleural cavity disease
	Pulmonary hypertension Cough syncope		
Peripheral vascular dysfunction	Vasovagal Carotid sinus hypersensitivity Postural hypotension Hyperventilation		
Metabolic	Hypoglycaemia Hypocalcaemia Hyperkalaemia		
Endocrine	Hypoadrenocorticism Hyperinsulinism Diabetes mellitus		
Haematological	Anaemia Polycythaemia		
Neurological	Cerebral emboli/thrombi Neoplasia Atherosclerosis		
Iatrogenic	Nitrates Beta blocking agents Prazosin Phenothiazine derivatives Anti-arrhythmic drugs ACE inhibitors Digitalis intoxication		

Table 9.1: Causes of syncope in the dog and cat.

Extracranial	
Toxins	
Metabolic disease	Hypoglycaemia
	Hypocalcaemia
	Hyperviscosity
	Hyperlipoproteinaemia
	Hepatic encephalopathy
	Electrolyte disturbances
	Uraemia
	Hyperosmolality
	Heat stroke
Intracranial	
Congenital	Hydrocephalus
malformations	Lissencephaly (Lhasa Apso)
Metabolic storage	
diseases	
Neoplasia	
Inflammatory disease	Infectious, e.g. FeLV, FIP,
	distemper, toxoplasma
	Granulomatous
	meningoencephalitis
Vascular disease	Haemorrhage
	Cerebral infarct
Trauma	
Dietary	Thiamine deficiency
Idiopathic epilepsy	

Table 9.2: *Causes of seizures in the dog and cat.*

the body, and frequently spread, resulting in a generalized convulsion.

Psychomotor seizures indicate an abnormality in the limbic system, and are characterized by paroxysmal episodes of abnormal behaviour, e.g. hysteria, rage, salivation and hallucinations.

Petit mal seizures and *presyncope* may be similar in presentation, and can be difficult to differentiate. Likewise, it may be difficult to distinguish a primary seizure from an epileptiform seizure secondary to prolonged hypoxia. See Table 9.2 for common causes of seizures in dogs and cats.

Narcolepsy/cataplexy

Typical features

- Flaccid collapse
- Often induced by excitement/eating
- Can be roused on stimulation.

Narcolepsy is a disorder of the brain characterized by recurring sudden attacks of sleep. The most common presenting sign in animals is cataplexy, i.e. brief episodes of muscle paralysis. Animals with narcolepsy typically have episodes in which they suddenly fall asleep, often when excited or during emotional stimulation. Eating is a common precipitating factor. The

attacks may last from a few seconds to several minutes. The animal appears unconscious or limp, although noise, shaking or other stimuli will rouse the animal. The episodes frequently occur many times a day.

Narcolepsy/cataplexy has been reported in many breeds (Mitler *et al.*, 1976) and is thought to be a hereditary condition in Dobermanns, Poodles and Labrador Retrievers. Signs are usually present before 6 months of age, but may develop in adult dogs (Foutz *et al.*, 1980).

Episodic weakness

This is a very broad term describing any brief period of weakness which may be related to rest, exercise, feeding, starvation or excitement. Presyncope, petit mal seizures and narcolepsy may be included in this category. The animal becomes weak and recovers after an undefined period. See Table 9.3.

Exercise intolerance

This is another common presenting symptom and is defined as an inability to exercise normally. Exercise intolerance may occur because of episodic weakness or syncope, but may also be due to lameness, obesity, pyrexia, excessive panting, or generalized weakness. See Table 9.4.

CONDITIONS CAUSING SYNCOPE, COLLAPSE AND EPISODIC WEAKNESS

Cardiac disorders

- Syncope
- Presyncope
- Episodic weakness
- Exercise intolerance

Cardiac disease may cause syncope, presyncope, episodic weakness or exercise intolerance because of insufficient cardiac output. Cyanotic congenital cardiac disease may also cause the same signs. A decrease in cardiac output may occur due to poor myocardial function, obstruction to outflow, arrhythmia or impaired filling of the heart. Clinical signs are frequently associated with exercise or excitement, where there is an inability to increase cardiac output in response to increased demand. Cardiac causes of syncope in dogs and cats are well documented in the literature (Beckett *et al.*, 1978; Bonagura and Ware, 1985; Fingland *et al.*, 1986; Sisson *et al.*, 1991; Kienle, 1994; Lehmkuhl *et al.*, 1994).

Respiratory disorders

- Episodic collapse
- Syncope
- Exercise intolerance

Endocrine	Insulinoma
	Hypoadrenocorticism
	Hypothyroidism
	Hyperadrenocorticism
	Diabetic ketoacidosis
	Phaeochromocytoma
Metabolic	Hypoglycaemia
	Hypokalaemia
	Hypocalcaemia
	Hyponatraemia
	Hyperglycaemia
	Hyperkalaemia
	Hypercalcaemia
	Hyperthermia
	Acidosis
	Shock
	Hepatic encephalopathy
Muscular	Polymyositis
	Muscular dystrophy
	Mitochondrial myopathy
	Hypokalaemic myopathy
	Myotonic myopathy
	Steroid myopathy
	Malignant hyperthermia
Skeletal	Degenerative joint disease
	Polyarthritis
	Panosteitis
	Hypertrophic osteodystrophy
	Bilateral anterior cruciate ligament rupture
Neuromuscular	Myasthenia gravis
	Botulism
	Peripheral polyneuropathies
Neurological	Seizures (see Table 9.2)
	Vestibular disease
	Cerebellar disease
	Sensory ataxia
	Narcolepsy/cataplexy
	Lysosomal storage disease
	Scottie cramp (Scottish Terriers)
	Episodic falling (Cavalier King Charles Spaniel)
	Cervical spondylopathy
	Intervertebral disc protrusion
	Discospondylitis
	Neoplasia
	Fibrocartilaginous emboli
	Spinal trauma
Haematological	Anaemia
	Polycythaemia
	Myeloproliferative disorders
Respiratory disease	(see Table 9.1)
Cardiovascular disease	(see Table 9.1)

Table 9.3: *Causes of episodic weakness/collapse in the dog and cat.*

Extracranial	
Cardiac disease	(see Table 9.1)
Respiratory disease	(see Table 9.1)
Skeletal disease	(see Table 9.3)
Neuromuscular disease	(see Table 9.3)
Neurological disease	(see Table 9.3)
Metabolic/endocrine disease	(see Table 9.3)
Generalized weakness	Chronic inflammation
	Chronic infection
	Chronic wasting
	Fever
	Nutritional deficiencies
	Parasitism
	Neoplasia
	Overwork
	Barbiturates
	Anticonvulsants
	Antihistamines
	Diuretics
	Vasodilators
	Antiarrhythmic agents
	Obesity
	Anaemia

Table 9.4: *Causes of exercise intolerance.*

Any cause of *hypoxia* may potentially lead to episodic collapse, syncope or exercise intolerance. Airway obstructive disease is particularly associated with syncope or collapse in dogs. *Pulmonary hypertension* and *pulmonary thromboembolism* are reported in humans to cause effort syncope due to obstruction to right ventricular outflow (Kapoor, 1992). *Cough syncope* is commonly reported, especially in dogs of small breeds with chronic pulmonary disease. The typical pattern is of loss of consciousness following a paroxysm of vigorous coughing; several mechanisms have been proposed (Lusk and Ettinger, 1988).

Peripheral vascular dysfunction

Several types of peripheral vascular dysfunction have been recognized in animals with normal cardiac function, which can result in syncope or presyncopal episodes.

Vasodepressor syncope

• Syncope

This is frequently associated with sudden extreme excitement. Often the animal is immobile leading up to the incident. This form of syncope is associated with a marked fall in total peripheral resistance which is not compensated by a rise in cardiac output. Vagally mediated bradycardia is a contributing factor. This is the mechanism of the common faint in humans, and may be the cause of syncope as seen in young Boxers (Fisher, 1971; Rush, 1993).

Postural hypotension

• Syncope

This form of syncope occurs on rising, and is associated with a fall in systolic and diastolic blood pressure. Blood volume depletion accounts for the postural hypotension associated with dehydration, excessive diuresis, anaemia, haemorrhage, hypoadrenocorticism and excessive gastrointestinal losses. Drug therapy may induce similar effects.

Carotid sinus hypersensitivity

• Syncope

Compression of the carotid sinus is associated with transient slowing of the heart and mild hypotension. In animals with carotid sinus hypersensitivity, this response is exaggerated and mild stimulation is followed by profound slowing of the heart rate and/or a marked diminution of arterial pressure. This syndrome is observed in brachycephalic breeds and is also observed in cases where neoplasia, inflammatory processes or tight collars stimulate the carotid sinuses (Ettinger and Barrett, 1995).

Hyperventilation syndrome

• Presyncope

Anxious or hyperexcitable pets may hyperventilate, causing over-aeration of the alveoli and a subsequent fall in arterial PCO_2 levels. Hypocapnia causes cerebral arterial vasoconstriction and peripheral vasodilatation, thus reducing cerebral perfusion. Presyncope is more common than complete loss of consciousness.

Many more types of syncope have been described in humans but to date have not been documented in animals, e.g. micturition syncope, defecation syncope, glossopharyngeal neuralgia, deglutition syncope and hysterical syncope (Lewis *et al.*, 1994).

Haematological disorders

• Weakness
• Exercise intolerance

Severe anaemia may cause hypoxia and resulting weakness, exercise intolerance and collapse. Frequently symptoms are associated with exercise or excitement.

Polycythaemia is also recognized as a cause of collapse secondary to increased viscosity of the blood.

Metabolic disorders

• Syncope
• Weakness
• Seizures

Numerous metabolic disorders may give rise to syncope, episodic collapse or exercise intolerance (see Table 9.3). Hypoglycaemia commonly causes episodic weakness or seizures (Dunn *et al.*, 1992). General weakness has been reported in dogs and cats with hypokalaemia (Dow *et al.*, 1987). Hyperkalaemia causes bradycardia, depression and neuromuscular weakness. Hypocalcaemic animals present with tetany and seizures, whilst hypercalcaemic animals show lethargy, central nervous system depression, muscle weakness and muscle fasciculations. Animals with hepatic encephalopathy due to hepatic insufficiency often have seizures precipitated by feeding high protein meals. Exercise-induced malignant hyperthermia has been described in the dog (Kirmayer *et al.*, 1984; Rand and O'Brien, 1987), and is characterized by hindlimb cramping and dyspnoea on exercise.

Endocrine disorders

• Syncope
• Episodic collapse
• Exercise intolerance

Numerous endocrine disorders may be associated with a variety of signs, depending on the cause (see Table 9.3), e.g. hypoadrenocorticism, hyperadrenocorticism, hypothyroidism, hypoparathyroidism, diabetic ketoacidosis, insulinoma and phaeochromocytoma. In some conditions, there may be more than one possible mechanism for the clinical signs, e.g. in hypoadrenocorticism, the signs may be secondary to hypovolaemia, hyponatraemia or hyperkalaemia. In hypothyroidism, collapse or exercise intolerance may be due to bradycardia or peripheral neuropathies. In other conditions, the mechanism is more straightforward, e.g. hypoglycaemia in insulinomas and tachyarrhythmias with phaeochromocytoma.

Muscular disorders

• Exercise intolerance
• Weakness
• Episodic collapse

Muscular disorders usually present with episodic collapse or weakness associated with exercise, and are not associated with changes in consciousness (Herrtage and McKerrell, 1996). Several conditions have been described (see Table 9.3).

Myopathies are usually bilaterally symmetrical, reflexes are preserved and muscle atrophy is seen. In Labrador Retriever myopathy, Golden Retriever myopathy, Irish Terrier X-linked myopathy and mitochondrial myopathy in Clumber Spaniels, animals present at a young age with exercise intolerance.

Myotonia is seen in young animals and is characterized by stiffness on rising, which improves with exercise. In some cases, generalized muscle spasm may cause collapse.

Myasthenia gravis has been reported in the dog and cat, and may be acquired or congenital (Palmer, 1980). The symptoms are of severe muscle weakness and fatigue on exercise, which improves on rest. The condition is frequently associated with dysphagia and regurgitation.

Scottie cramp is an inherited condition seen in young Scottish Terriers, characterized by cramp on exercise or excitement (Meyers *et al.*, 1969). Episodes are of short duration and full recovery occurs within 15 seconds.

Neurological disorders

- Seizures
- Ataxia
- Weakness

Seizures cause episodic collapse. They may be primary, or secondary to metabolic disturbances, e.g. hypoglycaemia or hypoxia.

Ataxic animals may occasionally show signs of collapse, which is not usually intermittent, depending on the cause.

The *peripheral neuropathies* usually present with ataxia or collapse on exercise. Initial presenting signs may be restricted to hindlimbs; however, involvement of the larynx, oesophagus and forelimbs may also occur.

Spinal disorders commonly present with pain, and ataxia with paresis. There may be evidence of motor and postural deficits, changes in muscle tone or alterations in local reflexes depending on the level of the lesion. See Table 9.3.

Skeletal disorders

- Exercise intolerance
- Weakness

Skeletal disorders may cause exercise intolerance, but are not associated with loss of consciousness. Pain is usually a feature, and may be elicited on palpation or manipulation. See Table 9.3.

DIAGNOSTIC APPROACH

The differential diagnosis list for syncope, episodic collapse and exercise intolerance is a long one. A very thorough investigative approach is required. It is important to characterize the *type of collapse*, as the possible causes of a collapsing episode associated with loss of consciousness are different from those of exercise intolerance. A detailed history and good physical examination are therefore vital. Routine and specialized investigative tests are frequently required.

History

A detailed description of the event is *vital*. The following information will help to differentiate syncope, presyncope, grand mal seizures, petit mal seizures, narcolepsy and episodic weakness:

- Presence or absence of consciousness
- Association with exercise, feeding, rest, excitement
- Duration of event
- Altered behaviour before or after episode
- Colour of mucous membranes during episode
- Frequency of episodes
- The pattern of episodes.

In some cases, it may be necessary to ask the owner to keep a diary and to teach the owner to observe mucous membrane colour, and to take heart rate, either with their hand or with a cheap stethoscope. In many cases, provocative testing may be indicated to help with diagnosis.

General history, including thirst, appetite, dysphagia, vomiting, urination, defecation, respiratory noises, weight loss or weight gain, may help point the investigation in a certain direction.

Physical examination

A thorough physical examination should be undertaken. The number of different body systems which may be responsible for syncope, episodic collapse and exercise intolerance cannot be overemphasized. Particular attention should be paid to the cardiac, respiratory, musculoskeletal and neurological systems. Any changes suggestive of an endocrine disorder should be noted.

Laboratory tests

Routine screening should include the following tests:

- Haematology
- Blood glucose
- Blood urea
- Liver enzymes (ALT, AP)
- Muscle enzymes (CPK, AST)
- Electrolytes (sodium, potassium, calcium, magnesium)
- Routine urinalysis.

In cases of episodic collapse, it is important to realize that serious abnormalities may only be present at the time of collapse. Where marginal abnormalities are noted, repeat sampling may be indicated or provocative testing with samples taken pre- and post-exercise or feeding, as indicated by the history (Darke, 1990).

Further laboratory tests

In some cases, the above screening tests may provide the diagnosis but in other cases further selected tests may be indicated.

- Glucose tolerance test
- Insulin/glucose ratio
- Liver function tests: bile acids, pre- and post-prandial ammonia levels, ammonia tolerance test, BSP clearance
- Adrenal function tests: ACTH stimulation, low dose dexamethasone suppression test
- Thyroid function tests: basal T4, TSH stimulation, T3 and T4 antibodies
- Renal function: blood urea and creatinine, inorganic phosphate, routine urine analysis, urine creatinine/protein ratio
- Blood gas analysis: resting, pre- and post-exercise.

Diagnostic imaging

Radiography
Radiography is important in the diagnosis of cardiac or respiratory tract disease. Inspiratory and expiratory films may be necessary in the diagnosis of tracheal collapse. Radiographs of the skull, spine, joints, or abdomen may be indicated depending on the clinical findings.

Contrast radiography such as angiography, portal venography, and myelography may be indicated in selected cases. Barium studies may be indicated in the investigation of peripheral neuropathies to check for megaoesophagus.

Ultrasonography
Doppler echocardiography is the technique of choice in the investigation of congenital and acquired cardiac defects. Abdominal ultrasonography may aid in the diagnosis of specific cases, e.g. hepatic disease, adrenal tumours, pancreatic tumours, renal disease.

Electrocardiography

Routine ECG
If a cardiac cause is suspected, then a multi-lead ECG with a long lead two rhythm strip (at least 3 minutes) is indicated. There may be evidence of a continuous arrhythmia or cardiac chamber enlargement. Frequently, the arrhythmias are intermittent; negative findings are inconclusive and warrant further investigation. A lead two rhythm strip may be repeated after a vagal manoeuvre or after exercise. If results are still negative, then further techniques are indicated.

Telemetry
Telemetry allows the animal to be exercised during ECG monitoring. There are no standardized regimens for exercise testing in dogs, and the animal is usually exercised until collapse or for a minimum of 15 minutes.

Holter monitor/event recorders
Continuous ambulatory ECG recordings (Hall *et al.*,

1991; Moise and Defrancesco, 1995) may be used to look for arrhythmic causes of syncope or presyncope. Occasionally, potentially lethal arrhythmias may be identified, even if the patient did not collapse. In examining recordings it is important to remember that while pauses of 3–6 seconds associated with clinical signs of weakness or syncope are diagnostic, the same pause in a sleeping animal may be normal. Likewise, ventricular or supraventricular arrhythmias must generally be sustained for more than 10 seconds to be considered responsible for clinical signs of weakness or syncope. An alternative is the Chiltern box (Brownlie, 1987); this is an event recorder which is worn by the animal and turned on if symptoms occur. It is not uncommon for animals to remain asymptomatic whilst wearing these devices, but on occasions very useful information is obtained.

Laryngoscopy/bronchoscopy/bronchoalveolar lavage
Laryngoscopy and bronchoscopy may be indicated in investigation of suspected upper respiratory tract obstruction, tracheal disease or pulmonary disease.

Additional routine tests
Electromyography, nerve conduction velocities, muscle and nerve biopsies may all be indicated in the investigation of suspected myopathies, myotonia, polymyositis and peripheral neuropathies.

Cerebrospinal fluid analysis may be required in some cases of seizures, and electroencephalography (EEG) may be helpful in cases of suspected narcolepsy.

Miscellaneous tests

Edrophonium response test
Edrophonium chloride (0.1–1.0 mg by slow i.v. injection) is the ultra-short-acting anticholinesterase used in the diagnosis of *myasthenia gravis*. Administration results in immediate dramatic improvement in the exercise tolerance in affected dogs. Oxygen should be available in case of respiratory difficulties.

Scottie cramp test
Administration of serotonin antagonists, e.g. *methysergide*, will induce episodes in affected dogs. The dose rate is 0.3 mg/kg given orally, and the dog is exercised 2 hours later.

Exercise testing for malignant hyperthermia
A short period of exercise in affected animals will induce the hyperlactacidaemia, hyperthermia, haemoconcentration and mild respiratory alkalosis normally only seen with prolonged strenuous exercise.

Immunological tests
Antibodies to acetylcholine receptors are suggestive of

acquired myasthenia gravis. Polymyositis cases may have a positive antinuclear or anti-muscle antibody test.

SUMMARY

The causes of syncope, episodic collapse and exercise intolerance are numerous. Appropriate case evaluation will provide a diagnosis in a high percentage of cases. A retrospective study by Cobb and Stepien (1994) showed that if no obvious diagnosis was evident after case evaluation, the clinical signs did not usually progress, and death associated with these conditions was very rare. These findings concur with the findings in human studies on syncope, which concluded that if no diagnosis was obtained after exhaustive tests in these patients, the prognosis regarding mortality and death was favourable (Kapoor, 1991).

REFERENCES

Beckett SD, Branch CE and Robertson BT (1978) Syncopal attacks and sudden deaths in dogs: mechanisms and etiologies. *Journal of the American Animal Hospital Association.* **14**, 378

Bonagura JD and Ware WA (1985) Atrial fibrillation in the dog; clinical findings in 81 cases. *Journal of the American Animal Hospital Association* **22**, 111

Brownlie SE (1987) Evaluation of the Chiltern box: a device for home electrocardiography. *Veterinary Record* **120**, 85

Cobb MA and Stepien RL (1994) A retrospective study of the outcome of 69 cases: undiagnosed syncope, collapse or exercise intolerance in dogs. *Proceedings of the Veterinary Cardiovascular Society*, Spring 1994. Birmingham, UK

Darke PGG (1990) Differential diagnosis of weakness and collapse. In: *Manual of Small Animal Endocrinology*, ed. M Hutchinson, p. 189. BSAVA, Cheltenham

Dow SW, LeCouter RA, Fettman MJ and Spurgeon TL (1987) Potassium depletion in cats; hypokalemic polymyopathy. *Journal of the American Veterinary Medical Association* **191**, 1563

Dunn JK, Bostock DE, Herrtage ME, Jackson KF and Walker MJ (1992) Insulin secreting tumours of the pancreas: clinical and pathological features of 11 cases. *Journal of Small Animal Practice* **34**, 325

Ettinger SJ and Barrett KA (1995) Weakness and syncope. Chapter 11.

In: *Textbook of Veterinary Internal Medicine*, 4th edn, ed. SJ Ettinger and EC Feldman, p. 50. WB Saunders, Philadelphia

Fingland RB, Bonagura JD and Myer CW (1986) Pulmonic stenosis in the dog: 29 cases (1975-1984). *Journal of the American Veterinary Medical Association* **189**, 218

Fisher EW (1971) Fainting in Boxers - the possibility of vaso-vagal syncope (Adams–Stokes attacks). *Journal of Small Animal Practice* **12**, 347

Foutz AS, Mitler MM and Dement WC (1980) Narcolepsy. *Veterinary Clinics of North America: Small Animal Practice* **10**, 65

Hall LW, Dunn JK, Delaney M and Shapiro LM (1991) Ambulatory electrocardiography in dogs. *Veterinary Record* **129**, 213

Herrtage ME and McKerrell, RE (1996) Episodic weakness. In: *Manual of Small Animal Neurology*, ed. SL Wheeler, p. 189. BSAVA, Cheltenham.

Kapoor WN (1991) Diagnostic evaluation in syncope. *The American Journal of Medicine* **90**, 91

Kapoor WN (1992) Hypotension and syncope. Chapter 30. In: *Heart Disease*, 4th edn, ed. E Braunwald, p. 875. WB Saunders, Philadelphia

Kienle RD, Thomas WP and Pion PD (1994) The natural clinical history of canine congenital subaortic stenosis. *Journal of Veterinary Internal Medicine* **8**, 423

Kirmayer AH, Klide AM and Purvance JE (1984) Malignant hyperthermia in a dog: case report and review of the syndrome. *Journal of the American Veterinary Medical Association* **185**, 978

Lehmkuhl LB, Ware WA and Bonagura JD (1994) Mitral stenosis in 15 dogs. *Journal of Veterinary Internal Medicine* **8**, 2

Lewis PR, Budoulas H, Schaal S and Weissler AM (1994) Diagnosis and management of syncope. In: *The Heart*, 8th edn, ed. RC Schlant, RW Alexander, RA O'Rourke, R Roberts and EH Sonnerblick, p. 927. McGraw Hill, New York

Lusk HR Jr and Ettinger SJ (1988) Cardiovascular syncope. In: *Canine and Feline Cardiology*, ed. PR Fox, p. 335. Churchill Livingstone, New York

Mitler MM, Soave O and Dement WC (1976) Narcolepsy in seven dogs. *Journal of the American Veterinary Medical Association* **168**, 1036

Meyers KM, Lund JE, Padgett G and Dickson WM (1969) Hyperkinetic episodes in Scottish Terrier dogs. *Journal of the American Veterinary Medical Association* **155**, 129

Moise NS and Defrancesco T (1995) Twenty-four hour ambulatory electrocardiography (Holter monitors). In: *Kirk's Current Veterinary Therapy XII*, ed. JD Bonagura, pp. 792-799. WB Saunders, Philadelphia

Palmer AC (1980) Myasthenia gravis. *Veterinary Clinics of North America: Small Animal Practice* **101**, 213

Rand JS and O'Brien PJ (1987) Exercise induced malignant hyperthermia in an English Springer Spaniel. *Journal of the American Veterinary Medical Association* **190**, 1013

Rush J (1993). Syncope - diagnosis and management. *Proceedings of the 11th Annual Forum of the American College of Internal Medicine*, Washington DC

Sisson D, Thomas WP, Woodfield J, Pion PD, Leuthy M and DeLellis LA (1991) Permanent transvenous pacemaker implantation in forty dogs. *Journal of Veterinary Internal Medicine* **5**, 322

Cardiac Murmurs and Abnormal Sounds

Paul R. Wotton

AUSCULTATION TECHNIQUE

Auscultation of the heart and lungs plays a fundamental role in the investigation of cardiovascular and respiratory diseases. A careful and complete examination should be carried out systematically in a quiet environment, with the patient gently restrained, preferably in a standing position. Dogs should be prevented from panting or barking, if necessary by gently holding the mouth closed. Cats can sometimes be prevented from purring by changing their position, gently blowing on the face or distracting their attention, e.g. by running water. If the patient is excessively excited, it may be necessary to re-evaluate the heart sounds later, when more relaxed. Sedation should be avoided, however, since, apart from any other considerations, this may introduce artefacts such as bradyarrhythmias or gallop sounds (see later). Extraneous sounds, such as those originating from respiration, gut activity, the effects of trembling or movement and the noise of the patient's hair against the diaphragm of the stethoscope, must be distinguished from true heart sounds. The whole cardiac area should be evaluated methodically, listening on both sides of the thorax at the cardiac apex, sternal border and base of the heart (Table 10.1). It is also of value to auscultate at the thoracic inlet, over the carotid arteries and, especially in cats, ventrally over the sternum where murmurs may radiate (see later) and where lung and other extraneous sounds may be less intrusive.

Both the bell and diaphragm of the stethoscope's chest-piece should be employed. The diaphragm selectively transmits *high* frequency sounds. The diaphragm also transmits louder sounds (because of its larger area), and it is used for general auscultation of the heart and lungs. The bell, which when applied *lightly* to the chest wall allows *lower* frequency components to be heard more clearly, is used to aid the detection of gallop sounds and low pitched murmurs. It is important to use a *good quality stethoscope* with comfortable, close fitting ear tips; the ear tubes should angle forwards. The tubing should not be excessively long (35–45 cm). In cats and small puppies, the small physical size of the heart, in addition to a rapid heart rate, makes the localization of heart sounds difficult. The use of a stethoscope with a *small chest piece* (e.g. an 'infant' or 'paediatric' stethoscope) may help considerably in these smaller patients.

The normal heart sounds – S1 and S2

The normal heart sounds arise as vibrations of the heart and great vessels, caused by the sudden acceleration or deceleration of blood at the beginning and end of each ventricular contraction. Blood flow through the heart is otherwise normally silent. These sounds are short in duration and thus are termed *transient sounds*. Only two transient sounds are normally heard in each cardiac cycle in cats and dogs; these are the *first* and *second heart sounds*.

The first heart sound (S1, described as 'lub') is

		Dog	**Cat**
Apex region	Left A-V (mitral) area	L 5th ICS at CCJ	L 5–6th ICS $^1/_4$ VD distance from sternum
	Right A-V (tricuspid) area	R 3—5th ICS near CCJ	R 4–5th ICS $^1/_4$ VD distance from sternum
Heart base	Aortic area	L 4th ICS above CCJ	L 2–3rd ICS, just dorsal to pulmonic area
	Pulmonic area	L 2—4th ICS at sternal border	L 2–3rd ICS, $^1/_3$–$^1/_2$ VD distance from sternum

L = left; R = right; A-V = atrioventricular; ICS = intercostal space; CCJ = costochondral junction; VD = ventrodorsal (adapted from Smith and Tilley, 1992).

Table 10.1: *Anatomical areas of auscultation in the dog and cat.*

longer in duration and lower pitched than the second heart sound, and is *most clearly* heard over the region of the palpable cardiac apex beat (normally over the 5th to 6th intercostal spaces at the level of the costochondral junction on the left, one to two intercostal spaces further cranially on the right – see Table 10.1), although it is usually audible over *all* areas of cardiac auscultation. At the cardiac apex, S1 may be louder, equal to or softer than the second heart sound. S1 is generated by events occurring at the start of the isovolumetric phase of ventricular systole (Figure 10.1). As the left (mitral) and right (tricuspid) atrioventricular (A-V) valves close and the ventricles start to contract, the A-V valves, chordae and papillary muscles suddenly come into a state of tension, generating vibrations which are heard as S1. The left A-V valve apparatus generates most of this energy, although the ejection of blood into the great vessels may also contribute. The first heart sound thus marks the start of ventricular systole and occurs just before the peripheral pulse, at or just after the R wave of the electrocardiogram (ECG) (Figure 10.2).

The second heart sound (S2, described as 'dup') is shorter and higher pitched than S1. It marks the termination of ventricular systole and occurs at or just after the T wave of the ECG (Figures 10.1 and 10.2). As the ventricles start to relax and intraventricular pressure begins to fall, the columns of blood in the aorta and pulmonary artery recoil, causing the semi-

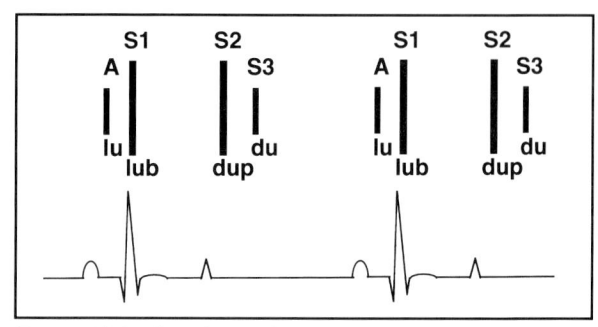

Figure 10.2: *The relationship of the normal and abnormal transient heart sounds to the ECG.*

lunar valves to close and producing the vibrations which are heard as S2. It is heard *most clearly* at the base of the heart on the left (left axilla, 2nd to 4th intercostal spaces), although again it is normally audible over all areas of cardiac auscultation. S2 is normally louder than S1 when listening at the heart base. The pattern of the normal heart sounds in dogs and cats may thus be represented as 'lub–dup, lub–dup, lub–dup, …'

Factors affecting the intensity of S1 and S2

The intensity of the heart sounds may be influenced by many factors, which may or may not affect S1 and S2 equally.

S1 and S2 may both be altered in intensity:

- *Reduced* in intensity by obesity of the patient, pleural or pericardial effusions, and reduced systolic function (e.g. hypothyroidism, dilated cardiomyopathy)
- *Increased* in intensity in thin patients and where the strength of ventricular contraction is increased (e.g. hyperthyroidism, anaemia, excitement or stress)
- *Beat-to-beat variations* in the loudness of the heart sounds may be caused by arrhythmias (e.g. ectopic beats and especially atrial fibrillation), and may also arise due to changes in cardiac rhythm and filling during the respiratory cycle.

S1 and S2 may change in their intensity relative to each other:

- *S1 is accentuated relative to S2* if the P-R interval decreases, and *vice versa*
- *S1 is diminished relative to S2* where volume overload alters the isovolumetric phase of ventricular systole (e.g. by left A-V regurgitation)
- *S2 is accentuated relative to S1* by pulmonary or systemic hypertension, and when left-to-right shunting occurs with congenital anomalies such as patent ductus arteriosus (PDA) and septal defects
- *S2 is reduced in intensity relative to S1* by premature (ectopic) beats. If the time available

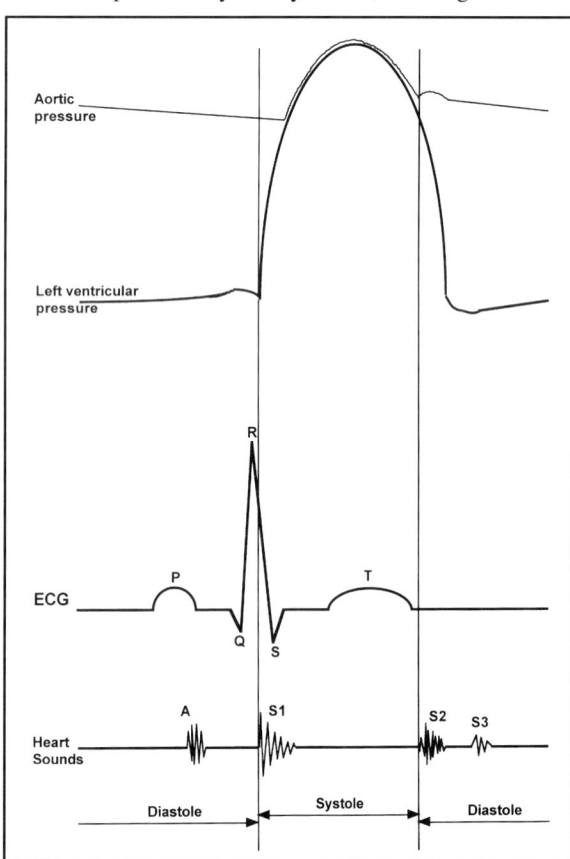

Figure 10.1: *The relationship of aortic and left ventricular pressures, ECG and heart sounds during one cardiac cycle.*

for diastole is very much shortened by the occurrence of a premature beat, ventricular filling may be so much reduced that the semilunar valves do not open during systole, S2 may be absent and S1 may become relatively louder.

ABNORMAL HEART SOUNDS

Gallop sounds

Other transient sounds may become audible which, in dogs and cats, almost invariably indicate the presence of disease. The *third heart sound* (S3) occurs at the end of the rapid ventricular filling phase of early diastole, just after S2, when the jets of blood flowing in from the atria impinge on the ventricular apex and produce vibrations (Figures 10.1 and 10.2). These vibrations may have enough energy to produce an audible sound in situations such as congestive heart failure of any cause, A-V valve or aortic regurgitation or high output states (e.g. severe anaemia, hyperthyroidism). S3 is best heard with the bell of the stethoscope at the cardiac apex, especially on the left. It is a low pitched sound, and, when audible in small animals is termed a *ventricular* or *protodiastolic gallop* sound ('lub–dup–du'). It may vary in intensity during the respiratory cycle and may be accentuated by exercise.

The *fourth heart sound* (S4), also called the *atrial sound* or 'A-sound', occurs just before S1 and arises, like S3, from the inflow of blood into the ventricles, in this case caused by atrial contraction (Figures 10.1 and 10.2). Transient closure of the A-V valves also contributes to the generation of this sound. S4 may become audible in similar situations to S3, especially where ventricular compliance is reduced (e.g. hypertrophic cardiomyopathy). Again, it is a low pitched sound, best heard using the bell of the stethoscope at the cardiac apex, and, when audible in small animals is termed an *atrial* or *presystolic gallop* sound ('lu-lub–dup'). Like S3, it may vary in intensity during the respiratory cycle and may be accentuated by exercise. Atrial sounds may also become audible during periods of second and third degree atrioventricular block.

The presence of audible S3 and S4 gallop sounds is considered to be *pathological in dogs and cats*. They are commonly heard in cases of heart disease and usually indicate the presence of ventricular myocardial disease or congestive heart failure, but may also occur with hypertension (systemic or pulmonary). They may be the only audible abnormality of heart sounds in some patients, for example in cases of cardiomyopathy. Gallop sounds are, however, occasionally heard in *normal* cats after sedation. S3 is heard more commonly than S4, but both gallop sounds may be audible in the same individual and they can be very loud. At high heart rates, particularly in cats, S3 and S4 may merge to form a *summation gallop* sound. It should be noted that S3 and S4 are frequently heard in horses and cattle, where they are considered to be normal.

Split sounds and clicks

Both S1 and S2 consist of right- and left-sided components, but these normally occur almost simultaneously and are too close (less than approximately 30 ms apart) to be differentiated by ear at the high heart rates commonly encountered in cats and dogs. However both may become audibly *split* (i.e. the left and right components are heard separately). Occasionally this is detected in normal animals (e.g. physiological splitting of S1 in large and giant breed dogs) but it is usually pathological. S1 may become split due to ventricular ectopic beats or bundle branch blocks, which cause *asynchronous activation* of the ventricles. Splitting of S2 ('lub–du.dup') may arise for similar reasons and also due to pulmonary or systemic hypertension, congenital arterio-venous shunts (e.g. septal defects, PDA), or congenital aortic or pulmonic valvular stenosis. The most commonly encountered cause of a split S2 is probably pulmonary hypertension, but even this is uncommon.

Short, high pitched sounds termed *clicks* may occur during systole, although they are not commonly detected. Early systolic clicks (also called ejection sounds) may arise due to congenital anomalies of the semilunar valves (e.g. valvular pulmonic stenosis) or systemic or pulmonary hypertension. These are heard most clearly at the heart base. Clicks occurring later in systole may arise as a consequence of A-V valve disease (endocardiosis, left A-V valve prolapse). These are heard most clearly at the left or right apex and may be very variable in occurrence and timing during systole. Clicks often have little or no immediate clinical significance.

It is not always possible to determine the presence or identity of abnormal transient sounds by auscultation alone, especially at fast heart rates. The technique of *phonocardiography*, where heart sounds recorded by a microphone are transcribed by a chart recorder simultaneously with an ECG, can be used to help in distinguishing these sounds.

Murmurs

Causes

Murmurs arise when the normal, silent, laminar flow of blood through the heart or blood vessels is disturbed, causing *turbulence*, vortices, and micro-bubble formation. If the vibrations so produced have sufficient energy they become audible as a *murmur*, and with even greater energy they may be *palpable* as a *thrill*. Disturbances in the pattern of blood flow may arise due to changes in blood viscosity, increased velocity of blood flow or, most commonly, changes in the shape of the chamber or vessel within which the blood is flowing.

Pathological murmurs

A murmur is described as pathological if it arises due to a defect of heart or blood vessel structure or function. Examples include:

- *Regurgitation* of blood back through an incompetent A-V valve during systole (e.g. due to congenital A-V valve dysplasia or acquired endocardiosis, endocarditis or chordal rupture; A-V valve incompetence may also arise *secondary* to dilatation of the valve annulus from some other cause, such as cardiomyopathy)
- Abnormal turbulent, high velocity blood flow through a *shunt* [e.g. ventricular septal defect (VSD), PDA]
- High velocity systolic flow through a *stenotic* outflow tract (e.g. congenital pulmonic or (sub-) aortic stenosis, aortic valve endocarditis)
- *High volume* flow through a *normal* valve or outflow tract ('*relative stenosis*', e.g. left-to-right shunting through an atrial septal defect leads to abnormal flow through the right A-V valve and pulmonary outflow tract).

Physiological and innocent murmurs

A murmur is described as *physiological* if it arises due to a change in blood viscosity or velocity of flow in the *absence* of any anatomical defects of the heart, e.g. in anaemia (if the haemoglobin level falls below approximately 6 g/dl), hypoproteinaemia, fever, hyperthyroidism, stress, etc. Murmurs may also arise following sedation. The term *innocent* or *functional* is used for the murmurs which may occur in the *absence of disease*, typically in puppies and kittens. These murmurs usually disappear as the animal matures beyond 16–24 weeks of age. Innocent murmurs may occur in adult (usually athletic) animals, where no structural defects or other abnormalities can be detected, although this is a matter of some controversy. Physiological murmurs are also sometimes called 'functional'.

Innocent and physiological murmurs are usually variable, soft to moderate in intensity (grades I or II, occasionally up to III: see later), localized, occur in early to mid systole and are heard most clearly at the heart base. It is possible, especially in kittens, to produce a murmur simply by compressing the thoracic wall during auscultation.

Some *extraneous sounds* may mimic heart murmurs. Blood flow in the carotid arteries may produce audible sounds, usually called '*bruits*', which are heard over the jugular furrow. Compression of adjacent lung tissue by the contractile movements of the heart may also produce bruits which are heard over the cardiac apex, and which vary with respiration. Pericarditis may *rarely* give rise to a 'friction rub', caused by the rubbing together of inflamed, dry pericardial membranes with each cardiac contraction. This usually disappears rapidly due to the formation of a pericardial effusion.

Classification of murmurs

Accurate descriptive classification of murmurs, especially their timing within the cardiac cycle and their point of maximum loudness, can give much information of clinical value.

Timing and duration

Systolic murmurs are by far the most common. They may occur in the early (protosystolic), middle or late part of systole, or may extend throughout it (holosystolic – Figure 10.3). If the murmur obscures the normal heart sounds, it is described as pansystolic. Simultaneous auscultation and palpation of the peripheral pulse or apex beat helps the clinician to determine the timing of a murmur within the cardiac cycle. A systolic murmur follows S1 and occurs at the same time as the apex beat or arterial pulse. Examples of systolic murmurs include left and right A-V valve regurgitation, aortic and pulmonic stenosis, VSD and functional murmurs (Table 10.2).

Diastolic murmurs are uncommon. They follow S2 and the arterial pulse, and may be short (protodiastolic)

Systolic	Regurgitant	Left A-V valvular regurgitation
		Right A-V valvular regurgitation
		Ventricular septal defect
	Ejection	(Sub-) aortic stenosis
		Pulmonic stenosis
		Tetralogy of Fallot (pulmonic stenosis)
		Atrial septal defect (relative *pulmonic stenosis*)
		Functional murmurs
Diastolic	Decrescendo	Aortic regurgitation
		Pulmonic regurgitation (rarely audible)
		Left A-V valvular stenosis (rare)
		Right A-V valvular stenosis (rare)
Continuous		Patent ductus arteriosus
		(other arterio–venous shunts)

Table 10.2: Murmur types and their causes (adapted from Gompf, 1988).

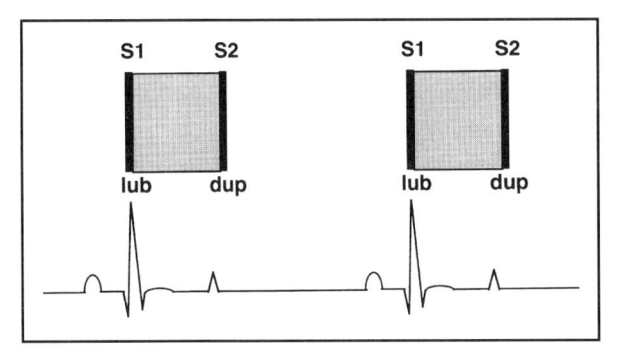

Figure 10.3: *Diagrammatic representation of a holosystolic (regurgitant) murmur.*

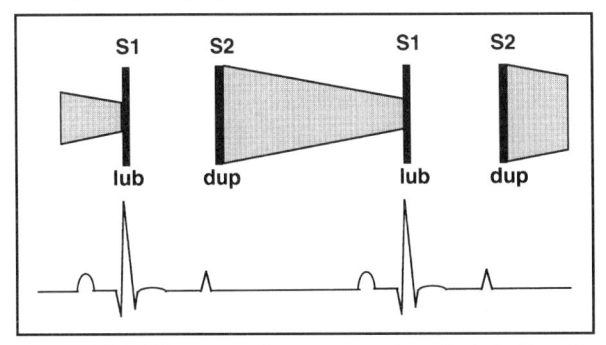

Figure 10.4: *Diagrammatic representation of a holodiastolic decrescendo murmur.*

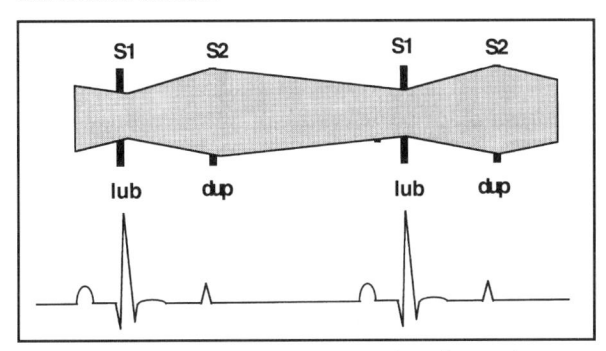

Figure 10.5: *Diagrammatic representation of a continuous murmur (PDA).*

or may last throughout diastole (holodiastolic – Figure 10.4). The most common example of a diastolic murmur is *aortic regurgitation*, e.g. due to congenital disease or endocarditis. Pulmonic regurgitation rarely produces an *audible* murmur. Left and right A-V valve stenoses (either absolute or relative), which may produce late diastolic murmurs, are rare.

Continuous murmurs extend throughout systole and into diastole, spanning S2 and generally peaking in intensity at S2; these murmurs are also not common. The most common example is PDA (Figure 10.5). This murmur characteristically waxes and wanes, being louder during systole, and is sometimes described as a 'machinery murmur'. Occasionally the murmur may not persist for the whole of diastole, for example if diastole is long due to a slow heart rate. There are other *rare* examples of continuous murmurs, usually caused by other forms of arterio-venous shunt. Combined aortic stenosis and incompetence (congenital, or acquired due to endo-

carditis) produces a systolic *and* diastolic 'to-and-fro' or 'see-saw' murmur, which may *sound* continuous, but S2 should be audible between the two compone VSD produces a similar sound.

Point of maximum intensity (PMI)

The point on the chest wall where a murmur or other abnormality is heard most clearly (and where the thrill, if present, is palpable) indicates the likely source of the sound from within the heart (Table 10.1). It should be realized that the PMI for each valve sound does *not* correspond to the anatomical position of the valve, but reflects radiation of these sounds within the heart (see Table 10.1).

Caudal cardiac area (apex region)

Left apex
Murmurs of left A-V valve regurgitation are best heard over the left apex.

Right apex
Murmurs of right A-V valve regurgitation are best heard over the right apex, at about the same level as the left A-V region.

VSD murmurs are also heard best over the right apex, but nearer the sternal border and more cranial than murmurs of right A-V regurgitation.

Cranial cardiac area (heart base)

Left base
Aortic stenosis murmurs and functional murmurs from the aortic outflow tract are best heard over the left heart base.

Pulmonic stenosis murmurs are slightly more cranial and ventral than aortic outflow murmurs. It is often difficult to distinguish the aortic and pulmonic valve areas clinically.

The murmur of PDA is best heard high in the left axilla.

Radiation

Murmurs may radiate away from their point of maximum intensity, particularly if loud or associated with cardiomegaly. The pattern of radiation may be very variable, depending on the cause of the murmur and the direction of the jet of turbulence.

The murmur of *left A-V regurgitation* may radiate dorsally and caudally or dorsally and cranially, and may also radiate across the chest to the right. A-V valve regurgitant murmurs may be clearly heard ventrally over the sternum in cats.

The murmur of *aortic stenosis* radiates to the right cranial thorax and may also radiate up the carotids, and rarely to the top of the cranium. The murmur of aortic regurgitation may radiate more caudally or variably.

The murmur of *pulmonic stenosis* may radiate

dorsally into the left axilla or across to the right cranial thorax, and sometimes up the carotids.

The murmur of *PDA* radiates to the thoracic inlet and right cranial thorax. The systolic component may radiate widely while the diastolic component is often much more localized.

It may be difficult to distinguish between radiation of murmurs and the multiple origin of murmurs. For example, if a systolic murmur is audible at the left apex in a case of PDA, this may represent radiation of the systolic component of the shunt murmur, or it may arise from left A-V regurgitation secondary to left ventricular dilation.

Character ('acoustic profile' or quality) and pitch
These are *subjective* assessments if made without access to phonocardiography.

Regurgitant murmurs are usually long (holosystolic) murmurs with a relatively uniform loudness throughout systole ('plateau' or 'band' shape – Figure 10.3). The murmur may be harsh, or it may have a high pitched or 'blowing' quality. They arise due to left A-V or right A-V regurgitation (due to any of the causes mentioned earlier under pathological murmurs), or VSD. Left A-V regurgitation tends to produce louder, higher pitched murmurs than right A-V regurgitation. Where A-V regurgitation is *secondary* to A-V valve ring stretching (e.g. dilated cardiomyopathy), or in *early* cases of valvular endocardiosis, a softer, shorter, early to mid-systolic, decrescendo murmur may occur.

Ejection murmurs are crescendo–decrescendo ('diamond shaped') in configuration, reaching maximum loudness in early to mid-systole (Figure 10.6). They arise due to outflow obstructions such as aortic (valvular or sub-valvular) or pulmonic stenosis, or hypertrophic cardiomyopathy. In these cases, the murmur is usually harsh and holosystolic, and the more severe the obstruction, the louder and longer the murmur usually is.

Functional murmurs are also ejection in type, but are softer and shorter, and may be lower in pitch.

Aortic regurgitation produces a decrescendo diastolic murmur, which may have a long, 'sighing' quality (Figure 10.4).

PDA produces a continuous, waxing and waning murmur with a harsh or 'rumbling' quality (Figure 10.5).

Musical murmurs (regurgitant or ejection types) may contain vibrations with one predominant frequency, but more commonly they contain a mixed spectrum of frequencies.

Intensity
Loudness of murmurs may be *subjectively* graded (out of six grades). Recording this in the patient's notes allows changes to be appreciated. Although *in general* louder equals more severe, loudness is *not always* correlated with severity. Some very loud regurgitant murmurs (e.g. across a small, restrictive VSD or where the pressure gradient between the left ventricle and atrium is large) have little haemodynamic significance. Conversely, some *soft* murmurs may be associated with *severe* disease, e.g. right A-V valve dysplasia or *advanced* left A-V regurgitation. The murmur of aortic stenosis is reduced in intensity by failure of myocardial function. The six grades of loudness are defined as follows:

- Grade I: very faint – not heard immediately
- Grade II: soft but heard immediately on commencing auscultation
- Grade III: moderate and equal in loudness to the normal (transient) heart sounds – most murmurs of clinical significance are grade III or louder
- Grade IV: loud, usually widespread, but no thrill is palpable
- Grade V: loud and associated with a palpable thrill
- Grade VI: very loud – audible with the stethoscope just held away from thorax, or audible without the use of a stethoscope.

Variability
The intensity of a murmur may vary from beat to beat, e.g. due to arrhythmias or with respiration. Murmur intensity may also be altered by heart rate, exercise and vasoactive drugs (including sedatives). The ejection murmur caused by dynamic outflow obstruction in hypertrophic cardiomyopathy may vary *markedly* with heart rate.

SUMMARY

A complete description of auscultatory findings should take account of the following points:

Normal heart sounds

- Intensity
- Audibility
- Variability
- Position
- Rate
- Rhythm
- Correlation with the peripheral pulse.

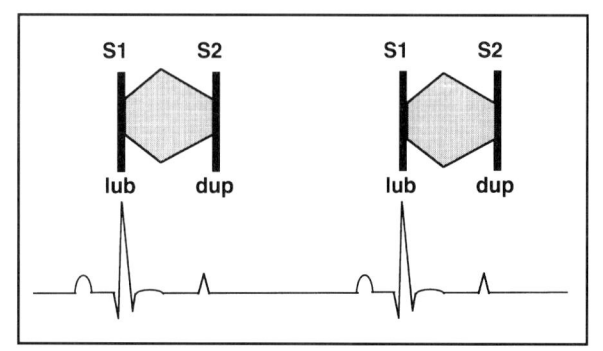

Figure 10.6: Diagrammatic representation of a holosystolic crescendo–decrescendo (ejection) murmur.

Abnormal rhythms

See Chapter 11.

Abnormal transient sounds

- Gallop sounds
- Split sounds
- Clicks.

Murmurs

- Timing and duration during the cardiac cycle
- Point or area of maximum intensity
- Radiation over the thorax
- Character (pitch, acoustic quality and configuration)
- Loudness (intensity)
- Variability (e.g. beat-to-beat changes in intensity or character).

Lung and airway sounds

- Accentuation or muffling of the normal airway and vesicular sounds
- Presence and distribution of any abnormal (adventitious) sounds.

REFERENCES

Gompf RE (1988) The clinical approach to heart disease: history and physical examination. In: *Canine and Feline Cardiology*, ed. P. R. Fox. Churchill Livingstone, New York

Smith Jr, FWK and Tilley LP (1992) *Rapid Interpretation of Heart Sounds, Murmurs and Arrhythmias: a Guide to Cardiac Auscultation in Dogs and Cats (Workbook and Audio Cassette)*. Lea & Febiger, Philadelphia.

Arrhythmias

Mike Martin

NORMAL CARDIAC RHYTHM

The *sinoatrial (SA) node* in the right atrium is normally the primary site of impulse formation, and is therefore the usual dominant 'pacemaker' of the heart. From the SA node, the impulse spreads to the rest of the atrial myocardium, and on to the ventricular myocardium via the *atrioventricular (AV) node, bundle of His, bundle branches* and *Purkinje fibres* (Figure 11.1). The SA node will speed up or slow down its rate of discharge according to the prevailing autonomic influence. If the SA node fails to discharge at a normal rate, the lower specialized conduction fibres are capable of depolarizing spontaneously at a slower rate.

'Arrhythmia' and 'dysrhythmia' are synonymous terms used in reference to abnormalities in the cardiac rhythm. Arrhythmia literally means 'absence of rhythm' and dysrhythmia means 'abnormal rhythm'. Arrhythmias can be broadly categorized into those with a predominantly slow rhythm – *bradyarrhythmias* and those with a fast rhythm – *tachyarrhythmias* (Table 11.1).

Bradyarrhythmias	Tachyarrhythmias
Sinus bradycardia	Sinus tachycardia
Sinus arrest & block	Ventricular pre-excitation
Atrial standstill	Ventricular premature
1st degree AV block	complexes and ventricular
2nd degree AV block	tachycardia
3rd degree AV block	Supraventricular
Escape rhythms	premature complexes
	and supraventricular
	tachycardia
	AV dissociation
	Ventricular fibrillation
	Atrial fibrillation and
	flutter

Table 11.1: List of arrhythmias discussed in this monograph. Sick sinus syndrome can present with a combination of bradyarrhythmias and tachycardias, e.g. brady–tachy syndrome.

ABNORMALITIES IN RATE

Sinus bradycardia
Sinus bradycardia is defined as *sinus rhythm at a heart rate less than normal for the species, breed and age of animal*. In dogs, normal heart rate is usually quoted as greater than 70 bpm, and greater than 140 bpm in cats.

ECG features
The P-QRS-T complexes are normal in appearance but at a lower rate (Figure 11.2).

Associated conditions

- Normal in physiologically fit dogs, some giant breed dogs
- Hypothyroidism
- Hyperkalaemia
- Increased intracranial pressure
- Some systemic diseases, e.g. uraemia
- Hypothermia
- Drugs such as tranquillizers (e.g. medetomidine, xylazine, acepromazine maleate) or antiarrhythmics (e.g. propranolol, digitalis)
- Heart failure in cats.

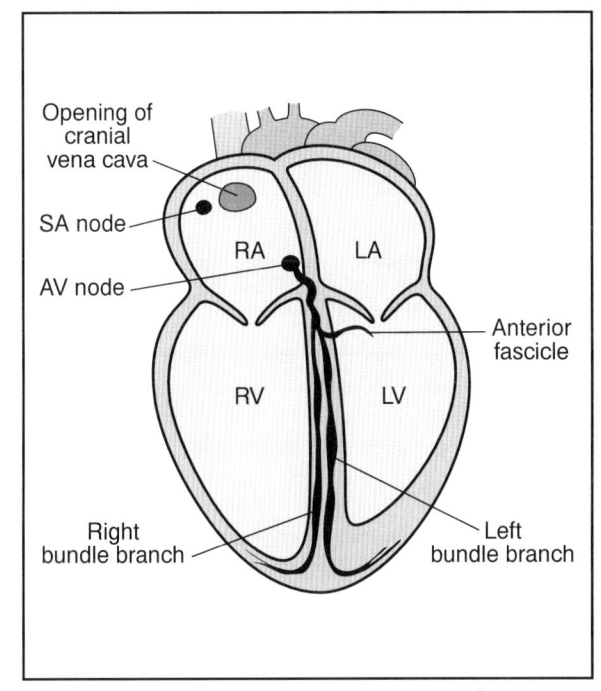

Opening of cranial vena cava

SA node

AV node

RA

LA

Anterior fascicle

RV

LV

Right bundle branch

Left bundle branch

Figure 11.1: The normal cardiac conduction pathways.

Management

Treatment is not usually required, as either the primary cause can be found, or there are no clinical signs. If the animal presents with weakness, lethargy or collapse and the primary cause is not found, treatment may initially be instituted with *atropine*, *glycopyrrolate* or *isoprenaline*.

It may be helpful to carry out an *atropine response test* to determine if the underlying cause is an increase in vagal tone. Atropine is administered at 20–40 µg/kg sc, and another ECG is recorded 30 minutes later. An increase in rate following atropine suggests a vagal mechanism. *Pacemaker* implantation (Table 11.2), although effective, is rarely necessary.

Sinus tachycardia

Sinus tachycardia is defined as sinus rhythm at a heart rate greater than normal for the species, breed and age of animal. Top of the normal quoted reference range

Complete (3rd degree) AV block
2nd degree Mobitz type II, persistent or intermittent
2nd degree Mobitz type I, with symptoms
Sinus bradycardia ± sinus arrest, with symptoms
'Tachy–brady' sick sinus syndrome, when anti-tachyarrhythmic drugs produce symptoms
Persistent atrial standstill (questionable)

Table 11.2: List of indications for permanent pacemaker implantation. These are generally symptomatic bradyarrhythmias.

for dogs is around 180 bpm, with 240 bpm in cats, although these figures may be rather high for the majority of normal, relaxed animals. Sinus tachycardia is a normal compensatory response in heart failure.

ECG features

The P-QRS-T complexes are normal in appearance, but at a faster rate than normal. The rhythm is usually regular, although there may be a slight variation in the R-R interval (Figure 11.3).

Associated conditions

- Pain
- Stress
- Excitement
- Pyrexia
- Shock
- Septicaemia
- Hyperthyroidism
- Drugs (e.g. atropine, hydralazine, adrenaline)
- Heart failure.

Management

Treatment should be aimed at the primary cause.

ABNORMALITIES IN THE CONDUCTION SYSTEM

Sinus arrest or block

This occurs as a result of the SA node failing to discharge (*sinus arrest*) or failure of conduction from an otherwise

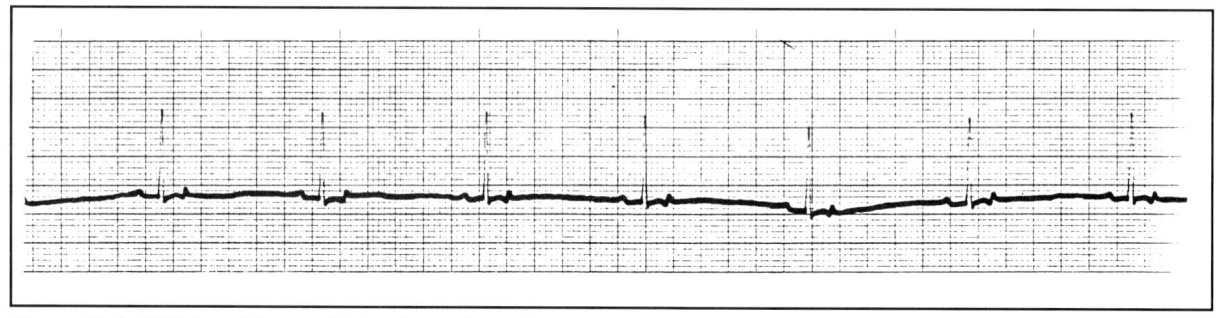

Figure 11.2: ECG from 13-year-old female Border Collie with sinus bradycardia (50/min) and first degree AV block (PR interval = 0.16 seconds) due to digoxin toxicity associated with renal failure. Lead II, 25 mm/s, 1 cm/mV.

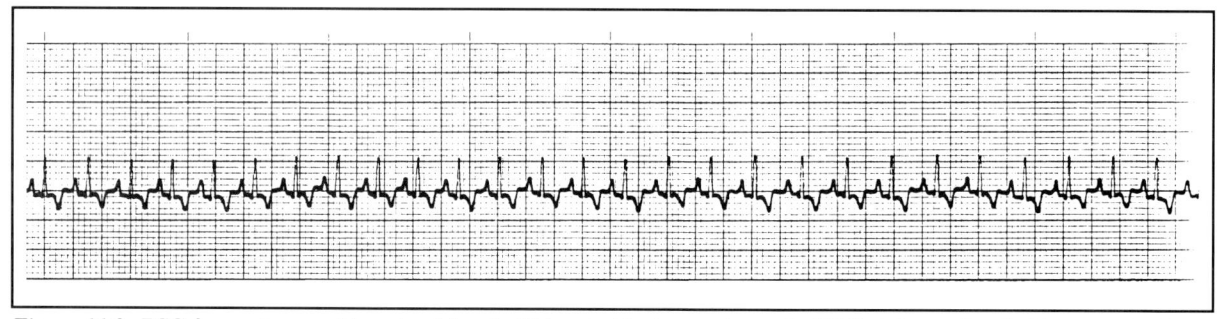

Figure 11.3: ECG from a 6-year-old neutered female Whippet with sinus tachycardia (200/min) associated with congestive heart failure. The bitch also had pleural effusion, which may explain the small R waves (0.6 mV). Lead II, 25 mm/s, 1 cm/mV.

regularly firing SA node (*sinus block*). A long period of sinus arrest (greater than 5–10 seconds at exercise, to 20–30 seconds at rest) may result in syncope.

ECG features
There is a pause in the rhythm with *no P-QRS-T complexes* (Figure 11.4). If the pause is twice the R-R interval, it suggests *sinus block*. If the pause is greater than two R-R intervals, it suggests *sinus arrest*. Long periods of arrest are often followed by escape complexes (see later).

Associated conditions

- Normal variation in brachycephalic breeds with exaggerated respiratory sinus arrhythmia
- Atrial pathology (e.g. fibrosis, dilation, cardiac neoplasia)
- Electrolyte imbalances, e.g. hyperkalaemia
- Hypothyroidism
- Thoracic surgical manipulation
- Drugs (see sinus bradycardia).

Management
Treatment is aimed at the primary cause and animals without clinical signs do not require treatment. As with sinus bradycardia, *atropine*, *glycopyrrolate* and *isoprenaline* may be used. If medical treatment is ineffective or it produces unacceptable side effects, then *pacemaker* therapy is indicated.

Sick sinus syndrome
Sick sinus syndrome is a term for a number of abnormalities of the SA node (i.e. sinus node dysfunction), including severe sinus bradycardia and severe SA block or arrest. However, many of these cases also have episodes of supraventricular tachycardias; this is termed the '*bradycardia–tachycardia syndrome*'. It is characteristic of this arrhythmia that during long periods of sinus arrest, there is failure of rescue *escape beats* (Hamlin *et al.*, 1972).

Clinical findings
There may also be alternating periods of bradycardia with a supraventricular tachycardia, either of which may result in weakness or syncope.

ECG features
These are quite variable, and include *persistent sinus bradycardia*, and *episodes of sinus arrest without escape beats*, sometimes following an atrial premature complex or there may be alternating periods of bradycardia with a supraventricular tachycardia.

Associated conditions
Sick sinus syndrome has been reported to occur most commonly in female Miniature Schnauzers at least 6 years of age (Tilley, 1992), and may therefore be idiopathic. It has not been recorded in cats.

Management
The treatment of choice for symptomatic cases is *pacemaker* implantation with or without antiarrhythmic drugs to control any tachycardias. Medical treatment alone is usually unsuccessful.

Atrial standstill
In atrial standstill there is an absence of any atrial activity due to a failure of atrial myocardial activation.

Clinical findings
Usually those of weakness, lethargy and syncope.

ECG features
These include an absence of P waves with a regular, slow (less than 60 per minute) escape rhythm with a supraventricular configuration. The QRS complexes are often of a relatively normal shape, although sometimes of prolonged duration (Figure 11.5). The sinus node continues to fire and its impulses are conducted by *internodal pathways* to the atrioventricular (AV) node. The escape rhythm is therefore a *sinoventricular rhythm* (Tilley, 1992).

Associated conditions

- *Persistent* atrial standstill (fascioscapulohumeral muscular dystrophy in English Springer Spaniels)
- *Temporary* atrial standstill (hyperkalaemia and digitalis toxicity)
- *Terminal* atrial standstill (in association with a 'dying' heart).

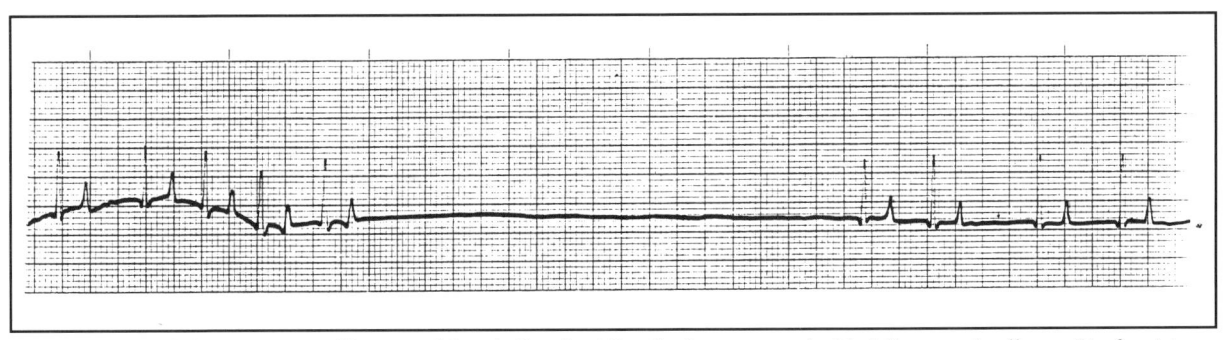

Figure 11.4: ECG from a 4-year-old neutered female Standard Poodle that presented with dullness and collapse. Biochemistry revealed a marked hyperkalaemia due to hypoadrenocorticism. There is a long period of sinus arrest (3.5 seconds). P waves are not clearly seen on this lead 2 tracing but were evident on precordial leads. Lead II, 25 mm/s, 1 cm/mV.

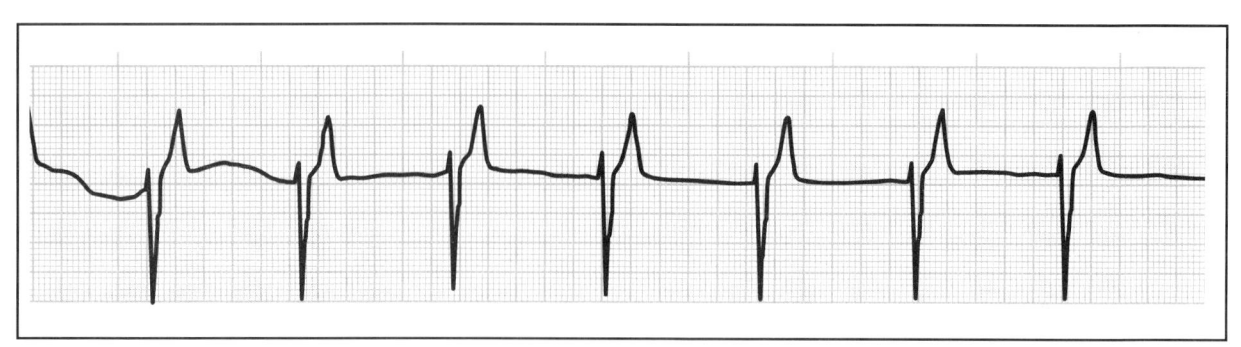

Figure 11.5: *ECG from a 1-year-old Cavalier King Charles Spaniel that presented with lethargy and weakness. The ECG shows idiopathic persistent atrial standstill. Note the absence of P waves (also absent on precordial chest leads) with a ventricular escape rhythm at 60/min. Atrial activity was demonstrated to be absent on echocardiographic examination. Lead II, 25 mm/s, 1 cm/mV.*

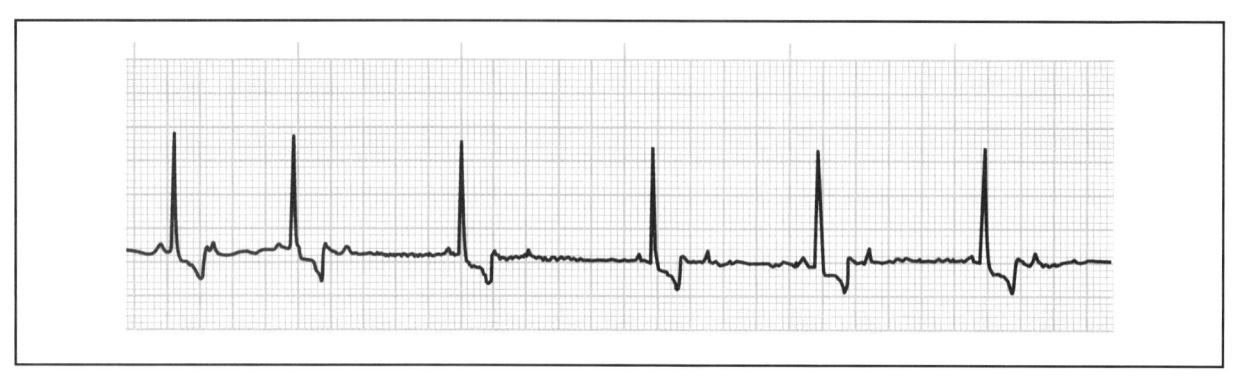

Figure 11.6: *ECG from a 12-year-old Yorkshire Terrier in which a bradycardia was detected on routine examination at annual vaccinations. There were apparently no significant clinical signs, although the dog had been gradually slowing up with 'old age'! The ECG shows second degree AV block (2:1 block). Lead II, 25 mm/s, 1 cm/mV.*

Management

Treatment is directed towards the primary cause described above. However, hyperkalaemia can be life-threatening, and needs prompt treatment, such as administration of a *saline infusion*. If the cause is due to hypoadrenocorticism (confirmed by an ACTH test), then a saline infusion can be given with dexamethasone iv, followed by oral administration of prednisolone and fludrocortisone acetate. More intensive therapy such as insulin can be instituted when an intensive therapy unit is available with the facility to monitor potassium levels frequently (Morgan, 1982).

With persistent atrial standstill without underlying heart disease permanent *pacemaker* implantation is a consideration, but is not always successful.

Atrioventricular (AV) block

AV block is a failure to conduct impulses normally through the AV node. It is also commonly known as 'heart block'. AV block may be partial (first or second degree block) or complete (third degree block).

First degree AV block

First degree AV block occurs when there is a delay in conduction through the AV node when the heart is in sinus rhythm. First degree block does not in itself cause any clinical problems.

ECG features: The P wave and QRS complexes are normal in configuration, but the PR interval is prolonged (Figure 11.6).

Associated conditions:

- May be normal at slow heart rates
- Drugs (especially digoxin, propranolol, procainamide)
- Hyperkalaemia
- Ageing changes in the AV node.

Management: Treatment should be aimed at the underlying cause.

Second degree AV block

Second degree AV block occurs when conduction intermittently fails to pass through the AV node.

Clinical findings: Cases of second degree AV block with a slow ventricular rate may present with weakness, lethargy or syncope. Auscultation reveals an intermittent pause in the heart's rhythm.

ECG features: The P wave is normal, but there is either an occasional or frequent failure (depending on severity) of conduction through the AV node, resulting in the absence of an associated QRS complex (Figure 11.6).

There are two sub-classifications of second degree AV block:

1. *Mobitz type I (Wenckebach phenomenon)*
   The P-R interval increases prior to the block.
2. *Mobitz type II*
   The P-R interval remains constant prior to the block, and the frequency of the block is usually constant, i.e. 2:1, 3:1 etc.
A. *Type A*; the QRS duration is normal, and the block is believed to be above the division of the bundle of His.
B. *Type B*; the QRS is prolonged, and the block is believed to be below the division of the bundle of His.

Mobitz type I is usually type A, and Mobitz type II is usually type B. Second degree AV block that is severe or advanced (i.e. block occurs frequently) is usually the Mobitz type II sub-classification, and may progress to complete AV block.

Associated conditions:

- High vagal tone (especially brachycephalic breeds) – often in association with sinus arrhythmia
- Idiopathic
- Older dogs with AV nodal fibrosis
- Hereditary stenosis of the bundle of His in the pug
- Drugs (e.g. digitalis toxicity, xylazine, medetomidine, atropine and quinidine)
- Hyperkalaemia.

Management: The treatment is aimed at the primary cause. In advanced and symptomatic cases of unknown cause, treatment may be attempted medically with parasympatholytic drugs (e.g. *atropine* or *glycopyrrolate*) or sympathomimetic drugs (e.g. *isoprenaline* or *terbutaline*). Some improvement is often seen. In those cases that are unresponsive to medical therapy or develop unacceptable side effects, then *pacemaker* implantation is indicated. In low-grade, asymptomatic second degree AV block, the animal should be examined at regular intervals to monitor for progression of the block.

Complete (third degree) AV block
Complete AV block occurs when there is a persistent failure of the impulse to be conducted through the AV node. A second pacemaker below the AV node, i.e. the area of block, discharges to control the ventricles with a rate of discharge that is slower than the SA node (Figure 11.7).

The second pacemaker may arise from:

- The *lower AV node* or *bundle branches* producing a normal QRS (junctional escape complexes) at approximately 60–70 per minute in dogs (higher rate in cats)
- *Purkinje cells* producing an abnormal QRS-T complex (ventricular escape complexes) at approximately 30–40 per minute in dogs (higher rate in cats).

Clinical findings: These may include weakness, lethargy, syncope or sudden death. The severity of the clinical signs is dependent upon the rate of the escape rhythm. A ventricular escape rhythm is usually associated with more marked clinical signs, with the possibility of sudden death. Generalized cardiomegaly is common in chronic cases with a slow ventricular response rate, and congestive heart failure may develop. On auscultation a characteristic finding is a very regular but slow heart rhythm, together with the palpation of a hyperdynamic femoral pulse. In some cases the more rapid atrial contraction sounds (S4) may be faintly audible.

ECG features: P waves can be seen at a regular and fast rate, and QRS-T complexes at a regular and slow rate, but independently of each other. This is best demonstrated by plotting out each P wave and each QRS complex on a piece of paper.

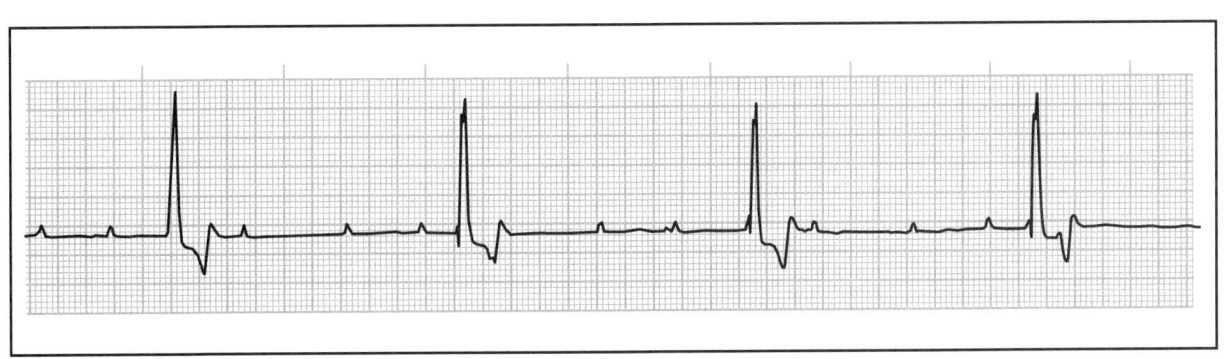

Figure 11.7: *ECG from a 6-year-old Labrador Retriever with recent onset lethargy and exercise intolerance. The ECG shows third degree (complete) AV block. The P wave rate is 100/min and the QRS rate is 30/min. Permanent pacemaker implantation is indicated in this case. Lead II, 25 mm/s, 1 cm/mV.*

Associated conditions:

- Cardiomyopathy
- Cardiac neoplasia
- Digitalis toxicity
- AV node fibrosis
- Endocarditis
- Electrolyte imbalance
- Hypothyroidism
- Lyme disease.

Management: Treatment with parasympathomimetic drugs is ineffective, and usually only results in an increase in the P wave rate. Sympathomimetic drugs (e.g. *isoprenaline* or *terbutaline*) may increase the rate of ventricular escapes in a few cases (Ettinger, 1969). Most cases will require *pacemaker* implantation.

Bundle branch blocks (intraventricular conduction defects)

The bundle of His divides into left and right bundle branches, supplying the left and right ventricles respectively. The left bundle branch further divides into anterior and posterior fascicles. Block may occur in one or more of these conduction tissues, and in a number of combinations. The most commonly seen conduction defects in dogs and cats are:

- Right bundle branch block (RBBB)
- Left bundle branch block (LBBB)
- Left anterior fascicular block (LAFB)

These result in abnormal depolarization patterns, as there will be a delay in depolarization of the part of the ventricles supplied by the affected conduction tissue.

Right bundle branch block

Right bundle branch block (RBBB) occurs due to failure/delay of impulse conduction through the RBB, and depolarization of the left ventricle occurs normally.

ECG features: Depolarization of the right ventricular mass occurs through the myocardial cell tissue, resulting in a very prolonged complex (>0.07 seconds). The QRS complex has a deep (negative) S in leads I, II, III, aVF and the left chest leads; and is positive in aVR, aVL and the right chest lead. The mean electrical axis is to the right. RBBB must be differentiated from a right ventricular enlargement pattern, which less commonly results in such a prolonged QRS duration.

Associated conditions: The right bundle branch is long and slender, thus vulnerable to damage. RBBB is commonly seen in dogs, but is of no haemodynamic significance unless the left bundle branch becomes damaged, when complete heart block may follow. It may be associated with congenital or acquired heart disease, neoplasia or *Trypanosoma cruzi* infection (not in UK).

Management: Treat any underlying disease.

Left bundle branch block

Left bundle branch block (LBBB) occurs due to failure of conduction through the LBB, and depolarization of the right ventricle occurs normally.

ECG features: Depolarization of the left ventricle is delayed, and occurs through the myocardial cell tissue resulting in a very prolonged complex (>0.07 seconds). There are positive complexes in leads I, II, III, aVF and the left chest leads; and negative in aVR, aVL and the right chest lead (Figure 11.8). LBBB must be differentiated from a left ventricular enlargement pattern, which is usually associated with increased R wave voltages.

Associated conditions: The left bundle branch is thick, and therefore a larger lesion is required to produce conduction block. It is therefore not commonly seen, but usually represents *severe underlying disease.* It can be associated with cardiomyopathy, congenital subaortic stenosis and ischaemia.

Management: Treat any underlying disease.

Left anterior fascicular block

Left anterior fascicular block occurs due to failure of conduction through the anterior fascicle of the LBB.

ECG features: LAFB results in a QRS complex with a normal duration and tall R waves in leads I and aVL, and deep S waves (>R wave) in leads II, III and aVF. The mean electrical axis is markedly to the left; approximately −60° in the cat. It is uncommon in the dog. It is often considered a relatively specific indicator of hypertrophic cardiomyopathy in the cat (although it can be seen with many heart diseases in cats). LAFB must be differentiated from ventricular pre-excitation and left ventricular hypertrophy.

Associated conditions: It can be associated with hypertrophic or restrictive cardiomyopathy, and electrolyte imbalance such as hyperkalaemia.

Management: Treat any underlying disease.

Ventricular pre-excitation

Ventricular pre-excitation occurs when the impulse from the SA node bypasses the AV node via an accessory conduction pathway to the ventricles (i.e. pre-excites the ventricles). The impulse conducted through the accessory pathway stimulates a portion of the ventricles with the rest of the ventricles being activated in the normal sequence through the AV node. There are believed to be three accessory pathways: Bundles of Kent, James fibres and Mahaim fibres.

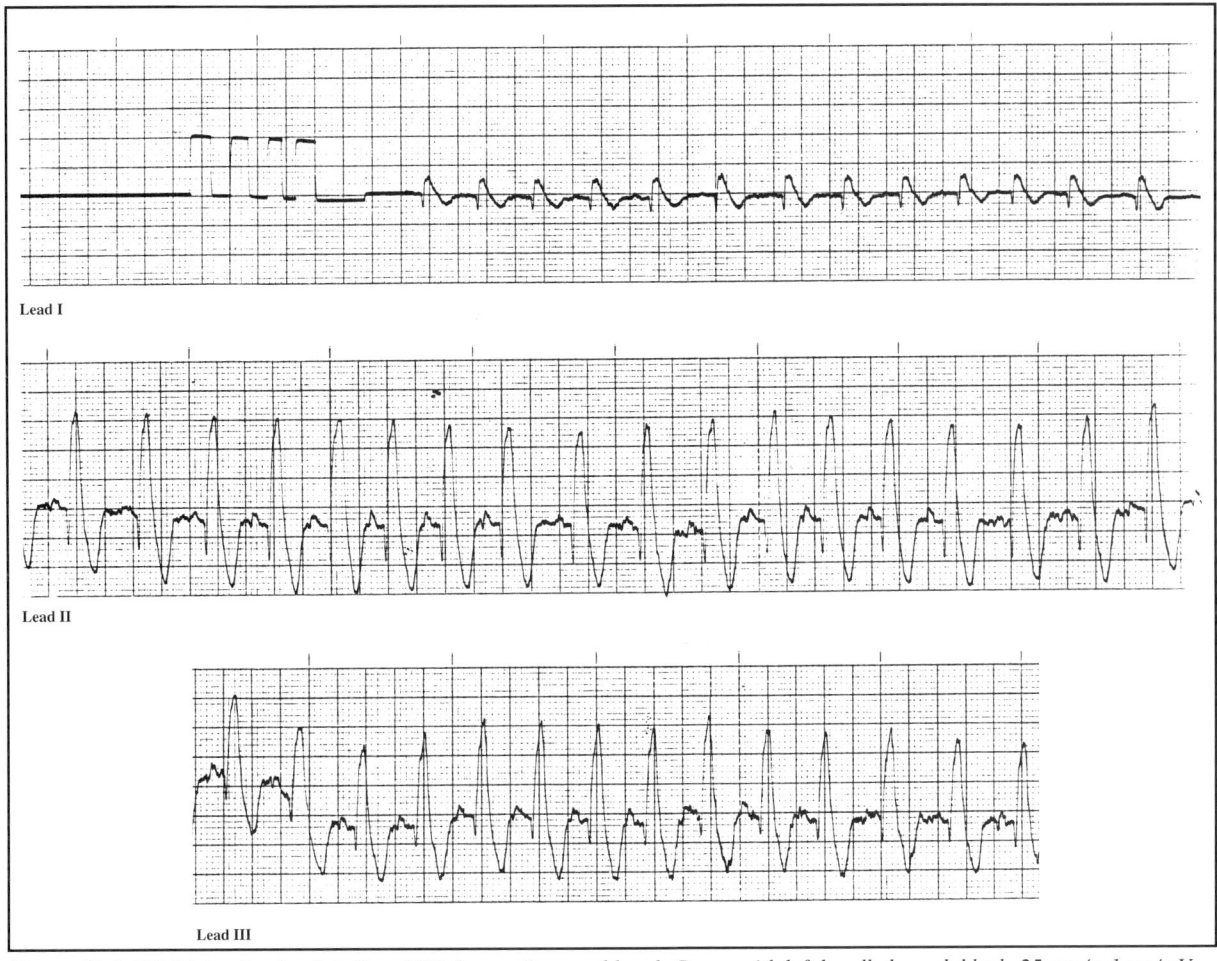

Figure 11.8: ECG (showing leads I, II and III) from a 7-year-old male Boxer with left bundle branch block. 25 mm/s, 1 cm/mV.

Wolff-Parkinson-White (WPW) syndrome

This syndrome consists of ventricular pre-excitation with episodes of paroxysmal supraventricular tachycardia.

Clinical findings

The heart rhythm (except with WPW syndrome) is unaffected, and is usually regular. WPW syndrome may cause weakness or syncope, as the supraventricular tachycardia is often in excess of 300 per minute. However, ventricular pre-excitation itself is not haemodynamically significant.

ECG features

The electrocardiographic characteristics (Hill and Tilley, 1985) are within the P-QRS-T complex itself. There is a short PR interval, a slur or notch (delta wave) in the upstroke of the R wave and a slight prolongation of the QRS complex. The associated supraventricular tachycardia may be of a narrow-complex or wide-complex form; and may be regular, or irregular if atrial fibrillation occurs.

Associated conditions

Pre-excitation may be present as a congenital lesion with or without structural heart disease.

Management

Asymptomatic ventricular pre-excitation requires no treatment. Treatment in symptomatic cases may be attempted with *vagal manoeuvres* (e.g. ocular or carotid sinus massage), *calcium channel blocking agents*, *beta blocking agents*, *lignocaine* or *quinidine*.

Digitalis, calcium channel blocking agents and beta blocking agents should be used with caution in WPW syndrome, as *slowing the AV node can exacerbate a re-entrant rhythm with accessory pathways*.

ABNORMALITIES DUE TO ECTOPIA

'Ectopia' literally means 'in an abnormal place'. With reference to the heart, this means outside the SA node, which is the dominant pacemaker. Ectopic beats arise as a result of various mechanisms (e.g. re-entry, abnormal automaticity, after-depolarizations) and a number of different causes (e.g. electrolyte imbalances, hypoxia, cardiac pathology). The reader is referred to Tilley (1992) for further details.

Terminology

The electrocardiographic interpretation of arrhythmias

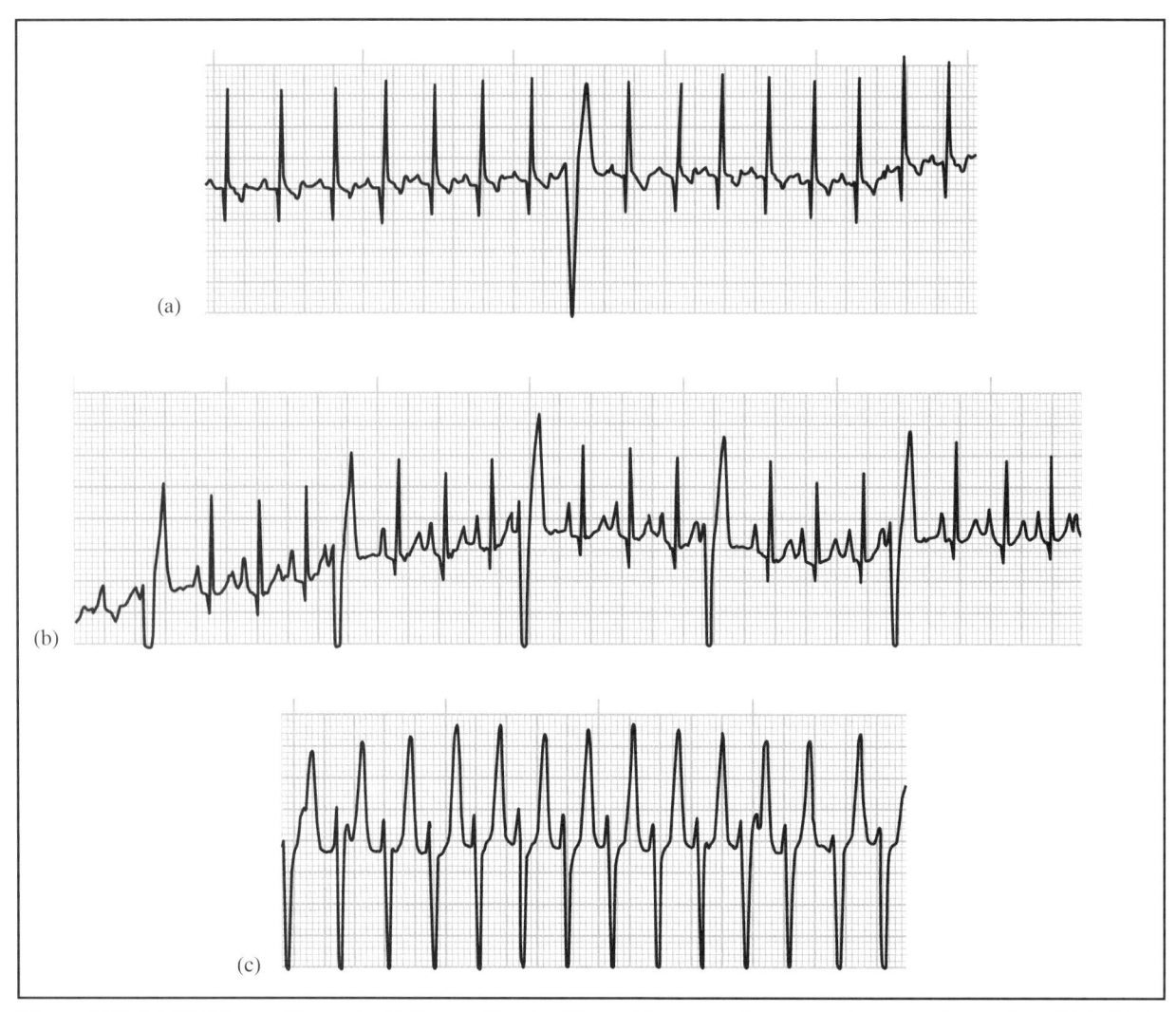

Figure 11.9: *(a) ECG from a 12-month-old German Shepherd Dog with a patent ductus arteriosus, cardiomegaly and left sided congestive heart failure. There is a single ventricular premature complex (VPC). Note also the tall R waves (3.2 mV) and underlying sinus tachycardia at 180/min. Lead II, 25 mm/s, 1/2 cm/mV. (b) ECG from a 12-month-old Great Dane with frequent ventricular premature complexes (VPCs). Lead II, 25 mm/s, 1 cm/mV. (c) ECG showing a sustained ventricular tachycardia at 220/min. Lead II, 25 mm/s, 1 cm/mV.*

due to ectopia requires an understanding of the terminology used. If this is accomplished, interpretation becomes relatively easy. The term 'beat' implies that there has been an actual contraction. In electrocardiography it is therefore more correct to use the term *complex* or *depolarization* to describe waveforms on the electrocardiograph.

Ectopic complexes may be classified as follows.

Site of origin
Ectopic complexes are either *ventricular* or *supraventricular*. Supraventricular ectopics may be sub-classified into *atrial* or *junctional* (junctional ectopics arise from the AV node or bundle of His).

Timing
Ectopic complexes that occur before the next normal complex would be expected are termed *premature*, and those that occur following a long period of asystole (e.g. sinus arrest) are termed *escape* complexes.

Similarity to each other
Those complexes which have a similar configuration to each other are referred to as *uniform* (although not necessarily unifocal), and those that are different to each other as *multiform*.

Number of ectopics
Premature ectopic complexes may occur singly, in pairs or in runs of three or more; the latter is referred to as a *tachycardia*. A tachycardia may be continuous, termed *persistent* or *sustained*; or intermittent, termed *paroxysmal*.

Frequency
A rhythm where premature complexes occur at a rate of one sinus complex to one ectopic complex is termed *bigeminy*, and one ectopic to two sinus complexes as *trigeminy*.

Ventricular premature complexes (VPCs) and ventricular tachycardia (VT)

Ventricular premature complexes (or depolarizations) arise from an ectopic focus or foci within the ventricular myocardium. Depolarization therefore occurs in a retrograde direction through the myocardium, and the impulse conducts from cell to cell (not within the conduction tissue). A run of three or more VPCs is termed *ventricular tachycardia (VT)*, and may occur if a *re-entry circuit* is set up within the ventricular myocardium. VT usually occurs at a rate in excess of 100 per minute (Figure 11.9c).

Clinical findings

On auscultation the normal rhythm is disturbed by premature beats, often followed by pauses. Pulse deficits are usually present, and the pulse may be very weak with VT. Single VPCs may not cause any clinical signs, but VT may result in weakness, syncope (and may lead to ventricular fibrillation and sudden death). Fast ventricular tachycardias are particularly serious, but slow ventricular tachycardias may be surprisingly well-tolerated.

ECG features

Since conduction is not from the AV node (and 'down' through the ventricles) *the QRS complex is usually wide (prolonged) and bizarre* in shape (Figure 11.9a,b). As a rule; VPCs that arise from the left ventricle have a negative QRS in lead II, and those from the right ventricle a positive QRS. The T wave of a VPC is usually opposite in direction to the QRS and large. Since the VPC occurs prematurely, a normal sinus depolarization arriving at the AV node will meet ventricles which are refractory, with the associated P wave usually hidden by the ventricular premature complex. The AV node (and consequently the ventricles) will not be stimulated again, until the next normal sinus discharge; thus there will be an apparent pause (*compensatory pause*) and the normal rhythm will not be disturbed, i.e. not *reset* (note that the depolarization wave of a VPC does not normally pass retrograde through the AV node to depolarize the atria).

Associated conditions

VPCs are a common finding in dogs and cats.

- Congestive heart failure
- Cardiomyopathy (particularly Dobermanns and Boxers)
- Myocarditis (e.g. traumatic)
- Endocarditis
- Hypoxia
- Acid–base imbalance
- Uraemia
- Gastric dilation–volvulus (Muir and Lipowitz, 1978)
- Pyometra
- Pancreatitis
- Splenic masses
- Drugs (digitalis, anaesthetics, atropine and isoprenaline).

VT, multiform VPCs and ventricular bigeminy are usually associated with severe underlying heart disease or a systemic disorder.

Management

Treatment of the primary underlying cause (e.g. control of congestive heart failure) will often reduce the number of VPCs. If ventricular tachycardia is considered life-threatening, treatment should be administered with *intravenous lignocaine* (initially: 2 mg/kg bolus in dogs and 0.5 mg/kg slowly in cats). Oral therapy (see Chapter 21) includes *procainamide*, *tocainide*, *mexiletine* or *propranolol* (propranolol is the preferred drug in cats). Refractory arrhythmias can often be treated by combining propranolol with one of the other drugs listed. The reader is referred to Ware and Hamlin (1989) for a more detailed review.

Supraventricular premature complexes (SVPCs) and supraventricular tachycardia (SVT)

Supraventricular premature complexes (or depolarizations) arise from an ectopic focus or foci above the ventricles. The ventricles are therefore depolarized normally, producing a *normally shaped QRS complex with a normal duration* (Figure 11.10a). Supraventricular premature complexes can be classified further into either atrial premature complexes or junctional premature complexes.

Clinical findings

SVPCs sound similar to VPCs on auscultation; i.e. 'extra' early beats interrupting the normal rhythm. The rate in SVT is often very rapid, with a sudden onset and offset. Pulse deficits may be present with SVPCs, and the pulse may be very weak with SVT. SVPCs do not usually result in clinical signs, but SVT may cause weakness, syncope or congestive heart failure.

ECG features

Atrial premature complexes (APC): These arise in the atria, thus producing an 'ectopic' P wave (referred to as a P′) that is abnormal in shape, being negative, positive or biphasic, and the P-R interval is often prolonged. The ectopic atrial depolarization may *reset* the SA node, such that the interval between the APC and the next sinus complex is the same as a normal R-R interval, i.e. there is *no compensatory pause* (sometimes referred to as having a *non-compensatory pause*). Occasionally, an atrial premature complex may occur so early that it meets the AV node when it is still refractory from the previous depolarization. In these occasions the P′ will not be followed by a QRS complex. If the AV node or the His–Purkinje system is in the relative refractory period (partially refractory) then the depolarization will be conducted with aberrancy (i.e. the QRS will be abnormal in shape, often with a right bundle branch block pattern).

Junctional premature complexes (JPC): These arise within the AV node or bundle of His. The depolarization wave spreads through the ventricles normally, but also retrogradely through the atria; thus producing a P′ wave that is abnormal in shape and usually negative in lead II. The P′ wave may occur before, during or after the associated QRS complex. If occurring before the QRS complex, the P′-R interval is usually shorter than normal and the SA node is reset (i.e. there is not a compensatory pause).

Supraventricular tachycardias (SVT): These are usually at a rate in excess of 160 per minute and fairly regular (Figure 11.10b). The P′ waves of a junctional tachycardia are usually negative in lead II and are sometimes seen in the preceding T wave. The differentiation of SVPCs into APCs or JPCs is difficult, and often of little clinical importance.

P′ waves must be differentiated from the variation in the P wave seen with a wandering pacemaker. SVPCs and SVT must also be distinguished from a marked sinus arrhythmia or a sinus tachycardia, respectively. With SVT, there is usually an abrupt start or finish to the rhythm, whereas with sinus arrhythmia and sinus tachycardia this is more gradual. Frequent SVPCs or an SVT can be a precursor to atrial fibrillation.

Associated conditions
SVPCs and SVT commonly occur secondary to atrial pathology, e.g. atrial stretching secondary to atrioventricular valve incompetence. Possible causes of atrial pathology include:

- Congenital/acquired atrioventricular valve disease
- Cardiomyopathy
- Congenital cardiac shunts
- Right atrial haemangiosarcoma
- Digitalis toxicity (often less than 160 bpm)
- Ventricular pre-excitation syndrome
- Hyperthyroidism in cats.

Management
Treatment should initially be aimed at the primary cause. Management of these conditions can often reduce the frequency of SVT to an acceptable level. Infrequent SVPCs do not generally compromise the cardiac output and therefore do not require treatment. *Vagal manoeuvres* (e.g. ocular or carotid sinus massage) may be tried in paroxysmal or sustained SVT. Occasionally, these will abruptly terminate an atrial tachycardia, and may be attempted with or without prior digitalization. In symptomatic cases of SVT the choice of drug is an *intravenous beta blocking agent* (e.g.

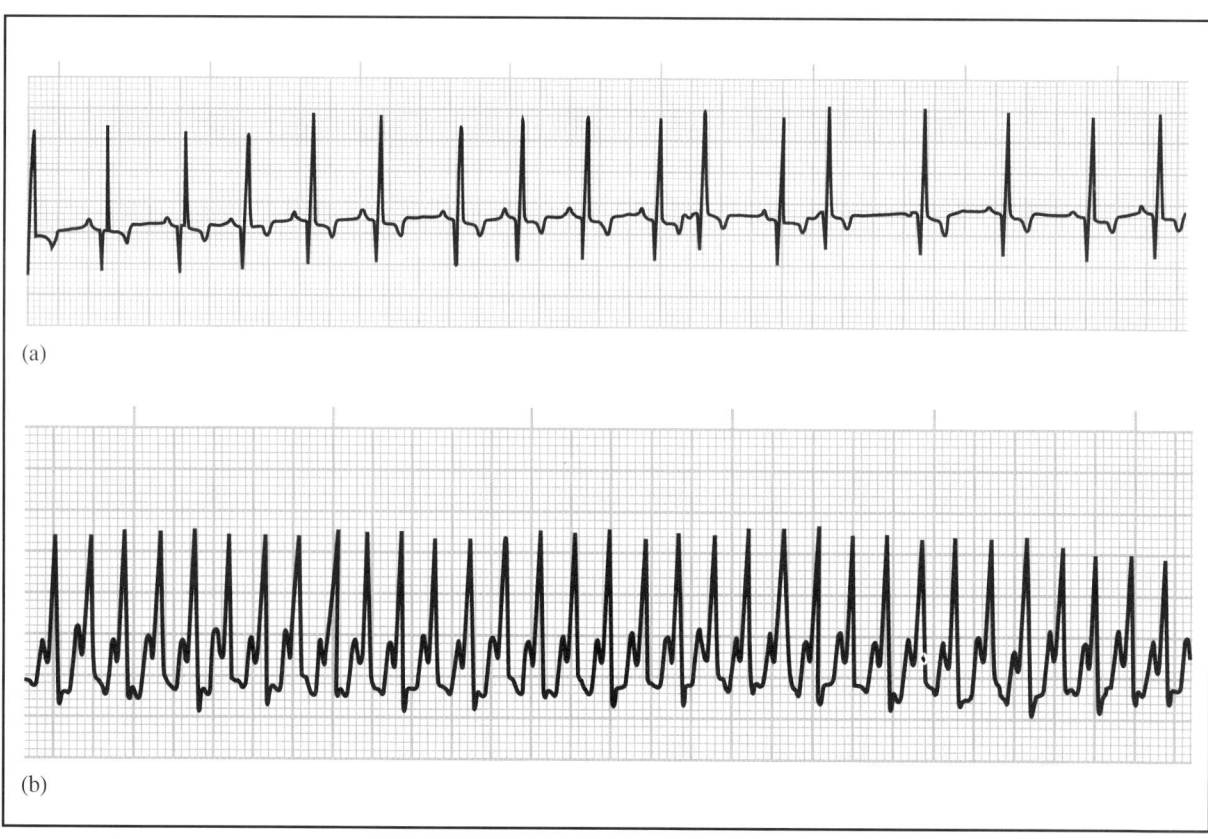

(a)

(b)

Figure 11.10: (a) ECG from a 12-year-old Cavalier King Charles Spaniel with AV valve endocardiosis and heart failure. Note the occasional supraventricular premature complex (SVPC) which appears to be preceded by an abnormally shaped P wave suggesting that these SVPCs can be further classified as atrial premature complexes (APCs). Lead II, 25 mm/s, 1 cm/mV. (b) ECG from a 6-year-old Dalmatian that presented with acute weakness. The ECG shows a sustained supraventricular tachycardia at 350/min. Lead II, 25 mm/s, 1 cm/mV.

esmolol) or *calcium channel blocking agent* (Kittleson *et al.*, 1988; Foodman and Macintire, 1989). If these are unavailable treatment may be attempted with intravenous *procainamide*. Lignocaine may be effective in some SVTs caused by an accessory pathway or re-entrant mechanism.

Oral therapy with *calcium channel blocking agents*, *beta blocking agents* or *digoxin* (drug of choice if there is ventricular myocardial failure) will often control supraventricular tachyarrhythmias. However, it should be remembered that digoxin can cause SVPCs or SVT, in which case it should be discontinued.

Escape rhythms

When the dominant pacemaker tissue (usually the SA node) fails to discharge for a long period, pacemaker tissue with a slower rate (junctional or ventricular escape) may discharge (Figure 11.5). This is commonly seen in association with the bradyarrhythmias (e.g. sinus bradycardia, sinus arrest, AV block). Escape complexes are sometimes referred to as *rescue beats*, because if they did not occur death would be imminent. Junctional escapes are fairly normal in shape (i.e. junctional ectopic), whereas ventricular escapes are abnormal and bizarre (i.e. ventricular ectopic). A continuous junctional escape rhythm occurs at a rate of 60–70 bpm in dogs, and a continuous ventricular escape rhythm occurs at a rate of less than 40 bpm. Either may be seen in complete AV block.

Management

Escape complexes or escape rhythms are commonly seen in association with bradyarrhythmias (e.g. sinus bradycardia, sinus arrest, AV block); treatment is therefore directed towards the underlying bradyarrhythmia.

AV dissociation

The term AV dissociation describes the situation when the atria and ventricles are depolarized by separate independent foci. This may occur due to several mechanisms:

- An accelerated ventricular rhythm (junctional or ventricular)
- Disturbed AV conduction
- Depressed SA nodal function.

ECG features

The ECG usually shows a ventricular rate that is very slightly faster than the atrial rate. The P waves may occur before, during or after the QRS complex. The P waves and QRS complexes are independent of each other with the QRS complexes appearing to 'catch up' on the P waves (Figure 11.11). Complete AV block is one form of AV dissociation, but AV dissociation does not mean there is AV block.

Associated conditions

- Anaesthesia (especially cats)
- Cardiomyopathy
- Electrolyte disturbances.

Management

Management will depend on the underlying cause of the AV dissociation (e.g. see junctional and ventricular tachycardia).

Fibrillation and flutter

Fibrillation means rapid irregular small movements of fibres, and *flutter* means to wave or flap quickly and irregularly. Fibrillation or flutter occurs by a mechanism termed *random re-entry* (the reader is referred to Tilley, 1992).

Ventricular fibrillation (VF)

This is a nearly always a terminal event associated with cardiac arrest. The depolarization waves occur randomly throughout the ventricles. There is therefore no significant co-ordinated contraction to produce any cardiac output. If the heart is observed or palpated, fine irregular movements of the ventricles are evident – likened to a 'can of worms'. VF may develop from ventricular tachycardia.

ECG features: Coarse (larger) or *fine* (smaller) rapid, irregular and bizarre movement with no recognizable waveforms or complexes.

Management: The causes are numerous, but similar to those of VPCs and VT. Treatment is essentially the initiation of *cardiopulmonary resuscitation*. However the success of this will depend on the extent of existing pathology and death is a common outcome.

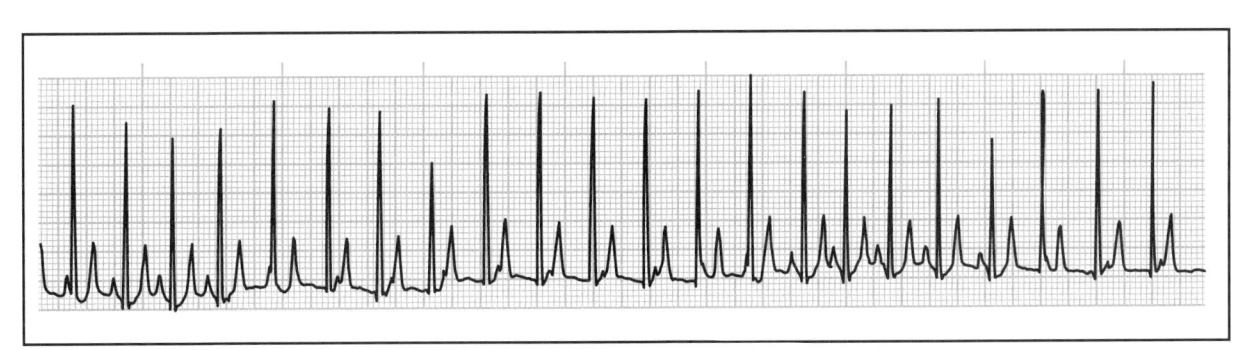

Figure 11.11: *ECG from a 7-year-old male Labrador Retriever with AV dissociation. Lead CV6LU, 25 mm/s, 1 cm/mV.*

Atrial fibrillation and flutter

In atrial fibrillation or flutter, depolarization waves occur randomly throughout the atria. These 'wavelets' of depolarization are conducted to the AV node and ventricles at a rate chiefly governed by the AV nodal conduction velocity, and refractory period. The likelihood of atrial fibrillation is influenced by the size of the atria, with larger atria predisposed. Atrial fibrillation is sometimes seen in giant breed dogs with no gross cardiac pathology – sometimes referred to as '*lone*' *AF*. Lone AF usually has a slow ventricular rate.

Clinical findings: The cardiac rhythm is completely chaotic on auscultation, and marked pulse deficits are usually present. Affected animals are often in congestive heart failure, and even giant breed dogs with lone AF often progress to dilated cardiomyopathy and heart failure.

Atrial flutter and fibrillation do not always have major haemodynamic effects, depending on the ventricular response rate. Loss of atrial contraction may reduce cardiac output by up to 20%. This may be compensated for by an increase in rate, but can be sufficient to cause onset of cardiac failure if cardiac output is already critically compromised.

ECG features of atrial flutter: Rapid and regular 'saw-toothed' type movements of the baseline, at a rate of 300–500 per minute. The QRS complex is normal, at a more normal and regular heart rate, often at a set ratio to the F waves. Atrial flutter is rare, probably because it quickly progresses to atrial fibrillation.

ECG features of atrial fibrillation: Atrial fibrillation (AF) is recognized by the irregular chaotic ventricular (i.e. QRS) rate and rhythm (i.e. chaotic R-R intervals). The QRS complexes usually vary in amplitude, and there are no consistently recognizable P waves preceding the QRS complexes (Figure 11.12a, b). Sometimes fine irregular movements of the baseline are seen as a result of the atrial fibrillation waves – referred to as '*f*' *waves*; however, these are frequently indistinguishable from baseline artefact (e.g. muscle tremor) in small animals. The ventricular rate in dogs and cats is nearly always fast, as most cases are in congestive heart failure and therefore there is a compensatory sympathetic drive (decreased AV nodal conduction time, reduced ventricular refractory period and therefore increased rate).

Associated conditions: Atrial fibrillation (Bonagura and Ware, 1986) or flutter usually occurs as a result of *dilation and stretching of one or both atria*, although primary atrial pathology can also be responsible (e.g. heart base tumours).

It is most commonly seen in medium to large breed dogs with dilated cardiomyopathy. It is uncommon in the cat, but is sometimes seen when there is severe left atrial dilation secondary to hypertrophic cardiomyopathy. It can also be seen in association with cardiac neoplasia, following pericardiocentesis or cardiac catheterization.

Management: Treatment is aimed at reducing the ventricular response rate to less than 150 to 160 bpm. *Digitalis* is the drug of choice to reduce the ventricular

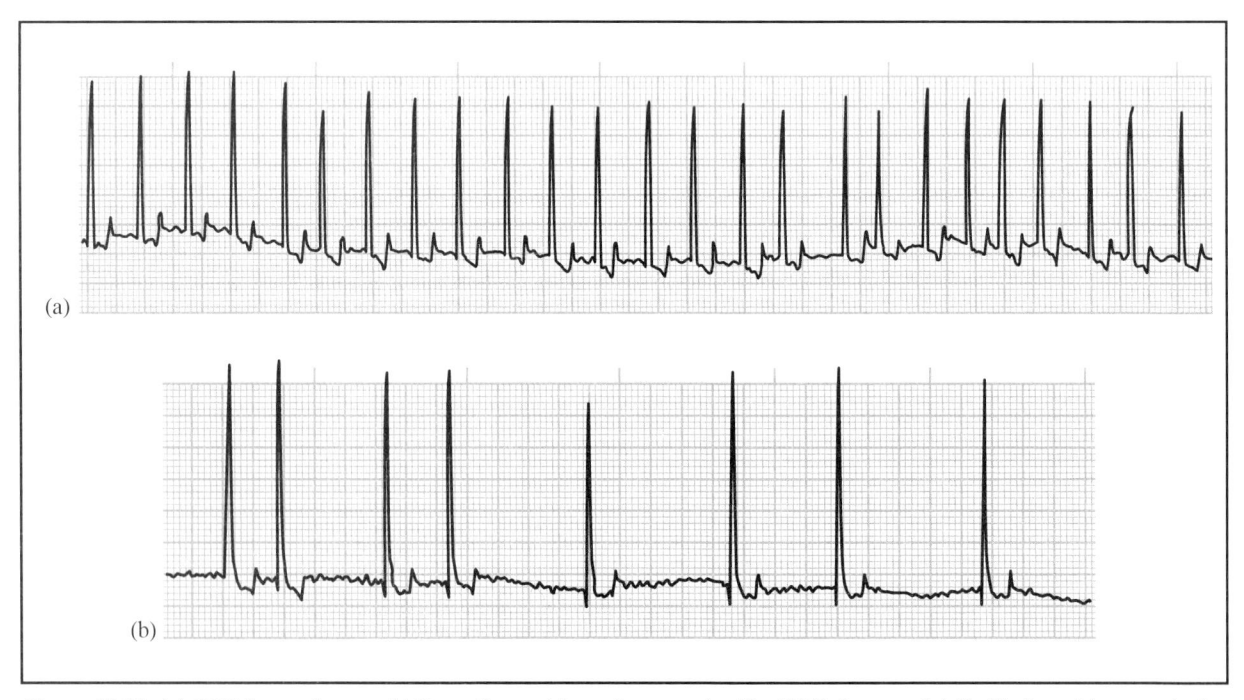

Figure 11.12: (a) *ECG from a 9-year-old Great Dane with cardiomyopathy. The ECG shows atrial fibrillation with a ventricular response rate of 180/min. Lead II, 25 mm/s, 1 cm/mV.* (b) *ECG from a 7-year-old Golden Retriever in which an arrhythmia was heard on routine examination; no other clinical signs were present. This ECG shows lone atrial fibrillation. Note the presence of f waves. Lead II, 25 mm/s, 1 cm/mV.*

rate in animals with ventricular myocardial failure (e.g. dilated cardiomyopathy). Additional anti-arrhythmic drugs may be required if digitalis alone does not reduce the rate adequately, such as calcium channel antagonist or β blocking agents. In cats with hypertrophic cardiomyopathy and animals with good ventricular function, the options include a *calcium channel blocking agent* or *beta blocking agent*.

Conversion of atrial fibrillation to sinus rhythm may be attempted in larger breed dogs if there is no cardiac pathology, but is pointless in cases with atrial enlargement (Robertson, 1970).

REFERENCES AND FURTHER READING

Anselmi A, Giurdiel O, Saurez JA and Anselmi G (1967) Disturbances in the AV conduction system in Chagas' myocarditis in the dog. *Circulation Research* **20**, 56

Bonagura JD and Ware WA (1986) Atrial fibrillation in the dog: clinical findings in 81 cases. *Journal of the American Animal Hospital Association* **22**, 111

Calvert CA, Chapman WL and Toal RL (1982) Congestive cardiomyopathy in Doberman Pinscher dogs. *Journal of the American Veterinary Medical Association* **181**, 598

Ettinger SJ (1969) Isoproterenol treatment of atrioventricular block in the dog. *Journal of the American Veterinary Medical Association* **154**, 398

Feldman EC and Ettinger SJ (1977) Electrocardiographic changes associated with electrolyte disturbances. *Veterinary Clinics of North America* **7**, 487

Foodman MS and Macintire D (1989) Reversal of atrial tachycardia with intravenous administration of verapamil in a dog. *Journal of the American Veterinary Medical Association* **194**, 800

Gross DR, Hamlin RL and Pipers FS (1973) Response of P-Q intervals to digitalis glycosides in the dog. *Journal of the American Veterinary Medical Association* **162**, 888

Hamlin RL, Smetzer DL and Breznock EM (1972) Sinoatrial syncope in miniature Schnauzers. *Journal of the American Veterinary Medical Association* **161**, 1023

Harpster N (1983) Boxer cardiomyopathy. In: *Current Veterinary Therapy: Small Animal Practice*, ed. RW Kirk, Vol 8, pp. 329–337. W.B. Saunders, Philadelphia

Hill BL and Tilley LP (1985) Ventricular pre excitation in seven dogs and nine cats. *Journal of the American Veterinary Medical Association* **187**, 1026

Kittleson M, Keane B, Pion P and Woodfield J (1988) Verapamil administration for acute termination of supraventricular tachycardia in dogs. *Journal of the American Veterinary Medical Association* **193**, 1525

Morgan RV (1982) Endocrine and metabolic emergencies – Part 1. *Compendium on Continuing Education for the Practising Veterinarian* **4**, 755

Muir WW and Lipowitz AJ (1978) Cardiac arrhythmias associated with gastric dilatation-volvulus in the dog. *Journal of the American Veterinary Medical Association* **172**, 683

Peterson ME, Keene B, Ferguson DC and Pipers FS (1982) Electrocardiographic findings of 45 cats with hyperthyroidism. *Journal of the American Veterinary Medical Association* **180**, 934

Robertson BT (1970) Correction of atrial flutter with quinidine and digitalis. *Journal of Small Animal Practice* **11**, 251

Tilley LP (1992) *Essentials of Canine and Feline Electrocardiography*, 3rd edn. Lea and Febiger, Philadelphia

Ware WA and Hamlin RL (1989) Therapy for ventricular arrhythmias. In: *Current Veterinary Therapy: Small Animal Practice*, ed. RW Kirk, Vol. 10, pp. 278-285. W.B. Saunders, Philadelphia.

Left Heart Failure

Malcolm A. Cobb

PATHOPHYSIOLOGY

An understanding of the determinants of cardiac output, the mechanisms involved in regulating arterial blood pressure and the haemodynamic changes commonly found in heart failure is essential to the understanding of the clinical signs associated with left heart failure and is helpful in formulating rational therapy.

Of the many causes of left heart failure in the dog and cat (listed in Table 12.1), *valvular disease* and *myocardial disease* are the most common. Both result in a fall in the effective forward stroke volume of the left ventricle which triggers a series of compensatory responses which can often result in the maintenance of systemic arterial blood pressure and cardiac output for months or even years, until late in the natural history of the primary disease condition (see Chapter 3).

The maintenance of an effective forward stroke volume in the face of a progressive primary disease condition is achieved at the expense of rising left ventricular diastolic, mean left atrial and pulmonary venous pressures. Eventually, pulmonary venous pressure rises to the point where the other Starling forces in the pulmonary capillaries are overwhelmed. Transudation of fluid occurs, initially into the interstitial space and later into the alveoli, forming pulmonary oedema. Thus, individuals with left heart failure usually show clinical signs which develop insidiously, and are referable to congestion and oedema ('backward' failure). Clinical signs resulting from a reduced cardiac output ('forward' failure) tend to become more apparent later in the disease process, when left ventricular systolic function deteriorates to the point where compensatory responses are no longer effective, and in fact contribute more and more to patient deterioration and incapacity.

Volume overload	Mitral valve disease
	endocardiosis
	endocarditis
	congenital dysplasia
	Aortic regurgitation
	endocarditis
	congenital valve disease
	Left to right shunts
	patent ductus arteriosus
	ventricular septal defect
	peripheral arteriovenous fistulae
Systolic pressure overload	Aortic/subaortic stenosis
	Systemic hypertension[*]
Myocardial disease	Dilated cardiomyopathy
	Hypertrophic cardiomyopathy
	Restrictive cardiomyopathy
	Secondary myocardial disease
	hyperthyroidism in cats
	toxicity, e.g. doxorubicin
	carnitine deficiency has been described as a cause of
	dilated cardiomyopathy in some families of dogs
Compliance (diastolic) failure	Myocardial diseases (see above)
Abnormalities of heart rate and/or rhythm	
High output failure (hyperkinetic circulation)	Hyperthyroidism
	Pregnancy[*]
	Pyrexia[*]
	Anaemia[*]

These conditions rarely cause failure alone; they may, however, contribute to the precipitation of signs of failure in a patient in which cardiac function is already compromised.

Table 12.1: *Causes of left heart failure.*

Heart failure has typically been described as right or left sided, but the common cardiac disease conditions tend to affect both sides of the heart. In addition, the right and left sides of the heart share an anatomical connection in the interventricular septum, and form part of a dual circulation which works in series. In the long term the output of the two sides must equal each other; consequently, biventricular failure is common.

The pulmonary venous circulation is less able to accommodate haemodynamic imbalances than the systemic venous circulation, as a result of a lower pressure and blood volume capacity. This fact and the effect of pulmonary oedema on respiratory function, mean that the clinical manifestations of left-sided cardiac failure tend to be recognized sooner and have more serious consequences than those associated with pure right-sided failure.

RECOGNITION OF LEFT HEART FAILURE

The signs exhibited vary according to the severity of the failure and the primary disease process. Typically, signs are initially apparent on exercise. Patients have limited cardiac reserve, and filling pressures increase with exercise as a result of elevation of sympathetic tone, and this makes venous congestion and oedema more likely.

The patient details ('signalment'), age, sex, breed etc., may alert the clinician to a particular condition (e.g. endocardiosis in small breeds) but should not be relied upon. Exacerbations and remissions of clinical signs may occur throughout the course of the disease. Individuals free of signs of heart failure, but with 'occult' disease may be identified on routine clinical examination (by the identification of a murmur, a gallop rhythm or an arrhythmia for example), or as a result of electrocardiographic, radiographic or echocardiographic examination.

History
A full medical history should be obtained from the owner. Findings common in patients with left heart failure are listed below.

Exercise intolerance or *lethargy.* This may be a result of poor muscle perfusion; probably accompanied by intrinsic skeletal muscle abnormalities associated with cardiac failure.

Dyspnoea, tachypnoea, or *orthopnoea* occur for one or more of the following reasons: increased lung stiffness due to pulmonary venous congestion or overt interstitial or alveolar oedema; pleural effusion or severe ascites if there is concurrent right heart failure; airway compression by the enlarged left heart or compromise of respiratory function as a result of gross cardiomegaly.

Coughing occurs as a result of bronchial compres-

sion by the enlarging left atrium (not necessarily associated with congestive cardiac failure), and/or airway irritation associated with the development of interstitial or alveolar oedema. Coughing may be exacerbated by exercise. Severe, acute pulmonary oedema may result in pink froth exiting the mouth or nose, or the expectoration of blood-tinged foam or froth (haemoptysis). Coughing is rare in cats with left heart failure.

Syncopal episodes in patients with left heart failure are usually the result of a sudden fall in cardiac output, or an inability to increase cardiac output on demand, for example during exercise. Syncope may occur as a result of a paroxysmal arrhythmia; it may occur associated with coughing ('tussive' syncope); or as a result of drug use, for example hypotension associated with the use of vasodilators or beta blocking agents, or electrolyte abnormalities associated with diuretic use.

Nocturnal restlessness may be a feature of the history as the hydrostatic effects of recumbency result in fluid accumulation in the lungs.

Sudden death is probably most common in dogs with dilated cardiomyopathy, but is a possibility in any patient with structural cardiac disease.

Anorexia and weight loss are common non-specific signs.

Physical examination
A full general physical examination should be performed on all patients. Findings frequently noted in patients with cardiac disease are listed below.

Cardiac murmurs may be found, with or without a palpable precordial 'thrill'.

Prominent or displaced apex beat may be present, resulting from ventricular dilation or hypertrophy. In cases of dilated cardiomyopathy, the apex beat may be weak as a result of poor stroke volume.

Pulmonary crackles may be heard on auscultation of the lung fields in patients with pulmonary oedema. Absence of audible crackles does not rule out pulmonary oedema, and the presence of adventitious lung sounds can be associated with primary lung disease; older dogs often have heart disease and chronic airway or lung disease.

Abnormal cardiac rate and rhythm. In the early stages of left heart failure, rate and rhythm are usually normal. As the underlying disease progresses, the heart rate usually increases and tachy- (or, less frequently, brady-) arrhythmias may develop.

Changes in pulse quality. A hyperkinetic pulse may be found in cases in which stroke volume is high and the pulse pressure wide, e.g. aortic regurgitation, patent ductus arteriosus, arteriovenous fistulae. *Hypokinetic* pulses may be found if stroke volume is low, for example in myocardial failure, outflow tract obstruction. Pulse deficits and irregularities of pulse amplitude may occur in patients with arrhythmias.

Gallop rhythms or sounds are usually heard only in individuals with cardiac failure; occasionally in the cat a gallop rhythm may occur physiologically associated with a high heart rate.

Pale mucous membranes may be evident if cardiac output is severely compromised and vasoconstriction is pronounced. Severe respiratory compromise in left heart failure may result in cyanosis as a result of pulmonary oedema.

The presence of ascites, pleural effusion, jugular vein distension or positive hepatojugular reflux suggests concurrent right heart failure (see Chapter 13).

Diagnosis

A tentative diagnosis is usually made based on the patient details, the history and the results of the physical examination. The extent to which the problem in an individual case is investigated is dependent on the wishes of the owner and on economic guidelines, which should be established early on. Diagnostic and therapeutic interventions should not be embarked upon without careful consideration of the risks involved and consideration of the cost:benefit ratio.

Ancillary diagnostic aids are commonly required to confirm the presence of cardiac disease, diagnose the cause of the disease more precisely, identify any complicating factors, and assess the severity of any cardiac failure.

Electrocardiography may show evidence of left atrial and/or left ventricular enlargement, an abnormal mean electrical axis, or morphological abnormalities of the P wave, QRS complexes or T wave/ST segment.

Arrhythmias are common, and an electrocardiographic diagnosis of any clinical abnormality of rate or rhythm is essential.

The ECG may be unremarkable, even when cardiac failure has developed.

Radiography will demonstrate progressive left-sided (or global) cardiomegaly as the disease progresses (Figure 12.1a). As cardiac failure develops, pulmonary venous congestion becomes evident (Figure 12.1b). Initially, an interstitial pattern confirms the development of pulmonary oedema; this may progress to an alveolar pattern (Figure 12.1c). In the dog, 'cardiogenic' pulmonary oedema is usually first seen to develop dorsally in the perihilar region in the plain lateral chest radiograph, and in the right diaphragmatic lobe in the plain dorsoventral chest radiograph. In the cat, the distribution tends to be more diffuse. Pleural effusion may be evident if there is concomitant right heart failure.

Echocardiography allows a definitive diagnosis to be approached. Two-dimensional echocardiography may identify anatomical cardiac lesions. M-mode echocardiography permits assessment of chamber size, global myocardial function and myocardial hypertrophy patterns. Doppler echocardiography will often allow identification of the source of a murmur, and assessment of the haemodynamic consequences of any valvular or myocardial disease.

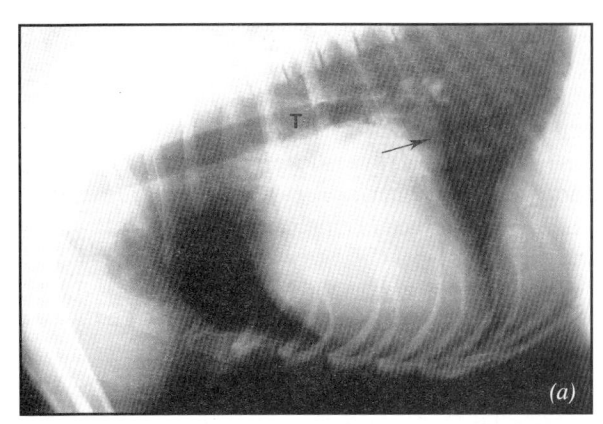

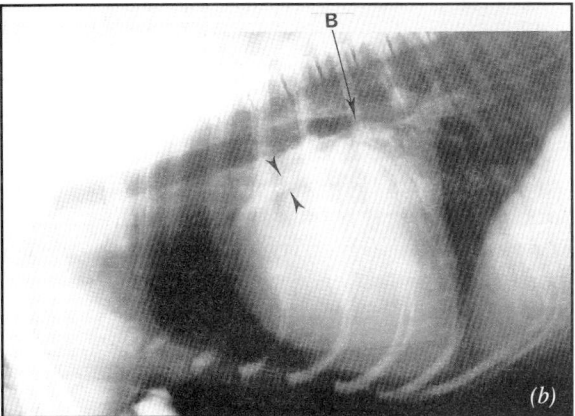

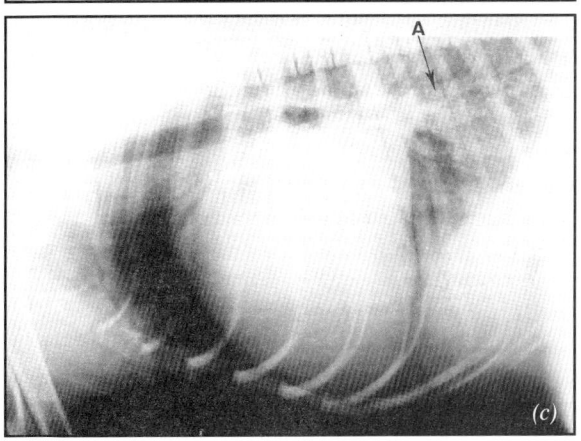

Figure 12.1: *Plain lateral chest radiographs of a dog at different stages in the development of left heart failure. (a) Left atrial enlargement, evident as straightening of the caudal border of the cardiac silhouette (arrow) and elevation of the distal trachea (T). (b) Compression of the airway above the enlarging left heart (B) and pulmonary venous congestion (arrowheads). (c) Marked left heart enlargement with pulmonary venous congestion, severe compression of the airway by the large left atrium and an alveolar filling pattern in the caudodorsal lung field (A) typical of cardiogenic pulmonary oedema in the dog.*

Routine laboratory tests may reflect the haemodynamic effects of cardiac failure on regional blood flow, the effects of any therapeutic agents or the presence of concurrent extracardiac disease. A thorough knowledge of the patient's metabolic condition is very useful, having important implications when pharmacological agents are used in treatment.

A 'stress leucogram' may be evident on a

haematological profile from patients with heart failure. Anaemia may precipitate 'high output' cardiac failure. Neutrophilia or monocytosis is often evident in endocarditis (see below).

There is commonly evidence of pre-renal azotaemia, particularly in patients with moderate or severe cardiac failure. Total protein/albumin may be slightly low; this may be a dilutional effect as water is retained, or due to reduced hepatic protein synthesis and reduced gastrointestinal absorption (particularly if there is concomitant right heart failure). Electrolyte level changes are often the result of treatment; however, in severe cardiac failure high aldosterone levels may result in marginal hypokalaemia, and excessive ADH secretion may result in hypochloraemia and hyponatraemia.

Some assessment of thyroid function may be indicated in individuals in which hyper- or hypothyroidism might be considered to be contributing to the disease state. Assessment of blood taurine, carnitine or growth hormone levels may be indicated in some patients with myocardial disease. Blood culture may be indicated in cases where bacterial endocarditis is suspected. Blood gas analysis or measurement of blood lactate concentration may be useful in some cases.

Blood pressure measurement may be indicated if arterial hypertension or hypotension is thought to be contributing to the clinical syndrome in an individual patient.

Cardiac catheterization. Pressure measurement and selective or non-selective angiography may be required in some cases to obtain a definitive diagnosis. Elevated pulmonary arterial or pulmonary capillary wedge pressure will be evident in congestive left heart failure.

Management

The complex physiological responses to the many causes of left heart failure mean that the clinical presentation of affected patients is not always the same. Successful management requires the individual assessment of each patient with respect to the primary cause, and the extent to which compensatory responses are contributing to the clinical signs in an individual patient.

In most cases it is not possible to treat the primary disease, and therapy which limits the degree of debility suffered by a patient as a result of the compensatory responses probably does nothing to alter the on-going pathological changes.

General therapeutic principles

- *Exercise.* When exercise intolerance becomes evident in a patient with heart disease, a regular daily exercise regime is instituted with which the patient can readily cope (exercise 'control'). Complete exercise restriction in mild cardiac failure may itself further compromise exercise tolerance.

- *A salt-restricted diet* may allow a reduction in the level of drug therapy required to control oedema in patients with congestive heart failure, although clinical trials documenting the efficacy of dietary salt restriction in patients with cardiac failure are currently lacking. Salty treats and sudden changes in diet are to be avoided. In more advanced cases, the most important dietary consideration is that the patient's appetite is maintained.

- *Diuretic therapy* encourages renal excretion of salt and water, reducing preload and helping to limit the development of oedema. Whenever diuretics are used it is often possible to titrate the dose to effect, using the lowest dose necessary to control pulmonary oedema. Refractory pulmonary oedema may resolve with combinations of different classes of diuretic.

- *Vasodilators* are used with increasing frequency in the management of congestive heart failure. Venodilation increases pooling of blood in the veins, reducing preload, and is often beneficial in patients with pulmonary oedema. Arterial dilation reduces afterload, improving forward flow and exercise tolerance and reducing mitral regurgitation, left atrial size and the tendency to cough.

- *Angiotensin converting enzyme (ACE) inhibitors* are balanced vasodilators producing both arterial dilation and venodilation as a result of the reduction in the circulating level of angiotensin II. They also reduce salt and water retention as a result of the consequent fall in the level of circulating aldosterone.

- Arrhythmias evident on physical examination need to be characterized with an ECG, and antiarrhythmics are used if indicated.

- Digoxin is introduced to control ventricular rate in supraventricular tachyarrhythmias, (especially atrial fibrillation), or if there is evidence of myocardial failure. Digoxin may help patients with left-sided heart failure through less specific effects mediated by the autonomic nervous system.

- Bronchodilators or cough suppressants may be indicated in some individuals, especially if concurrent small airway disease is present.

The progressive nature of the disease processes resulting in left heart failure allows a clinical categorization of the degree of failure according to the extent of the patient's disability. Traditionally, the intensity of the treatment required has been determined by the clinical category into which a patient is put. Although not entirely satisfactory (an alternative classification for small animal patients with cardiac failure has recently been proposed; Anon, 1992), the New York Heart Association (NYHA) functional heart failure classification (Anon, 1964) is used in a modified form to provide a useful guide to the management of left heart failure in the dog and cat (Table 12.2).

Defining criteria	Management
NYHA class one: heart disease with no clinical signs Objective evidence of heart disease on physical examination (usually detection of a murmur/arrhythmia) in the *absence* of associated clinical signs Chest radiography is often unremarkable; may be left-sided cardiomegaly	No therapy indicated, client informed & regular reassessment advised. Discuss prognosis & signs to watch for with owner Ideally a *definitive diagnosis* obtained to assess the likelihood of disease progression, allows a more accurate prognosis to be offered Weight control in overweight individuals Any arrhythmia characterized with ECG
NYHA Class two: mild heart failure Objective evidence of heart disease on physical examination, clinical signs of cardiac failure develop with exercise or excitement Chest radiography may demonstrate enlargement of the cardiac silhouette, there may be evidence of pulmonary venous congestion	Controlled exercise Salt-restricted diet traditionally introduced; maintain if tolerated and considered beneficial Low dose of diuretic if necessary to control pulmonary oedema Arrhythmias characterized with ECG, antiarrhythmics used if indicated Digoxin introduced if there is evidence of myocardial failure to control ventricular rate in supraventricular arrhythmias, especially atrial fibrillation (if present); for 'autonomic' effects Angiotensin converting enzyme (ACE) inhibitor often introduced
NYHA Class three: moderate heart failure Objective evidence of heart disease on physical examination; clinical signs occur in the course of normal physical activity but not at rest Obvious evidence of left-sided cardiomegaly and left heart failure on chest radiographs	Exercise control, may benefit from hospitalization to stabilize Maintain or introduce dietary salt restriction, if considered beneficial Diuretics are used to control oedema ACE inhibitor maintained or introduced Arrhythmias characterized with an ECG and antiarrhythmics used if indicated Digoxin maintained or introduced if indicated
NYHA class four: advanced heart failure Objective evidence of heart disease on physical examination; clinical signs are present even at rest Diagnosis usually evident on consideration of the history and the results of physical examination Therapy to stabilize the patient often necessary before investigations are completed Chest radiographs demonstrate cardiomegaly, often generalized, pulmonary venous congestion and pulmonary oedema	*Remove any precipitating cause* Hospitalization and strict cage rest Supply O_2 if 'hands off' supply available Intravenous frusemide to reduce preload (combination of different classes of diuretic may be necessary) Careful introduction of vasodilator, e.g. a venodilator such as glyceryl trinitrate (ointment or patches), a balanced vasodilator such as nitroprusside* may help relieve signs of congestive failure ACE inhibitor maintained or introduced Sedation (opiate usually recommended) may help Arrhythmias characterized with an ECG, antiarrhythmics used if indicated Inotropes are indicated in myocardial failure, digoxin or dobutamine*, digoxin for 'autonomic' effects Life-threatening pleural effusion (or severe ascites) may require drainage *Use of these drugs requires continuous ECG and blood pressure monitoring.

***Table 12.2:** NYHA functional classification of patients with left heart failure.*

Patient follow-up

Follow-up is essential to determine the efficacy of a therapeutic regime, to help avoid acute decompensation (see below), to ensure compliance with the overall management regime and to assess the patient for side-effects, toxicity or idiosyncratic reaction to drugs used. The frequency of check-ups is determined by severity (functional class), the patient's stability, and economic guidelines established by the owner. It may be neces-sary to take blood samples to assess renal and hepatic function and electrolyte levels. Radiography, echocardiography or ECGs may also be indicated.

Acute decompensation

A number of factors can contribute to the development of cardiac failure in hearts already compromised; for example, the development of a tachyarrhythmia in a patient with subclinical dilated cardiomyopathy may

Arrhythmias	Bradyarrhythmias Tachyarrhythmias

Reduced contractility	Negative inotropes
	        -beta adrenergic blocking agents
	        -anti-arrhythmic drugs
	        -calcium channel blocking agents
	Anaesthetic agents
	Myocardial toxins
	        -doxorubicin

Volume overload	Intravenous fluid administration Corticosteroid use
Concurrent systemic disease	Thromboembolism Sepsis Neoplasia Hypertension
Non-compliance with therapy/sudden changes in management	e.g. sudden intake of a high salt load or an increase in the level of exercise
Progression of the underlying disease	e.g. rupture of chordae tendineae in dogs with endocardiosis

Table 12.3: *Factors commonly precipitating left heart failure.*

be enough to precipitate overt clinical cardiac failure (Table 12.3).

In patients which suffer acute decompensation, the fall in cardiac output may be too acute for compensatory salt and water retention to occur. Consequently, while many patients may present in severe congestive left heart failure, signs referable to a low cardiac output and hypotension ('forward' failure) may predominate. Presenting signs in these cases include:

- Syncope
- Hypothermia, cold extremities
- Lethargy, exercise intolerance
- Mucous membrane pallor, prolonged capillary refill time
- Mental dullness
- Poor pulse volume
- Azotaemia.

Of the many causes of left heart failure in the dog and cat listed in Table 12.1, valvular disease and myocardial disease are the most common (Buchanan, 1992) and these two conditions and bacterial endocarditis will be discussed in detail. Other cardiac diseases which may result in left heart failure are discussed elsewhere in this manual.

DEGENERATIVE VALVULAR DISEASE (ENDOCARDIOSIS)

Endocardiosis is the result of an idiopathic myxomatous degeneration of the atrioventricular valves which leads to valvular insufficiency. The aetiology is unknown. Grey–white, smooth, glistening nodules or plaque-like thickening of the valve cusps are usually first seen in the areas of cusp apposition, but may also be seen at the base of the valve (Figure 12.2). As the pathology extends, the valve cusps become distorted and shrunken, and the chordae tendineae are often

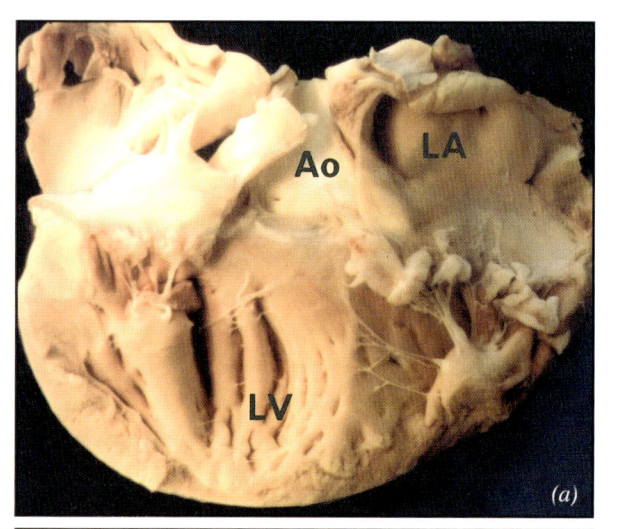

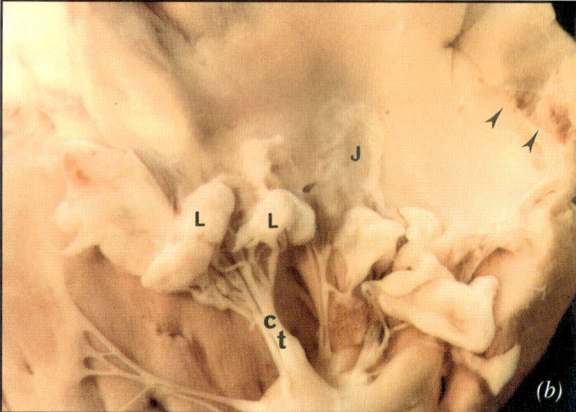

Figure 12.2: *(a) Heart from an aged small breed dog that died of congestive left heart failure, opened to show the left ventricle (LV), left atrium (LA) and aorta (Ao). The leaflets of the mitral valve are grossly distorted by endocardiosis lesions. Note that the leaflets of the aortic valve are unaffected. (b) Close up of one of the mitral valve leaflets seen in (a). Note the severe endocardiosis lesions (L) which are distorting the mitral valve leaflets, and the thickening of the chordae tendineae (ct). There is also a jet lesion (J) evident in the wall of the left atrium and a tear (arrowheads) in the left atrial endocardium.*

Courtesy of R.A. Hammond; specimen courtesy of Dr J.B.A. Smyth.
(b) Reproduced from Gorman (1998) with the permission of Blackwell Science.

thickened near their attachment to the valve (Whitney, 1974; Buchanan, 1977). The lesions are most frequently seen on the left atrioventricular valve, often in association with less severe lesions of the right atrioventricular valve; the semilunar valves are rarely affected. Physical irritation of the endocardium of the left atrium results in 'jet lesions' developing in the wall of the left atrium at the site of impact of regurgitant blood flow. Endocardiosis lesions are frequent incidental post-mortem findings in older dogs.

Histologically, lesions include a degeneration of the lower layer of valvular connective tissue (the *fibrosa*), and a thickening of the upper layer (the *spongiosa*) as a result of deposition of excessive extracellular matrix (glycosaminoglycans) along with fibroblastic proliferation and lipid deposition. The valvular lesions of endocardiosis develop over many years. Early on, they cause few detectable signs. Eventually, valvular distortion resulting from the disease process can lead to valvular insufficiency and heart failure in some (but not all) affected individuals.

Endocardiosis represents the most common cause of cardiac failure in the dog, but is extremely rare in cats. The frequency of valvular disease increases with advancing age; consequently, clinical signs tend to be seen in middle-aged and older dogs. It is seen with greatest frequency in smaller breeds of dog, especially the Cavalier King Charles Spaniel (Beardow and Buchanan, 1993), Poodle, Chihuahua, Cocker Spaniel and Yorkshire Terrier. Occasionally larger breeds are affected.

Pathophysiology
The insufficient mitral valve complex allows a significant proportion of the stroke volume to re-enter the left atrium during ventricular systole, resulting in an elevation of left atrial pressure and volume and a fall in the effective forward ventricular stroke volume. The fall in cardiac output results in activation of the compensatory mechanisms; increases in blood volume and venous return contribute to the volume-overloading of the left heart. Left-sided cardiomegaly develops as a result of eccentric ventricular hypertrophy. Initially myocardial function remains good, and the end-systolic volume remains within normal limits. Total stroke volume (forward plus regurgitant stroke volume) goes up, compensating for the regurgitation so that there is no significant rise in the end-diastolic pressure in the ventricle, atrium or pulmonary veins. Progressive cardiac enlargement subsequently results in further distortion of the components of the atrioventricular valve apparatus, so that regurgitation gets worse and the left atrium gets bigger. Eventually, the compensatory mechanisms required to maintain effective forward blood flow result in an increase in the pulmonary capillary pressure to a level which overwhelms the other Starling forces within the capillaries, and pulmonary oedema develops. Finally the myocardium also

fails, and this contributes to progression of the disease.

Complications of mitral valve disease include the rupturing of diseased chordae tendineae. The resulting sudden increase in regurgitant volume occurs before left atrial compliance can increase, which in turn results in a fast, sustained rise in left atrial pressure and the acute development of signs of left-sided cardiac failure. Another rare complication is the rupturing of the left atrial wall at the site of any jet lesions, resulting in peracute development of haemopericardium.

History
Typical presenting signs include exercise intolerance, dyspnoea, coughing, nocturnal restlessness, lethargy and anorexia. Syncope may sometimes occur, and weight loss may be seen particularly with advanced disease.

Clinical signs
Patients typically present with signs of left heart failure as detailed above. Specific features associated with endocardiosis include a *systolic murmur* which is auscultated over the left cardiac apex. The murmur of mitral regurgitation associated with valvular endocardiosis typically increases in intensity, duration and radiation as the disease progresses over a period of months or years; eventually a precordial thrill may be palpable. A murmur is also frequently heard over the right hemithorax either as a result of radiation of the mitral murmur or as a result of concomitant tricuspid regurgitation.

Diagnosis
A tentative diagnosis can often be made based on the identification of a systolic murmur (frequently detected at a routine examination) audible over the left cardiac apex, typically in small and medium-sized dogs.

Electrocardiography. There may be evidence of left atrial or left ventricular enlargement (wide P waves or tall R waves, respectively). Arrhythmias are common, especially in more advanced cases; electrocardiographic findings frequently include supraventricular premature complexes, sinus or atrial tachycardia or other supraventricular tachycardias such as atrial fibrillation (usually in more advanced cases). Ventricular arrhythmias do occur, but are seen less commonly than in patients with dilated cardiomyopathy.

Thoracic radiography will demonstrate progressive left-sided (or global) cardiomegaly as the disease progresses, with pulmonary venous congestion and finally an interstitial or alveolar pulmonary pattern seen as congestive left heart failure develops. A definitive diagnosis of mitral insufficiency can be made by left-sided *cardiac catheterization* and *angiography*.

Echocardiography. Two-dimensional echocardiography will identify more advanced valvular endocardiosis lesions, along with progressive left atrial and left ventricular enlargement. M-mode echocardiography permits assessment of chamber size and global myocardial function. Left ventricular volume overload will induce eccentric left ventricular hypertrophy. In the early stages of the disease, myocardial function remains good; consequently end-systolic volume is usually normal. The left ventricle may appear to be hyperdynamic as a result of the large total stroke volume (increased end-diastolic volume with a normal end-systolic volume). However, as the disease progresses, myocardial failure may become evident. At this stage, differentiating primary myocardial disease with secondary valvular insufficiency from primary valvular disease with secondary myocardial failure can be difficult. Colour-flow or spectral Doppler echocardiography will identify a systolic regurgitant jet in the left atrium.

Management

Successful management (Table 12.4) requires individual assessment of each patient with respect to severity, and adjustment of the therapeutic regime according to response, as described above in Table 12.2.

Prognosis

Patients with compensated mitral insufficiency may be free of clinical signs for years. However, the disease is progressive, and once cardiac failure develops the outlook is poor. Careful management can extend the comfortable life of some patients with mild or moderate failure for years, but sudden death or acute decompensation may develop at any time.

CANINE DILATED CARDIOMYOPATHY

Cardiomyopathies are diseases of the myocardium associated with cardiac dysfunction (Anon, 1995). Dilated cardiomyopathy (DCM) probably represents a common end-stage of myocardial failure resulting from a wide variety of insults to the myocardium; the offending primary cause is no longer apparent at presentation. Although myocardial function may be compromised in a number of diseases, a primary cause for the myocardial failure is rarely identified in patients with DCM. (Feline myocardial disease is dealt with in Chapter 19).

DCM is characterized by impaired ventricular function and a gradual dilation of one (typically the left) or both ventricles. Isolated right-sided DCM is rare. Like

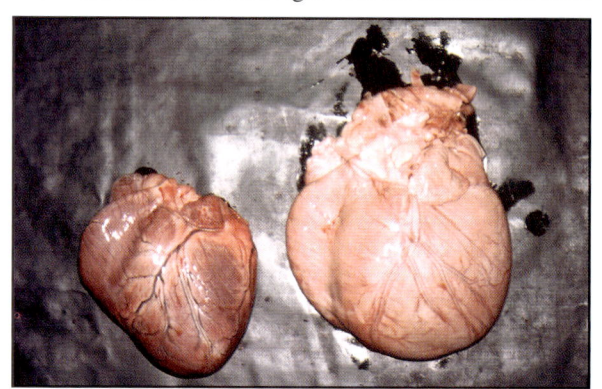

Figure 12.3: *Severe cardiac enlargement due to dilated cardiomyopathy in a Great Dane (right) compared with the heart from an unaffected Great Dane of the same age (left).*
Reproduced from Gorman (1998) with the permission of Blackwell Science.

Asymptomatic patients with endocardiosis	• Make definitive diagnosis • Assess severity of disease (e.g. with thoracic radiographs) • Reassess regularly for evidence of decompensation • Control obesity if necessary • Advise the owner about likely progression of the disease
Mild failure	• Sodium-restricted diet is traditionally introduced; maintain if considered helpful • Exercise control • A diuretic is usually introduced – dose titrated to effect • ACE inhibitor is often introduced • Anti-arrhythmic medication indicated if arrhythmias are contributing to the clinical syndrome
Moderate failure	• Maintain sodium-restricted diet (if in use and considered helpful) and exercise control • Diuretic dose increased as necessary, titrated to effect; may require combination of diuretics • Regular checks of renal function and electrolyte levels are advisable • ACE inhibitor introduced or maintained • Digoxin introduced to control ventricular rate in supraventricular tachyarrhythmias such as atrial fibrillation, and to augment contractility if myocardial failure is evident • Anti-arrhythmic medication indicated if arrhythmias are contributing to the clinical syndrome
Severe failure	• Remove any precipitating factor • Cage rest • Intravenous frusemide (may require a combination of diuretics) • Vasodilators (e.g. topical glyceryl trinitrate, ACE inhibitor or intravenous sodium nitroprusside) • Oxygen administration, if 'hands off' administration is possible (e.g. O_2 cage) • Sedation (opiate) may help in some cases • In refractory cases with significant element of myocardial failure, digoxin or intravenous dobutamine may improve cardiac output • Arrhythmias require ECG diagnosis and may need appropriate management • Monitoring of renal function and electrolyte levels is advisable

Table 12.4: *Therapeutic regimes for endocardiosis.*

the valvular degeneration seen in endocardiosis, evidence suggests that in DCM, insidious left ventricular dysfunction progresses gradually over a period of years with mild left ventricular dysfunction and frequently cardiac arrhythmias evident for months, or even years before congestive cardiac failure develops (Brownlie, 1991; Calvert, 1992).

On post mortem, the heart is pale, soft and flabby (Figure 12.3), exhibiting a variable degree of enlargement and dilation, usually of all four chambers; although the disease process may affect the left side predominantly. The ventricular walls appear thin, but eccentric hypertrophy is invariably present. Thinning and atrophy of the papillary muscles and trabeculae are usually evident and there may be coexistent valvular endocardiosis, especially in the smaller breeds. The circumference of the atrioventricular valve orifice is usually enlarged. Scattered pale foci representing areas of necrosis or fibrosis may be evident grossly.

Microscopically, the histopathological findings are variable and non-specific. There are scattered areas of myocyte hypertrophy and degeneration, and varying degrees of myocardial necrosis as well as areas of interstitial oedema and fibrosis. Medial hyperplasia is evident in some of the intramyocardial arterioles; cellular myocardial infiltrates are rarely described, and much of the myocardium will often appear normal (Van Vleet *et al.*, 1981; Sandusky *et al.*, 1984).

DCM is primarily a disease of young and middle-aged dogs, although a wide range of age groups may be affected from 6 months old to older than 10 years. DCM affects particularly medium, large or giant breeds, and has been described in most of the common breeds. Breed differences in clinical presentation and progression of the disease suggest that different causes and/or genetic factors play a role. Frequently affected breeds include:

- Dobermann – typically acute-onset left-sided failure, ventricular tachyarrhythmias, short clinical course, high incidence of sudden death (Calvert *et al.*, 1982)
- Boxer – principally affects left side, high incidence of ventricular tachyarrhythmias, longer clinical course (Harpster, 1983)
- Spaniels – Cocker and Springer (Staaden, 1981) – principally left-sided heart failure, may have a longer clinical course than many breeds
- Giant breeds, especially Irish Wolfhound, St Bernard, Great Dane, Newfoundland – often present with a subclinical arrhythmia (usually atrial fibrillation) that is well tolerated for months or years before congestive cardiac failure develops (Brownlie, 1991).

The degree and extent of systolic dysfunction varies; chamber dilation and reduced systolic function are usually evident prior to the onset of clinical signs. The disease is invariably progressive. Patients may apparently develop acute, severe myocardial failure with signs of reduced tissue perfusion and hypotension.

Pathophysiology

DCM is primarily a disease of myocardial dysfunction and poor cardiac output. As a result of reduced myocardial contractility, stroke volume falls and left ventricular end-systolic diameter and volume increase. The fall in cardiac output leads to activation of compensatory salt and water retention. As a result of this volume overload, end-diastolic diameter and volume increase, and eccentric ventricular hypertrophy develops. The resulting cardiomegaly allows a normal stroke volume and end-diastolic pressure to be maintained initially. As cardiac enlargement and myocardial hypertrophy develop, there is distortion of the components of atrioventricular valve apparatus, compromising atrioventricular valve function, which contributes to the progressive development of cardiac failure. With time, as contractility continues to deteriorate and blood volume increases, the ability of the heart to hypertrophy becomes limited. Consequently, the diastolic pressure within the ventricle and therefore the atrium and pulmonary veins and capillaries increases and pulmonary oedema develops. Finally, cardiac output may become so inadequate that signs of 'forward' failure become evident.

History

There is often no previous history of cardiac disease, and the onset of clinical signs is often apparently acute (1–3 weeks). Commonly reported historical features include anorexia and weight loss, and reduced exercise tolerance with lethargy or weakness. Respiratory signs such as dyspnoea and coughing are often present, or affected animals may present with syncope. Ascites may be present with concomitant right heart failure. Alternatively, the initial sign may be sudden death, or affected animals may die suddenly at any point in the clinical course.

Clinical signs

Patients typically present with signs of left heart failure as detailed above. Specific features associated with DCM are listed below.

Soft systolic murmurs due to secondary valvular incompetence are often heard in the region of the atrioventricular valves.

Arrhythmias are common; both supraventricular tachyarrhythmias such as atrial fibrillation and/or ventricular arrhythmias are frequently described. Bradyarrhythmias have been described in cardiomyopathic Dobermanns (Calvert *et al.*, 1996).

Gallop rhythms may be heard on auscultation.

A reduced apex beat may be present as a result of the poor stroke volume.

A hypokinetic pulse may be associated with a poor stroke volume.

Weight loss may occur in dogs with mild to moderate heart failure due to DCM.

Diagnosis

A tentative diagnosis is usually made based on the patient details, the history and the results of the physical examination.

Electrocardiography. There may be electrocardiographic evidence of left atrial and/or left ventricular enlargement or conduction abnormalities. Changes in QRS complex morphology are common. Arrhythmias are frequently identified; electrocardiographic findings include supraventricular premature complexes, sinus or atrial tachycardia, atrial fibrillation (common in giant breed dogs with DCM), as well as ventricular premature complexes and ventricular tachycardia (often a feature of DCM in the Dobermann and the Boxer). Long-term arrhythmia-monitoring or ambulatory electrocardiography (Holter monitoring) may help to identify paroxysmal arrhythmias not detected on routine electrocardiography. Ambulatory electrocardiography may also be indicated in patients exhibiting syncopal episodes, and in breeds in which the primary disease is commonly complicated by life-threatening arrhythmias. Weakness and syncope associated with brady-arrhythmias have been described recently in cardiomyopathic Dobermanns following detection with ambulatory electrocardiography (Calvert *et al.*, 1996).

Radiography will demonstrate progressive left-sided (or global) cardiomegaly as the disease progresses. Cardiomegaly may be difficult to appreciate in some cases of acute-onset left heart failure, especially in deep-chested breeds. As cardiac failure develops, pulmonary venous congestion becomes evident and an interstitial and finally an alveolar pattern confirm the development of pulmonary oedema. Pleural effusion may be evident if there is concomitant right heart failure.

M-mode echocardiography permits accurate assessment of chamber size and global myocardial function, allowing a definitive diagnosis to be made (Figure 12.4). Cardiac chamber dimensions are usually above the upper limits of normal, and end-systolic diameter is increased as a result of reduced myocardial contractility. There is a secondary increase in end-diastolic diameter, and eccentric myocardial hypertrophy as a result of volume-overloading. E point-to-septal separation (EPSS) is often increased and left ventricular shortening fraction is depressed (Lombard, 1984). *Doppler echocardiography* will allow identification of secondary systolic atrioventricular valvular regurgitation, and can be used to assess the haemodynamic consequences of the myocardial disease.

Management

As with all cases of left heart failure, each DCM patient requires individual assessment of the severity of the disease and adjustment of the therapeutic regime according to response as described in Table 12.2. General therapeutic guidelines however, are detailed in Table 12.5.

Prognosis

The prognosis seems to vary according to the breed and the severity of the disease at presentation. Patients (especially giant breed dogs) identified as a result of the discovery of an arrhythmia may remain compensated and free of clinical signs for years. Once cardiac failure develops, however, the outlook is poor. Most patients die or are put to sleep within 6–12 months of the development of overt cardiac failure, although with careful management some patients will survive for years. In all cases, sudden death or acute decompensation is possible.

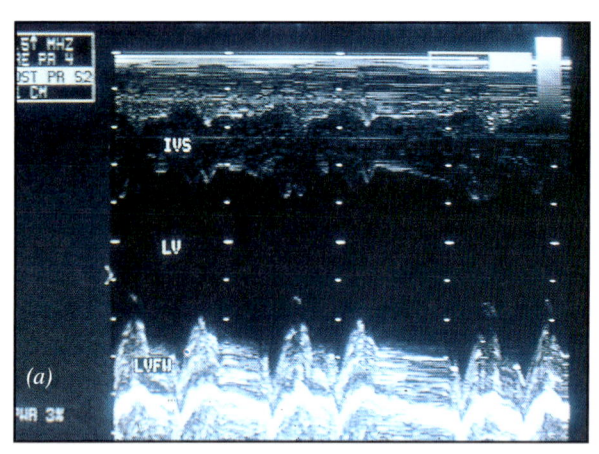

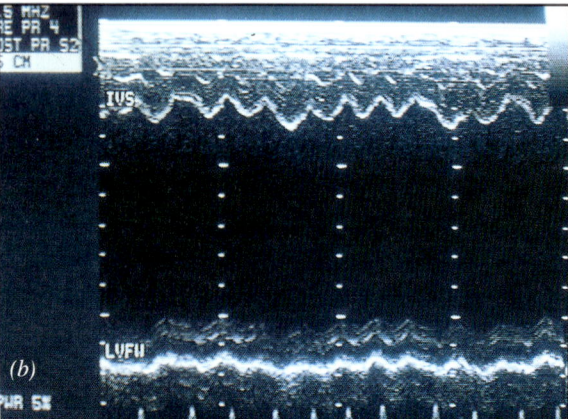

Figure 12.4: *M-mode echocardiographic images of (a) a normal dog and (b) a dog of the same breed with dilated cardiomyopathy at the level of the left ventricle. The left ventricle (LV) of the dog affected with DCM is dilated and the left ventricular free wall (LVFW) and interventricular septum (IVS) are hypomotile, compared with the normal dog.*

Reproduced from Gorman (1998) with the permission of Blackwell Science.

BACTERIAL ENDOCARDITIS

Bacterial endocarditis (BE) is a term used to describe bacterial infection of the heart valves or mural endocardium following transient or persistent bacteraemia.

Asymptomatic patients	· Definitive diagnosis is made
	· Assess severity of disease
	· Regular reassessment for evidence of decompensation is advisable
	· Breeds or individuals in which a deficiency can be documented (e.g. carnitine or taurine) may benefit from supplementation
	· ECG diagnosis of any arrhythmia
	· Discuss prognosis and likely progression of the disease with the owner
Mild cardiac failure	· Exercise control
	· A low-salt diet may be considered helpful
	· A diuretic is normally introduced – titrate to effect
	· A positive inotrope (e.g. digoxin) to improve systolic function is usually introduced. Digoxin is often indicated for the control of the ventricular rate in atrial fibrillation. In cases where this does not provide sufficient control of the heart rate, an additional negatively chronotropic agent such as a beta blocking agent or a calcium channel blocking agent may be required
	· An ACE inhibitor is often introduced
	· In those cases in which ventricular arrhythmias are a significant factor in the disease, specific arrhythmic therapy may be required
	· Monitoring renal function and electrolyte levels is advisable
Moderate cardiac failure	· Maintain exercise control. Maintain low-salt diet if considered helpful
	· Higher doses of diuretic (may require combination of diuretics)
	· ACE inhibitor
	· Digoxin
	· Anti-arrhythmics if indicated
	· Monitor renal function and electrolyte levels
Severe failure	· Remove any precipitating factor
	· Cage rest
	· Intravenous frusemide (may require combination of diuretics), titrate to effect
	· Vasodilators (e.g. topical nitroglycerine, ACE inhibitor or intravenous sodium nitroprusside
	· Oxygen administration, if 'hands off' administration is possible
	· Sedate (opiate) may help some cases
	· Maintain or introduce digoxin
	· Intravenous dobutamine may help improve cardiac output
	· Anti-arrhythmics if indicated
	· Monitor renal function and electrolyte levels if possible

Table 12.5: Therapeutic regimes for dilated cardiomyopathy.

Such transient bacteraemias are likely to occur occasionally in normal individuals, without causing any deleterious effects. The disease is said to be more common in medium and large breed male dogs.

Pathophysiology

The bacteria involved are typically normal inhabitants of the skin or the urogenital or gastrointestinal tracts; these sites are considered to be the primary source of the organisms involved in many cases. Other portals of entry are thought to be wounds (traumatic and surgical), catheters and chronic septic conditions.

Some bacteria are better able to adhere to the endocardium than others; the endocardium is infected by direct extension from the blood stream and the affected regions are usually normal prior to infection. Diseased valves (especially cases of subvalvular aortic stenosis) are said to be more susceptible to infection, but pre-existing valve damage is not a prerequisite for infection. The presence of circulating agglutinating antibody may increase the likelihood of endocardial colonization as a result of clumping circulating organisms. Some cases may result from the colonization of acellular, non-bacterial fibrin thrombi attached to the valves or mural endocardium.

Two syndromes are generally recognized. The acute form is characterized by a rapidly progressive, ulcerative septic condition; with rapid tissue destruction and necrosis. It is associated with large numbers of bacteria, and an acute local inflammatory response consisting mainly of neutrophil polymorphs. More commonly, a subacute or chronic form is seen, characterized by the development of a friable vegetation with evidence locally of necrosis associated with an attempt at repair.

Colonization of a valve or an area of the endocardium by bacteria results in ulceration, platelet aggregation on exposed collagen and the formation of vegetations consisting of bacterial colonies in a fibrin-platelet thrombus. Valvular lesions may spread to involve the local mural endocardium or the chordae tendineae which may rupture. In the case of lesions affecting the aortic valve, the sinus of Valsalva and coronary arteries may also become involved, and septic myocardial emboli may result in destruction of sections of the conducting system or myocardial infarction and consequently, the development of arrhythmias (Boswood, 1996).

In chronic cases, the vegetations organize (sometimes even undergoing hyalinization or calcification), resulting in the distortion of affected valves and valvular insufficiency, occasionally with coexisting valvular stenosis.

Because of the friable nature of the vegetations, pieces of variable size frequently break off, and septic or aseptic thromboembolism may occur with metastatic spread to other organs. The consequences of these events are determined by the degree of vascular obstruction, the organ affected and the availability of a collateral circulation. Secondary immune-mediated disease is common.

In the dog, the mitral or aortic valves (or both) are the most commonly affected. Tricuspid and pulmonic valve lesions are rare.

HISTORY

Rarely, the history may suggest previous or current bacterial infection, or an opportunity for bacteria to gain access to the circulation such as via catheterization, the use of immunosuppressive medication, or recent surgery. However, usually the history is vague, non-specific, and suggestive of systemic infection or inflammation rather than cardiac disease. Typical historical findings in cases of BE include anorexia, malaise, and lethargy. Shaking is a common feature, as is weight loss. Lameness is sometimes present, and may be variable or shifting. Some animals present with syncope, abdominal pain or even neurological signs.

Clinical signs
Clinical signs may be referable to:

- Sepsis and bacteraemia
- Thromboembolic disease and metastatic infection
- Valve lesions and the development of heart failure
- Secondary immune-mediated disease.

Patients rarely present with signs of cardiovascular disease; presenting signs in most cases are usually secondary to recurrent long-standing bacteraemia, and are therefore generally non-specific, often variable, and chronic or intermittent; making frequent re-examination worthwhile (Elwood *et al.*, 1993). Typical findings on physical examination include:

- Poor physical condition
- Weakness
- Persistent or recurrent pyrexia
- Joint swelling or pain, spinal pain
- Petechiation or haemorrhage
- Abdominal pain
- Neurological signs
- Arrhythmia.

A heart murmur developing in an individual in which none had been previously detected is suggestive of BE, especially if accompanied by other signs consistent with the disease. The characteristics of such murmurs (timing, character, grade etc.) may vary between examinations, and they must be differentiated from physiological murmurs associated with any concurrent pyrexia or anaemia. Signs of overt congestive heart failure are rare. Secondary thromboembolic

and/or immune-mediated disease is common. Whether extracardiac septic foci are the primary source of the infection or the result of metastatic spread can be difficult to determine. Common secondary findings at post-mortem include:

- Renal infarction, abscessation, pyelonephritis, glomerulonephropathy
- Central nervous system abscessation, encephalitis, meningitis
- Joint swelling, polyarthritis; septic or immune complex
- Discospondylitis, osteomyelitis or myositis
- Vasculitis, small vessel occlusion
- Evidence of disseminated intravascular coagulation (DIC)
- Splenic and/or gastrointestinal infarction.

Diagnosis
Definitive diagnosis is difficult. The occurrence of fever, a murmur (especially a murmur not previously identified in an individual or a murmur with variable characteristics) and evidence of embolic disease in an individual are, however, suggestive of BE. The disease is expensive and often unrewarding to investigate and treat, and the extent of the investigation and treatment in an individual case will frequently be subject to financial constraints. The history, findings on physical examination and the results of urinalysis and routine haematology and biochemistry as detailed below may alert the clinician to the possibility of BE, particularly if a high index of suspicion is maintained. If possible, an attempt should be made to obtain a definitive diagnosis.

Blood culture is indicated in order to document the presence of bacteraemia and identify the organism(s) involved and their sensitivity to antimicrobials. The more samples that are taken, the greater the likelihood of identifying the organism involved. Ideally, at least four samples are taken. Recommendations concerning the timing of the sampling vary; sampling three or four times at least 1 hour apart, if possible from different sites, is likely to be as good a protocol as any. Skin preparation at the venepuncture site is as for surgery, and samples should be incubated aerobically and anaerobically. Growth of the same organism from two or more samples is very suggestive of bacteraemia. Any site suspected of being the primary source of a bacteraemia, e.g. the urinary tract, should also be cultured.

Haematology. Evidence of chronic inflammatory disease is most commonly evident, with leucocytosis as a result of a mature neutrophilia, often accompanied by a monocytosis. A neutrophilia accompanied by a left shift may be seen in cases of acute, ulcerative BE. There is often evidence of a mild non-regenerative anaemia of chronic disease; occasionally a secondary autoimmune haemolytic anaemia develops. Thrombocytopenia may be evident in cases which develop DIC or secondary immune-mediated thrombocytopenia.

Clinical biochemistry. Chronic inflammation may result in an elevation of total protein due to an elevation of serum globulin; albumin levels may be low if there is significant haemorrhage, renal or gastrointestinal protein loss or reduced hepatic protein synthesis. There may be biochemical evidence of dysfunction in organs affected by embolization or metastatic infection, e.g. renal insufficiency, elevated muscle enzyme levels.

Urinalysis. Urinary tract infections may be primary or secondary. Renal infarction is common, and there may be pyuria, haematuria, and evidence of cells and casts in the sediment. Significant proteinuria may accompany secondary glomerulonephropathy.

Joint fluid/cerebrospinal fluid analysis may demonstrate septic or aseptic joint or meningeal inflammation in animals showing suspicious clinical signs.

Tests for immune-mediated disease. Tests for antinuclear antibodies, Coomb's tests etc. are sometimes positive.

Electrocardiography. Abnormalities of rate and rhythm are common and require electrocardiographic documentation. Abnormal complex size or configuration may suggest chamber enlargement or conduction abnormalities.

Radiography is often indicated, e.g. joint or spinal radiography. Chest radiographs may be necessary to document cardiomegaly, overt or impending congestive cardiac failure.

Echocardiography, especially two-dimensional, is very useful for the demonstration of vegetations and the secondary effects of valvular damage (volume overload and chamber dilation, chordae tendineae rupture, flail valve leaflets etc.; Lombard and Buergelt, 1983). Doppler echocardiography will assist in identifying malfunctioning, diseased valves and allow assessment of their haemodynamic significance.

Cardiac catheterization and angiography may be required to demonstrate any valvular or endocardial lesions and give an indication of the haemodynamic consequences of such lesions.

In some cases, definitive diagnosis is only obtained at post-mortem examination.

Management

1. Treat any active infection:
   - Long courses of high doses of bactericidal antibiotics are indicated
   - Begin once blood sampling for culture is completed if index of suspicion is high
   - A useful antibacterial combination for use while culture results are pending and in culture-negative individuals is *ampicillin*, combined with an *aminoglycoside* (monitor renal function) or a quinolone such as *enrofloxacin*
   - Treat intravenously if possible for the first 7 days
   - Change anti-bacterial if indicated by blood culture results
   - Follow up with a 6-week course of non-aminoglycoside oral antibiotics, and if possible and practical check efficacy with follow-up blood cultures.
2. Identify and deal with any potential portals of entry (abscesses, pyometra etc.).
3. Consider and treat as necessary any cardiac complications, e.g. arrhythmias, overt congestive cardiac failure.
4. Consider and treat as necessary any extra-cardiac complications.
5. Frequent reassessment of the patient for signs of improvement or the development of further complications.

Prognosis

Always guarded, the prognosis is determined by the virulence of the organism involved, the haemodynamic effects of any valve damage, and the severity of any extra-cardiac complications. Even if the primary infection is controlled, permanent valve damage is to be expected. The prognosis seems to be especially poor if the disease is associated with large vegetations, overt congestive cardiac failure, evidence of DIC or severe tachyarrhythmias. Prophylactic antibiotic treatment is indicated if significant bacteraemia is likely, especially in the patient with pre-existing valvular disease.

REFERENCES AND FURTHER READING

Anon (1964) Criteria Committee, New York Heart Association. In: *Diseases of the Heart and Blood Vessels. Nomenclature and Criteria for Diagnosis, 6th edn*, ed. Little, Brown and Co, Boston

Anon (1992) *Recommendations for the Diagnosis and the Treatment of Heart Failure in Small Animals.* International Small Animal Cardiac Health Council

Anon (1995) Report of the 1995 World Health Organization/International Society and Federation of Cardiology task force on the definition and classification of cardiomyopathies. *Circulation* **93**, 841

Beardow A W and Buchanan J W (1993) Chronic mitral valve disease in Cavalier King Charles Spaniels: 95 cases (1987-1991). *Journal of the American Veterinary Medical Association* **203**, 1023

Boswood A. (1996) Resolution of dysrhythmias and conduction abnormalities following treatment for bacterial endocarditis in a dog. *Journal of Small Animal Practice* **37**, 327

Brownlie SE (1991) An electrocardiographic survey of cardiac rhythm in Irish Wolfhounds. *Veterinary Record* **129**, 470

Buchanan JW (1977) Chronic valvular disease (endocardiosis) in dogs. *Advances in Veterinary Science and Comparative Medicine* **21**, 75

Buchanan JW (1992) Causes and prevalence of cardiovascular disease. In: *Current Veterinary Therapy XI*, ed. RW Kirk and JD Bonagura. WB Saunders, Philadelphia

Calvert CA (1992) Update: canine dilated cardiomyopathy. In: *Current Veterinary Therapy XI*, ed. RW Kirk and JD Bonagura. WB Saunders, Philadelphia

Calvert CA, Chapman WL and Toal RL (1982) Congestive cardiomyopathy in Doberman Pinscher dogs. *Journal of the American Veterinary Medical Association* **181**, 598

Calvert CA, Jacobs GJ and Pickus CW (1996) Bradycardia-associated episodic weakness, syncope and aborted sudden death in cardiomyopathic Doberman Pinschers. *Journal of Veterinary Internal Medicine* **10**, 88

Elwood CM, Cobb MA and Stepien RL (1993) Clinical and echocardiographic findings in 10 dogs with vegetative bacterial endocarditis. *Journal of Small Animal Practice* **34**, 420

Gorman NT (1998) *Canine Medicine and Therapeutics, 4th edn.* Blackwell Science, Oxford

Harpster N K (1983) Boxer cardiomyopathy. In: *Current Veterinary Therapy VIII*, ed. RW Kirk. WB Saunders, Philadelphia

Lombard CW (1984) Echocardiographic and clinical signs of canine dilated cardiomyopathy. *Journal of Small Animal Practice* **25**, 59

Lombard CW and Buergelt CD (1983) Vegetative bacterial endocarditis in dogs: echocardiographic diagnosis and clinical signs. *Journal of Small Animal Practice* **24**, 325

Sandusky GE, Capen CC and Kerr KM (1984) Histological and ultrastructural evaluation of cardiac lesions in idiopathic cardiomyopathy in dogs. *Canadian Journal of Comparative Medicine* **48**, 81.

Staaden RS (1981) Cardiomyopathy of English Cocker Spaniel. *Journal of the American Veterinary Medical Association* **178**, 1289

Van Vleet JF, Ferrans VJ and Weirich WE (1981) Pathologic alterations in congestive cardiomyopathy of dogs. *American Journal of Veterinary Research* **42**, 416

Whitney JC (1974) Observations on the effect of age on the severity of heart valve lesions in the dog. *Journal of Small Animal Practice* **15**, 511

Right Heart Failure

Virginia Luis Fuentes

PATHOPHYSIOLOGY

Although left heart failure may have more catastrophic consequences than right heart failure, the function of both ventricles is interdependent. The two ventricles share an interventricular wall, and pericardial restraint can enable distortion of one chamber to affect the function of the other. The type of congestive signs seen will reflect which ventricle has failed; left ventricular failure will result in pulmonary venous congestion, whereas right ventricular failure leads to systemic venous congestion. Often both ventricles will be affected, either because of a pathological process common to both ventricles (e.g. dilated cardiomyopathy) or because a rise in left atrial pressures can lead to a rise in pulmonary arterial pressures, resulting in right heart failure.

The right heart has been compared to a bellows, and in some ways acts as a simple conduit between the venous system and the lungs. The right heart is a low-pressure system compared with the left, and is more vulnerable to compression with any rise in intrapericardial pressure. The geometry of the right ventricle is also very sensitive to changes in intraventricular pressure and volume. The normal right ventricle 'wraps around' the left ventricle, with a crescent-shaped cross-section compared with the circular cross-section of the left ventricle. With volume or pressure overload of the right ventricle (e.g. tricuspid regurgitation or pulmonic stenosis, respectively), the ventricle may dilate (volume overload) or develop concentric hypertrophy (pressure overload). In either case, the shape of the right ventricle will be altered, distorting the tricuspid valve apparatus and causing or exacerbating tricuspid regurgitation.

An increase in right atrial pressures will be transmitted to the systemic veins. Systemic capillaries are more leaky than pulmonary capillaries, and peripheral venous congestion leads to hepatic enlargement. *Ascites* may develop, or *pleural effusion*; even *chylothorax* may be a sequel. In severe, long-standing right heart failure, mesenteric hypertension may lead to gut

Pericardial disease	congenital	peritoneo–pericardial diaphragmatic hernia
		pericardial cysts
	neoplastic	right atrial haemangiosarcoma
		heart base tumour
		lymphoma
	inflammatory	idiopathic pericardial haemorrhage
		feline infectious peritonitis
		purulent pericarditis
		constrictive pericarditis
	traumatic	left atrial rupture
Myocardial disease	primary	dilated cardiomyopathy
		hypertrophic cardiomyopathy
		restrictive cardiomyopathy
	secondary	hyperthyroidism
		taurine deficiency
Acquired valvular disease		endocardiosis
Congenital disease		pulmonic stenosis
		tricuspid dysplasia
Pulmonary hypertension	pulmonary vascular disease cor pulmonale	heartworm disease severe primary respiratory disease
Arrhythmias	bradyarrhythmias tachyarrhythmias	3rd degree atrioventricular block sustained supraventricular tachycardia

Table 13.1: Causes of right heart failure.

oedema and impairment of gastrointestinal function. *Cardiac cachexia* (loss of body fat and muscle mass associated with heart failure) is more common in right heart failure than in left heart failure. Although frequently seen in humans and cattle, cardiac causes of subcutaneous oedema are uncommon in dogs and cats. It may occur in the presence of hypoalbuminaemia, or with severe, chronic right heart failure with marked fluid retention.

Output failure may also arise from right heart failure; adequate filling of the left heart depends on normal right ventricular output. On a beat-to-beat basis, the balance between the ventricles is maintained by Starling's Law: a fall in right ventricular output will lower left ventricular filling pressures, and left ventricular output will drop correspondingly. Right ventricular outflow tract obstruction may prevent a normal rise in cardiac output with exercise, just as with left ventricular outflow tract obstruction. With both causes of outflow tract obstruction, the clinical result may be syncope.

CAUSES OF RIGHT HEART FAILURE

Causes of right heart failure are listed in Table 13.1.

RECOGNITION OF RIGHT HEART FAILURE

The key features of right heart failure are *jugular distension*, *ascites*, *pleural effusion* and *hepatomegaly*.

Presenting signs of right heart failure

The commonest presenting signs of right heart failure include abdominal distension (caused by ascites), dyspnoea (caused by pleural effusion) and syncope or exercise intolerance (poor right ventricular output on exercise). Additional signs may include inappetence and weight loss. Subcutaneous oedema is unusual.

Physical findings in right heart failure

Most physical signs of right heart failure are referable to backwards failure of the right ventricle.

Jugular veins

A rise in right atrial pressures is transmitted to the venae cavae and peripheral veins. This can be detected on physical examination as distended jugular veins. The finding of distended jugular veins with ascites is highly indicative of right heart failure, as it will not be seen with other causes of ascites. Abnormal jugular pulsation may be seen in tricuspid regurgitation with right heart failure, and the pulsation may extend far up the neck, even with the head raised. Jugular pulsation should only be seen up to a point that is at the same horizontal level as the right atrium in normal animals.

Hepatojugular reflux may be demonstrated in animals with mildly elevated right atrial pressures. A normal right atrium can accommodate an increased volume of blood without transmitting increased pressure to the systemic veins. One can increase the volume of blood returning to the right heart by applying pressure to the cranial abdomen and displacing hepatic venous blood into the caudal vena cava. If the right atrial pressures are already slightly elevated, the increase in venous return may result in a temporary distension of the jugular veins, which collapse again when the cranial abdominal pressure is removed.

Ascites

Ascites may develop with congestion of the hepatic veins (generally a modified transudate). Ascites is seen more often in dogs with right heart failure than in cats.

Hepatomegaly

The liver may be palpably enlarged in right heart failure. With chronic systemic venous congestion, splenomegaly may also be found.

Pleural effusion

Pleural effusion is more common in cats than dogs with right heart failure. As with ascites, it is generally a modified transudate.

Subcutaneous oedema

Subcutaneous oedema is not often seen with right heart failure, but when it does occur, it is usually seen in the limbs, brisket, prepuce and ventral abdomen.

Radiography

Right heart failure can be recognized on radiographs as pleural effusions and ascites (see Chapter 5(i)). Pleural effusions will be seen as interlobar fissures, with scalloping of ventral lung borders on lateral views. Ascites leads to poor abdominal contrast and a 'ground glass' appearance (Figure 13.1). The caudal vena cava is usually widened (Lehmkuhl *et al.*, 1997), and hepatomegaly may be evident.

Ultrasonography

Ultrasonography will confirm the presence of pleural and peritoneal fluid, but will also demonstrate dilated hepatic veins, which can help to distinguish ascites due to right heart failure from other causes. Echocardiography is helpful for determining the underlying cause of right heart failure, and readily demonstrates pericardial effusions.

Management of right heart failure

As with all therapy of cardiac disease, the underlying cause must be addressed. This is particularly important with pericardial disease, in which the usual principle of diuretic therapy for abnormal fluid accumulation is not

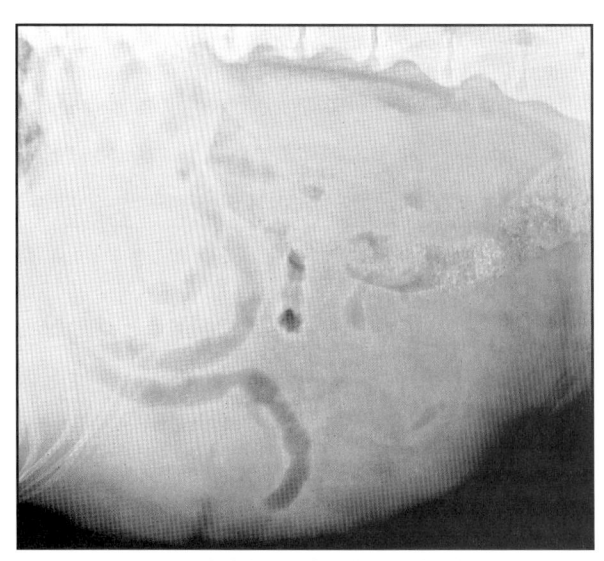

Figure 13.1: *Lateral abdominal radiograph of a German Shepherd Dog with biventricular congestive cardiac failure, showing poor abdominal contrast due to ascites.*

only ineffective, but also potentially harmful. With pericardial effusions resulting in congestive failure, the only effective treatment is to drain the effusion. It is also important to differentiate a pericardial effusion that is the result of right heart failure, from a pericardial effusion that is the cause of right heart failure. The former is not likely to result in cardiac tamponade.

In mild right-sided congestive heart failure due to valvular or myocardial disease, the same principles are followed as with left heart failure (see Chapter 12). The severity of the problem dictates the degree of aggression with therapy. Whilst attempting to deal with the underlying problem, additional therapy may include diuretics for ascites and pleural effusion, exercise and sodium restriction, and possibly angiotensin converting enzyme (ACE) inhibitors if appropriate.

Management of refractory ascites in valvular or myocardial disease can be very frustrating. Although severe ascites may not be as life-threatening as severe pulmonary oedema, affected animals often have poor appetites and may experience discomfort associated with hepatic and visceral congestion. Cardiac cachexia is common. Absorption of medication may be reduced, compromising the efficacy of therapy still further. As always, the ideal solution is to correct the underlying problem. With pulmonic stenosis this may be possible, although the presence of severe congestive failure increases the risk of invasive procedures. With DCM and endocardiosis it is generally necessary to rely on medical treatment:

- Administer drugs parenterally where possible, particularly diuretics
- Drain pleural effusions if severe and causing dyspnoea
- Consider sequential nephron blockade, i.e. using more than one type of diuretic (e.g. frusemide and a potassium-sparing diuretic such as

spironolactone); however, monitor effects for dehydration, prerenal azotaemia, hypotension and hypokalaemia (loop diuretics)
- Reduce activation of the renin–angiotensin–aldosterone system (i.e. ACE inhibitors)
- Do not drain ascitic effusions unless absolutely necessary for the animal's welfare: repeated drainage can lead to further loss of serum protein and hypoproteinaemia will exacerbate right heart failure
- Feed palatable, high density diets but avoid high salt levels (or consider a low salt diet).

PERICARDIAL DISEASE

General features

Pericardial disease leads to right heart failure by restricting filling of the right side of the heart. The pericardium is a relatively incompliant fibrous sac, and the pericardial space normally contains only a few millilitres of serous fluid. A sudden effusion into the pericardial space results in a marked increase in pericardial pressure, as the pericardium cannot stretch. Raised intrapericardial pressures impede right atrial filling and may actually lead to collapse of the right atrium. A further rise in pericardial pressures may even collapse the right ventricle. If blood cannot enter the right atrium, systemic venous pressures will rise. Restriction of filling of the right side of the heart due to pericardial compression is known as *cardiac tamponade*. Gradual pericardial effusions may be better tolerated, as the pericardium may stretch with time. Indeed, several litres may sometimes accumulate in idiopathic pericardial effusions in giant breeds. The severity of cardiac tamponade is dependent on intra-pericardial pressures rather than volume. Types of pericardial effusions are listed in Table 13.2.

It should be noted that a small pericardial effusion might be one of the possible effects of right heart failure, although this is unlikely to become so severe as to cause cardiac tamponade.

Haemorrhagic	idiopathic pericardial haemorrhage intrapericardial neoplasia trauma coagulopathy ruptured left atrium
Transudates	right heart failure hypoproteinaemia intrapericardial neoplasia peritoneo–pericardial diaphragmatic hernia
Exudates	feline infectious peritonitis infection foreign body

Table 13.2: *Types of pericardial effusion.*

Clinical signs

Presenting signs of pericardial disease are typical of right heart failure, but will depend on the rapidity with which the effusion has developed as well as its volume. Animals with acute cardiac tamponade may present with severe weakness and hypotension. Symptomatic animals usually have ascites and exercise intolerance, although small or chronic effusions may not result in any clinical signs. Vague signs such as lethargy and inappetence are common (Berg and Wingfield, 1984).

Diagnosis

Physical examination: Apart from signs of right heart failure (including jugular distension), the apex beat is less pronounced than normal and the heart sounds may be muffled. *Pulsus paradoxicus* may be present (where the strength of the pulse decreases in inspiration).

ECG: Electrical alternans may be seen, where the QRS complex voltages alter from beat to beat (Figure 13.2). This tends to be seen only in large effusions, and reflects swinging of the heart within the pericardium (which 'changes' the electrical axis from beat to beat). QRS voltages may also be small.

Radiography: The heart is characteristically large and round, with no evidence of left atrial enlargement (Figure 13.3). The cardiac outline may be sharper than normal, although this may be obscured if there is any pleural effusion present. If a small effusion has developed acutely, the cardiac outline may not be very enlarged (Figure 13.4). Pneumopericardiography can be employed to image cardiac masses in the absence of echocardiography. The pericardial effusion is drained, and room air (or ideally, CO_2) is injected into the pericardial space as negative contrast to highlight any pericardial masses. Pneumopericardiograms can be difficult to interpret, and have been largely superseded by echocardiography.

Echocardiography: Pericardial effusions are readily

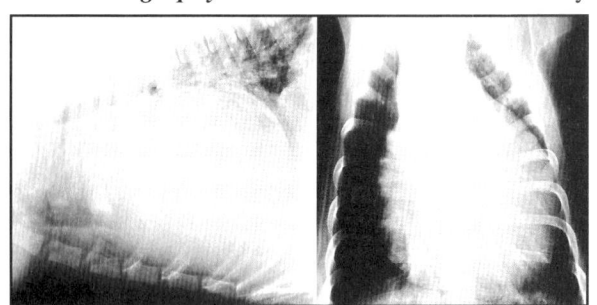

Figure 13.3: *Lateral and dorsoventral radiographs of a 2-year-old St Bernard with idiopathic haemorrhagic pericardial effusion, showing generalized cardiomegaly and a globose cardiac silhouette on both views.*

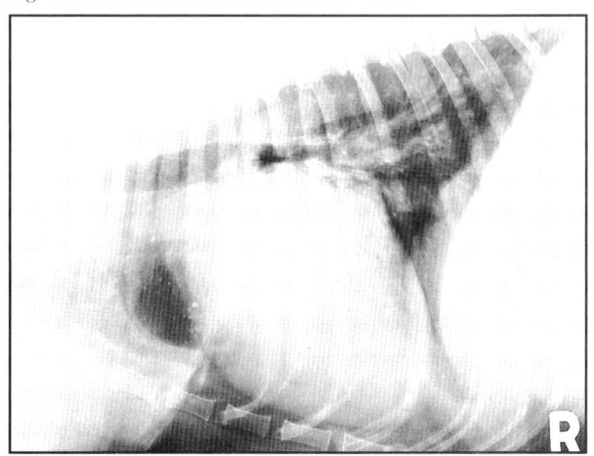

Figure 13.4: *Lateral radiograph of an 11-year-old Afghan Hound with a large chemodectoma. The dog presented with tamponade with a comparatively small volume of pericardial effusion.*

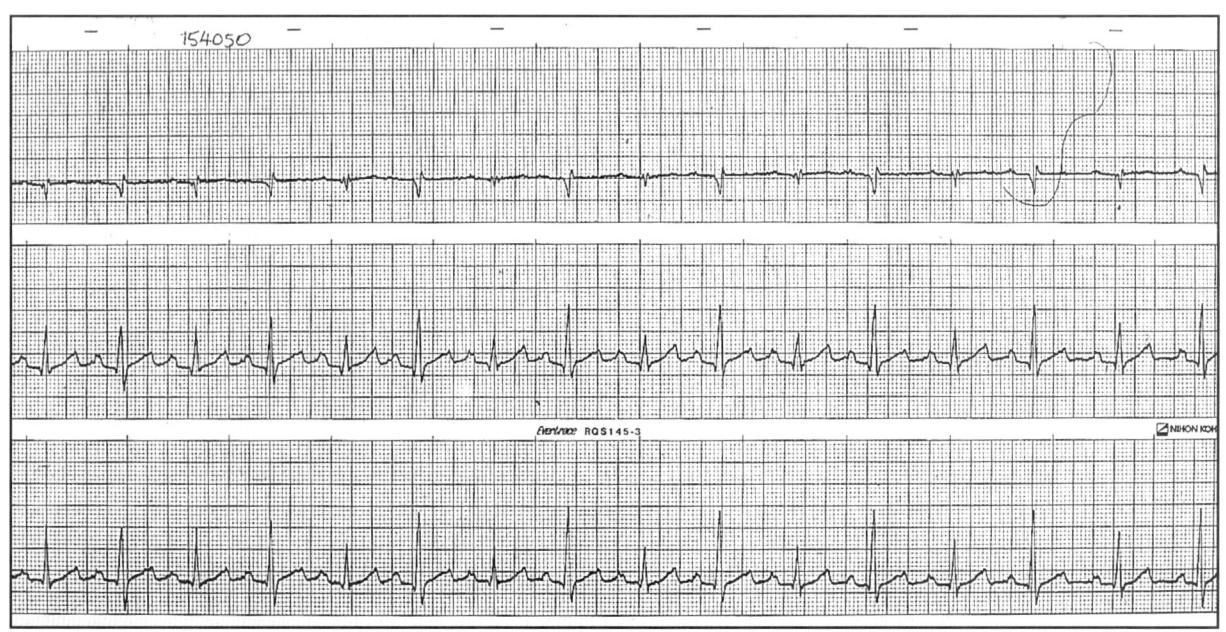

Figure 13.2: *Lead II electrocardiogram from a dog with a large pericardial effusion, showing alternating amplitude of the QRS complex (1 cm/mV, 50 mm/s).*

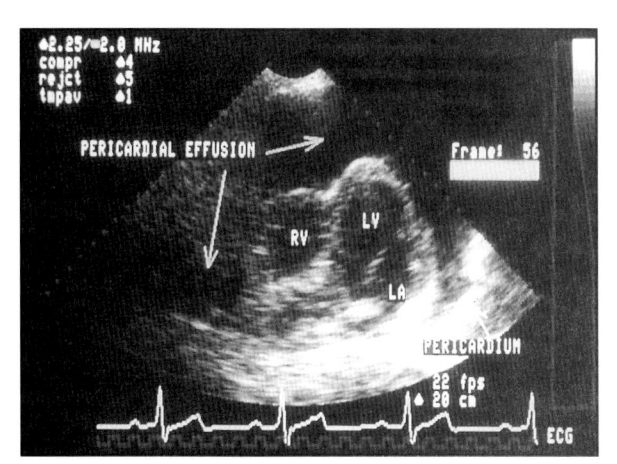

Figure 13.5: Two-dimensional echocardiogram of the St Bernard in Figure 13.3, showing a large pericardial effusion surrounding the heart. LA, left atrium; LV, left ventricle; RV, right ventricle.

confirmed with echocardiography as a hypoechoic space between the pericardium and heart (Figure 13.5). Collapse of the right atrium may be imaged, as well as a pendulum-like swinging of the heart within the pericardial space (responsible for electrical alternans). It is important to search carefully for signs of cardiac or pericardial masses, as this will have important implications for prognosis.

Magnetic resonance imaging (MRI): Although not widely available, excellent resolution of cardiac structures can be obtained with MRI. It is probably the most sensitive technique for the identification of cardiac tumours.

Fluid analysis: Samples of pericardial fluid should always be collected for analysis, including culture and sensitivity, packed cell volume estimation, and cytology. It can be extremely difficult to distinguish neoplastic from benign effusions, although it has been suggested that inflammatory effusions may have a lower pH (6.5 or less) compared with neoplastic or non-inflammatory effusions (pH around 7.5) (Edwards, 1996). It is unusual to obtain a diagnosis on cytology, with the possible exception of feline lymphoma.

Management
If there is any question of cardiac tamponade, then the effusion should be drained. Although diuretics are generally indicated for congestive heart failure, they are not advisable in pericardial effusions, as they reduce cardiac preload. They will therefore decrease filling of the right heart, and worsen any collapse of the right atrium, decreasing cardiac output further. Similarly, vasodilators may exacerbate any hypotension.

Drainage may be carried out without sedation or general anaesthesia, particularly if the animal is in a collapsed state. The details are covered in Chapter 29. After (and sometimes during) drainage, a rapid clinical improvement may be seen. Diuresis is often immedi-

ate, as the improvement in ventricular filling restores cardiac output and renal perfusion. The heart rate usually slows noticeably, and the QRS complexes may become larger. Occasionally with rapid drainage of large effusions, the sudden increase in left heart filling may result in pulmonary oedema (Shenoy *et al.*, 1984). This does not usually occur with large dogs, as it is difficult to drain the effusion quickly enough.

Although diuretics can be given after drainage to eliminate ascites, this is often unnecessary provided the pericardial effusion does not recur.

Subsequent management will depend on the underlying cause. Every effort should be made to check for the presence of tumours. If the pericardial effusion recurs, a second drainage can be attempted, although a recurrence would generally be an indication for surgical exploration and pericardiectomy.

Haemorrhagic effusions
Haemorrhagic effusions are most commonly idiopathic or neoplastic in origin.

Idiopathic pericardial haemorrhage
Idiopathic pericardial haemorrhage, also known as benign pericardial effusions or idiopathic sterile pericarditis, may result in variable volumes of haemorrhagic pericardial fluid (Gibbs *et al.*, 1982). The aetiology is unknown, although immune-mediated mechanisms and viral infections have been suggested as causes. The epicardium often shows marked thickening and inflammatory changes, although these may be secondary rather than causal. The condition is common, particularly in Golden Retrievers and St Bernards. There is no specific age or sex predisposition.

Diagnosis: It can be extremely difficult to distinguish idiopathic haemorrhagic effusions from neoplastic effusions, as mentioned above. Cytological examination often fails to distinguish between idiopathic and neoplastic effusions, although pH changes may provide an indication. Echocardiographic examination usually shows an otherwise normal heart apart from the effusion.

Management: The effusion must be drained (see Chapter 29). Idiopathic effusions may recur in over 50% of cases (Thomas, 1989), and it is advisable to explore the pericardium surgically if this happens. If no neoplasms are identified at an exploratory pericardotomy, then a subtotal pericardiectomy may be performed to allow any further effusion to drain directly into the chest. The subsequent prognosis is usually good, although some St Bernards may subsequently develop dilated cardiomyopathy.

Intrapericardial neoplasia
Tumours which can result in pericardial effusion include right atrial haemangiosarcoma, chemodectoma,

lymphoma, mesothelioma and metastatic carcinoma (Cobb and Brownlie, 1992).

Right atrial haemangiosarcoma

The right atrium is one of the more common sites for the development of haemangiosarcomas, and the typical pericardial effusion produced by these tumours is haemorrhagic. Metastasis to the lungs may be present by the time of diagnosis, and masses are often also present in the liver or spleen. German Shepherd Dogs (and Golden Retrievers) are particularly predisposed, and older dogs are more likely to be affected.

Diagnosis: Presenting signs are the same as with idiopathic effusions. The radiographic appearance is the same, although sometimes pulmonary metastases or splenic masses may also be visualized. Echocardiography may be helpful in identifying cardiac masses, and abdominal ultrasonography may detect concurrent splenic or hepatic masses. Cytology of pericardial fluid is usually unhelpful.

Management: Treatment is fairly hopeless. Drainage relieves signs of tamponade, but the effusion always recurs. Drainage holes produced by balloon dilatation of the pericardium may allow drainage via a less invasive technique than sub-total pericardectomy (Cobb *et al.*, 1996). Metastasis usually occurs within months of diagnosis.

Chemodectoma

Chemodectomas are also known as heart base tumours, paragangliomas or aortic body tumours. These are slow growing but invasive tumours which usually envelop the base of the aorta and pulmonary artery. They may be found as incidental findings, or may result in a serous or haemorrhagic pericardial effusion which can lead to cardiac tamponade. They tend to occur in older brachycephalic (or even crossbred) dogs.

Diagnosis: Again, the presenting signs in symptomatic dogs are the same as in other pericardial effusions. Sometimes a mass may be suspected from plain radiographs, where the trachea may be elevated over the cranial heart base. A chemodectoma may be suspected if an effusion is serous rather than haemorrhagic. Echocardiography will usually enable the mass to be visualized (Figure 13.6). Cytology is sometimes helpful.

Management: It is rarely possible to resect a chemodectoma completely, but a subtotal pericardiectomy will allow any effusion to drain directly into the chest, thereby relieving clinical signs. Animals thus treated may survive for over a year after diagnosis (Wykes *et al.*, 1986).

Left atrial rupture

This appears to be an uncommon cause of pericardial

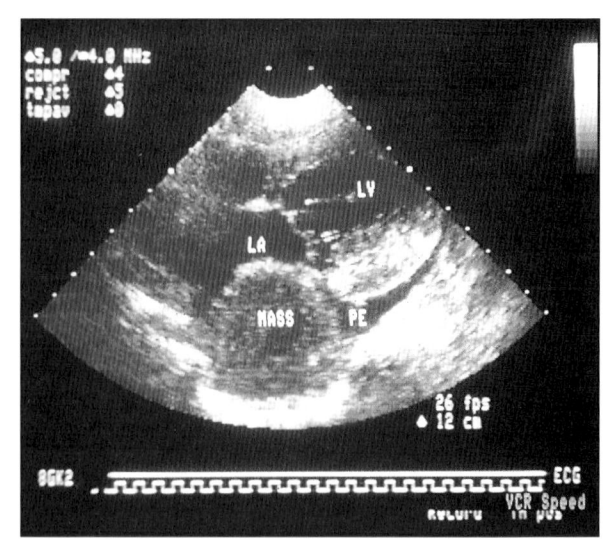

Figure 13.6: *Two-dimensional echocardiogram of the Afghan in Figure 13.4, showing a large chemodectoma (mass). LA, left atrium; LV, left ventricle; PE = pericardial effusion.*

haemorrhage, but is reported in small breed dogs with advanced mitral regurgitation (Buchanan, 1972). Jet lesions affecting the endocardium of the left atrium may eventually lead to splitting of the left atrial wall, resulting in a sudden dramatic bleed into the pericardium. The pericardial pressure rises abruptly. The prognosis is guarded. Similar effects may occur with other traumatic causes of cardiac rupture.

Pericardial transudates

Serous effusions may be found as an effect of right-sided heart failure. Pericardial effusions may also be seen in cats with feline infectious peritonitis (FIP); the specific gravity and protein content of the fluid are usually high. The type of effusion produced by chemodectomas and lymphomas is variable. Renal failure has been recorded as a cause of serous pericardial effusions, although it appears to be a very uncommon cause in small animals (Madewell and Norrdin, 1975).

Purulent pericardial effusions

These are also very uncommon, although they may develop from direct penetrating injuries, foreign bodies or haematogenous spread (Luis Fuentes *et al.*, 1991). In some cases of bacterial pericarditis, the effusion may be haemorrhagic, as with benign pericardial effusions or neoplastic causes. Effective drainage and aggressive antimicrobial therapy is indicated for septic pericarditis. Foreign bodies may be difficult to identify without surgical exploration, and pericardectomy is usually required.

Congenital abnormalities

Peritoneo–pericardial diaphragmatic hernia (PPDH)

This is a congenital anomaly where there is direct connection between the peritoneum and the pericardial space. Abdominal contents may herniate into the pericardium (see Chapter 14).

Pericardial defects: Congenital absence or partial absence of the pericardium is rare in small animals. It does not usually result in clinical signs, and is difficult to diagnose.

Pericardial cysts: Pericardial cysts are also uncommon, although they may result in signs of right heart failure. The cardiac silhouette may be abnormal on radiography, and diagnosis can be achieved with echocardiography or pneumopericardiography. Successful surgical excision has been reported (Sisson *et al.*, 1993).

Constrictive pericardial disease

Constrictive pericarditis is rare, but may be underdiagnosed. The pericardium adheres to the epicardium, or the visceral pericardium (epicardium) alone restricts filling of both ventricles. The result may be raised diastolic pressures in the atria and ventricles, which may all end up at the same pressure in mid- to end-diastole. The aetiology is unknown, but it is thought that constrictive pericardial disease may be a sequel to a variety of inflammatory pericardial conditions (Thomas *et al.*, 1984). Constrictive pericarditis is rare in dogs, and extremely rare in cats.

Diagnosis: Affected animals usually present with signs of right heart failure. Occasionally gallop sounds may be present, or heart sounds may be muffled. The heart may be slightly enlarged on radiography. ECG changes include small QRS complexes and prolonged P waves. Diagnosis is not straightforward. Intracardiac pressure recordings show an early diastolic fall in ventricular pressure followed by an abrupt rise and plateau in mid-diastole. Doppler echocardiography has proved helpful in human restrictive pericardial disease, but has not been reported in small animals.

Management

Pericardectomy will usually relieve clinical signs, although sometimes the visceral pericardium is also affected, increasing the technical difficulty and risk.

OTHER CAUSES OF RIGHT HEART FAILURE

Myocardial disease

Both primary and secondary myocardial diseases commonly result in biventricular failure or left heart failure. Isolated right heart failure is uncommon.

Dilated cardiomyopathy

Some dogs with dilated cardiomyopathy may have more dramatic signs of right heart failure than left heart failure (see Chapter 12), and cats with dilated cardiomyopathy (DCM) often have pleural effusions (see Chapter 19). Virtually all animals with DCM have concurrent left heart failure, although a form of right ventricular cardiomyopathy has been described (Simpson *et al.*, 1994).

Restrictive cardiomyopathy: Cats with restrictive cardiomyopathy often have signs of right and left heart failure, and both atria are usually dilated (see Chapter 19). Pleural effusion is more common than ascites.

Acquired valvular disease

Endocardiosis

Although endocardiosis affects both atrioventricular valves, it usually affects the mitral more severely than the tricuspid valve, and signs are predominantly those of left-sided heart failure. However, in advanced cases, ascites is relatively common. This may be because the tricuspid valve is also severely affected (and a precordial thrill will often be palpated over the right apex beat as well as on the left); or raised pulmonary capillary pressures may lead to raised pulmonary arterial pressures, pulmonary hypertension and right ventricular failure. It is not unusual for dyspnoea associated with pulmonary oedema to improve following the development of right heart failure, as the fall in right heart output reduces preload and left heart filling pressures. Nevertheless, the appearance of right heart failure is ominous, as it usually signals advanced disease.

Congenital conditions

Pulmonic stenosis may lead to right heart failure and ascites, or syncope may be the predominant sign.

Tricuspid dysplasia produces the same haemodynamic disturbances as tricuspid endocardiosis. Ascites may be very marked, although pleural effusions or even chylothorax may be present (see Chapter 14).

Arrhythmias

Signs of right-sided heart failure may be more obvious than signs of left heart failure in bradyarrhythmias and tachyarrhythmias. This may relate to neurohormonal activation and excessive retention of sodium and water.

Cor pulmonale

Respiratory disease can lead to pulmonary hypertension, which can in turn have cardiac effects, which is termed cor pulmonale. This is mediated by the same mechanism responsible for optimizing ventilation-perfusion ratios: pulmonary hypoxic vasoconstriction. Pulmonary arterioles will vasoconstrict in the presence of hypoxia, thus reducing perfusion of unventilated areas of lung. Chronic hypoxia can thereby lead to chronically raised pulmonary arterial pressures. Any effective loss of pulmonary vascular units will produce the same response. The heart responds as it would to any pressure overload, and the right ventricle becomes dilated and hypertrophied. In extreme cases, right heart failure may even follow (although this is unusual in dogs apart from heartworm disease). Cor pulmonale can also refer to the cardiac effects of pulmonary hypertension associated with pulmonary emboli; the cardiac effects tend to be more acute than with primary respiratory disease. Secondary intimal changes may occur in the pulmonary arterial vasculature irrespective of the primary cause of pulmonary hypertension (McFadden and Braunwald, 1992).

Clinical findings

The clinical presentation will depend on the cause. Acute pulmonary thromboembolism usually results in sudden onset dyspnoea, often with minimal radiographic changes. Conditions which might theoretically lead to chronic cor pulmonale include any conditions leading to alveolar hypoventilation. Conditions commonly associated with cor pulmonale in man (e.g. chronic bronchitis) may only rarely have similar effects in dogs, with the most severe changes being limited to right heart enlargement. Severe cor pulmonale and right heart failure may only be seen in dogs with severe heartworm disease. Physical findings include right-sided systolic murmurs of tricuspid regurgitation, and a split second heart sound. Ascites, jugular distension and hepatomegaly may be seen with advanced heartworm disease. Radiography may demonstrate right-sided enlargement, and the main pulmonary artery is usually dilated with widened and truncated peripheral pulmonary arteries.

Management must address the underlying cause. The use of vasodilators such as hydralazine and nifedipine has been reported for treatment of cor pulmonale in humans, but there can also be significant side-effects (McFadden and Braunwald, 1992).

Heartworm disease

The nematode *Dirofilaria immitis* is endemic in parts of southern Europe, the USA, Africa, Asia, Australia, and Japan. It may occasionally be encountered in the UK in imported dogs. A variety of mosquitoes may act as vectors, depending on the location.

Life cycle

Female mosquitoes ingest microfilariae (L1) from infected dogs. Within 3 weeks the microfilariae will develop into infective third-stage larvae, when they can be transmitted to dogs by a bite from the host mosquito. The L3 stage larvae migrate through the new canine host, developing into L4 stage larvae. By 100 days post-infection, the adult stage heartworms (L5) reach the vascular system. These adult worms congregate in the pulmonary arteries, and usually produce microfilariae 6 months after the original infection with

L3 larvae. The clinical effects relate to damage to the endothelial surface of the pulmonary arteries. Intimal proliferation, villous hypertrophy, thrombosis and obstruction by worms are all factors which can decrease the number of patent vascular units. This can increase hypoxic vasoconstriction and lead to pulmonary hypertension.

Dead worms can cause even more exaggerated responses, as well as marked inflammation in the surrounding lung parenchyma. Immune-mediated reactions may also result in allergic pneumonitis in occult infections. Thromboembolic disease and disseminated intravascular coagulation are possible complications.

Clinical effects

Small numbers of adult worms may cause occasional coughing, or no clinical signs at all. Thoracic radiographs show few (or no) pulmonary artery changes. Moderately affected dogs may cough more frequently or show exercise intolerance. Radiography will usually show enlargement of pulmonary lobar arteries. Severely affected dogs may be presented with ascites and signs of severe right heart failure. Exercise intolerance, syncope, weight loss and haemoptysis may all occur. Radiography shows marked lobar artery widening. Caval syndrome is a life-threatening complication of severe heartworm disease, where acute physical obstruction of the tricuspid valve occurs due to the presence of a tangled mass of worms.

Diagnosis

Microfilariae can be detected by direct blood smear, concentration tests (e.g. modified Knott's test), and serological tests. Radiography is useful for estimating the severity of disease. Echocardiography may demonstrate adult worms in the right ventricle and right atrium in very severe cases, as well as the indirect effects on the right heart.

Management

Dogs in endemic regions can be protected by prophylactic therapy with *diethylcarbamazine* or *ivermectin*. Treatment for animals positive for microfilariae previously relied on the adulticide *thiacetarsamide*. Thiacetarsamide may result in direct toxicity, and *melarsomine hydrochloride* is now the adulticide of choice (Knight, 1995). This is given as two deep intramuscular injections 24 hours apart (at 2.5 mg/kg for each dose). Animals with serious pulmonary artery disease have a high rate of complications, which can be reduced with *aspirin* and cage-rest. The prognosis for mildly affected animals is excellent, but poor for animals with severe clinical signs using standard therapy. Newer treatment regimes may offer higher survival rates. Corticosteroids may be indicated for inflammatory lung complications, and heparin is used in the prevention or treatment of pulmonary thromboembolism.

REFERENCES

Berg RJ and Wingfield W (1984) Pericardial effusion in the dog: a review of 42 cases. *Journal of the American Animal Hospital Association* **20**, 721-730

Buchanan JW (1972) Spontaneous left atrial rupture in dogs. *Advances in Experimental Medicine and Biology* **22**, 315-334

Cobb MA and Brownlie SE (1992) Intrapericardial neoplasia in 14 dogs. *Journal of Small Animal Practice* **33**, 309-316

Cobb MA, Boswood A, Griffin GM, and McEvoy FJ (1996) Percutaneous balloon pericardiotomy for the management of malignant pericardial effusion in two dogs. *Journal of Small Animal Practice* **37**, 549-551

Edwards NJ (1996) The diagnostic value of pericardial fluid pH determination. *Journal of the American Animal Hospital Association* **32**, 63-67

Gibbs C, Gaskell CJ, Darke PGG, and Wotton PR (1982) Idiopathic pericardial haemorrhage in dogs: a review of fourteen cases. *Journal of Small Animal Practice* **23**, 483-500

Knight DH (1995) Guidelines for diagnosis and management of heartworm (*Dirofilaria immitis*) infection. In: Kirk's *Current Veterinary Therapy. XII edn*, ed. JD Bonagura and RW Kirk, pp 879-887. WB Saunders, Philadelphia

Lehmkuhl LB, Bonagura JD, Biller, DS and Hartman, WM (1997) Radiographic evaluation of caudal vena-cava size in dogs. *Veterinary Radiology and Ultrasound* **38**, 94-100

Luis Fuentes V, Long KJ, Darke PGG and Burnie AG (1991) Purulent pericarditis in a puppy. *Journal of Small Animal Practice* **32**, 585-588

Madewell BR and Norrdin RW (1975) Renal failure associated with pericardial effusion in a dog. *Journal of the American Veterinary Medical Association* **167**, 1091-1093

McFadden ER and Braunwald E (1992) Cor pulmonale. In: *Heart Disease. A Textbook of Cardiovascular Medicine, 4th edn*, ed. E Braunwald, pp 1581-1601. WB Saunders, Philadelphia

Shenoy MM, Dhar S, Gittin R, Sinha AK and Sabado M (1984) Pulmonary edema following pericardiotomy for cardiac tamponade. *Chest* **86**, 647-648

Simpson KW, Bonagura JD and Eaton KA (1994) Right-ventricular cardiomyopathy in a dog. *Journal of Veterinary Internal Medicine* **8**, 306-309

Sisson D, Thomas WP, Reed J, Atkins CE and Gelberg HB (1993) Intrapericardial cysts in the dog. *Journal of Veterinary Internal Medicine* **7**, 364-369

Thomas WP (1989) Pericardial disorders. In: *Textbook of Veterinary Internal Medicine: Diseases of the Dog and Cat, 3rd edn*, ed. SJ Ettinger, pp 1132-1150. WB Saunders, Philadelphia

Thomas WP, Reed JR, Bauer TG and Breznock EM (1984) Constrictive pericardial disease in the dog. *Journal of the American Veterinary Medical Association* **184**, 546-553

Wykes PM, Rouse GP and Orton EC (1986) Removal of five canine cardiac tumors using a stapling instrument. *Veterinary Surgery* **15**, 103-106

Congenital Heart Disease

Joanna Dukes McEwan

INTRODUCTION

Careful and systematic auscultation is one of the most effective techniques for the detection of congenital heart disease. History and a thorough clinical examination will assist in formulating a differential diagnosis list (Table 14.1). The signalment, murmur characteristics, site of precordial impulse (left versus right sided), the presence of a precordial thrill, the colour of mucous membranes, the pulse quality and any signs of heart failure may all help in obtaining a sensible list of differentials. Radiographic assessment of the pulmonary circulation is also useful in refining the differential diagnosis list. A number of useful reviews on congenital heart disease are available (Bonagura, 1987, 1989; Fox, 1988; Matic, 1988; Olivier, 1988; Darke, 1989; Bonagura and Darke, 1995).

CONGENITAL CARDIOVASCULAR DEFECTS WITH NON-CARDIAC SIGNS

Vascular ring anomalies usually result in regurgitation of food immediately after eating, usually at the time of weaning on to solid foods (Figure 14.1). These pups

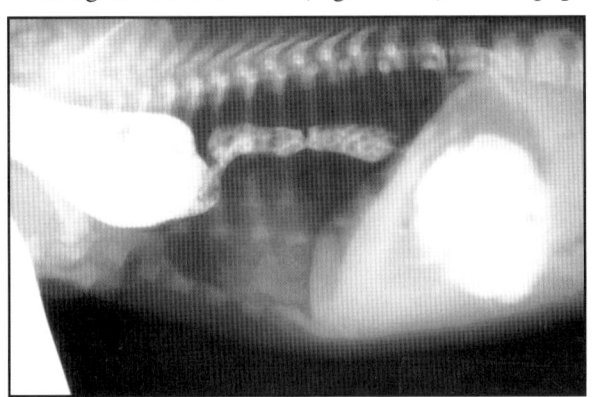

Figure 14.1: Lateral thoracic radiograph from a 6-week-old female Jack Russell Terrier with regurgitation of solid foods since weaning. Barium sulphate mixed with canned food was fed and the subsequent radiograph indicates megaoesophagus cranial to the heart base, with a relatively normal oesophagus coursing caudally from the heart to the stomach. A persistent right aortic arch was confirmed at thoracotomy with oesophageal entrapment between the heart base, the pulmonary trunk and the ligamentum arteriosum.

are usually markedly stunted compared with litter mates. A persistent right aortic arch is the most common cause, and surgical correction is possible (Eyster *et al.*, 1993).

Pericardial defects such as peritoneal–pericardial diaphragmatic hernias may result in gastrointestinal disturbance, without the presence of heart murmurs (see Chapter 18).

Some *vascular abnormalities* may result in other systemic signs without a heart murmur, such as portosystemic shunts with signs of hepatic encephalopathy.

Murmurs in puppies and kittens

After the detection of a heart murmur, further investigation will be required to confirm the diagnosis should the owner wish to take things further. Some owners will obviously opt to return the pup or kitten to the breeder, especially if a murmur is detected in a pre-purchase examination. It is important to obtain a definitive diagnosis in order to give a prognosis and discuss any therapeutic intervention.

Puppies and kittens may have *innocent flow murmurs* – these tend to be low grade (Ware, 1995), and usually disappear by 14–16 weeks of age (Bonagura, 1989). For the breeder, the possible inheritance of an identified congenital cardiac defect has to be considered. The findings for some of the common congenital cardiac defects are described below.

PATENT DUCTUS ARTERIOSUS (PDA)

Incidence

This condition is usually reported in the veterinary literature as being the most common congenital cardiac defect in the USA (Patterson, 1971). However, in some recent USA surveys (Buchanan, 1992), it appears that aortic stenosis has increased in prevalence. From the only nationwide UK survey of congenital heart disease in dogs, PDA appears to be less common than pulmonic stenosis and aortic stenosis; 20% of dogs diagnosed with congenital cardiac disease had PDA (Matic, 1993). PDA is the only congenital cardiac defect where there is a distinct sex predisposition

	Patent Ductus Arteriosus	Aortic Stenosis	Pulmonic Stenosis	Ventricular Septal Defect	Mitral Dysplasia	Tricuspid Dysplasia	Tetralogy of Fallot
PMI of murmur	Left base 2nd–3rd I/C space	Left base 3rd–4th I/C space	Left 3rd I/C space costochondral junction	Right 4th I/C space	Left 5th I/C space	Right 4th I/C space	Left 3rd I/C space, also right 4th I/C space
Radiation	Dorsally and to right side	To right side and thoracic inlet	Dorsally	Left 5th I/C space – typically a *diagonal murmur*	Left apex, to right side	To left side	Dorsally. Also to left apex
Timing of murmur	Systolic – diastolic continuous	Mid- or holo-systolic	Mid- or holo-systolic	Holo- or pan-systolic	Holo- or pan-systolic	Holo- or pan-systolic	Mid- or holo-systolic
Character of murmur	Waxing/Waning so-called *machinery murmur*	Crescendo–decrescendo (diamond shaped) ejection murmur	Crescendo–decrescendo (diamond shaped) ejection murmur	Plateau shaped or decrescendo murmur	Plateau shaped	Plateau shaped	Crescendo–decrescendo (diamond shaped) ejection murmur
Pulse quality	May be rapidly collapsing *(tapping or waterhammer pulse)*	May be weak and slowly rising	Normal	Usually normal. May be rapidly rising 'tapping'	Usually normal. May be 'tapping'	Normal	Usually normal
Mucous membrane colour	Pink	Pink	Pink	Pink	Pink	Pink	Cyanotic
Precordial impulse	Left	Left	Possibly right	Left	Left	Possibly right	Possibly right
Radiographic evidence of pulmonary overcirculation	*Yes*	*No*	*No (often apparent hypo-perfusion)*	*Yes if significant L–R shunting*	*No*	*No*	*No. Hypovascular lung fields*

Table 14.1: *Deriving a differential diagnosis from clinical examination.*

Abbreviations: *PMI = point of maximal intensity of heart murmur, I/C = intercostal, L–R = left to right*

for females (3:1), regardless of breed (Buchanan, 1992). An autosomal dominant mode of inheritance has been suggested (Patterson, 1968).

Predisposed breeds include Maltese, Pomeranians, Shetland Sheep Dogs, English Springer Spaniels, Bichon Frise, Poodles, Yorkshire Terriers, Collies and German Shepherd Dogs (Patterson, 1971; Buchanan, 1992). In the UK survey (Matic, 1993), German Shepherd Dogs, Border Collies and their crosses, and Cavalier King Charles Spaniels were predisposed. Cats also may have PDA, although it is not common in this species (Fox, 1988; Johnston and Eyster, 1995).

Pathophysiology

PDA is a condition where the normal ductus arteriosus of the fetus fails to close after birth (Noden and DeLahunta, 1985a). There is therefore a vascular connection between the descending aorta and the distal pulmonary trunk (Figure 14.2). As there is a pressure gradient between these two vessels throughout the cardiac cycle, blood will shunt from the aorta into the pulmonary artery (left to right) throughout systole and diastole. This results in overcirculation of the lung fields, and volume overloading of the left atrium and left ventricle. This may progress to left-sided heart failure. Secondary mitral incompetence sometimes develops as a result of the left ventricular dilation. In some cases of untreated long-standing PDA, myocardial failure occurs secondary to the chronic volume overload of the left ventricle. The left atrium may become very enlarged and allow the establishment of atrial fibrillation.

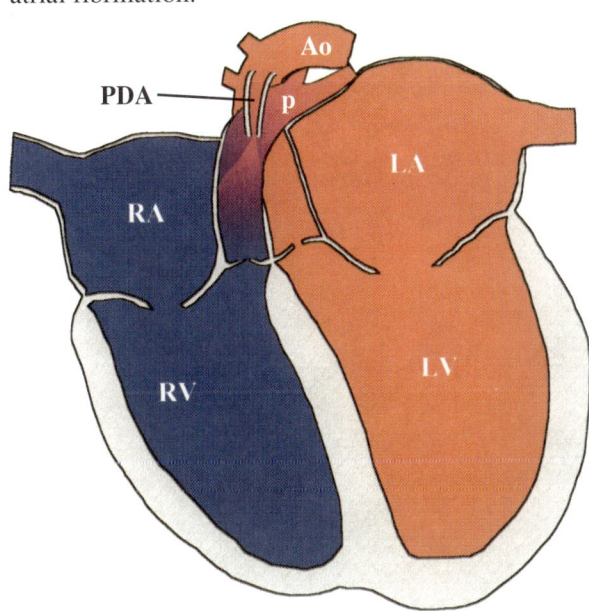

Figure 14.2: Schematic diagram of patent ductus arteriosus. The ductus remains as a vascular connection between the descending aorta and the distal pulmonary trunk. There is a continuous left-to-right shunt of blood throughout systole and diastole giving the characteristic waxing and waning continuous murmur. RA = right atrium; LA = left atrium; RV = right ventricle; LV = left ventricle; P = pulmonary trunk; Ao = aorta; PDA = patent ductus arteriosus.

Right-to-left shunting PDAs

The flow in PDA may sometimes shunt from right to left. This occurs when pulmonary hypertension is present. If the pulmonary artery pressure exceeds the aortic pressure, blood will flow from the pulmonary circulation to the systemic circulation. This-right-to left shunting results in de-oxygenated blood passing to the caudal parts of the body only, as the brachiocephalic trunk and left subclavian artery emanate from the ascending aorta, prior to the ductus. This can result in a differential cyanosis; the caudal mucous membranes of the vulva or prepuce should be checked if this is suspected.

Actual change from left-to-right to right-to-left shunting of the shunt is not well documented in the literature (Bonagura, 1989). It is more likely that the right-to-left shunting PDA is a separate form with associated pulmonary hypertension, perhaps secondary to prematurity or neonatal hypoxia with retained fetal vasculature (Eyster *et al.*, 1993). It must be emphasized that right-to-left shunting PDAs are very rare.

History

The murmur is usually detected at pre-vaccination veterinary examination. Some puppies are presented with left-sided heart failure with pulmonary oedema. Occasionally, observant owners will actually detect the precordial thrill themselves. In some animals, the murmurs may go undetected until adulthood, especially if puppies are only superficially auscultated.

Clinical examination

The murmur is heard with maximal intensity far forward at the left heart base, and may be very localized; this area must be carefully auscultated. It is a continuous murmur waxing in systole and waning through diastole; sometimes called a 'machinery' murmur. It is often very loud and associated with a precordial thrill. The systolic component may radiate extensively to the right base and the thoracic inlet, and a separate systolic murmur of mitral regurgitation may be detected further caudally. Because of the run-off of the systemic circulation through the ductus, the femoral pulse is often rapidly collapsing and appreciably *hyperkinetic*; a so-called 'water-hammer' pulse. Signs of left-sided heart failure may be detected with shortness of breath, coughing and adventitious respiratory sounds.

In the very rare right-to-left shunting PDA, as well as the caudal cyanosis, a soft systolic murmur may be detected or there may be no murmur.

Establishing the diagnosis

The murmur and clinical signs, especially in a bitch or predisposed breed, is almost pathognomonic of a PDA. However, it is wise to confirm the diagnosis prior to subjecting the patient to surgery to exclude other congenital defects, such as an aortico-pulmonary win-

Patent Ductus Arteriosus	
Radiography	• LA enlargement (2–3 o'clock) • LV enlargement • dilated pulmonic trunk on DV view (1–2 o'clock) • dilated descending aorta (12–1 o'clock) the 'ductus bump' (Figure 14.3) • pulmonary overcirculation • ± pulmonary oedema
Electrocardiography	• wide P waves (P mitrale) • tall R waves (> 3.0 mV in dogs) • various arrhythmias are possible – most commonly atrial fibrillation
2D and M-mode Echocardiography	• LA enlargement • LV dilation with eccentric left ventricular hypertrophy • dilated main pulmonary trunk • hyperkinetic LV initially, subsequent myocardial failure in long-standing cases with reduced fractional shortening (<29%) • ductus may be imaged with difficulty between main pulmonary arteries and descending aorta
Doppler Echocardiography	• diastolic turbulent flow in main pulmonary artery • continuous turbulent flow at bifurcation of pulmonary trunk and in descending aorta • ductus may be easily imaged with colour flow mapping • mitral regurgitation is common

Table 14.2: Ancillary investigations in PDA.

dow or persistent left cranial vena cava (Eyster, 1993). Table 14.2 gives the pertinent findings from ancillary investigations.

Management options

PDA can be cured surgically by double ligation of the ductus (see Chapter 27), and so it is important to recognize affected animals early before left-sided heart failure and irreversible myocardial damage result. Patients with right-to-left shunting PDAs are not candidates for surgery.

Most dogs will develop left-sided heart failure and myocardial failure before they reach middle age (Bonagura, 1989) (Figure 14.3). An experienced cardiothoracic surgeon operating on uncomplicated cases can achieve a high success rate and very low mortality (Buchanan, 1994). Some PDAs may close spontaneously, although this is not well documented in the literature.

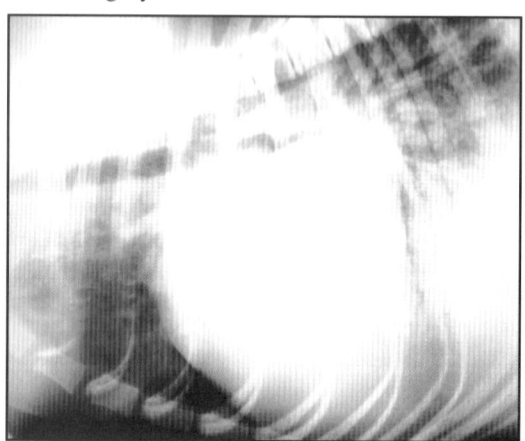 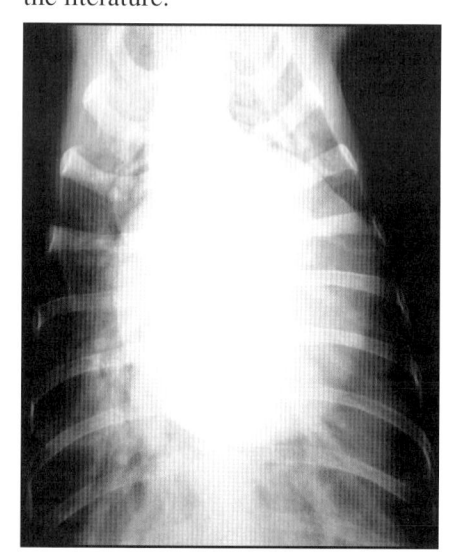

Figure 14.3: These radiographs were obtained from a mature German Shepherd Dog with patent ductus arteriosus and clinical signs of left-sided congestive heart failure. The lateral thoracic film shows marked left atrial and left ventricular enlargement. The lung fields appear hypervascular. Cranial lobar pulmonary arteries and veins are both enlarged, and pulmonary venous distension is most marked. There is a generalized mixed (interstitial and alveolar) pulmonary infiltration consistent with pulmonary oedema which is predominantly perihilar, although the alveolar infiltrate is well illustrated by the presence of air bronchograms in the cranial lobes. The dorsoventral thoracic film confirms the left atrial and left ventricular enlargement and the pulmonary changes described above. Additionally, the classical 'triple knuckle' is seen between 12 o'clock and 3 o'clock with a bulge on the descending aorta (12–1 o'clock), a pulmonary artery bulge (1–2 o'clock) and a left auricular appendage bulge (2–3 o'clock).

If there is heart failure at the time of presentation, it should be managed with *diuretics*, and *arteriodilators* or *angiotensin converting enzyme (ACE) inhibitors* to reduce the myocardial wall stress. Digoxin may be indicated with atrial fibrillation and myocardial failure. Surgery can be contemplated once the congestive signs are controlled, but is associated with increased risk compared with uncomplicated cases. Surgery in older dogs carries a higher risk, as the ductus and dilated pulmonary arteries are very friable.

Recently, less invasive techniques for occluding the ductus have been tried in dogs, such as transcatheter placement of intravascular coils (Snaps *et al.*, 1995).

AORTIC STENOSIS

Incidence

There appears to be a genuine increase in the prevalence of aortic stenosis, in both the USA and the UK. It is particularly prevalent in certain breeds, especially Boxers in the UK, and Golden Retrievers and Newfoundlands in North America (Buchanan, 1992; Kienle *et al.*, 1994). It is a condition with a broad spectrum of severity, from the severely incapacitated dog to the dog which is essentially normal and active, with a low grade murmur. It was the most commonly diagnosed congenital cardiac defect in the UK survey (Matic, 1993), with Boxers, Golden Retrievers and German Shepherd Dogs the most commonly affected breeds. Aortic stenosis was also reported as the most common congenital heart defect in Swedish dogs (Tidholm, 1997). An autosomal dominant mode of inheritance has been proposed in Newfoundlands (Patterson, 1968; Pyle *et al.*, 1976). In cats, a more uniform severity is recognized (Stepien and Bonagura, 1991).

Aortic stenosis may be valvular, subvalvular or more rarely, supravalvular. The commonest form in dogs is subvalvular (subaortic stenosis), where the lesions usually consist of fibrous bands (Levitt *et al.*, 1989). These may range from a complete circumferential band resulting in severe stenosis; to a small crescentic area in the left ventricular outflow tract, which may not cause any clinical problems. These mild lesions may be difficult to detect on two dimensional echocardiography. However, Doppler echocardiography demonstrates turbulent flow in the left ventricular outflow tract, with elevated blood flow velocities. The lesion may progress as the animal matures (Nakayama *et al.*, 1996).

A dynamic form of subaortic stenosis has also been described, perhaps similar to hypertrophic (obstructive) cardiomyopathy (Sisson, 1992; Buoscio *et al.*, 1994).

Aortic stenosis breed schemes

The British Boxer Breed Council operates a testing scheme for breeding Boxers, where RCVS Cardiology certificate and diploma holders auscultate Boxers over 12 months for the presence of a murmur. In Boxers, it is recommended that dogs with grade 2/6 or louder are not used for breeding unless passed by Doppler echocardiography (aortic velocity <2.0 m/s). The Newfoundland clubs in the UK also operate a heart testing scheme, although definite guidelines about breeding are not yet established.

Innocent 'flow' murmurs

The main differential diagnosis for low grade midsystolic murmurs over the left heart base are 'flow' murmurs. The innocent physiological murmurs occurring in puppies disappear by 20 weeks of age. The existence of 'innocent ejection murmurs' in adult dogs, such as those found in athletic horses, is controversial. Most low intensity 'ejection' murmurs appear to occur in breeds predisposed to aortic stenosis, and this is a grey area as far as breeding programmes are concerned.

Pathophysiology

The aortic stenosis lesion increases impedance to left ventricular ejection (Figure 14.4). The resultant increased afterload results in concentric myocardial hypertrophy (in proportion to the pressure overload and the degree of stenosis). Unfortunately, the coronary capillary vascular bed is unable to compensate for

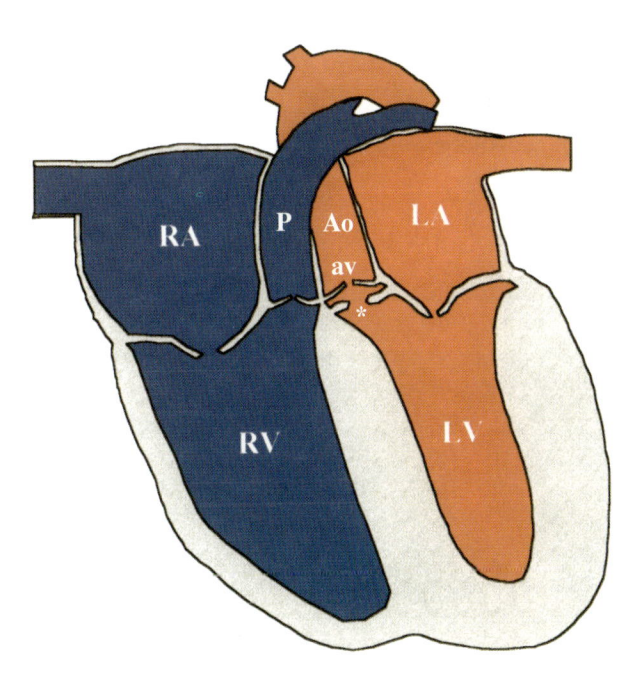

Figure 14.4: *Schematic diagram of aortic stenosis. This is usually in the form of a fibrous ring or crescent in the left ventricular outflow tract below the aortic valve (subaortic stenosis). This causes increased impedance to left ventricular ejection (increased afterload). A compensatory concentric left ventricular hypertrophy occurs to minimize left ventricular wall stress. RA = right atrium; LA = left atrium; RV = right ventricle; LV = left ventricle; P = pulmonary trunk; Ao = aorta; av = aortic valve; * = site of subvalvular ring in left ventricular outflow tract.*

the degree of hypertrophy. The increased systolic pressures also compromise coronary perfusion (particularly of the subendocardium), and the resulting myocardial ischaemia can lead to ventricular arrhythmias. Exertional syncope may result, although there is also a risk of sudden death in dogs with severe aortic stenosis. Myocardial failure and/or congestive cardiac failure are less common sequelae in long-standing cases of severe aortic stenosis (O'Grady *et al.*, 1989; Kienle *et al.*, 1994).

History

The murmur should be detectable at initial veterinary examination. Patients may be presented with a history of exercise intolerance, or syncope. Sometimes sudden death is the first indication of the problem, if the murmur has been missed.

Clinical examination

The classical signs of aortic stenosis are of a left-sided mid-systolic crescendo–decrescendo murmur at the left base, radiating to the right base and thoracic inlet. High grade murmurs are accompanied by a precordial thrill. The grade of the murmur usually correlates with the severity of the stenosis in fixed obstructions. The femoral pulse may be discernibly weak.

There is a spectrum of severity, and some dogs will have a very localized low grade mid-systolic murmur

Aortic Stenosis	
Radiography	• cardiac silhouette may be unremarkable • LV enlargement may be recognized • ± post-stenotic dilatation of ascending and descending aorta
Electrocardiography	• may be unremarkable • tall R waves • ± S-T segment depression indicating myocardial hypoxia • ± notched QRS complexes • ventricular ectopia due to myocardial hypoxia/ischaemia
2D and M-mode Echocardiography	• may find no abnormality in mild cases • concentric left ventricular hypertrophy • anatomical abnormalities of the LV outflow tract and aortic valve may be recognized – e.g. a fibrous ridge in the LV outflow tract (Figure 14.5a) • ± post-stenotic dilatation of ascending aorta
Doppler Echocardiography	• maximal aortic velocities > 2.0 m/s are arbitrarily defined as aortic stenosis • peak velocities (from different windows) are important in determining pressure gradient and prognosis – the subcostal view is usually more informative (Lehmkuhl and Bonagura, 1994) • turbulent high velocity aortic flow (Figure 14.5b) • aortic insufficiency is common

Table 14.3: Ancillary investigations in aortic stenosis.

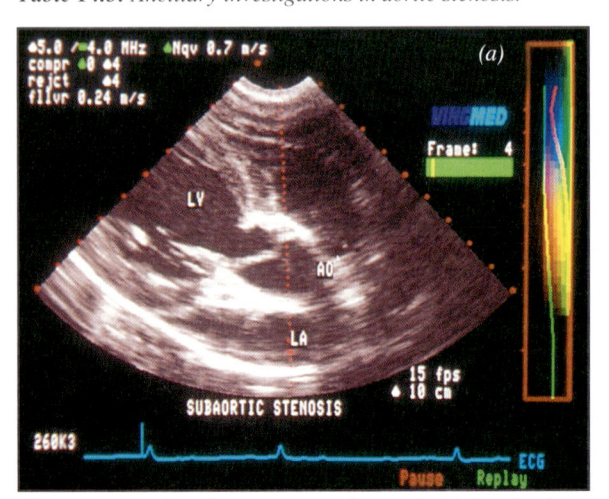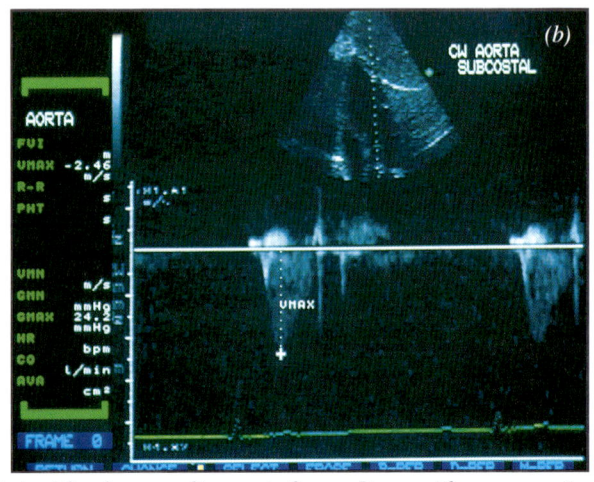

Figure 14.5: (a) Right parasternal long axis '5 chamber' view optimized for the ascending aorta from a Boxer with severe aortic stenosis. A distinct echogenic ridge is evident proximal to the aortic valves in the left ventricular outflow tract. LA = left atrium, LV = left ventricle, Ao = aorta. (b) Subcostal view of the heart optimized for the ascending aorta in a Newfoundland with mild aortic stenosis, with a spectral continuous wave (CW) aortic outflow Doppler trace. The peak velocity of 2.46 m/s is consistent with mild disease.
(a) Courtesy of Anne French.

audible far forward at the left base, without any radiation. This area may not be auscultated routinely and should be carefully examined, especially in puppies of predisposed breeds. This murmur is not distinguishable from innocent 'puppy murmurs' on auscultation, unless accompanied by a precordial thrill.

Establishing the diagnosis

Table 14.3 and Figure 14.5 give the pertinent findings from ancillary investigations.

Management options

The requirement for treatment will depend on the severity of the stenosis. This can be assessed by measuring the systolic pressure gradient across the stenosis; severe cases will usually have a pressure gradient in excess of 100 mmHg, whereas mild cases usually have a gradient of <50 mmHg. Mild cases do not require treatment; most severe cases are managed medically. Exertion should be avoided in severe cases. Patients with ventricular arrhythmias are controlled with *anti-arrhythmic drugs*. Patients with concentric left ventricular hypertrophy should be managed with *β-blockade* or *calcium channel antagonists*, to reduce myocardial oxygen consumption and help prevent myocardial ischaemia (Lehmkuhl and Bonagura, 1995). Calcium channel antagonists are coronary vasodilators, so may be more effective; although whether this is true in the setting of very high myocardial wall stress is debatable. Arterial vasodilators are contraindicated, as they will increase the pressure gradient across the aortic valve.

Surgical correction of various types has been described, but valvuloplasty has not been particularly effective in the long term (Eyster, 1993; Eyster *et al.*, 1993).

PULMONIC STENOSIS

Incidence

In a recent UK survey (Matic, 1993), pulmonic stenosis was overtaken in prevalence by aortic stenosis and PDA. The UK breeds reported were the Cocker Spaniel, Miniature Schnauzer and Boxer; in contrast with English Bulldogs, Mastiffs, Samoyeds and Miniature Schnauzers in the USA (Buchanan, 1992). An autosomal dominant mode of inheritance has been reported in Beagles (Patterson, 1968). It is not common in cats, although it is recognized in association with other congenital cardiac defects.

Pathophysiology

Pulmonic stenosis is a condition where there is a stenosis of the pulmonic valve (subvalvular and supravalvular lesions are also described) (Olivier, 1988). This causes a pressure overload of the right ventricle, and right ventricular hypertrophy results (Figure 14.6).

As patients get older, the right ventricular hypertrophy may cause infundibular narrowing of the right ventricular outflow tract to exacerbate the pressure gradient, sometimes with a dynamic component (Olivier, 1988). The higher the pressure gradient across the stenotic area, the worse the prognosis (Fingland *et al.*, 1986). Severe or long-standing cases may progress to right-sided heart failure.

History

The murmur is usually detected at primary veterinary examination. Affected animals may be asymptomatic, or be presented after syncopal episodes or with ascites.

Clinical examination

Classically, the murmur is left sided, cranial (third intercostal space) and ventral, radiating dorsally. The murmur is a typical mid-systolic ejection-type crescendo–decrescendo murmur (Figure 14.7). High grade murmurs may have precordial thrills palpable, and the murmur may radiate extensively. If there is significant right ventricular hypertrophy, the precordial impulse in thin deep-chested breeds may be more pronounced over the right hemithorax. Pulse quality is usually good.

If right-sided heart failure has developed, there may be distended jugulars, hepatomegaly and ascites, with positive hepatojugular reflux.

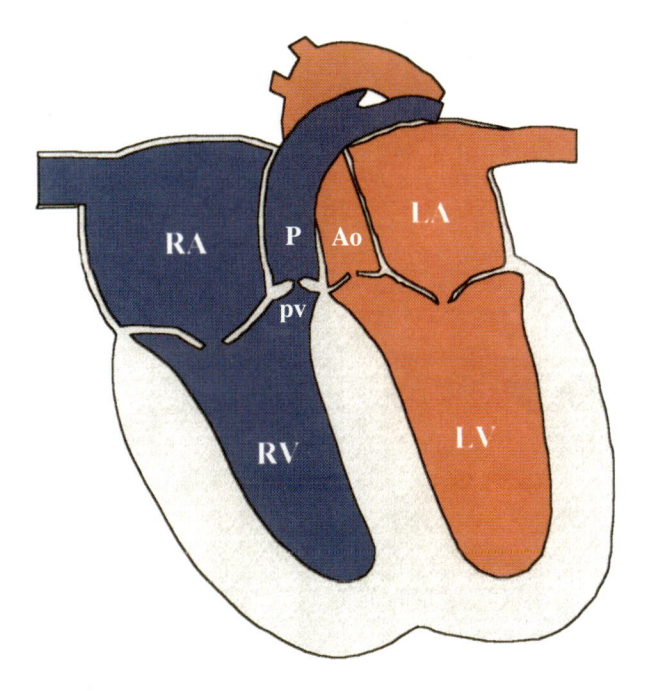

Figure 14.6: *Schematic diagram of pulmonic stenosis. There is increased afterload on the right ventricle due to the stenotic pulmonic valve. Secondary right ventricular hypertrophy occurs, which may cause further dynamic right ventricular outflow tract (infundibular) obstruction, exacerbating the pressure gradient across this area. RA = right atrium; LA = left atrium; RV = right ventricle; LV = left ventricle; P = pulmonary trunk; Ao = aorta; pv = pulmonic valve.*

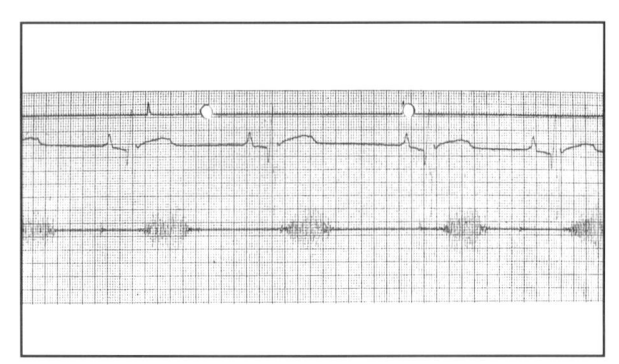

Figure 14.7: Simultaneous lead II ECG and phonocardiogram recorded from the ventral 3rd intercostal space from a patient with pulmonic stenosis. Mixed frequency recordings are obtained and timed against the ECG (top trace below second markers). The holosystolic murmur is crescendo–decrescendo or 'diamond shaped' as illustrated in the outline. Note also the deep S waves in the lead II ECG, indicative of right ventricular hypertrophy.

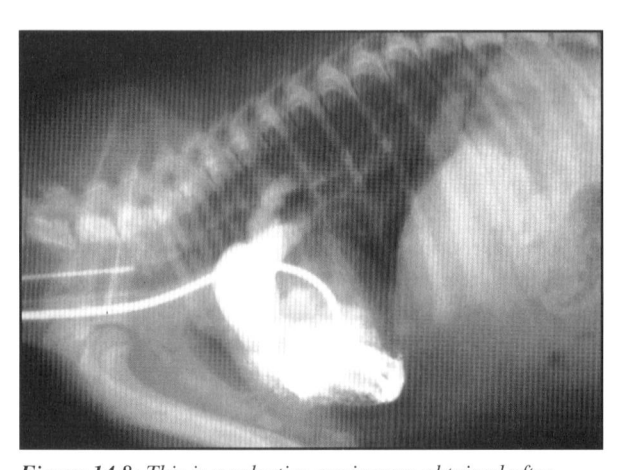

Figure 14.8: This is a selective angiogram obtained after right ventricular catheterization of an anaesthetized patient with pulmonic stenosis. Minimal contrast remains in the right ventricle, but the infundibulum and the stenotic pulmonic valve are outlined. There is massive post-stenotic dilatation of the pulmonary trunk and main pulmonary arteries – the resulting 'cap' overlying the trachea can also be visualized.

Establishing the diagnosis

Table 14.4 and Figures 14.7–14.10 give the pertinent findings from ancillary investigations.

Management options

Various surgical techniques have been described, from manually dilating the affected area, to *patch graft techniques* (Orton and Monnet, 1994) (see Chapter 27). The initial treatment of choice is *balloon valvuloplasty* (McIntosh Bright *et al.*, 1987; Brownlie *et al.*, 1991; Martin *et al.*, 1992; Thomas, 1995). This is minimally invasive, although repeat procedures may be required. Patients with pressure gradients of >50 mmHg and symptomatic patients are candidates for balloon valvuloplasty, although the best results are obtained in cases where the valve leaflets are fused. Surgical correction should be considered in cases where balloon valve dilatation has failed or there is severe infundibular hypertrophy (Bonagura, 1989).

VENTRICULAR SEPTAL DEFECT (VSD)

Incidence

Ventricular septal defect is not common in dogs, but is common in cats. In dogs in the USA, the Bulldog is most commonly reported as being affected (Buchanan, 1992). In the UK, West Highland White Terriers, and Cocker Spaniels were most commonly reported in the recent survey (Matic, 1993).

Pathophysiology

The lesion is usually in the high, membranous part of the interventricular septum (Figure 14.11). Because of the systolic pressure gradient between the left and right ventricles, left-to-right shunting of blood occurs through systole, although some degree of right-to-left shunting can occur with very large defects. Small defects offer

Pulmonic Stenosis	
Radiography	• RV enlargement (may cause apex tipping on the lateral view) • post-stenotic dilatation of the pulmonary trunk (may appear as a 'cap' overlying trachea on lateral view) • normal/underperfused pulmonary vasculature • may appear normal if mild lesion • angiography will confirm the diagnosis (Figure 14.8)
Electrocardiography	• deep S waves in leads I, II, III and a VF (Figure 14.7) • right axis deviation (> + 100° dogs or > 180° cats) in the frontal plane • ± ventricular ectopics (right ventricular origin)
2D and M-mode Echocardiography	• RV hypertrophy (Figure 14.9) • interventricular septum has flat or paradoxical motion (Figure 14.10) • abnormal pulmonic valve leaflets • ± post-stenotic dilatation of pulmonary trunk
Doppler Echocardiography	• high velocity and turbulent flow across the pulmonic valve • ± tricuspid regurgitation

Table 14.4: Ancillary investigations in pulmonic stenosis.

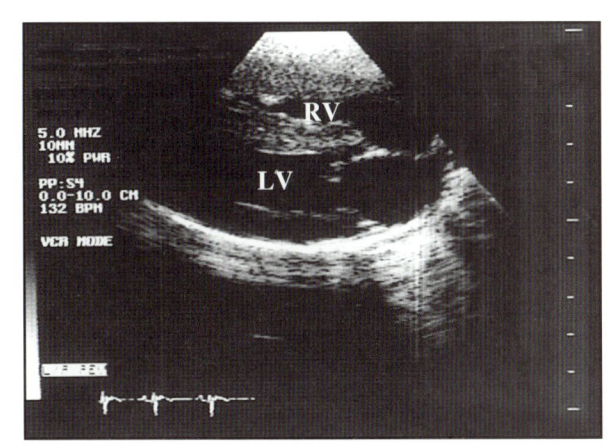

Figure 14.9: Two-dimensional echocardiogram. This is a right parasternal long axis four-chamber view obtained from a patient with pulmonic stenosis. The interventricular septum is thick and bulging into the left ventricle. The right ventricular freewall is also hypertrophied and imaged in the near field. RV = right ventricle; LV = left ventricle.

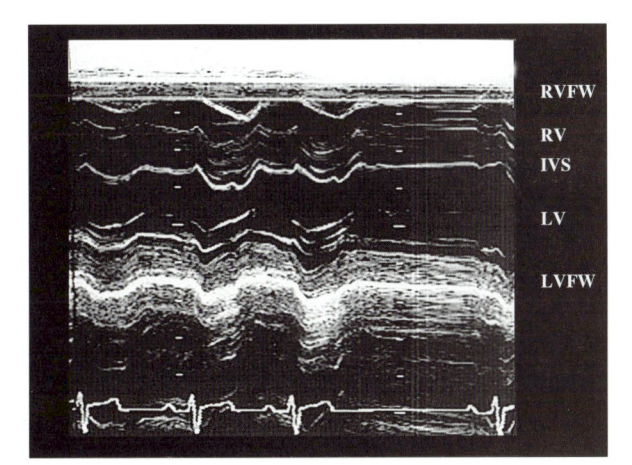

Figure 14.10: M-mode echocardiogram. This was obtained from the right parasternal position in a patient with pulmonic stenosis. The right ventricular freewall can be imaged and is hypertrophied. The interventricular septum is moving paradoxically – parallel with left ventricular freewall movement instead of oppositely. This is because right ventricular pressure exceeds left ventricular pressure. RVFW = right ventricular freewall; RV = right ventricle; IVS = interventricular septum; LV = left ventricle; LVFW = left ventricular freewall.

high resistance to left-to-right flow (high pressure gradients maintained between left and right ventricles); and loud murmurs are generated. These are called *restrictive VSDs*, and are unlikely to become haemodynamically significant (Olivier, 1988). Larger defects offer less resistance to the shunt; these are haemodynamically significant, and are associated with quieter murmurs.

With significant left-to-right shunting, right ventricular volume overload occurs with pulmonary overcirculation. Pulmonary venous blood returns to the left atrium and left ventricle, so these chambers are volume overloaded as well.

Various sequelae are described:

• Some VSDs may close spontaneously (Breznock, 1973)

• Left-sided heart failure may result from the left-sided volume overload
• Eisenmenger's physiology may develop, where chronic overcirculation of the pulmonary vasculature results in pulmonary hypertension. It is not clear if the increased pulmonary vascular resistance is reactive, or present from birth in dogs. Whatever the mechanism of pulmonary hypertension, the resulting increased right ventricular systolic pressures cause some right-to-left shunting, and cyanosis may become evident (Olivier, 1988; Bonagura, 1989; Eyster *et al.*, 1993). This syndrome is usually acquired before the age of 6 months (Bonagura and Darke, 1995).

History
A murmur is usually detected at primary vaccination. Stunting, signs of exercise intolerance or left-sided heart failure may occur.

Clinical examination
Typically, the murmur is louder on the right craniosternal hemithorax (as the blood shunts to the right side). The murmur is typically plateau-shaped and holosystolic, but may be decrescendo or blowing. The murmur is also heard on the left side, more caudally, giving a 'diagonal' murmur. The grade of the murmur is approximately inversely correlated with the size of the defect; louder murmurs, possibly with precordial

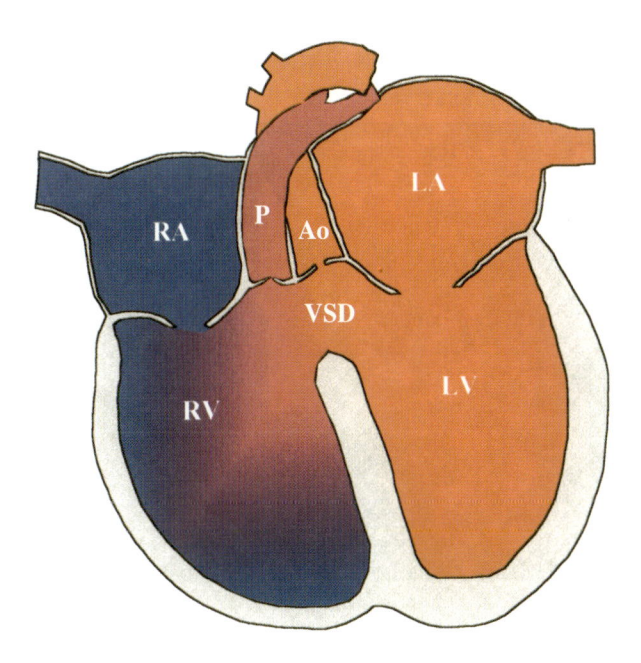

Figure 14.11: Schematic diagram of ventricular septal defect. There is a systolic pressure gradient between the left and right ventricles allowing left to right shunting across the defect. The right ventricle and pulmonary vasculature, left atrium and left ventricle are therefore volume overloaded. RA = right atrium; LA = left atrium; RV = right ventricle; LV = left ventricle; P = pulmonary trunk; Ao = aorta; VSD = ventricular septal defect.

Ventricular Septal Defect (VSD)	
Radiography	• LV enlargement • ± LA enlargement • RV enlargement • pulmonary overcirculation if significant L–R shunting
Electrocardiography	• may be unremarkable • tall R waves • ± wide P waves • deep Q waves I, II, II & a VF ± right axis deviation if pulmonary hypertension present
2D and M-mode Echocardiography	• LA enlargement • LV enlargement (eccentric hypertrophy) • RV dilation • hyperkinetic LV • may image VSD in membranous part of septum below aortic valve and septal leaflet of tricuspid valve in 5-chamber long axis view (Figure 14.12)
Doppler Echocardiography	• spectral or colour flow Doppler should be used to interrogate the RV side of the area described above • turbulent high velocity flow is identified • the velocity of blood flow across the VSD should be measured to assess the pressure gradient; the higher the velocity, the better the prognosis • mitral regurgitation is common • tricuspid regurgitation is not common but can be used to assess right ventricular pressures

Table 14.5: Ancillary investigations in ventricular septal defects.

thrills, are associated with smaller defects and a better prognosis. Where there is significant left-to-right shunting, a hyperkinetic pulse may be detected. A separate murmur of relative pulmonic stenosis may be detected, caused by increased blood flow across a normal pulmonic valve.

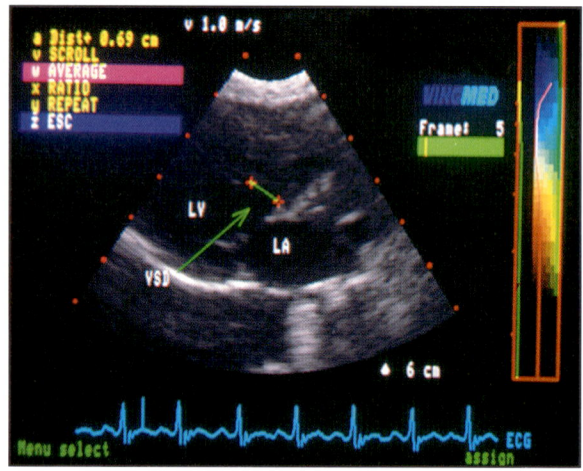

Figure 14.12: A right parasternal long axis view from a kitten with a large ventricular septal defect, which can be imaged and measured on the two-dimensional echocardiogram. LA = left atrium; LV = left ventricle; VSD = ventricular septal defect.
Courtesy of Virginia Luis Fuentes.

Establishing the diagnosis
Table 14.5 and Figure 14.12 give the typical results from ancillary investigations.

Management options
The only surgical technique suggested (without cardio-pulmonary bypass facility) is *pulmonary artery banding* (see Chapter 27). This technique is used palliatively to protect the pulmonary vascular bed.

If left-sided heart failure has developed, then restricted exercise and dietary sodium; *diuretics*, and *ACE inhibitors* are indicated. If significant right-to-left shunting and polycythaemia are present, then phlebotomy may be required. Many cases of uncomplicated VSD are small restrictive defects which need no special management or treatment.

MITRAL DYSPLASIA

Incidence
The atrioventricular valve dysplasias appear to be becoming more common in dogs. Mitral dysplasia is the most common congenital defect in cats (Liu, 1977). In the UK it is reported in Bull Terriers, German Shepherd Dogs, Cavalier King Charles Spaniels and Springer Spaniels (Matic, 1993). In the literature, Bull Terriers, Great Danes and German Shepherd Dogs are reported (Buchanan, 1992).

Pathophysiology
The defect is usually associated with mitral incompetence. Mitral regurgitation results in volume overloading of the left atrium and left ventricle, as in acquired

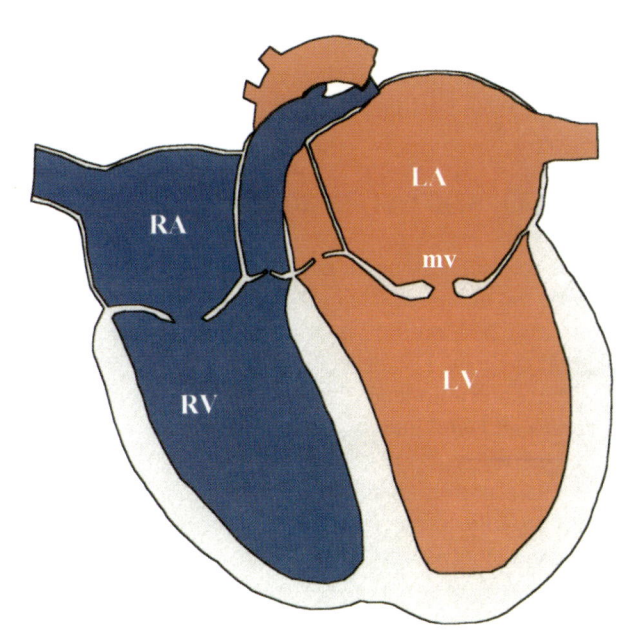

Figure 14.13: Schematic diagram of mitral dysplasia. The dysplastic changes affecting the mitral valve may also affect the papillary muscles and the chordae tendinae and typically result in mitral incompetence. Mitral regurgitation causes left atrial and left ventricular volume overload. RA = right atrium; RV = right ventricle; LA = left atrium; LV = left ventricle; mv = mitral valve.

mitral valve disease. Left-sided heart failure usually results. Occasionally (especially in Bull Terriers) the dysplastic mitral valve apparatus is also stenotic, and enormous left atrial enlargement is recognized (Lehmkuhl *et al.*, 1994; Dukes McEwan, 1995) (Figure 14.13). There is some suggestion that cats and some dogs may 'out-grow' the lesion (Hamlin and Harris, 1969).

History
A systolic murmur should be recognized at primary veterinary examination. Coughing (dogs only), dys-

pnoea and exercise intolerance may be the presenting signs reported by the owner.

Clinical examination
The murmur is typically most intense over the mitral valve area, and can be holo- or pansystolic. It may be of variable grade and radiate extensively if loud (Table 14.1). The murmur does not correlate well with the severity of the lesion. Atrial fibrillation, other supraventricular arrhythmias, sinus tachycardia and adventitious respiratory sounds may be identified if the patient is in left-sided heart failure.

Establishing the diagnosis
Table 14.6 and Figures 14.14 and 14.15 give the typical results from ancillary investigations.

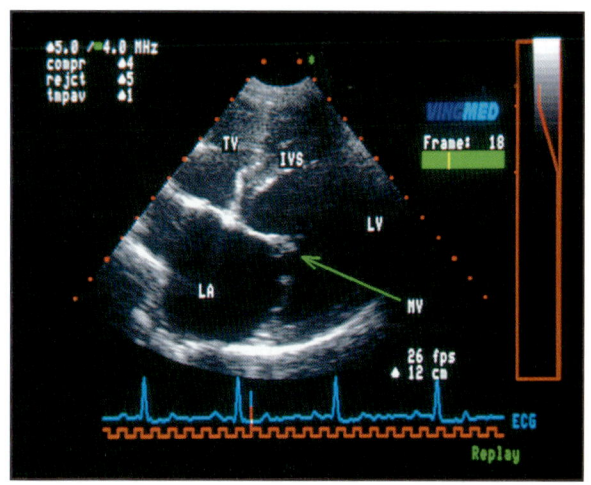

Figure 14.14: Right parasternal long axis 4-chamber view of a heart from a Bull Terrier with mitral dysplasia. The thickened mitral valve leaflets can be appreciated with the 'hooked' appearance of the anterior leaflet typical of mitral stenosis. LA = left atrium, LV = left ventricle, MV = mitral valve, IVS = interventricular septum, TV = tricuspid valve.
Courtesy of Dr P. G. G. Darke.

Mitral Dysplasia	
Radiography	• LA enlargement • LV enlargement • pulmonary venous congestion and pulmonary oedema if left-sided heart failure
Electrocardiography	• ± wide P waves • ± tall R waves • ± arrhythmias such as atrial fibrillation
2D and M-mode Echocardiography	• LA enlargement • LV dilation • dysplastic mitral valve apparatus may be recognized, e.g. thick mitral valve leaflets, short chordae tendineae, large papillary muscles (Figures 14.14 and 14.15) • abnormal M-mode mitral valve motion may be appreciated if mitral stenosis present
Doppler Echocardiography	• mitral regurgitation • increased velocity mitral inflow • ± abnormal mitral inflow spectral signal with mitral stenosis (rare)

Table 14.6: Ancillary investigations in mitral dysplasia.

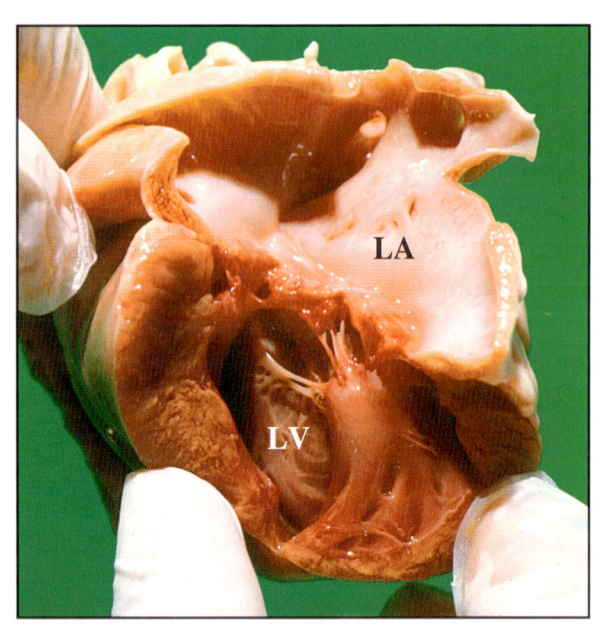

Figure 14.15: Heart from a Bull Terrier puppy euthanased due to lethal acrodermatitis. The dog had concurrent mitral dysplasia with both stenosis and incompetence of the mitral valve demonstrated by Doppler echocardiography. The mitral valve is thickened, the papillary muscles are large with short thick chordae tendineae and enormous left atrial enlargement is apparent. LA = left atrium; LV = left ventricle.
Courtesy of Dr H. Thompson.

Management options

The condition is managed as for acquired mitral regurgitation associated with endocardiosis, with diuretics and ACE inhibitors. Vasodilators are contraindicated if there is any mitral stenosis.

TRICUSPID DYSPLASIA

This has been reported in the literature in Labrador Retrievers, Weimaraners and other large breeds of dog (Moise, 1995). It is a fairly common congenital defect in cats (Liu, 1977). The condition is associated with tricuspid incompetence and may progress to right-sided heart failure (Figures 14.16 and 14.17). Ebstein's

anomaly is a form where the tricuspid valve is malpositioned in the right ventricle (Eyster *et al.*, 1993). Tables 14.1 and 14.7 list the typical findings.

ATRIAL SEPTAL DEFECT (ASD)

These are uncommon in cats and dogs, and isolated defects are not usually haemodynamically significant. They may be identified in association with other congenital defects. The defects are classified depending on the embryological development of the septum (Noden and DeLahunta, 1985b). Because the pressures between the two atria are similar (effectively there is a common atrium), no murmur is heard. Shunting is usually left to right, and a murmur of relative pulmonic stenosis may be detected.

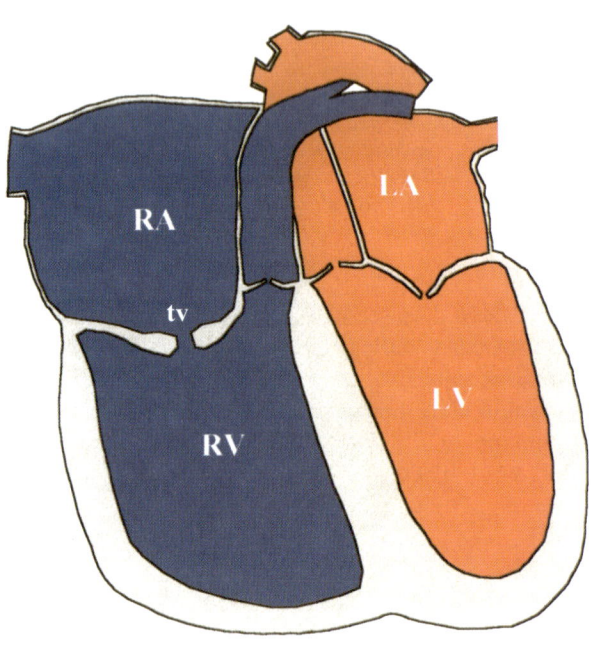

Figure 14.16: Schematic diagram of tricuspid dysplasia. The abnormal tricuspid valves are incompetent and tricuspid regurgitation results in volume overload of the right atrium and right ventricle. RA = right atrium, RV = right ventricle, LA = left atrium, LV = left ventricle, tv = tricuspid valve.

Tricuspid Dysplasia	
Radiography	• RA enlargement • RV enlargement
Electrocardiography	• ± tall P waves • deep Q waves in I, II, III & aVF ± right axis deviation • ± supraventricular arrhythmias
2D and M-mode Echocardiography	• RA enlargement • RV dilation • ± abnormal appearance of tricuspid valve apparatus (Figure 14.17)
Doppler Echocardiography	• tricuspid regurgitation

Table 14.7: Ancillary investigations in tricuspid dysplasia.

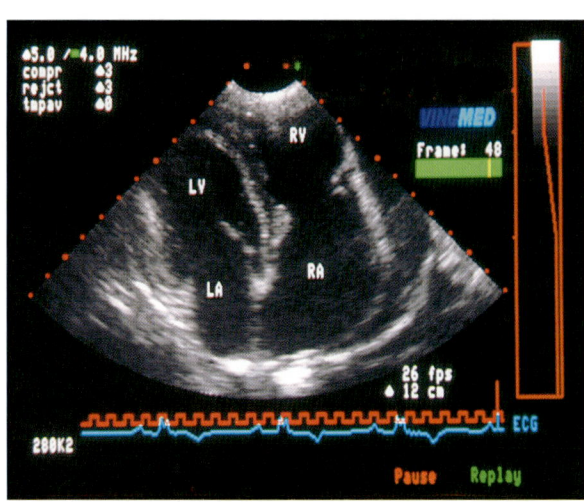

Figure 14.17: *Left apical four-chamber 2D echocardiogram of a Labrador Retriever with tricuspid dysplasia, showing dilated right chambers and abnormal tricuspid leaflets. RA = right atrium; LA = left atrium; RV = right ventricle; LV = left ventricle*

Courtesy of Virginia Luis Fuentes.

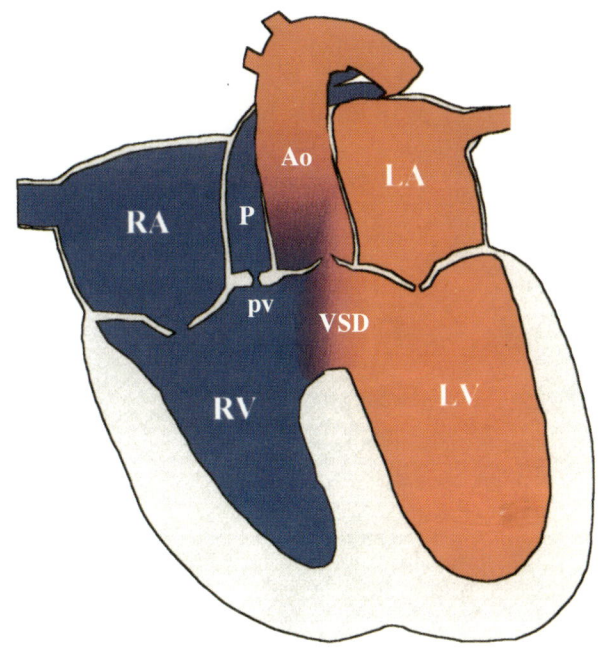

Figure 14.18: *Schematic drawing of tetralogy of Fallot. This consists of right ventricular outflow obstruction with a secondary right ventricular hypertrophy. There is also a subaortic ventricular septal defect which is usually large and a dextraposed (over-riding) aorta. Right-to-left flow through the VSD results in desaturated blood entering the aorta and cyanosis, hypoxia and polycythaemia. RA = right atrium; LA = left atrium; RV = right ventricle; LV = left ventricle; P = pulmonary trunk; Ao = aorta; pv = pulmonic valve; VSD = ventricular septal defect.*

TETRALOGY OF FALLOT

This is the most common of the cyanotic congenital defects. It is not common in small animals. Pulmonic stenosis, overriding aorta and ventricular septal defect are present, due to abnormal development of the conotruncal system (Noden and DeLahunta, 1985b). Right ventricular hypertrophy is secondary to the pulmonic stenosis, often with a hypoplastic pulmonary trunk. Patients are usually presented by owners with stunting, cyanosis and severe exercise intolerance. It is most commonly reported in the literature in Golden Retrievers, Wire Haired Fox Terriers, Labrador Retrievers, Siberian Husky and Toy Poodle (Ringwald and Bonagura, 1988; Buchanan, 1992). The Keeshond has been shown to have an autosomal dominant mode of inheritance with variable penetrance (Patterson, 1968). Typical findings are detailed in Tables 14.1 and 14.8 and Figures 14.18 and 14.19.

ENDOCARDIAL CUSHION DEFECT (PERSISTENT COMMON ATRIOVENTRICULAR CANAL)

This is a common cause of cyanotic congenital heart disease in cats (Fox, 1988). It is an embryological developmental defect of endocardial cushions resulting in a low atrial septal defect, a high ventricular septal defect, and atrioventricular valvular abnormalities (Noden and DeLahunta, 1985b; Eyster, 1993).

Tetralogy of Fallot	
Radiography	• RV enlargement • hypovascular lung fields
Electrocardiography	• deep S waves in I, II, III & aVF • right axis deviation
2D and M-mode Echocardiography	• RV hypertrophy • Flat interventricular septum or paradoxical septal motion • ventricular septal defect imaged if large enough • over-riding aorta (overlying VSD) (Figure 14.19) • pulmonary trunk often hypoplastic – can be difficult to locate
Doppler Echocardiography	• pulmonic stenosis – high velocity and turbulent pulmonic flow • ventricular septal defect – low velocity flow shunting right to left

Table 14.8: *Ancillary investigations in tetralogy of Fallot.*

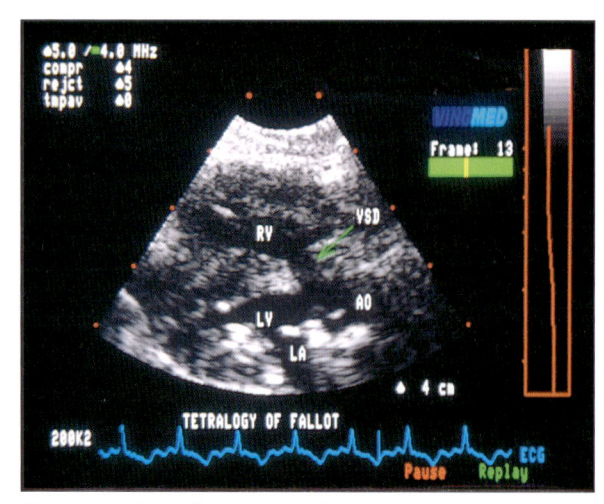

Figure 14.19: *Right parasternal long axis 2D echocardiogram of a 6-year-old cat with tetralogy of Fallot, showing right ventricular hypertrophy, a large ventricular septal defect and an over-riding aorta. AO = aorta; LA = left atrium; RV = right ventricle; LV = left ventricle; VSD = ventricular septal defect.*

Courtesy of Virginia Luis Fuentes.

Endocardial fibroelastosis

This condition occurs in cats (Liu, 1977; Fox, 1988) and dogs (Lombard and Buergelt, 1984). A familial incidence is recognized in Burmese cats (Fox, 1988). It is a post-mortem diagnosis but may be suspected in patients with myocardial failure. It appears to be very uncommon.

REFERENCES

Bonagura JD (1987) Congenital heart disease. Chapter 1. In: *Contemporary Issues in Small Animal Practice. No. 7. Cardiology*, p. 1. Churchill Livingstone, New York

Bonagura JD (1989) Congenital heart disease. Chapter 74. In: *Textbook of Veterinary Internal Medicine. 3rd edn*, ed. SJ Ettinger, p. 976. WB Saunders, Philadelphia

Bonagura JD and Darke PGG (1995) Congenital heart disease. Chapter 93. In: *Textbook of Veterinary Internal Medicine, 4th edn*, ed. SJ Ettinger and EC Feldman, p. 892. WB Saunders, Philadelphia

Breznock EM (1973) Spontaneous closure of ventricular septal defects in the dog. *Journal of the American Veterinary Medical Association* **162**, 399

Brownlie SE, Cobb MA, Chamber J, Jackson G and Thomas S (1991) Percutaneous balloon valvuloplasty in four dogs with pulmonic stenosis. *Journal of Small Animal Practice* **32**, 165

Buchanan JW (1992) Causes and prevalence of cardiovascular disease. In: *Kirk's Current Veterinary Therapy*, ed. RW Kirk and JD Bonagura, p. 647. WB Saunders, Philadelphia

Buchanan JW (1994) Patent ductus arteriosus. *Seminars in Veterinary Medicine and Surgery. (Small Animal)* **9**, 168

Buoscio DA, Sisson D, Zachary JF and Luethy M (1994) Clinical and pathologic characterization of an unusual form of subvalvular aortic stenosis in four Golden Retriever puppies. *Journal of the American Animal Hospital Association* **30**, 100

Darke PGG (1989) Congenital heart disease in dogs and cats. *Journal of Small Animal Practice* **30**, 599

Dukes McEwan J (1995) Mitral dysplasia in Bull Terriers. *The Veterinary Annual* **35**, 130

Eyster GE (1993) Basic cardiac surgical procedures. Chapter 60. In: *Textbook of Small Animal Surgery, 2nd edn*, ed. D Slatter, p. 893. WB Saunders, Philadelphia

Eyster GE, Gaber CE and Probst M (1993) Cardiac disorders. Chapter 58. In: *Textbook of Small Animal Surgery, 2nd edn*, ed. D Slatter, p. 856. WB Saunders, Philadelphia

Fingland RB, Bonagura JD and Myer CW (1986) Pulmonic stenosis in the dog: 29 cases (1975-1984). *Journal of the American Veterinary Medical Association* **189**, 218

Fox PR (1988) Congenital feline heart disease. In: *Canine and Feline Cardiology*, ed. PR Fox, p. 391. Churchill Livingstone, New York

Hamlin RL and Harris SG (1969) Mitral incompetence in Great Dane pups. *Journal of the American Veterinary Medical Association* **154**, 790

Johnston SA and Eyster GE (1995) Patent ductus arteriosus. In: *Kirk's Current Veterinary Therapy XII. Small Animal Practice*, ed. JD Bonagura, p. 830. WB Saunders, Philadelphia

Kienle RD, Thomas WP and Pion PD (1994) The natural clinical history of canine congenital subaortic stenosis. *Journal of Veterinary Internal Medicine* **8**, 423

Lehmkuhl LB and Bonagura JD (1994) Comparison of transducer placement sites for Doppler echocardiography in dogs with subaortic stenosis. *American Journal of Veterinary Research* **55**, 192

Lehmkuhl LB and Bonagura JD (1995) CVT update: canine subvalvular aortic stenosis. In: *Kirk's Current Veterinary Therapy XII. Small Animal Practice*, ed. JD Bonagura, p. 822. WB Saunders, Philadelphia

Lehmkuhl LB, Ware WA and Bonagura JD (1994) Mitral stenosis in 15 dogs. *Journal of Veterinary Internal Medicine* **8**, 2

Levitt L, Fowler JD and Schuh JCL (1989) Aortic stenosis in the dog: a review of 12 cases. *Journal of the American Animal Hospital Association* **25**, 357

Liu SK (1977) Pathology of feline heart diseases. *Veterinary Clinics of North America. Small Animal Practice* **7**, 341

Lombard CW and Buergelt CD (1984) Endocardial fibroelastosis in four dogs. *Journal of the American Animal Hospital Association* **20**, 271

McIntosh Bright J, Jennings J, Toal R and Hood ME (1987) Percutaneous balloon valvuloplasty for treatment of pulmonic stenosis in a dog. *Journal of the American Veterinary Medical Association* **191**, 995

Martin MWS, Godman M, Luis Fuentes V, Clutton RE, Haigh A and Darke PGG (1992) Assessment of balloon pulmonary valvuloplasty in six dogs. *Journal of Small Animal Practice* **33**, 443

Matic SE (1988) Congenital heart disease in the dog. *Journal of Small Animal Practice* **29**, 743

Matic SE (1993) Survey of congenital heart disease in dogs. Paper given from accumulated data of the Veterinary Cardiovascular Society. *Veterinary Cardiovascular Society Meeting*, April 1st

Moise NS (1995) Tricuspid valve dysplasia in the dog. In: *Kirk's Current Veterinary Therapy XII. Small Animal Practice*, ed. JD Bonagura, p. 813. WB Saunders, Philadelphia

Nakayama T, Wakao Y, Ishikawa R and Takahashi M (1996) Progression of aortic stenosis detected by continuous wave Doppler echocardiography in a dog. *Journal of Veterinary Internal Medicine* **10**, 97

Noden DM and DeLahunta A (1985a) Cardiovascular system I. Blood and arteries. Chapter 11. In: *The Embryology of Domestic Animals: Developmental Mechanisms and Malformations*, p. 211. Williams & Wilkins, Baltimore

Noden DM and DeLahunta A (1985b) Cardiovascular system II. Heart. Chapter 12. In: *The Embryology of Domestic Animals: Developmental Mechanisms and Malformations*, p. 231. Williams & Wilkins, Baltimore

O'Grady MR, Holmberg DL, Miller CW and Cockshutt JR (1989) Canine congenital aortic stenosis: a review of the literature and commentary. *Canadian Veterinary Journal* **30**, 811

Olivier NB (1988) Congenital heart disease in dogs. In: *Canine and Feline Cardiology*, ed. PR Fox, p. 357. Churchill Livingstone, New York

Orton EC and Monnet E (1994) Pulmonic stenosis and subvalvular aortic stenosis: surgical options. *Seminars in Veterinary Medicine and Surgery (Small Animal)* **9**, 221

Patterson DF (1968) Epidemiologic and genetic studies of congenital heart disease in the dog. *Circulation Research* **23**, 171

Patterson DF (1971) Canine congenital heart disease. Epidemiology and etiological hypothesis. *Journal of Small Animal Practice* **12**, 263

Pyle RL, Patterson DF and Chacko S (1976) The genetics and pathology of discrete subaortic stenosis in the Newfoundland dog. *American Heart Journal* **92**, 324

Ringwald RJ and Bonagura JD (1988) Tetralogy of Fallot in the dog. Clinical findings in 13 cases. *Journal of the American Animal Hospital Association* **24**, 33

Sisson D (1992) Fixed and dynamic subvalvular aortic stenosis in dogs. In: *Kirk's Current Veterinary Therapy XI. Small Animal Practice*, ed. RW Kirk and JD Bonagura, p. 760. WB Saunders, Philadelphia

Snaps FR, McEntee K, Saunders JH and Dondelinger RF (1995) Treatment of patent ductus arteriosus by placement of intravascular coils in a pup. *Journal of the American Veterinary Medical Association* **207**, 724

Stepien RL and Bonagura JD (1991) Aortic stenosis: clinical findings in six cats. *Journal of Small Animal Practice* **32**, 341

Thomas WP (1995) Therapy of congenital pulmonic stenosis. In: *Kirk's Current Veterinary Therapy XII. Small Animal Practice*, ed. JD

Bonagura, p. 817. WB Saunders, Philadelphia

Tidholm A (1997) Retrospective study of congenital heart defects in 151 dogs. *Journal of Small Animal Practice* **38**, 94

Ware WA (1995) Abnormal heart sounds and heart murmurs. Chapter 17. In: *Textbook of Veterinary Internal Medicine, 4th edn*, ed. SJ Ettinger and EC Feldman, p. 86. WB Saunders, Philadelphia

Laryngeal Disorders

Richard A.S. White

FUNCTIONAL ANATOMY OF THE LARYNX

Anatomical structure

The larynx is a semirigid fibroelastic cylinder separating the upper and lower respiratory tracts, the structural basis of which are three major and two smaller hyaline cartilages (Figure 15.1). The larger cartilages include the spoon-shaped epiglottis positioned most rostrally, behind which are found the horseshoe-shaped thyroid cartilage and the circular cricoid cartilage. The thyroid and cricoid cartilages occupy fixed positions relative to each other by virtue of their firm attachment at the cricothyroid articulation although the thyroid is capable of some limited movement in a rostrodorsal plane. This 'chassis' provides the rigid base necessary for movement of the other cartilages. The epiglottis hinges in a rostrocaudal plane about its base which is in contact with the thyroid cartilage. The smaller, paired arytenoid cartilages articulate with the cricoid cartilages on their medial aspect and are capable of a swinging lateromedial movement about the crico-arytenoid articulations. Interposed between the arytenoids and lying rostral to the lamina of the cricoid are the interarytenoid and the sesamoidean cartilages, which bind the arytenoids to the dorsal aspect of the cricoid. The larynx is supported rostrally by its attachment to the hyoid apparatus – the thyrohyoid membrane and caudally by its attachment to the trachea (Evans and Christensen, 1979).

Two paired ligaments are found within the lumen of the laryngeal cylinder – the vocal ligaments which extend from the vocal processes of the arytenoids to the ventral midline and the vestibular ligaments which extend from the cuneiform process to the ventral midline (Figure 15.2). The larynx is lined with a stratified mucosa, folds of which protrude into the lumen of the cylinder over these ligaments – these are, respectively, the vocal and vestibular folds. The resultant crypts formed between the two folds are the laryngeal ventricles. The ventricles are absent in feline species. The diamond-shaped opening within the laryngeal lumen, delineated by the arytenoids dorsally and the vocal folds ventrally, is termed the rima glottidis (Figure 15.3) and is the narrowest point separating the upper and lower airways. The diameter of the rima is determined by the position and length of the vocal folds which in turn are dependent on the position of the arytenoid cartilages and to a lesser extent on that of the thyroid cartilage. Dorsolateral movement of the arytenoids about their cricoid articulation pulls the vocal folds apart thereby widening the rima (Figure 15.4). Medial movement reduces the diamond-shape of the rima to a slit-like opening or completely closes it. Cranial to the rima is the wider opening of the larynx, the aditus laryngis, which is delineated by the corniculate processes of the arytenoids, the epiglottis and the ary-epiglottic folds.

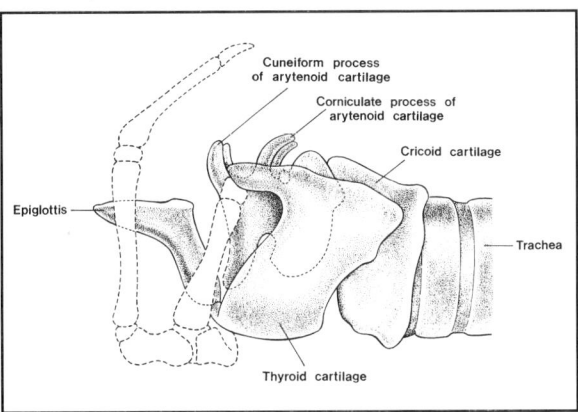

Figure 15.1: Diagrammatic representation of the cartilages of the canine larynx. © RAS White.

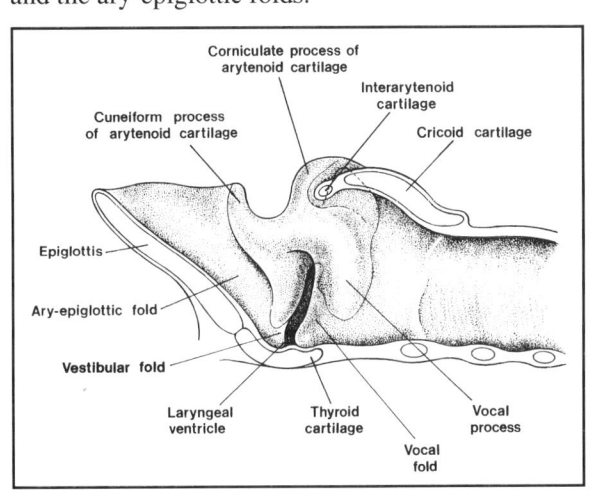

Figure 15.2: Diagrammatic representation of the sagittal view of the canine larynx. © RAS White.

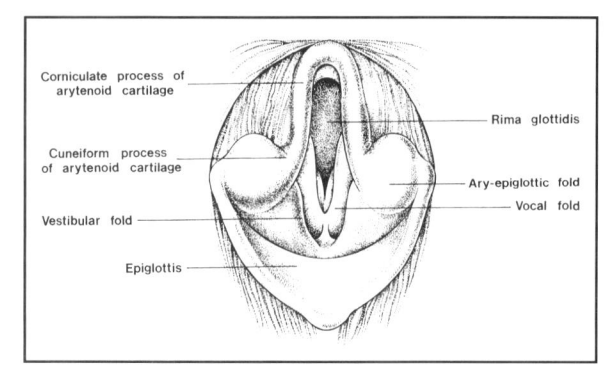

Figure 15.3: *Oral view of the canine larynx.* © *RAS White.*

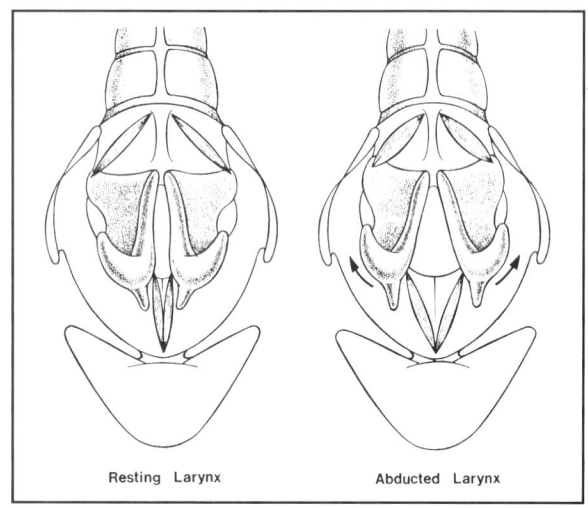

Figure 15.4: *Schematic representation of glottic function during resting and inspiratory (abducted) phases of respiration.*

Redrawn from Wykes PM (1983) Canine laryngeal diseases. I. Anatomy and disease syndromes. Compendium on Continuing Education for the Practicing Veterinarian 5, 8–15, with permission.

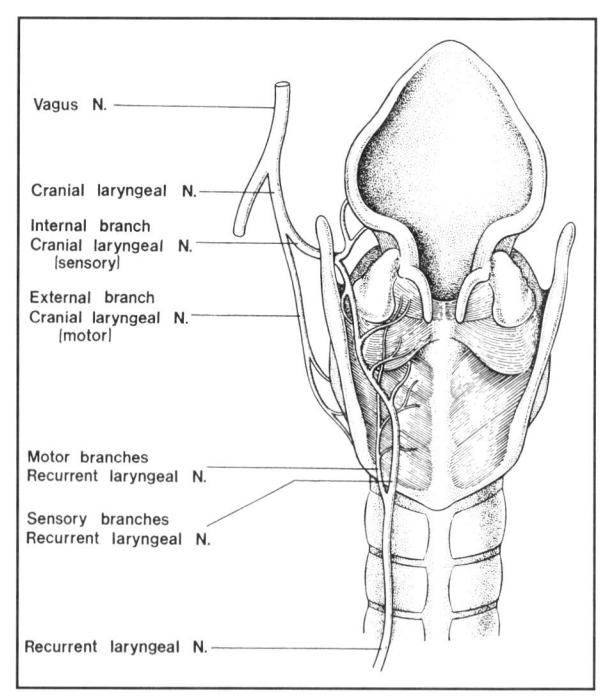

Figure 15.5: *Innervation of the canine larynx.*

Redrawn from Wykes PM (1983) Canine laryngeal diseases. I. Anatomy and disease syndromes. Compendium on Continuing Education for the Practicing Veterinarian 5, 8–15, with permission.

The larynx has both extrinsic and intrinsic muscles. The extrinsic muscles function in concert with the hyoid apparatus to vary the position and angle of the larynx. The intrinsic muscles of the larynx are responsible for controlling glottic diameter and can be broadly divided into the constrictors and dilators, depending on their primary function. They contain type I and II fibres providing both rapid and sustained contractile function (Braund *et al.*, 1988). The majority of the intrinsic muscles are associated with glottic constriction (adduction) of the rima and include the cricothyroid, lateral cricoarytenoid, transverse arytenoid ventricular and thyroarytenoid muscles. The latter of these is the most important in terms of constricting function. Only the dorsal cricoarytenoid muscle is concerned purely with dilation (abduction) of the rima. This muscle originates on the dorsal aspect of the cricoid cartilage and inserts on the muscular process of the arytenoid. Its contraction rotates the arytenoid laterally over the articulation with the cricoid (Figure 15.4).

The larynx is innervated by the vagus via the cranial and caudal laryngeal nerves (Figure 15.5). The cranial laryngeal nerves are concerned primarily with sensory function and provide innervation to the mucosal lining of the larynx via their internal branches. The sole exception to the sensory function of the external branches is the motor innervation to the cricothyroid muscles. The caudal (recurrent) laryngeal nerves arise from the vagal branches at the thoracic inlet, the right looping behind the subclavian artery and the left behind the aorta before heading rostrally to the lateral surface of the larynx. They provide motor innervation to all the intrinsic muscles of the larynx with the exception of the cricothyroid muscle.

The vascular supply of the larynx originates from the external carotid artery via the cranial laryngeal artery. The cranial laryngeal vein drains to the external maxillary vein.

LARYNGEAL FUNCTION

The larynx performs a valve-like role at the junction of the upper and lower respiratory tracts and its major functions can be summarized as:

- Protection of the lower respiratory tract from inhalation of debris
- Control of airway diameter during the respiratory cycle
- Phonation.

Airway protection

Prevention of aspiration is the result of a two-fold reflex mechanism. Firstly, during the swallowing phase the epiglottis hinges about its base and is 'flipped' backwards over the aditus to direct the food upwards and over the larynx into the lateral food channels, thereby preventing aspiration. The epiglottis provides a tight seal at the level of the ary-epiglottic fold and the whole process occurs in conjunction with rostral movement of the larynx and caudal movement of the tongue. Secondly, glottic protection is also provided by the intrinsic muscles of the larynx which adduct the vocal folds and arytenoid cartilages sealing off the rima tightly during swallowing. This may also occur in response to stimulation of the cranial laryngeal nerves by any food or liquid debris passing beyond the aditus.

Control of airway diameter

During the resting phase of the respiratory cycle, the arytenoids and vocal folds lie in a passive or 'neutral' midline position such that the rima is a narrow slit (Figure 15.4). Contraction of the dorsal cricoarytenoid muscles during inspiration causes the arytenoids to rotate quickly in a dorsolateral direction, dilating the rima to accommodate the inward flow of air. On expiration, the vocal folds move passively towards the midline slowing the outward air flow. During prolonged or heavy exercise, the rima may remain dilated during both the inspiratory and expiratory phases to minimize resistance to continued air flow.

Phonation

Barking or meowing is a glottic function and is the result of vibration of the vocal folds as air flows over them. The tone and pitch of the bark or meow are determined by the speed and amplitude of the vibrations which in turn are governed by air-flow rate and the length of the vocal cords. Vocal fold characteristics are governed primarily by tone in the vocalis and cricothyroid muscles.

DISEASES OF THE LARYNX

Laryngeal paralysis

Pathophysiology

Laryngeal paralysis is the failure of arytenoid movement during the respiratory cycle. The absence of abducting function affecting one or both arytenoids during the inspiratory phase with consequent narrowing of the rima results in an increased resistance to air flow through the larynx (Amis *et al.*, 1986). Air flow becomes turbulent due both to the increased resistance which necessitates a higher flow rate through the rima and to the movement of air over the fixed vocal fold(s). The concomitant reduction in intralaryngeal pressure may narrow the rima still further contributing to additional air flow resistance. This airway obstructive condition is encountered with some frequency in dogs (Cook, 1964; O'Brien *et al.*, 1973; Venker-van Haagen *et al.*, 1978; Lane, 1982; Gaber *et al.*, 1985; LaHue, 1989; White, 1989; Ross *et al.*, 1991) and is occasionally seen in cats (Schaer *et al.*, 1979; Hardie *et al.*, 1981; White *et al.*, 1986; White, 1994).

Aetiology

Paralysis of the vocal folds through failure of arytenoid function most often results from disease or damage to the innervation of the intrinsic muscles of the larynx. Much less frequently it may occur through disease involving the dorsal cricoarytenoid muscles themselves.

Idiopathic laryngeal paralysis (ILP): By far the majority of dogs with laryngeal paralysis fall into this category. ILP has a marked predisposition for medium to large breeds which in the UK includes such breeds as Labrador Retrievers, Afghan Hounds, Irish Setters, Pointers and some giant dogs (Lane, 1982; White, 1989). The male is affected two or three times more frequently than the female and the average age of the affected dog is usually greater than 10 years (Lane, 1982; Gaber *et al.*, 1985; Greenfield, 1987; LaHue, 1989; White 1989). The underlying cause of ILP still remains unclear. The suggestion that the condition may arise more frequently in hypothyroid dogs remains largely unsubstantiated (Harvey *et al.*, 1983; Gaber *et al.*, 1985; LaHue, 1989; White, 1989). The condition has also been reported as part of a laryngeal paralysis–polyneuropathy (LPP) complex in which affected dogs manifest signs of a generalized neuropathy, including motor deficits involving the rear limbs (O'Brien *et al.*, 1973; Gaber *et al.*, 1985; Dyer *et al.*, 1986; LaHue, 1989; Burbidge *et al.*, 1993). Demyelination and remyelination and also axonal degeneration involving the intrinsic laryngeal and appendicular peripheral nerves have been recorded in these dogs (O'Brien *et al.*, 1973; Gaber *et al.*, 1985).

Congenital: Laryngeal paralysis has been reported as an inherited congenital disease in the Bouvier des Flandres and the Siberian Husky (Venker-van Haagen *et al.*, 1978; Venker-van Haagen, 1980; Venker-van Haagen *et al.*, 1981; O'Brien and Hendriks, 1986a,b). The disease is transmitted as an autosomally dominant trait in the Bouvier (Venker-van Haagen *et al.*, 1981), affecting the male more frequently, and may be unilateral or bilateral. Degenerative changes are found both peripherally in the laryngeal nerves and centrally in the nucleus ambiguus. Selective breeding has now significantly reduced the incidence of this condition in Europe. More recently, a LPP complex has been recorded in the Dalmatian affecting dogs under the age of 6 months and presenting as a diffuse, generalized polyneuropathy distinct from that found in the Bouvier and Husky (Braund *et al.*, 1989; Braund *et al.*, 1994). Electromyographic abnormalities are present in laryngeal, facial, oesophageal and distal appendicular muscles and axonal degeneration is found affecting the laryngeal and appendicular nerves. A significant number of these dogs also have megaoesophagus. Most dogs with inherited laryngeal paralysis are presented as young pups and are rarely suitable for treatment.

Traumatic: Injuries to the neck or cranial thorax may bruise, or even sever the laryngeal innervation. Pharyngo-oesophageal trauma and 'big dog/little dog' confrontations resulting in crush injuries to the cervical region are probably the most important causes in this respect (White and Lane, 1988; Salisbury *et al.*, 1990).

Neoplastic: Tumour infiltration of the caudal laryngeal nerve may disrupt normal conduction function (Obradovich *et al.*, 1992). Amongst the more common tumours causing this presentation are malignancies of the thyroid gland and cranial mediastinal masses such as lymphomas and thymomas. Lymphomatous infiltration of the laryngeal nerve has also been recorded in the cat (Schaer *et al.*, 1979).

Iatrogenic: Any surgical intervention in the cervical region or rostral thorax which involves dissection of the caudal laryngeal nerves may result in their temporary dysfunction through neuropraxia or, more seriously, in permanent paralysis. Although many surgeries may potentially result in this complication the most notable procedure in this category is reconstruction of the trachea which necessitates separation of the nerves from their tracheal course and may give rise to this complication (White, 1989).

Cats: The aetiology of laryngeal paralysis in the cat is unknown, although it has been recorded as part of a generalized neuropathy (Hardie *et al.*, 1981; White *et al.*, 1986).

Clinical presentation

ILP typically has a prolonged and insidious onset and the clinical signs associated with it may predate presentation by months or even years. *Inspiratory stridor* is the major and consistent finding in all patients and results from the accelerated, turbulent air flow over the fixed vocal fold(s) (O'Brien *et al.*, 1973; Lane, 1982; White, 1989).

Exercise intolerance occurs frequently, although this sign is less obvious in some dogs which appear to tailor their exercise function to the reduction in their respiratory capacity (O'Brien *et al.*, 1973; Lane, 1982; Wykes, 1983; Greenfield, 1987; White, 1989). Severe cases will exhibit degrees of cyanosis and syncope, possibly progressing to asphyxiation. These signs are frequently exacerbated by a warm environment and although dogs may present at any time of the year many are presented during the summer months. Excitement, car travel, anxiety and stress also tend to promote the signs.

Dysphonia, or change in the character of the bark, is a very useful diagnostic pointer but is only found in approximately half of dogs with ILP (O'Brien *et al.*, 1973; Lane, 1982; White, 1989). *Dysphagia* or *cough* whilst eating or drinking is occasionally encountered, although *aspiration* leading to lower respiratory tract infection and coughing is probably less common than has previously been suggested (Greenfield, 1987; Greenfield and Dye, 1993). The symptoms of some patients may be exacerbated or precipitated by the presence of other coexisting respiratory disease, for instance, primary lung tumours.

Many of the above features are also common to cases of laryngeal paralysis caused by non-idiopathic conditions. The consistent presenting sign in cats with laryngeal paralysis is a whistling inspiratory stridor (Schaer *et al.*, 1979; Hardie *et al.*, 1981; White *et al.*, 1986; White, 1994).

Diagnosis

In many cases the presenting *signalment* may help the clinician to reach a presumptive diagnosis. A 10-year-old, male Labrador Retriever with a prolonged history of exercise intolerance and stridorous breathing should raise a significant index of suspicion.

Auscultation over the larynx even in the resting dog should allow detection of the earliest inspiratory stridor. This high-pitched, whistling respiratory noise should become more audible during exercise but care should be taken not to over-stress the patient and precipitate an obstructive crisis merely for the purposes of diagnosis.

A complete *physical examination* should be performed in all cases, and in cases of non-idiopathic paralysis a search should be made for possible causes (e.g. thoracic mass). Thoracic radiographs should be taken at this stage to assess if any aspiration pneumonia is present which, until satisfactorily resolved, may temporarily preclude progression to the next diagnostic step.

Laryngeal paralysis is a failure of dynamic function and hence a definitive diagnosis can only be made by observing this function or lack of it. In most instances this is done by means of *laryngoscopy*. In some dogs, it may be possible to inspect laryngeal function under sedation but in most a light plane of anaesthesia is more satisfactory. A deep plane of anaesthesia will paralyse the intrinsic laryngeal muscles and remove all laryngeal movement preventing a meaningful assessment of function. Laryngoscopy is therefore best performed either during induction of light anaesthesia or in the recovering patient as the laryngeal reflexes return. Arytenoid abduction is reduced or absent during the inspiratory phase in dogs with laryngeal paralysis (Figure 15.6). Most cases of ILP are affected bilaterally, although it is common for one side to be more severely affected than the other and asymmetric abduction may occur. Care should be exercised when evaluating arytenoid movement, since paralysed vocal folds often show paradoxical movement (i.e. move apart passively due to the expiratory air flow). It is essential, therefore, that each phase of the respiratory cycle is identified preferably by an assistant, whilst the

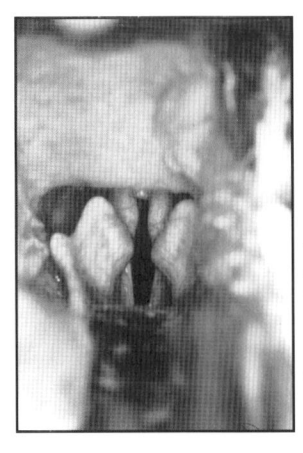

Figure 15.6: Laryngeal paralysis: laryngoscopic appearance of rima during inspiratory phase of respiration. Both arytenoids and vocal folds lie passively in the midline indicating bilateral paralysis.

larynx is observed. In some dogs, the mucosa overlying the corniculate process of the paralysed arytenoid cartilage(s) is often hyperaemic due to the turbulent air flow over the mucosal surface.

The use of *ultrasonographic examination* of the canine larynx has recently been described (Bray *et al.*, 1998). Movement of the arytenoid and vocal folds during the respiratory cycle could be identified, and this gives rise to the possibility of recognizing laryngeal dysfunction using this technique. The non-invasive nature of ultrasonographic examination of the larynx coupled with the ability to perform it in unanaesthetized patients are attractive advantages of this approach.

Respiratory function measurement techniques have been described in the investigation of laryngeal paralysis. The patient's hypoxic (i.e. low PaO_2) status can be quantified by *blood gas analysis* (Love *et al.*, 1987). The abnormal air flow versus volume pattern can be identified by tidal breathing flow volume loop (*TBFVL*) studies (Amis and Kupershoek, 1986; Amis *et al.*, 1986). It is doubtful if these measurements add materially to the assessment of an individual clinical case which can be gained by careful auscultation and laryngoscopy but they do permit a more objective analysis of the problem for research purposes.

Electromyography, nerve conduction velocity and *histological* studies have been used to demonstrate abnormalities in the laryngeal nerves and intrinsic muscles (Steiss and Marshall, 1988; LaHue, 1989; Braund *et al.*, 1994; Gaber *et al.*, 1985).

Laryngeal eversion/collapse syndrome (LECS)

Pathophysiology

Chronic respiratory diseases resulting in turbulent air flow and abnormal negative pressures in the lower respiratory tract or abnormal cartilage structure can initiate a progressive and degenerative sequence of events within the upper airway which eventually result in obstruction of the rima. In the early stages, the mucosal lining of the larynx and pharynx becomes oedematous and chronically thickened. This process also involves the mucosa within the laryngeal

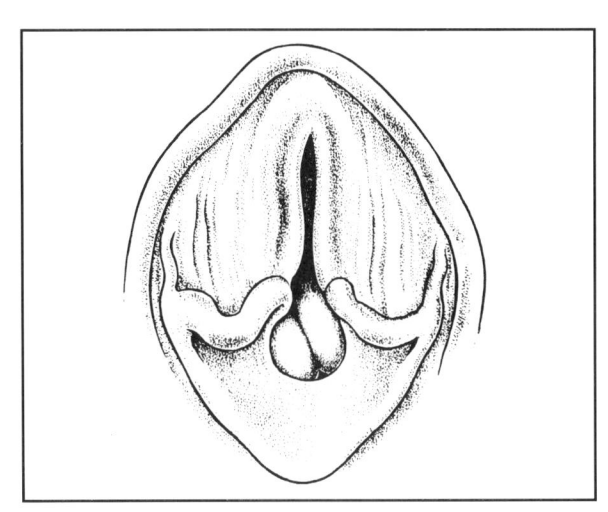

Figure 15.7: Laryngeal eversion: the mucosa of the laryngeal saccules are everted in front of the vocal folds. © *RAS White.*

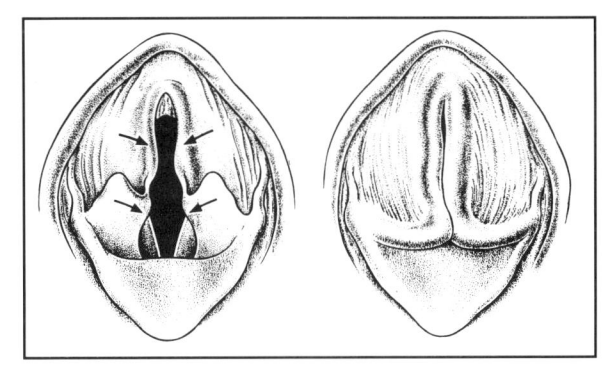

Figure 15.8: Laryngeal collapse: the rima becomes progressively obscured by the collapsing corniculate and cuneiform processes of the arytenoid cartilages. The epiglottis may also collapse towards the rima. © *RAS White.*

ventricles and the saccules are consequently forced to evert into the ventral rima (Figure 15.7) (Harvey, 1982a). As the condition progresses the laryngeal cartilages begin to lose their structural rigidity and collapse towards the midline. The leading and lateral edges of the epiglottis roll inward and the cartilage folds dorsally towards the glottic opening (Harvey, 1982b). The weaker regions of the arytenoids, including the cuneiform processes, collapse medially drawing the corniculate processes with them (Lane, 1982) (Figure 15.8). The rima is progressively narrowed by these processes and in the final stages is completely occluded. The early changes involving the saccules and pharyngeal tissue are often reversible and may be resolved by prompt management of the underlying problem. Changes involving the cartilages are, however, more permanent and, once clinically evident, laryngeal collapse is a difficult condition to manage.

Aetiology

Airway obstruction syndromes: The development of LECS is most often associated with concurrent upper airway obstruction syndrome. It is frequently encountered in the brachycephalic dogs in which the overlarge soft palate, stenotic nares and hypoplastic nasal sinuses are responsible for upper airway turbulence. It is unclear, however, whether it is this airway turbulence during the inspiratory phase or the presence of abnormally weak laryngeal cartilages which are unable to resist deformation during the expiratory phase that allow the problem to develop. LECS may also be encountered as the sequel to other obstructive airway conditions such as tracheal collapse and hypoplasia.

Congenital: Laryngeal collapse is seen as an infrequent presentation in young English Bull Terriers during the first year of life (White, R.A.S., unpublished data). There is some indication that a congenital cartilaginous anomaly resulting in a weak, non-rigid larynx rather than airway obstruction may underlie the condition.

Clinical presentation
Laryngeal obstruction due to collapse results in stridorous breathing and severely restricted exercise ability. In the brachycephalic dog, the onset of these signs is insidious and often difficult to separate from those caused by the remainder of the obstructive airway syndrome. Ongoing exercise intolerance following surgical management of the overlarge soft palate and tonsils and the stenotic nostrils, however, should alert the clinician to the possibility of degenerative laryngeal changes.

Diagnosis
Dogs with laryngeal collapse have severely obstructive upper airway function. Auscultation directly over the larynx should enable the stridorous turbulence to be detected but in brachycephalic dogs, it may be difficult to distinguish this from the accompanying stertor. Laryngeal inspection in mildly affected dogs will reveal the glistening pea-like, everted laryngeal saccules immediately in front of the vocal folds whilst in more advanced cases the rima will be obscured by the inverting epiglottis and arytenoids (Figure 15.7).

Laryngeal trauma

Pathophysiology/aetiology
Laryngeal trauma is uncommon in small animal species, due to the relatively protected position of the larynx compared with that of humans or the larger species. External trauma may result from bite wounds, choke chain injuries and occasionally, crush injuries from road accidents (Nelson, 1993). Compressive injuries such as these may fracture or dislocate the laryngeal cartilages and hyoid bones obstructing the airway. Additionally, there may be neurogenic damage, particularly in the case of cervical bite wounds resulting in paralysis of the vocal folds. Damage directly to the laryngeal mucosa, epiglottis and arytenoids may be seen in stick penetration injuries

(White and Lane, 1988). In the acute phase of laryngeal trauma, the airway may be obstructed due to haemorrhage, oedema or dislocations and fractures of the cartilages. More long-term complications include fibrosis of the cartilage articulations which prevent normal arytenoid function and glottic stenosis resulting from the development of intralaryngeal scar tissue.

Clinical presentation
Injuries involving the larynx are clinically evident due to the obstruction of the airway. Patients may have laboured respiratory patterns, stridor, cyanosis and asphyxiating syncope. Occasionally, there may be subcutaneous emphysema due to air leaking into the perilaryngeal tissues.

Diagnosis
Inspection of the cervical region may reveal obvious penetrating wounds or cervical swellings may be evident on palpation. Auscultation will reveal stridorous laryngeal sounds. Radiography may demonstrate hyoid fractures or variations in the normal relationship of the laryngeal cartilages. Air may be present in the perilaryngeal tissues. Laryngoscopy should be performed to assess the severity of the airway obstruction and detect the presence of paralysis.

Laryngeal stenosis

Pathophysiology/aetiology
Disease or injury involving the mucosal lining of the larynx may result in the development of either scar tissue or proliferating granulation tissue which narrows the glottic opening. Intralaryngeal surgical interventions are particularly implicated in the development of scar tissue (Peterson *et al.*, 1987; Matushek and Bjorling, 1988; Nelson, 1993) and occasionally it may result from traumatic intubation of the larynx. A proliferating granulomatous form of laryngitis has been recorded as a cause of stenosis (O'Brien and Harvey, 1983).

Clinical presentation
Dogs with laryngeal stenosis will have reduced exercise tolerance and stridorous breathing.

Diagnosis
Laryngeal auscultation will confirm the presence of stridor. Laryngoscopy will allow inspection of the scar or proliferating tissue within the rima. Surgically induced lesions most often involve the vocal fold sites whereas granulomatous lesions may affect the arytenoid cartilages (O'Brien and Harvey, 1983).

Laryngeal neoplasia

Epidemiology and incidence
Tumours of the larynx are rare in the dog and cat (Beaumont, 1979; Wheeldon, 1982; Wykes, 1983;

White, 1991), but a variety of histological types have been reported (Table 15.1).

	Dog	Cat
Benign	Oncocytoma Chondroma	
Malignant	Squamous cell carcinoma Adenocarcinoma Chondrosarcoma Osteosarcoma	Lymphoma Squamous cell carcinoma

Table 15.1: *Histology of laryngeal neoplasia.*

Little is known of the epidemiology of tumours in this site, although lymphoma seems to be common in the cat. There is no apparent breed predilection but males may be at greater risk. Secondary tumours or local extension of other primary tumours, most notably thyroid carcinomas, are occasionally seen.

Aetiology

The aetiology of most laryngeal tumours is unclear. In humans, these tumours are frequently encountered and may be related to inhalation of the carcinogens associated with smoking.

Clinical presentation

Symptoms are the result of upper airway obstruction and failure of laryngeal function such as is found in laryngeal paralysis. Early signs include respiratory stridor, exercise intolerance, dysphonia and hoarseness, dysphagia and cough. More advanced lesions cause serious respiratory obstruction with episodes of cyanosis and syncope.

Diagnosis

Auscultation over the laryngeal region may localize the source of the respiratory stridor but direct inspection under general anaesthesia is the only means of confirming the presence of the lesion. This should be undertaken with great care since the upper airway may be obstructed to a considerable degree by the tumour and prior preparation should be made to pass a narrow endotracheal tube or if necessary to perform tracheostomy intubation. Biopsy should also be performed with caution because of the risk of haemorrhage which may be aspirated. Radiography plays little role in the diagnosis of the primary tumour but a search for metastatic extension should be made.

REFERENCES

Amis TC and Kupershoek C (1986) Tidal breathing flow-volume loop analysis for clinical assessment of airway obstruction in conscious dogs. *American Journal of Veterinary Research* **47**, 1002-1006

Amis TC, Smith MM, Gabe, CE and Kupershoek C (1986) Upper airway obstruction in canine laryngeal paralysis. *American Journal of Veterinary Research* **47**, 1007-1010

Beaumont PR (1979) Mast cell sarcoma of the larynx in the dog: a case report. *Journal of Small Animal Practice* **20**, 19-25

Braund KG, Steiss JE, Marshall AE, Mehta JR, Toivio-Kinnucan M and

Amling A (1988) The canine larynx - I. Morphology and morphometry of intrinsic laryngeal muscles in normal adult dogs. *American Journal of Veterinary Research* **49**, 2105-2110

Braund KG, Steinberg HS, Shores A, Steiss JE, Mehta JR, Toivio-Kinnucan M and Amling KA (1989) Laryngeal paralysis in immature and mature dogs as one sign of a diffuse polyneuropathy. *Journal of the American Veterinary Medical Association* **194**, 1735-1740

Braund KG, Shores A, Cochrane S, Forrester D, Kwiecien JM and Steiss JE (1994) Laryngeal paralysis-polyneuropathy complex in young Dalmatians. *American Journal of Veterinary Research* **55**, 534-542

Bray JP, Lipscombe VJ, Rudorf H and White RAS (1998) Ultrasonographic examination of the pharynx and larynx of the normal dog. *Veterinary Radiology* (in press)

Burbidge HM, Goulden BE and Jones BR (1993) Laryngeal paralysis in dogs: an evaluation of the bilateral arytenoid lateralisation procedure. *Journal of Small Animal Practice* **34**, 515-519

Cook WR (1964) Observations on the upper respiratory tract of the dog and cat. *Journal of Small Animal Practice* **5**, 309-329

Dyer KR, Duncan ID, Hammang JP *et al.* (1986) Peripheral neuropathy in two dogs: correlation between clinical, electrophysiological and pathological findings. *Journal of Small Animal Practice* **27**, 133-146

Evans HE and Christensen GC (1979) *Miller's Anatomy of the Dog*, 2nd edn. WB Saunders, Philadelphia

Gaber CE, Amis TC and LeCouteur A (1985) Laryngeal paralysis in dogs: a review of 23 cases. *Journal of the American Veterinary Medical Association* **186**, 377-380

Greenfield CL (1987) Canine laryngeal paralysis. *The Compendium of Continuing Education for the Practising Veterinarian* **9**, 1011-1020

Greenfield CL and Dye JA (1993) Laryngeal paralysis and collapse. In: *Disease Mechanisms in Small Animal Surgery*, ed. MJ Bojrab, 2nd edn, pp. 371-375. Lea and Febiger, Philadelphia

Hardie EM, Kolata RJ, Stone EA *et al.* (1981) Laryngeal paralysis in three cats. *Journal of American Veterinary Medical Association* **179**, 879-882

Harvey CE (1982a) Upper airway obstruction. 3: Everted laryngeal saccule surgery in brachycephalic dogs. *Journal of the American Animal Hospital Association* **18**, 545-547

Harvey CE (1982b) Upper airway obstruction. 4: Partial laryngectomy in brachycephalic dogs. *Journal of the American Animal Hospital Association* **18**, 548-550

Harvey HJ, Irby NL and Watrous BJ (1983) Laryngeal paralysis in hypothyroid dogs. In: *Current Veterinary Therapy VIII*, ed. RW Kirk, pp. 694-697. WB Saunders, Philadelphia

LaHue TR (1989) Treatment of laryngeal paralysis in dogs by unilateral cricoarytenoid laryngoplasty. *Journal of American Animal Hospital Association* **25**, 317-324

Lane JG (1982) Obstructions of the upper respiratory tract. In: *ENT and Oral Surgery of the Dog and Cat*, pp. 80-102. Wright PSG, Bristol

Love S, Waterman AE and Lane JG (1987) The assessment of corrective surgery for canine laryngeal paralysis by blood gas analysis: a review of thirty-five cases. *Journal of Small Animal Practice* **28**, 597-604

Matushek KJ and Bjorling DE (1988) A mucosal flap technique for correction of laryngeal webbing. Results in four dogs. *Veterinary Surgery* **17**, 318-320

Nelson WA (1993) *Upper Respiratory System*. In: *Textbook of Small Animal Surgery*, ed. D Slatter, 2nd edn, pp. 733-776. WB Saunders, Philadelphia

Obradovich JE, Withrow SJ, Powers BE *et al.* (1992) Carotid body tumors in the dog: eleven cases (1978-1988). *Journal of Veterinary Internal Medicine* **6**, 96-101

O'Brien JA, Harvey CE, Kelly AM and Tucker JA (1973) Neurogenic atrophy of the laryngeal muscles of the dog. *Journal of Small Animal Practice* **14**, 521-532

O'Brien JA and Harvey CE (1983) Diseases of the upper airway. In: *Textbook of Veterinary Internal Medicine*, ed. SJ Ettinger, pp. 692-722. WB Saunders, Philadelphia

O'Brien JA and Hendriks J (1986a) Inherited laryngeal paralysis analysis in the Husky cross. *Veterinary Quarterly* **8**, 301-302

O'Brien JA and Hendriks J (1986b) Inherited laryngeal paralysis in the Husky cross. In: *Textbook of Veterinary Internal Medicine*, ed. SJ Ettinger, pp. 692-722. WB Saunders, Philadelphia

Peterson SL, Smith MM and Senders CW (1987) Evaluation of stented laryngoplasty for correction of cranial glottic stenosis in four dogs. *Journal of the American Veterinary Medical Association* **191**, 1582-1584

Ross JT, Matthiesen DT, Noone KE and Scavelli TA (1991) Complications and long-term results after partial laryngectomy for the treatment of idiopathic laryngeal paralysis in 45 dogs. *Veterinary Surgery* **20**, 169-173

Salisbury SK, Forbes S and Blevins WE (1990) Peritracheal abscess associated with tracheal collapse and bilateral laryngeal paralysis in a dog. *Journal of American Veterinary Medical Association* **196**, 1273-1275

Schaer M, Zaki FA, Harvey HJ *et al.* (1979) Laryngeal hemiplegia due to neoplasia of the vagus nerve in a cat. *Journal of American Medical Association* **174**, 513-515

Steiss JE and Marshall AV (1988) Electromyographic evaluation of conduction time and velocity of the recurrent laryngeal nerves of clinically normal dogs. *American Journal of Veterinary Research* **44**, 1533-1536

Venker-van Haagen AJ (1980) *Investigations Of The Pathogenesis of Hereditary Laryngeal Paralysis in the Bouvier*. PhD Thesis. Proefschrift University, Utrecht, Netherlands

Venker-van Haagen AJ, Hartmann W and Goedegebuure SA (1978) Spontaneous laryngeal paralysis in young Bouviers. *Journal of the American Animal Hospital Association* **14**, 714-720

Venker-van Haagen AJ, Bouw J and Hartman W (1981) Hereditary transmission of laryngeal paralysis in Bouviers. *Journal of the American Animal Hospital Association* **17**, 75-76

Wheeldon ED (1982) Neoplasia of the larynx in the dog. *Journal of the American Veterinary Medical Association* **180**, 642-647

White RAS (1989) Unilateral arytenoid lateralisation: an assessment of technique and long term results in 62 dogs with laryngeal paralysis. *Journal of Small Animal Practice* **30**, 543-549

White RAS (1991) The respiratory system. In: *BSAVA Manual of Small Animal Oncology*, ed. RAS White, pp. 281-295. BSAVA, Cheltenham

White RAS, Littlewood JD, Herrtage ME *et al.* (1986) Outcome of surgery for laryngeal paralysis in four cats. *Veterinary Record* **118**, 103-104

White RAS and Lane JG (1988) Pharyngeal stick injuries in the dog. *Journal of Small Animal Practice* **28**, 13-35

White RN (1994) Unilateral arytenoid lateralisation for treatment of laryngeal paralysis in four cats. *Journal of Small Animal Practice* **35**, 455-458

Wykes PM (1983) Canine laryngeal diseases. I. Anatomy and disease syndromes. *Compendium of Continuing Education for the Practising Veterinarian* **5**, 8-13

Tracheobronchial Disease

Virginia Luis Fuentes

INTRODUCTION

Tracheobronchial disease generally results in *coughing*, although dyspnoea may occur if the airways are obstructed. Tracheobronchial diseases are common in both dogs and cats. A number of diseases will affect both the tracheobronchial tree and the pulmonary parenchyma, but this chapter will be restricted to diseases which primarily affect the airways (see Chapter 17 for diseases of the pulmonary parenchyma).

ANATOMY

The trachea extends from the larynx to the carina, and is made up of 35–45 C-shaped cartilages, with a dorsal annular ligament joining each cartilage. At the carina, the airway divides into two mainstem bronchi, and several generations of subdivisions give rise to progressively smaller bronchi. The smallest subdivisions are termed bronchioles, and the diameter of these can be varied by smooth muscle in the walls, which is under autonomic control. Cartilage provides rigidity in the main airways and cartilaginous bronchi, and most airway resistance occurs here rather than at the membranous bronchioles. There is always a compromise between airway resistance and anatomical dead space, as the bronchi do not contribute to gas exchange. The membranous bronchioles lead on to the respiratory bronchioles and alveoli, where gas exchange takes place.

The mucosa comprises a layer of pseudostratified ciliated columnar epithelium, with mucus-secreting glands in the submucosa. The cilia and mucus form the mucociliary escalator, which wafts particles and debris out of the tracheobronchial tree into the main airways, from where it can be coughed up or swallowed. The airway mucosa contains irritant receptors that will result in coughing when stimulated (see Chapters 2 and 8).

CLINICAL EFFECTS OF TRACHEO-BRONCHIAL DISEASE

The key presenting signs with tracheobronchial disease are coughing and dyspnoea. Tracheobronchial conditions are listed in Table 16.1.

Tracheal	tracheal collapse
	tracheal hypoplasia
	Oslerus osleri
	tracheal masses
	tracheal foreign bodies
	tracheal stenosis
Tracheobronchial	acute infectious tracheobronchitis
	acute tracheobronchitis
	chronic tracheobronchial syndrome
	tracheobronchial compression
	broncho-oesophageal fistulae
Bronchial	chronic bronchitis
	bronchiectasis
	bronchial foreign bodies
	feline bronchial disease
	primary ciliary dyskinesia
Bronchial/pulmonary parenchymal	bronchopneumonia
	pulmonary infiltrates with eosinophils
	smoke inhalation

Table 16.1: *Tracheobronchial diseases.*

Coughing in tracheobronchial disease may be caused by mechanical stimulation (foreign bodies, left atrial enlargement) or by inflammatory disease (acute infectious tracheobronchitis, chronic bronchitis). Irritant receptors are stimulated by inflammatory mediators, and mucous production may stimulate mechanoreceptors.

Dyspnoea in tracheobronchial disease is mainly associated with airway obstruction; if this affects the extrathoracic trachea the dyspnoea is usually inspiratory, whereas obstruction of the intrathoracic tracheobronchial tree causes expiratory dyspnoea. Airway obstruction may be intraluminal (*Oslerus (Filaroides) osleri* nodules, excess mucus) or extraluminal (hilar lymphadenopathy, extraluminal neoplasia). Bronchoconstriction may cause dyspnoea in cats with bronchial disease; the airway obstruction thus produced may cause wheezing. Bronchoconstriction may also lead to air trapping, where air can enter the lungs but cannot easily escape.

Diagnosis

Radiography can be useful for tracheal disease, particularly if fluoroscopy is available. Mild bronchial disease may result in only minor radiographic changes, although severe bronchial disease will often lead to a prominent bronchial pattern. Radiographs will often help to suggest the cause of extraluminal airway compression.

Bronchoscopy is probably the single most useful investigative technique for tracheobronchial disease. Direct imaging of the airway structure and mucosal surface is helpful in the diagnosis of most forms of tracheobronchial disease, and bronchoscopy may also be of value therapeutically in the removal of foreign bodies.

TRACHEAL DISEASES

Tracheal collapse

Tracheal collapse is a common condition of small and toy breed dogs (particularly Yorkshire Terriers). Affected dogs are usually middle aged or older, although it has been described as a congenital problem. The tracheal cartilages are abnormal or degenerate, so that the individual rings become flattened rather than C-shaped, with the dorsal membrane becoming redundant. The extent of the affected trachea may include the cervical trachea all the way through to the mainstem bronchi, although the problem is often most obvious at the thoracic inlet. Typically, the cervical trachea collapses during inspiration, and the intrathoracic trachea collapses during expiration, when the intrapleural pressure is elevated. Collapse of the cervical trachea may be exacerbated by laryngeal obstruction. Concurrent laryngeal paralysis has been reported, but is most likely to develop following surgery and iatrogenic damage (White, 1995). The underlying abnormalities of the cartilage matrix include deficiencies of glycoproteins and glycosaminoglycans and hypocellularity (Dallman *et al.*, 1985). It has been suggested that this is a congenital problem (Done and Drew, 1976), although clinical signs are most common later in life. Some authors believe that additional exacerbating factors are necessary in order for affected animals to become symptomatic (White and Williams, 1994). The dynamic obstruction may itself cause mucosal inflammation by mechanical irritation and subsequent oedema formation. Failure of the mucociliary escalator may contribute to lower airway disease.

Clinical signs

The presenting history is usually of a chronic 'goose-honk' cough, and/or intermittent bouts of acute dyspnoea with respiratory noise. The latter should not be confused with bouts of 'reverse sneezing' (see Chapter 7). The dyspnoea may be associated with cyanosis and a variety of inspiratory and expiratory sounds, often with an expiratory grunt. Excitement and tracheal pressure may trigger bouts of coughing, although the clinical course will often wax and wane. In general, it

is a progressive condition. On physical examination it may be possible to palpate the lateral borders of the collapsed cervical trachea as sharp edges. Mitral valve disease is also common in breeds predisposed to tracheal collapse, so that many affected dogs will have a murmur of mitral insufficiency. In the absence of concurrent left heart failure, sinus arrhythmia may be marked. Lung sounds may be confusing, although a 'snap' may be heard associated with complete collapse of the intrathoracic tracheal walls. The liver is often palpably enlarged, although abdominal effort with breathing may make this difficult to appreciate.

Diagnosis

The diagnosis may be strongly suspected based on history, signalment and physical examination.

Radiography of the cervical and thoracic trachea may demonstrate collapse or widening of the trachea, depending on the site and phase of respiration (Figure 16.1). Ideally, both inspiratory and expiratory films should be obtained. A tangential rostrocaudal view of the cervicothoracic trachea has also been described (O'Brien *et al.*, 1966). Sometimes suspicion may be alerted by an abnormally wide or irregular trachea, caused by billowing of the dorsal tracheal membrane. Fluoroscopy will demonstrate phasic collapse in time with respiration, which can be helpful when trying to assess the extent of the affected airway.

Bronchoscopy will also demonstrate clearly the extent of the problem, and has been used as the basis of a grading system (Hedlund and Tangner, 1983).

Management

Tracheal collapse can be successfully managed medically in the early stages. White and Williams (1994) proposed that management should be aimed at controlling exacerbating factors, rather than employing surgical techniques to correct the underlying tracheal collapse. In their study of 100 cases of tracheal collapse, 71% remained asymptomatic after a year of

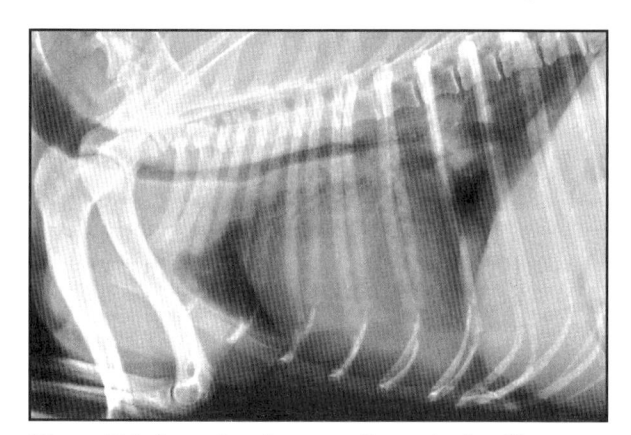

Figure 16.1: *Lateral expiratory radiograph of an 11-year-old Yorkshire Terrier with tracheal collapse. Note the narrowing of the intrathoracic trachea, and widening of the cervical trachea.*

medical treatment alone. Therapy included prednisolone, weight reduction, and avoidance of cigarette smoke or use of collars. Bronchodilators and cough suppressants have also been suggested as adjunct therapy (Hedlund, 1991). Sedation can be very helpful during acute bouts of dyspnoea. A variety of surgical techniques have been described for the management of tracheal collapse (see Chapter 26). Many techniques have been associated with serious complications, such as tracheal necrosis. Extraluminal prosthesis techniques appear to be the most successful, although there are few reports of long-term outcome (Buback *et al.*, 1996). Fewer complications and a more favourable outcome are more likely with dogs under 6 years of age and when arytenoid lateralization is carried out at the time of surgery.

Tracheal hypoplasia

Tracheal hypoplasia is one component of brachycephalic airway obstruction, together with stenotic nares, elongated soft palate, and everted laryngeal saccules. The trachea may be narrowed along its entire length. The tracheal cartilages are small and rigid, and are often closed dorsally. In conjunction with the other features of brachycephalic airway obstruction, tracheal hypoplasia may lead to critical airway obstruction. Affected animals are also believed to be predisposed to lower respiratory tract infections. Other congenital abnormalities reported with tracheal hypoplasia include megaoesophagus (which could also be responsible for lower respiratory tract infections), and cardiac abnormalities (such as pulmonic and aortic stenoses) (Coyne and Fingland, 1992).

Clinical signs

English Bulldogs are the most commonly affected breed, with Boston Terriers also being predisposed. Presenting signs include dyspnoea, stridor, exercise intolerance and syncope. To a large extent, the severity of signs depends on the severity of any exacerbating problems, such as elongated soft palate. In the absence of other congenital abnormalities, tracheal hypoplasia may be well tolerated.

Diagnosis

The diagnosis may be suspected based on breed, presenting signs and physical examination. Definitive diagnosis is usually based on radiographic examination, and various measurements of the trachea relative to other thoracic structures have been suggested as objective measures of abnormal diameter. The ratio of tracheal diameter to the thoracic inlet appears to be the most sensitive and reliable (Coyne and Fingland, 1992). The thoracic inlet distance (TI) is measured from the ventral aspect of the first thoracic vertebra at the level of the first rib to the junction of the first rib with the manubrium. The tracheal diameter (TD) is measured at the same level as the thoracic inlet. In Coyne's study

(1992) bulldogs with tracheal hypoplasia had a mean TD/TI ratio of < 0.1, whereas the mean ratio in unaffected bulldogs was > 0.14. However, there was no significant difference in tracheal diameter between affected dogs that were dyspnoeic and affected dogs that were not dyspnoeic.

Management

Management is based on correcting concurrent problems, such as stenotic nares and elongated soft palate. In Coyne and Fingland's study (1992), 60% were asymptomatic 6 months after diagnosis.

Oslerus osleri

Oslerus osleri (formerly *Filaroides osleri*) is a nematode that produces nodules in the tracheal lining. The males are about 5 mm long, and the females 10–15 mm. Transmission is via saliva from an infected dam to her pups, and does not require an intermediate host. After ingestion of the larvae, they travel in the bloodstream to the lungs where the larvae develop within nodules in the tracheal mucosa.

Clinical signs

Oslerus osleri infection is most often seen in young, kennelled dogs. Coughing with inspiratory noise and dyspnoea are the most common presenting signs.

Diagnosis

If the tracheal nodules are large, they may be visible on radiographs (see Figure 5.2). They are often clearly visible in the thoracic trachea on bronchoscopy as nodules or raised areas 1–5 mm in diameter. Tracheal washes may yield eggs or larvae, as may faecal samples.

Management

Fenbendazole has proved effective, at 50 mg/kg PO once daily for 7 days. Clinical signs will usually improve, and even the nodules may reduce in size with successful therapy.

Tracheal stenosis

Tracheal stenosis generally follows some form of traumatic insult such as tracheostomy or other tracheal surgery, foreign bodies, or following pressure damage from cuffed endotracheal tubes. Presenting signs include inspiratory dyspnoea and exercise intolerance. The diagnosis may be suspected based on a suggestive history and is usually confirmed with radiography and/or endoscopy. Tracheal resection may be necessary for successful management (Lau *et al.*, 1980).

Tracheal trauma

Trauma to the trachea may include penetrating wounds, fracture of tracheal cartilages, or tracheal avulsion. Tracheal avulsion has been reported following trauma resulting in hyperextension of the neck (White and Milner, 1995). The trachea usually ruptures just cranial to the carina, although generally the tracheal lumen is not breached, being maintained by an intact tracheal adventitia. Clinical signs are often delayed following the traumatic incident, and may be related to subsequent stenosis. Surgical repair often results in a successful outcome.

Tracheal masses

Tracheal compression may result from extratracheal space-occupying lesions, such as cranial mediastinal tumours or heart base tumours. Intraluminal tracheal space-occupying lesions include haematomas (e.g. warfarin toxicity) or granulomas. Neoplasms reported to affect the trachea include osteochondroma in young dogs and leiomyoma, adenocarcinoma, osteosarcoma and chondrosarcoma in older dogs (Bell, 1987). In cats, histiocytic lymphoma, squamous cell carcinoma and adenocarcinoma have been reported (Bell, 1987). Clinical signs are usually related to coughing or dyspnoea from airway obstruction. Radiography will often highlight the lesion and endoscopy can be invaluable, although animals with severe airway obstruction must be handled with extreme care. The prognosis following surgical resection for osteochondroma is good; for other tumours the prognosis is variable.

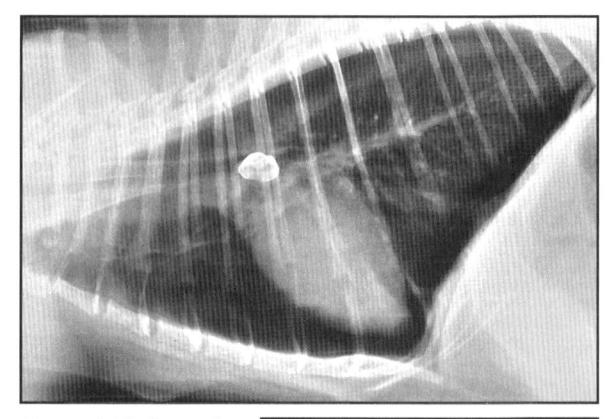
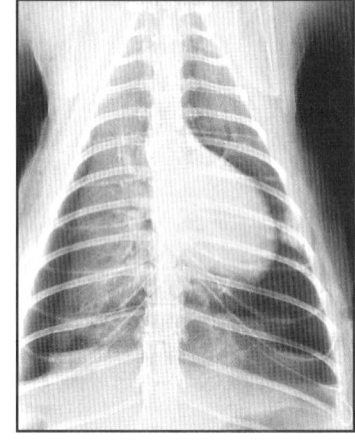

Figure 16.2: Lateral and dorsoventral radiographs of a cat with a foreign body (a metallic bell) lodged in the carina. Signs of air-trapping and a pneumothorax are also present.
Courtesy of Dr B. Stanley.

TRACHEOBRONCHIAL DISEASES

Tracheobronchial foreign bodies

Inhaled foreign bodies may lodge in the trachea, or more distally in the bronchial tree. Teeth and small stones may be sufficiently large to go no further than the carina, whereas plant materials such as grass awns often wedge in a smaller bronchus. The left caudal lobe bronchus is the most common site, as this continues on from the trachea in an almost straight line. With obstructive tracheal foreign bodies, the main presenting sign may be dyspnoea with respiratory noise. With bronchial foreign bodies, coughing is more likely. The coughing may be very sudden in onset, so that the owner may be able to identify precisely the day on which clinical signs began. Haemoptysis may occur in some cases. Tracheal foreign bodies in cats are more common than might be expected, considering the briskness of the laryngeal reflex in this species (Figure 16.2). Bronchial foreign bodies are most common in working dogs and gundogs. Undetected bronchial foreign bodies of plant origin may initiate local inflammatory changes that may progress to abscessation with perforation of the bronchus. Plant awns may continue to migrate, and cause recurrent pneumonic signs, pyothorax, or infection in more distant sites.

Diagnosis

Tracheal foreign bodies are often readily diagnosed with radiography. Bronchial foreign bodies are less likely to be radiodense, and a localized but poorly marginated pulmonary infiltrate may be the only change on thoracic radiographs (see Figure 5.19). Diagnosis usually requires endoscopy, although accumulations of purulent material may obscure the offending foreign body; localized airways containing pus should be meticulously explored using suction. With perforating or migrating foreign bodies, surgical exploration may be required.

Management

Bronchoscopy is the ideal technique for retrieval of tracheobronchial foreign bodies. For tracheal foreign bodies, rigid bronchoscopes may be more useful than fibreoptic scopes, as they allow better airway maintenance and can be used with large grasping forceps. Occasionally they can also be used for retrieval of proximal bronchial foreign bodies in the right caudal lobe bronchus, although flexible scopes are more often used. Plant material may be very friable, and repeated attempts may be necessary to remove the entire foreign body. The complication rate with surgical removal is very much higher than with endoscopic removal, and it is worth persisting with bronchoscopy if available. Appropriate antibiotics are used for any secondary bacterial infection.

Acute tracheobronchitis

Canine infectious tracheobronchitis, or 'kennel cough' is probably the most common respiratory disease of dogs. As with the common cold in humans, a number of different infectious agents can be responsible. The main agents are canine adenovirus (CAV) type 2, canine parainfluenza virus and *Bordetella bronchiseptica*. Additional agents that may be involved include canine adenovirus type 1, reoviruses, herpesvirus and mycoplasma species. Canine distemper virus may also cause respiratory signs, which may appear similar in those cases that only suffer a mild transient infection. Transmission occurs where infected animals are in close contact with susceptible animals, or via aerosol or fomite transmission.

History

Younger animals are more susceptible, and careful questioning usually reveals a history of recent kennelling, dog training classes, showing, or other situations involving mixing with new dogs. The main presenting sign is coughing, which is exacerbated by excitement or exercise. Nasal discharge is occasionally present, and affected dogs generally remain bright and alert.

Physical examination

Coughing is very readily elicited, and pyrexia is usually mild and transient.

Diagnosis

Diagnosis is usually based on history and clinical signs. Tracheal washes may yield increased numbers of neutrophils, and culture and sensitivity may be useful with bacterial infections. Virus isolation may allow identification of the specific cause in a major outbreak, but such investigations are not generally carried out in individual cases.

Management

Canine infectious tracheobronchitis is usually self-limiting, with clinical signs abating within 10 days. Most cases do not require medical therapy, and will improve with rest. When there are systemic signs, or coughing fails to improve after 2 weeks, in may be worthwhile obtaining tracheal washes to identify infection with *Bordetella bronchiseptica*. Treatment with amoxycillin, potentiated sulphonamides, tetracyclines or enrofloxacin may all be effective depending on sensitivity results. Cough suppressants such as butorphanol may be helpful, providing the cough is not productive; if there is any doubt it is safer not to use them.

Prevention

Prevention measures that help to reduce the incidence of acute tracheobronchitis include vaccinating against canine adenovirus 2, canine parainfluenza and *Bordetella*. The latter is available as an intranasal vaccine, which stimulates local mucosal immunity. In kennels, strict attention should be paid to hygiene, ventilation, and mixing of dogs. Coughing dogs should be isolated from other dogs.

Chronic tracheobronchial syndrome

Sometimes it is difficult to determine an underlying cause of chronic coughing in dogs. Corcoran *et al.* (1992) suggested that in canine cases of chronic coughing where pathological changes are minimal, the term 'chronic tracheobronchial syndrome' might be used. Nevertheless, every effort should always be made to find an underlying cause: chronic bronchitis, bronchial foreign bodies, pulmonary infiltrates with eosinophils, bronchial compression, or neoplasia should always be ruled out in any chronic coughing dog. When coughing continues after an episode of acute tracheobronchitis, washes should always be obtained to rule out persistent infection with *Bordetella bronchiseptica*. It has been postulated that the mechanism in chronic tracheobronchial syndrome may be associated with hypersensitivity of lung irritant receptors following infection with *Bordetella bronchiseptica* (Corcoran *et al.*, 1992).

Tracheobronchial compression

The mainstem bronchi may be particularly vulnerable to compression from extrinsic masses, and coughing due to bronchial compression in this region is common (Figure 16.3). Left atrial enlargement is a frequent cause of coughing in dogs (but not cats) with cardiac disease. Enlargement of the tracheobronchial lymph nodes may also compress the mainstem bronchi, although the direction of compression is usually different. Heart base tumours are an additional cause of extrinsic compression.

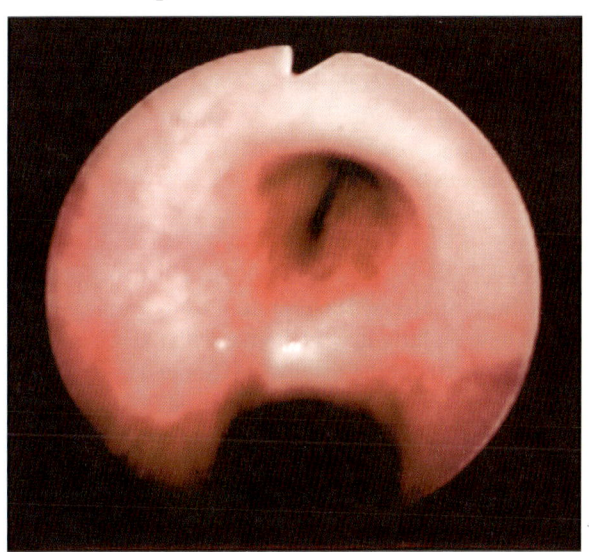

Figure 16.3*: Bronchoscopic view of the carina, showing compression of the left mainstem bronchus (top) by an enlarged left atrium.*

Courtesy of Brendan Corcoran.

BRONCHIAL DISEASES

Chronic bronchitis

Chronic bronchitis is a progressive inflammatory disorder of the bronchi, which results in chronic coughing, excess production of mucus and ventilation-perfusion mismatching. Wheeldon *et al.* (1974) adapted definitions of chronic bronchitis in humans to define chronic bronchitis in dogs, concluding that chronic bronchitis is a condition where chronic or recurrent cough occurs on most days of 2 consecutive months in the preceding year, when other bronchopulmonary diseases have been excluded. Although excess production of mucus was not included in the definition because of difficulties in the clinical recognition of this feature, they regarded mucous gland hypertrophy and excessive mucous secretion as essential characteristics, as in humans. This definition has been adopted and subsequently used by other authors (Padrid *et al.*, 1990). In humans, chronic bronchitis is associated with smoking, environmental pollutants and bacterial infections. The aetiology of naturally occurring chronic bronchitis has not been established in dogs. Padrid *et al.* (1990) did not find evidence of bacterial infection in the majority of one series of cases. Airway histopathological changes include bronchial epithelial thickening with squamous metaplasia, infiltration of the mucosa with neutrophils and mononuclear cells, and goblet cell hyperplasia.

Older dogs are more likely to be affected. Although small breed dogs were over-represented in Pirie and Wheeldon's study in 1976, Padrid *et al.* (1990) reported over half the dogs in their series to be over 15 kg. Breeds reported to be at increased risk include Poodles, terriers and Shetland Sheepdogs (Padrid and Amis, 1992).

Some dogs may become hypoxaemic with severe chronic bronchitis, although CO_2 retention does not appear to be as common as in affected humans. Radioaerosol scanning has demonstrated abnormal distribution of ventilation in affected dogs, as well as abnormalities in tidal breathing expiratory flow (Padrid *et al.*, 1990).

History
By definition, affected dogs present with chronic coughing. The coughing may be worse with exercise, or on getting up after being recumbent. Some dogs will also be exercise intolerant. It is not usually possible to verify the production of excess mucus on the basis of history, although owners may report gagging or retching at the end of a bout of coughing.

Physical examination
Some dogs will have audible wheezes, and most dogs will have inspiratory or even expiratory crackles on auscultation. These may be more audible with deeper breaths. The expiratory phase of respiration may be markedly prolonged. One of the important differentials for chronic bronchitis is mitral valve disease, although a murmur will invariably be present with this condition. If a cardiac murmur is noted, radiography is indicated to rule out left atrial enlargement as a cause of mainstem bronchial compression. In other cases,

mitral regurgitation may coexist with chronic bronchitis. Typically, the heart rate will be normal and sinus arrhythmia will be present with chronic bronchitis.

Diagnosis
Radiography will frequently reveal changes that include an increase in peribronchial markings (Figure 16.4), and sometimes ill-defined interstitial pulmonary infiltrates. Some affected dogs will have normal thoracic radiographs, and it can be difficult to distinguish mild pathological changes from 'normal' age-related changes in older dogs. Bronchiectasis may be seen in severely affected cases. Right-sided cardiomegaly may be present, but this is secondary to the primary respiratory abnormality and should not be confused with primary cardiac disease.

Bronchoscopy is invaluable in helping to exclude other causes of chronic coughing such as airway foreign bodies, as well as demonstrating the typical findings of chronic bronchitis, such as roughening of the airway mucosa and excessive production of airway mucus. Bronchial cytology usually reveals neutrophils to be the predominant cell type, although eosinophils have also been reported (Padrid *et al.*, 1990). Bacterial cultures may be negative, although cases that are complicated by bronchopneumonia will yield growth of significant organisms.

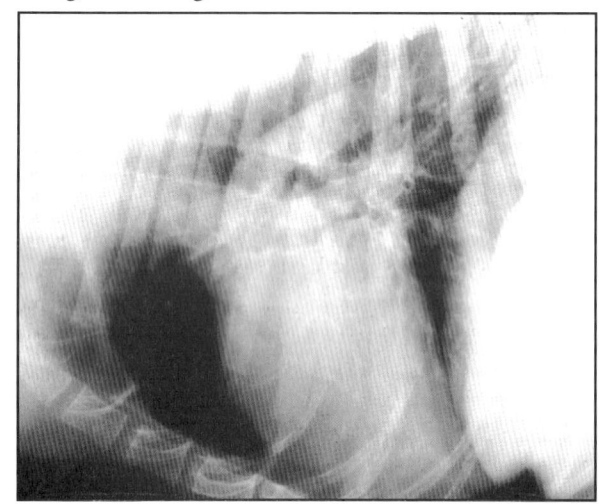

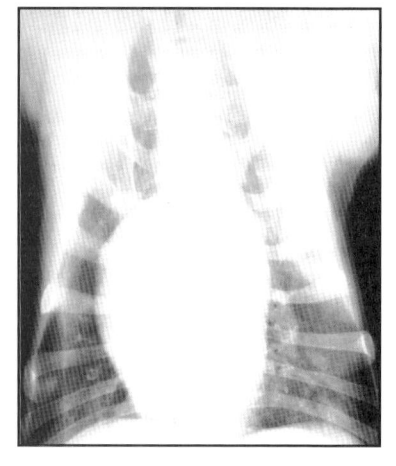

Figure 16.4*: Lateral and ventrodorsal view of an 11-year-old Dobermann with chronic bronchitis. An increase in bronchial markings is evident.*

Pulmonary function testing is not used much clinically, but has been used to demonstrate improvement in expiratory flow rates following therapy (Padrid and Amis, 1992).

Management
Whilst a clinical response and improvement in tidal expiratory flow have been demonstrated with bronchodilator therapy (Padrid *et al.*, 1990), corticosteroids are usually the mainstay of treatment. The minimum effective dose of prednisolone should be used. The combination of corticosteroids and bronchodilators may be synergistic (see Chapter 22). Antibiotics are not usually helpful, unless there is bronchiectasis or complications with bronchopneumonia. The condition is progressive and incurable, and control of coughing and exercise intolerance may be very difficult. Owner education is an important part of management.

Bronchiectasis
Bronchiectasis is usually a complication of chronic bronchitis, characterized by dilation and destruction of the muscular and elastic parts of the bronchial walls. Bronchiectasis may also occur following bronchial foreign bodies (see Figure 5.19). The dilation may be cylindrical, varicose or saccular, and is associated with pooling of mucus and ineffective mucus clearance. Tubular, dilated bronchial markings may be seen on radiographs.

Feline bronchial disease
Feline bronchial disease differs somewhat from canine bronchial disease, and is covered in Chapter 19.

Bronchopneumonia
The term bronchopneumonia is often used with reference to an infective process affecting the bronchi and lung parenchyma. It refers more to the anatomical site of the pathology than the actual cause, although the changes may overlap with other causes of bacterial pneumonia. Bronchopneumonia will occur with extension of bronchial infection to involve the pulmonary parenchyma. It is a potential complication of any purulent airway infection. The clinical signs, diagnosis and management are the same as for bacterial pneumonia (see Chapter 17).

Pulmonary infiltrates with eosinophils
Pulmonary infiltration with eosinophils (PIE) is the primary characteristic of a group of pulmonary conditions that includes the eosinophilic pneumonias discussed in Chapter 17. The underlying aetiology remains obscure, and the term PIE may be used for any condition where there is an eosinophilic infiltrate of the lungs (Corcoran *et al.*, 1991). PIE is believed to represent a hypersensitivity response, although the responsible antigen is rarely found.

History
Coughing is usually the major presenting sign, with varying degrees of dyspnoea or exercise intolerance. Anorexia and weight loss are occasionally seen.

Physical examination
Auscultation may be normal, or may reveal crackles or wheezes. Some affected animals are pyrexic.

Diagnosis
The radiographic appearance is variable, with changes including interstitial, bronchial or alveolar patterns. The diagnosis is made based on bronchial or bronchoalveolar lavage cytology, which yields a predominantly eosinophilic inflammatory response. Sometimes the eosinophilic reaction may be more evident on more direct sampling techniques, such as fine needle aspirates or lung biopsies. Peripheral blood does not always demonstrate a circulating eosinophilia, although a basophilia is sometimes evident.

Management
Providing parasitism and infectious agents are ruled out, management is usually based on prednisolone (1–2 mg/kg bid initially). Medication can be tapered off in some cases, whilst in others it may be necessary to continue with the minimum effective dose to control clinical signs.

Primary ciliary dyskinesia
Primary ciliary dyskinesia is a rare congenital condition characterized by abnormal microtubule arrangement in ciliary axonemes. This can result in abnormal ciliary motility, which may have clinical consequences for the respiratory mucociliary escalator, the paranasal sinuses, the middle ear and spermatozoa. It has been reported in a number of dogs, both with and without situs inversus (Carrig *et al.*, 1974; Hoover *et al.*, 1989). The combination of primary ciliary dyskinesia, situs inversus, chronic sinusitis, and bronchiectasis is known as Kartagener's syndrome. Poor mucous clearance resulting from abnormal ciliary motility often leads to chronic bronchitis or even bronchopneumonia.

History
Affected dogs may show signs from less than a few weeks of age, although some dogs are not presented until early adult life. Chronic coughing is the most common presenting sign, sometimes with dyspnoea. Nasal discharge may also be evident. Weight loss may be noted with bronchopneumonia. Male infertility is a feature of human ciliary dyskinesia.

Physical examination
Pulmonary auscultation may reveal abnormalities such as crackles and wheezes. Animals with bronchopneumonia may be febrile. The cardiac apex beat may be more prominent on the right if situs inversus is present.

Diagnosis

Radiography may show abnormalities consistent with chronic bronchitis: increased bronchial markings and a diffuse interstitial infiltrate. Bronchiectasis may also be observed. Radiography of the nasal chambers may reveal increased radiodensity of the nasal cavities and frontal sinuses, with blurring of the turbinate pattern.

Bronchoscopy is helpful in demonstrating the presence of increased quantities of mucus or mucopurulent material in the airways. Mucosal changes may also be seen. Bronchoscopy may permit collection of tracheal mucosal biopsies, which may allow a definitive diagnosis to be made when these are examined by electron microscopy.

Electron microscopy can be used to examine ciliary morphology in tracheal or bronchial mucosa. The number and arrangement of microtubules may be abnormal in over 50% of cilia, as opposed to only 2% in normal dogs (Wilsman *et al.*, 1982; Hoover *et al.*, 1989; Kipperman *et al.*, 1992). However, respiratory infections may directly damage ciliary microtubular orientation, so that electron microscopy abnormalities may be secondary rather than causal.

Management

Management is much the same as for chronic bronchitis or bronchopneumonia due to other causes. Repeated courses of antibiotics may be necessary, as the defective mucociliary transport predisposes to recurrent infections. The prognosis is guarded.

REFERENCES

Bell FW (1987) Neoplastic diseases of the thorax. *Veterinary Clinics of North America: Small Animal Practice* **17**, 387-409

Buback JL, Boothe HW and Hobson HP (1996) Surgical treatment of tracheal collapse in dogs: 90 cases (1983-1993). *Journal of the American Veterinary Medical Association* **208**, 380-384

Carrig B, Suter PF, Ewing GO and Dungworth I (1974) Primary dextrocardia with situs inversus, associated with sinusitis and bronchitis in a dog. *Journal of the American Veterinary Medical Association* **164**, 1127-1134

Corcoran BM, Thoday KL, Henfrey JI, Simpson JW, Burnie AG, and Mooney CT (1991) Pulmonary infiltration with eosinophils in 14 dogs. *Journal of Small Animal Practice* **32**, 494-502

Corcoran BM, Luis Fuentes V and Clarke CJ (1992) Chronic tracheobronchial syndrome in eight dogs. *Veterinary Record* **130**, 485-487

Coyne BE and Fingland RB (1992) Hypoplasia of the trachea in dogs: 103 cases (1974-1990). *Journal of the American Veterinary Medical Association* **201**, 768-772

Dallman MJ, McClure RC and Brown EM (1985) Normal and collapsed trachea in the dog: scanning electron microscopy study. *American Journal of Veterinary Research* **46**, 2110-2115

Done SH and Drew RA (1976) Observations on the pathology of tracheal collapse in dogs. *Journal of Small Animal Practice* **17**, 783-791

Hedlund CS (1991) Tracheal collapse. *Problems in Veterinary Medicine* **3**, 229-238

Hedlund CS and Tangner CH (1983) Tracheal surgery in the dog. *Continuing Education for the Practising Veterinarian* **5**, 738-751

Hoover JP, Howard-Martin MO and Bahr RJ (1989) Chronic bronchitis, bronchiectasis, bronchiolitis, bronchiolitis obliterans, and bronchopneumonia in a Rottweiler with primary ciliary dyskinesia. *Journal of the American Animal Hospital Association* **25**, 297-304

Kipperman BS, Wong VJ and Plopper CG (1992) Primary ciliary dyskinesis in a Gordon Setter. *Journal of the American Animal Hospital Association* **28**, 375-379

Lau RE, Schwartz A and Buergelt CD (1980) Tracheal resection and anastomosis in dogs. *Journal of the American Veterinary Medical Association* **176**, 134-139

O'Brien JA, Buchanan JW and Kelly DE (1966) Tracheal collapse in the dog. *Journal of the American Veterinary Radiology Society* **7**, 12-20

Padrid P and Amis TC (1992) Chronic tracheobronchial disease in the dog. *Veterinary Clinics of North America - Small Animal Practice* **22**, 1203-1229

Padrid PA, Hornof WJ, Kurpershoek CJ and Cross CE (1990) Canine chronic bronchitis. A pathophysiologic evaluation of 18 cases. *Journal of Veterinary Internal Medicine* **4**, 172-180

Wheeldon EB, Pirie HM, Fisher EW and Lee R (1974) Chronic bronchitis in the dog. *Veterinary Record* **94**, 466-471

White RAS and Milner HR (1995) Intrathoracic tracheal avulsion in three cats. *Journal of Small Animal Practice* **36**, 343-347

White RAS and Williams JM (1994) Tracheal collapse in the dog - is there really a role for surgery - a survey of 100 cases. *Journal of Small Animal Practice* **35**, 191-196

White RN (1995) Unilateral arytenoid lateralization and extra-luminal polypropylene ring prostheses for correction of tracheal collapse in the dog. *Journal of Small Animal Practice* **36**, 151-158

Wilsman NJ, Farnum CE, and Reed DK (1982) Variability of ciliary ultrastructure in normal dogs. *American Journal of Anatomy* **164**, 343-352

Pulmonary Parenchymal Disorders

Richard A. Squires

INTRODUCTION

In order to carry out its primary function of gas exchange, the pulmonary parenchyma must expose a huge surface area of highly vascular, delicate tissue to the environment. This necessity imposes substantial risks to health, but the normal respiratory system is superbly well adapted to deal with these risks. Inhaled air is filtered, warmed and humidified by the upper respiratory tract. Small particles that evade filtration in the convoluted air channels of the nasal cavities are likely to be trapped in airway mucous secretions, and cleared from the tracheobronchial tree by the co-ordinated sweeping action of cilia present on the luminal surface of airway epithelial cells (the so-called 'mucociliary escalator'). Larger particles may be forcefully coughed up. The relatively few small particles that reach the alveoli are phagocytosed by alveolar macrophages and subsequently cleared from the lungs.

In the alveoli, surface tension must be controlled to prevent collapse of the air spaces. Air must come into exquisitely intimate contact with blood circulating from the right heart. Both ventilation and perfusion of the lungs must be sufficient to ensure adequate gas exchange.

Such a complex and highly evolved system is prone to attack or failure at several levels. Inherited diseases may be associated with absence or dysfunction of essential components of the system. Inhaled infectious agents may overwhelm the defence mechanisms and invade the pulmonary parenchyma. Aspirated or inhaled toxins may provoke an excessive inflammatory response, leading to lung injury. Infectious agents, tumour cells, blood clots or fat may be transported to the lungs in blood, to infect cells or to lodge as emboli in the pulmonary vasculature. This may be associated with vascular obstruction, tumour growth, abscess formation, pneumonia or death.

This chapter will focus upon specific disorders of the pulmonary parenchyma. Most of the conditions that will be described cause coughing, abnormally increased respiratory effort, or both (see Chapters 7 and 8). In mildly affected patients, increased respiratory effort may be apparent only after exercise. In severely affected patients, mucous membrane cyanosis and 'air hunger'

will be present at rest. Careful history-taking, physical examination and good quality chest radiographs are usually essential for diagnosis. Systemically ill patients should be further evaluated by assessment of routine haematology, serum chemistry profile and urine analysis. Additional diagnostic tests that are useful in some patients with pulmonary parenchymal disease include arterial blood gas analysis, trans-tracheal aspiration, bronchoscopy, bronchoalveolar lavage, thoracic and abdominal ultrasonographic examination, pulmonary angiography, pulmonary function testing, percutaneous fine needle aspiration lung biopsy and faecal parasitological examination. The value of these ancillary tests will be mentioned, where appropriate, under each disease heading.

CONGENITAL AND DEVELOPMENTAL DISORDERS

Diverse congenital abnormalities of the cardiorespiratory system may lead to pulmonary parenchymal manifestations. For example, severe congenital cardiac abnormalities cause pulmonary oedema. Primary ciliary dyskinesia causes failure to clear inhaled particles, leading to bronchitis, bronchiectasis and bronchopneumonia. These disorders are discussed elsewhere in this volume.

Congenital emphysema

Congenital lobar emphysema (Herrtage and Clarke, 1985) and multilobar bullous emphysema (Tennant and Haywood, 1987) have been described in young puppies. These conditions, which have not been described in kittens, are characterized by worsening dyspnoea and cyanosis, beginning shortly after birth. Diagnosis is by radiography, which shows hyperlucency and hypovascularity of affected lung tissue and compression atelectasis of adjacent unaffected tissue (see Figure 17.1). In some cases, multiple air-filled bullae are evident radiographically. The cause of congenital emphysema is uncertain. It is likely that there are different causes for the lobar and multilobar forms. Abnormal, flattened bronchi may act as one-way valves in some cases of lobar emphysema, leading to hyperinflation. Inherited disorders of collagen or elastin synthesis, or unregulated protease activity may cause multilobar bullous emphysema. In cases of lobar emphysema, early lung lobectomy may be curative.

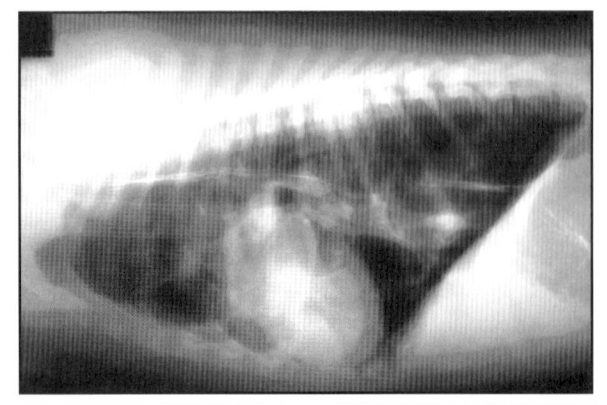

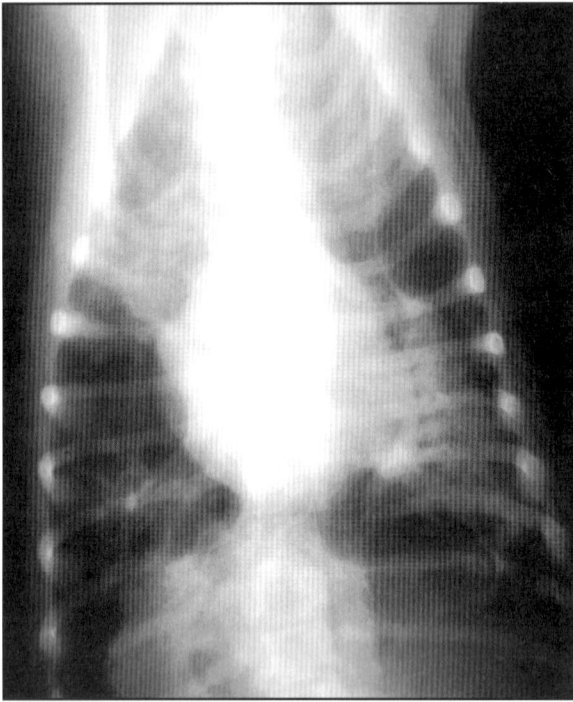

Figure 17.1: Lateral and dorsoventral radiographs of the thorax of a puppy with pulmonary multilobar bullous emphysema. Multiple air-filled bullae are evident. The caudal part of the left cranial lung lobe shows compression atelectasis. Barium contrast material is visible in the oesophagus. These radiographs are of the same case reported by Tennant and Haywood (1987).

INFECTIOUS PULMONARY DISEASES

Although certain viruses, fungi and protozoa can infect the pulmonary parenchyma of dogs, bacteria are by far the most important of the infectious causes of pulmonary inflammation, or pneumonia, in this species. In cats, bacterial pneumonia is less commonly encountered. Bacterial pneumonia is often complicated by the presence of concurrent bronchial infection and inflammation; the combination of disorders is termed bronchopneumonia (for a review of infectious pneumonia, see Roudebush, 1992).

Bacterial pneumonia

Aetiology
Bacterial pneumonia is relatively common in small animal patients. The bacteria that most frequently cause pneumonia are familiar to veterinarians: *Escherichia coli*, *Pseudomonas*, *Klebsiella*, staphylococci, *Pasteurella*, *Bordetella bronchiseptica*, and α- and β-haemolytic streptococci. A predisposing cause for development of bacterial pneumonia can be identified in most patients.

Underlying causes of bacterial pneumonia include:

- Immunosuppression
- Aspiration of saliva or food
- Inhalation of foreign bodies
- Disorders associated with failure to clear airway mucus.

Recumbent, severely ill, large breed dogs frequently develop bacterial pneumonia in the intensive care setting.

History: Careful attention to history-taking is important when trying to identify an underlying cause for bacterial pneumonia. There may be a history of regurgitation or upper respiratory stridor. A previous diagnosis of Cushing's disease, diabetes mellitus or immunosuppressive viral infection (feline leukaemia virus, feline immunodeficiency virus, canine distemper virus) may have been made. Immunosuppressive drugs (for example glucocorticoids or antineoplastic drugs) may have been administered.

Physical examination: Clinical signs usually include fever, anorexia, increased respiratory rate and effort, and may also include productive coughing. Crackles and wheezes may be heard on pulmonary auscultation, especially in the ventral lung fields.

Radiography: Thoracic radiographs typically show an alveolar pattern in the cranial ventral lung fields (see Figure 17.2). Prominent air bronchograms may be evident. Other areas of the lungs are less frequently involved. Thoracic radiographs of patients with bronchopneumonia show a mixed pulmonary radiographic pattern, with alveolar, bronchial and interstitial components.

Haematology: Routine haematological examination typically shows neutrophilia with a left shift. Conversely, neutropenia may be present in some immunosuppressed patients, and in occasional patients with severe, fulminant disease. Anaemia of chronic disease (non-regenerative) may be present in patients with chronic pneumonia.

Diagnosis should be confirmed by trans-tracheal aspiration before antibiotic therapy is started. Microbiological examination of the aspirated fluid will help

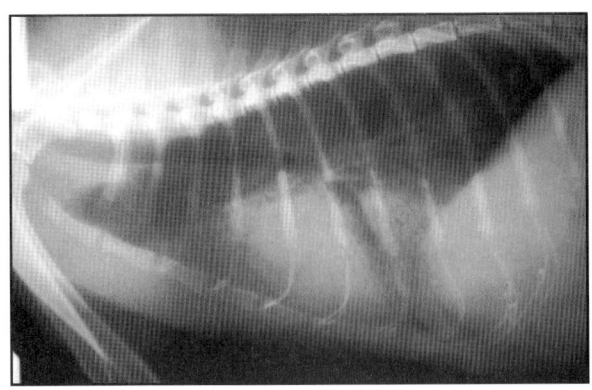

Figure 17.2: Lateral radiograph of the thorax of a cat with ventral pneumonia. The ventral lung fields show an increase in radio-opacity and air bronchograms.

to confirm the diagnosis, identify the causative organism and guide therapy. Ideally, both aerobic and anaerobic bacterial cultures and antibiotic sensitivity determination should be carried out. Cytological examination of the aspiration fluid will reveal numerous neutrophils, some of which may contain intracellular bacteria (see Figure 17.3). A predominance of eosinophils, mast cells or abnormal lymphoid cells; or negative bacterial culture results should prompt consideration of alternative diagnoses.

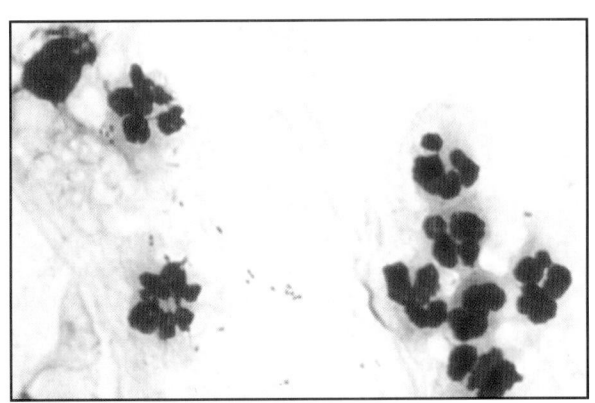

Figure 17.3: Cytological preparation of transtracheal wash fluid from a dog with bacterial bronchopneumonia. Bacteria are present both extracellularly and within neutrophils.
Courtesy of Dr Peter MacWilliams.

Management
Efforts should be made to identify and if possible, to eradicate any underlying cause for the pneumonia. If the underlying cause cannot be immediately eradicated, it should be managed as effectively as possible. Antibiotic therapy should be started immediately after transtracheal aspiration has been done. Trimethoprim/sulphadiazine (15 mg/kg bid by mouth) or amoxicillin/clavulanic acid (13.75 mg/kg bid by mouth) are good empirical selections, which can be given while awaiting bacterial culture and antibiotic sensitivity determination results. Severely ill patients will require intravenous crystalloid fluid therapy to maintain systemic and airway hydration. Intravenous antibiotic therapy is appropriate in such patients. In patients with normal renal function, a combination of ampicillin sodium (20 mg/kg i.v. qid) and

amikacin (15 mg/kg i.v. or s.c. sid) can be given while awaiting culture and sensitivity results. These drugs should not be mixed in a syringe. Supplemental oxygen can be provided to severely affected patients by means of an intranasal tube or a sealed oxygen cage.

Lower airway hydration can be optimized by aerosol inhalation therapy (see Chapter 21). Maintenance of airway hydration is important for normal function of the mucociliary escalator. A nebulizer that produces particles between 0.5 and 3.0 µm in diameter should be used to generate an aerosol of 0.9% sodium chloride solution. The patient should breathe the vapour for 30–45 minutes, several times a day. After each period of inhalation, chest wall coupage, gentle exercise or tracheal palpation should be used to encourage expectoration.

Bronchodilator therapy may be of some small benefit in the management of bacterial pneumonia. Glucocorticoids, diuretics and antitussives are contraindicated.

VIRAL, FUNGAL AND PROTOZOAL INFECTIONS

Viruses
Canine distemper virus (CDV) infection is associated with multisystemic disease and immunosuppression. In severe cases, there is clinically significant involvement of the lower respiratory tract. Lower respiratory epithelial cells are infected haematogenously, or by direct extension of infection from the upper respiratory epithelium. Secondary bacterial pneumonia is a frequent complication of severe CDV infection. Diagnosis is usually based upon a history of exposure to the virus, inadequate vaccination and the typical signs of multisystemic disease. Occasional vaccinated animals will succumb to the disease. Thoracic radiographs show an interstitial pattern or evidence of secondary bacterial pneumonia. Treatment consists of supportive care and management of secondary bacterial pneumonia, if it is present. Specific anti-viral therapy is not recommended. Prognosis is poor for these severely ill patients. Those patients that survive the acute multisystemic illness may subsequently develop neurological manifestations of distemper.

Canine parainfluenza virus, canine adenovirus-2 and, to a lesser extent, *canine adenovirus-1, canine herpesvirus* and *canine reoviruses* have been associated with upper respiratory tract disease. Only in severely immunocompromised dogs would these agents be expected to contribute to clinically significant lower respiratory tract disease.

Cats infected with *feline calicivirus* usually manifest upper respiratory tract signs, but the virus can also cause interstitial pneumonia. No specific treatment is available. Patients should be supported, monitored and, if appropriate, treated for secondary bacterial pneumonia. The *feline infectious peritonitis virus* can cause a dry or non-effusive form of disease characterized by multisystemic granuloma formation. Pulmonary granulomas may form, but are usually clinically inapparent. *Feline leukaemia virus*, by causing immunosuppression, may promote the development of pneumonia due to other infectious agents.

Fungi

Systemic mycoses are infrequently encountered in the United Kingdom. Occasional immunocompromised cats may succumb to *cryptococcal pneumonia*, although *Cryptococcus* more typically causes upper respiratory, ocular, lymphoid and central nervous system lesions. Diagnosis can usually be made by examination of cytological specimens taken from affected tissues. Treatment with a combination of amphotericin B and flucytosine, or with one of the newer oral azole drugs is recommended (itraconazole, 5 mg/kg bid by mouth, mixed in with fatty food).

Protozoa

Toxoplasma gondii and *Pneumocystis carinii* may cause pneumonia in immunodeficient dogs and cats. Diagnosis is usually confirmed by cytological or histopathological examination of tissues obtained by percutaneous transthoracic needle aspiration of affected lung. Therapy with potentiated sulphonamides can be tried, but is unlikely to be successful in the absence of an intact host immune system.

Parasitic infection of the lungs

The pulmonary parenchyma may be invaded by primary lung parasites, or may suffer damage when intestinal nematode larvae migrate through lung tissue. Larval migration by *Toxocara canis* may cause pneumonia in young animals.

Aelurostrongylus abstrusus is the commonest primary lungworm of cats. It infects the pulmonary parenchyma and small airways. Infection does not usually cause clinical signs, but when signs are present, they resemble allergic bronchitis. Definitive diagnosis depends upon repeated parasitological examination of faeces by the Baermann technique. Alternatively, an eosinophilic inflammatory response and characteristic larvae may be found by transtracheal aspiration. Prolonged treatment with fenbendazole (25–50 mg/kg by mouth bid for 14 days; Hawkins *et al*, 1989) is usually curative.

Other lungworms are relatively uncommon and of little clinical significance (Hawkins *et al*, 1989).

IDIOPATHIC INFLAMMATORY DISORDERS

Eosinophilic and granulomatous pneumonias

This is a heterogeneous and relatively poorly understood group of uncommon disorders. In each of these disorders, *inflammatory cells infiltrate the pulmonary parenchyma*. The inflammatory infiltrates are often massive and the reason for the accumulation of cells is not usually apparent. Infiltrates may be composed predominantly of eosinophils (as in eosinophilic pneumonia and pulmonary infiltrates with eosinophilia) or of mononuclear cells (as in pulmonary granulomatosis of systemic lupus erythematosus (SLE)). Some disorders that were previously classified as granulomatous (such as pulmonary lymphomatoid granulomatosis) have recently been reclassified as neoplastic (Berry *et al.*, 1990). It is likely that there is progression from inflammatory to neoplastic disease in some of these patients.

Clinical signs

Affected dogs are typically presented for weight loss, inappetance and chronic, progressive, dry cough; and, in severe cases, for increased respiratory effort. Other signs, referable to an underlying disease (such as SLE) may be present. Pulmonary auscultation is usually unremarkable, although harshness, crackles and wheezes may be heard.

Diagnosis

Thoracic radiographs show increased interstitial markings with multiple, sometimes coalescing areas of pulmonary consolidation or infiltration. These lesions resemble metastatic pulmonary neoplastic masses, except that they may contain air bronchograms and may be poorly marginated. Hilar lymphadenopathy is frequently present. Routine haematological examination typically (but not invariably) shows peripheral blood eosinophilia in patients with eosinophilic disorders. Transtracheal aspiration, or percutaneous transthoracic aspiration of a pulmonary infiltrate should show an abundance of normal eosinophils in these cases. A mixture of mononuclear and polymorphonuclear inflammatory cells will be found in cases of mononuclear granulomatous disease.

Management

Efforts should be made to discover and remove any possible underlying cause for these inflammatory lesions. Infectious, parasitic, autoimmune, drug-related, vaccine-related, and neoplastic causes should be considered. Unfortunately, in most cases an underlying cause is not identified. Treatment with prednisolone (2 mg/kg by mouth bid) should be started without delay. Prognosis is good for patients with eosinophilic pneumonia and fair for patients with other forms of granulomatous pneumonia.

Idiopathic pulmonary fibrosis

In humans, idiopathic pulmonary fibrosis is a chronic alveolar inflammatory disorder characterized by the presence of excessive numbers of alveolar macrophages and neutrophils. In this disorder alveolar macrophages (and perhaps neutrophils) are thought to release damaging inflammatory mediators; probably as a consequence of stimulation by immune complexes. The macrophage-derived mediators stimulate fibroblast proliferation, collagen synthesis and scar formation.

Clinical signs
West Highland White Terriers are prone to a form of pulmonary fibrosis, which resembles idiopathic pulmonary fibrosis of humans (Cogan and Carpenter, 1989; and personal observations). Older dogs of both sexes are affected. There is usually a history of several days of increased respiratory rate and effort. Air hunger and mucous membrane cyanosis are often evident at the time of presentation.

Diagnosis
Absolute polycythaemia is usually present, and suggests that subclinical hypoxaemia has been present for a prolonged period. Thoracic radiographs typically show a marked, diffuse interstitial pulmonary pattern.

Management
Treatment with oxygen supplementation, cage rest and frusemide may provide temporary improvement. Glucocorticoid therapy does not seem to be of benefit. Colchicine (0.025 mg/kg per day) may help to arrest progressive fibrosis, but is likely to be helpful only in early cases.

TOXINS, TRAUMA AND INHALATION INJURIES

Paraquat poisoning
Ingestion of small quantities of the bipyridilium contact herbicide paraquat causes multisystemic, often fatal toxicity in mammals (Darke *et al*, 1977; O'Sullivan, 1989). In dogs, respiratory toxic effects of the compound are most prominent. The toxin accumulates in lung tissue where free radicals are formed, lipid peroxidation is induced and nicotinamide adenine dinucleotide phosphate is depleted. This produces diffuse alveolitis and subsequent fulminant, obliterating pulmonary fibrosis.

Clinical signs
Dogs may be exposed to the toxin by ingestion of a poisoned carcass or by malicious dosing. Mild vomiting and dullness usually occur shortly after ingestion. Thereafter, progressively worsening respiratory distress develops over a few days to several weeks. Eventually cyanosis and extreme respiratory distress develop. Euthanasia is usually necessary at this advanced stage.

Diagnosis
Thoracic radiographs show disproportionately mild interstitial and alveolar infiltrates, compared with the severity of the dyspnoea. About a quarter of patients develop pneumomediastinum. This may be due to pulmonary barotrauma, caused by the severe dyspnoea. The toxin can cause detachment of alveolar and bronchiolar epithelial cells from basement membrane, which may further predispose to air leakage from lung into the mediastinum. Azotaemia, dehydration, neutrophilia, and monocytosis develop as the condition progresses. Diagnosis is usually based upon compatible clinical signs, radiographic findings and a history of possible exposure to the toxin. An attempt should be made to confirm the diagnosis by toxicological examination of urine. Important differential diagnoses are pulmonary embolism and acute infectious pneumonia.

Management
Treatment consists of oxygen supplementation, cage rest and stress avoidance. Frusemide is usually given, but should be avoided in dehydrated patients. Other therapies of uncertain efficacy that have been recommended recently include high dose cyclophosphamide and dexamethasone, niacin, taurine, vitamin E and colchicine, *N*-acetyl cysteine, hyperbaric hypoxia and haemoperfusion. It is unlikely that these therapies will be helpful unless they are instituted shortly after toxin ingestion. If a patient is presented within hours of known ingestion, thorough gastric lavage and instillation of Fuller's earth or activated charcoal, and cleansing enemas should be carried out.

Smoke inhalation
Smoke inhalation can cause *direct thermal* and *chemical injury* to respiratory structures (Saxon and Kirby, 1992). In addition, *carboxyhaemoglobin formation*, as a consequence of carbon monoxide inhalation, substantially reduces the oxygen-carrying capacity of blood.

Clinical signs
Affected patients are usually presented with a known history of exposure to a fire. There may be cutaneous burns and/or corneal opacification. Increased respiratory effort may be apparent at the time of presentation, or may develop and worsen in the hours following exposure. If thermal injury has caused upper airway swelling, there may be life-threatening upper respiratory obstruction, sufficient to require emergency tracheostomy.

Diagnosis
Thoracic radiographs are helpful in monitoring progress, but often show worsening evidence of pathology during the first 24–48 hours. A mixed radiographic pattern, with bronchial, interstitial and alveolar components is usually present. In severe cases, there is progression to a severe, generalized alveolar pattern.

Management

Initial management of dyspnoeic patients consists of *humidified 100% oxygen* administration (to clear carbon monoxide from the body), cage rest and careful monitoring of cardiorespiratory function. *Bronchodilator therapy* may be helpful. The routine use of short-acting glucocorticoids is not recommended. Maintenance of systemic hydration and airway humidification are important. Antibiotic therapy should only be started if there is evidence of secondary bacterial pneumonia. Prognosis depends mainly upon the severity of the inhalation injury.

Near-drowning

Kittens and puppies are more prone to drowning and near-drowning than are adult animals. Affected patients are usually presented on an emergency basis, immediately after water submersion. At presentation, there may be increased respiratory effort or respiratory arrest, hypothermia, and unconsciousness.

The clinical features in near-drowning are quite variable, and depend upon several factors (Farrow, 1983):

Dry- versus wet-drowning: A minority of patients become unconscious and cease respiratory efforts before inhalation of water occurs. They are thought to asphyxiate due to *laryngospasm*. Since no water is aspirated, patients with this so-called 'dry drowning' do not sustain primary pulmonary injury and are excellent candidates for successful resuscitation, if they are rescued in time. Most drowning patients aspirate contaminated water into their lungs, which causes extensive damage.

Fresh water versus seawater: Aspiration of fresh water damages alveolar lining cells, inactivates pulmonary surfactant and predisposes to alveolar collapse, decreased pulmonary compliance, and ventilation–perfusion mismatching. Water is drawn osmotically across the alveolar wall into alveolar capillaries. Dilutional hyponatraemia and plasma hypoosmolality develop and may lead to cellular swelling, haemolysis and cerebral oedema.

Conversely, seawater is hypertonic to plasma; hence aspiration of seawater tends to cause influx of body fluids into the alveoli. Fulminant, refractory pulmonary oedema usually develops.

Cold water versus warm water: Occasional small animal patients may survive a prolonged period (at least 8 minutes; Farrow, 1983) of submersion in very cold water. Children have been documented to survive even longer. Prolonged survival after cold water submersion can occur because hypothermia is associated with reduced tissue oxygen demand; and because blood is diverted from peripheral tissues to the brain and coronary circulation during cold water immersion.

Management

Management of near-drowned patients requires initial cardiopulmonary resuscitative efforts, as needed; followed by close monitoring and efforts to optimize cardiorespiratory function, neurological status, rectal temperature, hydration status, serum electrolytes and urine output. Sequential arterial blood gas and pH measurements are helpful in defining the extent of pulmonary injury and in guiding therapy. Oxygen supplementation is almost invariably required. Endotracheal intubation and mechanical assisted ventilation with positive end-expiratory pressure (PEEP) may be required to optimize arterial blood gas values. In cases of severe metabolic acidosis, sodium bicarbonate (1-2 mEq/kg i.v.) can be given, once adequate ventilation has been established. Bronchodilator therapy may be helpful. Glucocorticoids should not be used. Antibiotic therapy should be started if there is evidence of secondary bacterial pneumonia.

Aspiration pneumonia

Aspiration of various fluids and solids can occur in situations other than near-drowning. Although aspirated material may directly obstruct airways, pulmonary inflammation and secondary bacterial infection are usually more important causes of morbidity.

An anaesthetized patient, or a patient with an abnormally reduced level of consciousness, is at particular risk for aspiration, unless its airway is properly secured by endotracheal intubation. In conscious patients, neuromuscular disorders of the pharynx, oesophagus and larynx markedly increase the probability of aspiration (see Figure 17.4). Saliva, drinking water, food, regurgitated material and vomitus may all be aspirated. Aspirated material is usually contaminated with bacteria, and may be caustic to pulmonary tissue (for example, acidic gastric contents). Aspiration may occur surreptitiously, without warning. It is therefore important to anticipate the possibility of aspiration in unconscious patients, and in patients with megaoesophagus, pharyngeal dysphagia, and laryngeal paralysis.

Iatrogenic aspiration is possible after oral dosing of various medications. Liquid paraffin, or mineral oil, is a particular culprit. It is often used by cat owners to treat suspected constipation in their pet(s). Excessive restraint, overdosing, excessively rapid dosing, overextension of the patient's neck during dosing, and the tasteless, non-irritating nature of liquid paraffin are likely to increase the probability of aspiration; even by a normal, healthy animal. Care should be taken to minimize the risk of iatrogenic aspiration after nasooesophageal or orogastric intubation for administration of liquid food, radiographic contrast material or activated charcoal. If in doubt about the position of the tube, a survey radiograph should be taken.

Clinical signs

Aspiration pneumonia causes clinical signs very similar to those caused by bacterial pneumonia (see earlier discussion). Occasionally, the onset of coughing and

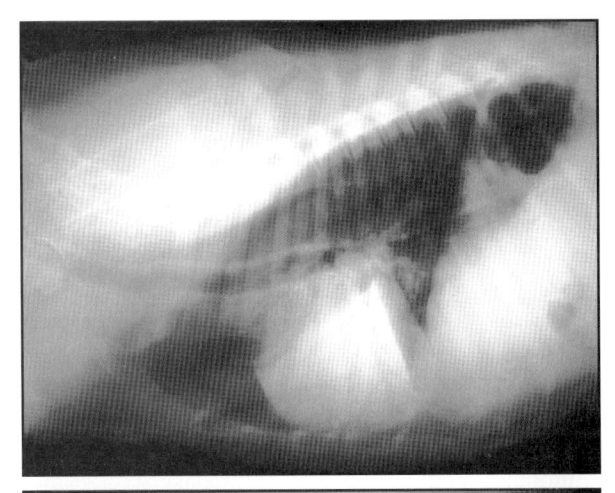

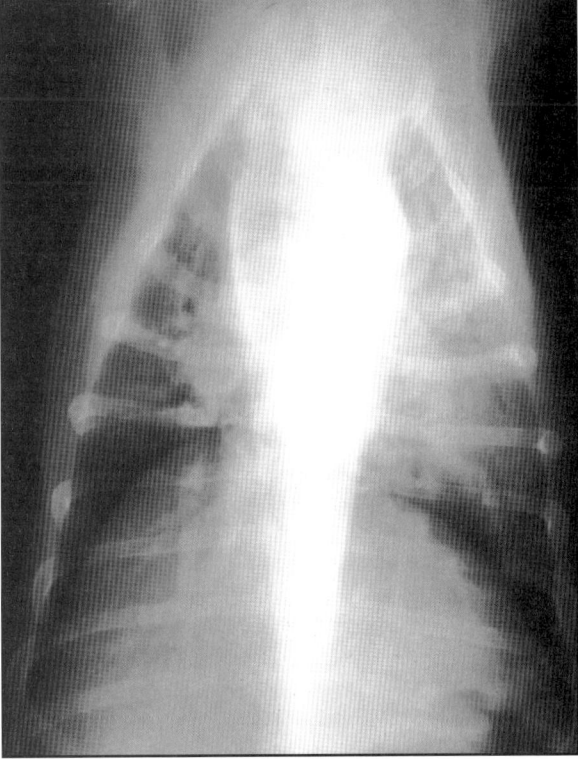

Figure 17.4: Lateral and dorsoventral radiographs of the thorax of a 12-year-old female spayed Irish Setter with a 2-month history of regurgitation and a recent onset of pyrexia. The radiographs show a gas-filled oesophagus and a prominent alveolar pattern in the ventral lung fields. Air bronchograms are evident, particularly in the lateral projection, superimposed on the heart. The diagnosis was aspiration pneumonia secondary to megaoesophagus.

Courtesy of University of Wisconsin-Madison School of Veterinary Medicine Radiology Department.

dyspnoea occurs very rapidly (within 1 or 2 hours) after an episode of vomiting, regurgitation, unconsciousness or oral dosing. More often, the patient is presented with signs typical of bacterial pneumonia and careful attention to history-taking reveals that aspiration is a likely predisposing cause.

Diagnosis

Thoracic radiographs typically show a severe bronchoalveolar pattern in the cranial and mid-ventral lung lobes. After acute aspiration, the severity of the radiographic abnormalities tends to lag behind the degree of respiratory compromise by about 24 hours. A more generalized, nodular interstitial pattern is seen in cats long after aspiration of liquid paraffin. This probably reflects a more chronic, granulomatous response to the foreign material. Transtracheal wash is indicated for patients with aspiration pneumonia, since secondary bacterial pneumonia is almost invariably present.

Management

Treatment should be aimed at preventing further aspiration, clearing any obstructing material from the upper airways, and correcting arterial blood gas abnormalities. Unconscious animals should have a cuffed endotracheal tube placed until laryngeal and pharyngeal reflexes return. Food and water should be temporarily withheld from animals with laryngeal, pharyngeal or oesophageal neuromuscular disease. Bronchoscopy and suctioning may be required to remove foreign material from the larger airways of some patients. Supplemental oxygen and mechanical ventilation with PEEP may be needed in severe cases. Broad spectrum antibiotic therapy can be started, pending the results of bacterial culture and sensitivity of the transtracheal wash fluid.

Pulmonary contusions

Traumatic injury to the lung may cause intrapulmonary haemorrhage and oedema. Such lesions, termed pulmonary contusions, may be caused by severe, blunt external trauma or by penetrating wounds (including bites). There is often a history of known trauma; for example, a road traffic accident, a fall from a height, a crush injury, attack by a large dog, or a gunshot wound.

Physical examination may reveal increased respiratory efforts, palpable fractured ribs, subcutaneous emphysema, penetrating wounds (often obscured by matted fur), pulmonary crackles and wheezes, or muffled lung sounds due to pulmonary consolidation. Pulmonary contusions are frequently complicated by the presence of a ruptured diaphragm, haemothorax and pneumothorax. Physical examination of traumatized patients should be gentle, but should encompass the whole body, so as to avoid missing lesions unrelated to the respiratory distress. Thoracic radiographs should be carried out with oxygen supplementation and minimal restraint. They usually show patchy areas of alveolar and interstitial disease. Sometimes diaphragmatic rupture cannot be ruled out by examination of the initial radiographs, because of pulmonary contusions. In this case, radiographs should be repeated after resolution of the contusions to ensure the presence of an intact diaphragm.

Management consists of cage rest and, in severe cases, oxygen supplementation. Treatment for hypovolaemic shock may be required by some patients. Short-acting glucocorticoid and bronchodilator therapy may be of some benefit. Patients with penetrating wounds should receive broad spectrum antibiotic therapy, after material from a wound has been obtained for bacterial culture and antibiotic sensitivity determination. Patients should be monitored for respiratory rate and effort, haemodynamic status and cardiac rhythm. Cardiac arrhythmias frequently develop post-trauma. Anti-arrhythmic therapy is not usually necessary but close monitoring is recommended.

Most patients with uncomplicated pulmonary contusions improve within one or two days. Failure to improve should prompt further diagnostic evaluations.

Pulmonary embolism

Embolism may be defined as the sudden blocking of an artery by a clot, or other material, that has been brought to the site of blockage by the flow of blood. In small animal practice, emboli most frequently lodge in the pulmonary arteries. Although pulmonary embolism may be caused by fat, air and fragments of infected debris; clots are by far the most frequent cause.

Thromboemboli

In hospitalized human patients, pulmonary thromboembolism is an important cause of morbidity and mortality. In the vast majority of cases, emboli arise from clots which form in large leg and pelvic veins (deep venous thromboses). In dogs, pulmonary thrombi are most frequently found as a complication of other illnesses (Dennis, 1991, 1993; see Table 17.1). It is not certain that embolism *per se* occurs in the majority of cases of canine pulmonary thrombosis. In some cases, clots may form in the pulmonary arteries, rather than being transported there. Pulmonary thromboembolism is relatively uncommon in cats. Regardless of their origins, large pulmonary arterial thrombi cause severe hypoxaemia and ventilation–perfusion mismatching by obstruction of blood flow.

Clinical signs: Patients are usually presented for severe respiratory distress, tachypnoea and cyanosis. They may adopt an 'air hunger' posture with outstretched neck, retracted lip commissures and, per-haps, open mouth breathing. There may be splitting of the second heart sound, due to acute pulmonary arterial hypertension; and the lungs may sound harsh or normal on auscultation. Oxygen supplementation causes little improvement.

Diagnosis: In many cases, initial thoracic radiographs are strikingly normal, in the face of severe dyspnoea. There may be hyperlucent areas within the lung fields or patchy alveolar infiltrates. Diagnosis is usually based upon compatible clinical signs, strikingly normal thoracic radiographs and (sometimes) the presence of a known predisposing risk factor. Contrast radiographic procedures (selective or non-selective pulmonary angiography) or pulmonary scintigraphy may help to confirm the diagnosis, but are done rarely because of the substantial risks involved in handling these very unstable patients.

Management: Rational therapy consists of cage rest, avoidance of stress, oxygen supplementation, and treatment of any underlying disease that might be contributing to a 'hypercoagulable state'. Establishment of adequate hydration and cardiac output is important to prevent blood stasis, but overhydration must be avoided. Heparinization of the patient (75 IU/kg s.c. tid) or transfusion with heparinized fresh or fresh frozen plasma may help to impede thrombus growth and encourage dissolution. Higher doses of heparin (200 IU/kg i.v., followed by 100–200 IU/kg s.c. qid) may have greater efficacy, but are associated with a greater risk of life-threatening haemorrhagic complications. Serial activated partial thromboplastin time measurements should be obtained if high dose heparin therapy is chosen; and the dose of heparin should be adjusted to maintain the APTT at 1.5–2.0 times normal. Controlled studies comparing the relative benefits of high dose heparin, low dose heparin, aspirin, warfarin, strepto-kinase and recombinant tissue plasminogen activator in the treatment of spontaneous canine pulmonary thromboembolism have not yet been published.

Other emboli

Fat may enter the circulation after fractures, crush injuries or major surgery. Fat emboli can lodge in the pulmonary arterial vasculature, causing severe dyspnoea or death. Fat may also embolize cerebral and myocardial vessels, contributing to morbidity and mortality.

Air may enter peripheral veins and circulate to the lungs to cause air bubble embolization. Air may be aspirated, injected or otherwise inadvertently administered through an intravenous catheter. Occasionally, pulmonary air embolism may result from the use of air for negative contrast radiographic procedures (for example, a pneumocystogram). For this reason, some veterinary practices use the highly soluble gas carbon dioxide rather than room air for these diagnostic pro-

Immune-mediated haemolytic anaemia

Severe protein-losing nephropathies
    glomerulonephritis
    amyloidosis

Disseminated intravascular coagulation
Hyperadrenocorticism
High-dose glucocorticoid therapy
Pancreatitis
Cardiac diseases
Sepsis
Various forms of neoplasia

Table 17.1: Disorders associated with the formation of pulmonary thrombi.

cedures. Most pulmonary air emboli produce no clinical signs. Large air emboli produce effects similar to those caused by thromboemboli.

'*Septic emboli*' may be found in patients with serious infections. Pulmonary valve bacterial endocarditis is a recognized cause of pulmonary embolization. The infected material that lodges in the pulmonary vasculature can cause multifocal bacterial pneumonia, pulmonary abscessation, haemoptysis and death.

Iatrogenic emboli arise when occasionally, an accident occurs during, or after intravenous catheterization, and a piece of catheter may be broken or sliced off and released into the circulation. Catheter fragments usually lodge in the heart or pulmonary arteries and may cause small-scale embolization. Although they frequently cause no apparent problems, these intravascular foreign objects may become infected haematogenously, or may predispose to larger scale thromboembolism.

Pulmonary neoplasia

Pulmonary neoplasia may arise from several sources:

- Primary lung neoplasia
- Metastatic neoplasia
- Spread from directly adjacent tissues
- Part of a multisystemic neoplastic process.

Primary lung neoplasia

Primary lung tumours are relatively uncommon in dogs and cats. The vast majority are *adenocarcinomas* (about 75%) or *other carcinomas* (about 20%; Ogilvie *et al.*, 1989). Mesenchymal tumours and tumours of mixed cell origin are rare.

Clinical signs

Patients with primary lung neoplasia are usually middle aged or older. They may be presented for chronic respiratory signs (dry cough, exercise intolerance, increasing tachypnoea and hyperpnoea). Some patients are presented for lameness due to hypertrophic pulmonary osteopathy, or metastasis of a lung tumour to a long bone. Others are presented for vague signs of inappetance, lethargy and depression. Occasionally, primary lung tumours are discovered as an incidental finding.

Diagnosis

Thoracic auscultation may reveal areas of increased, decreased or abnormal lung sounds. Heart sounds may be muffled or found in an abnormal position, if a large mass has displaced the heart. Thoracic radiographs usually show an increase in pulmonary interstitial markings and one or more discrete pulmonary soft tissue masses (see Figure 17.5). The right caudal lung lobe is more commonly affected than other lobes. There may be multiple pulmonary masses as a consequence of metastatic and local spread of a primary lung tumour to other parts of the lung. Sometimes pleural effusion may be present, obscuring the underlying pulmonary parenchymal disease.

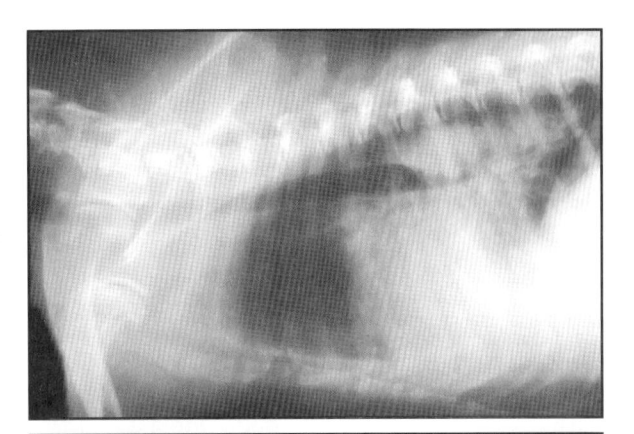
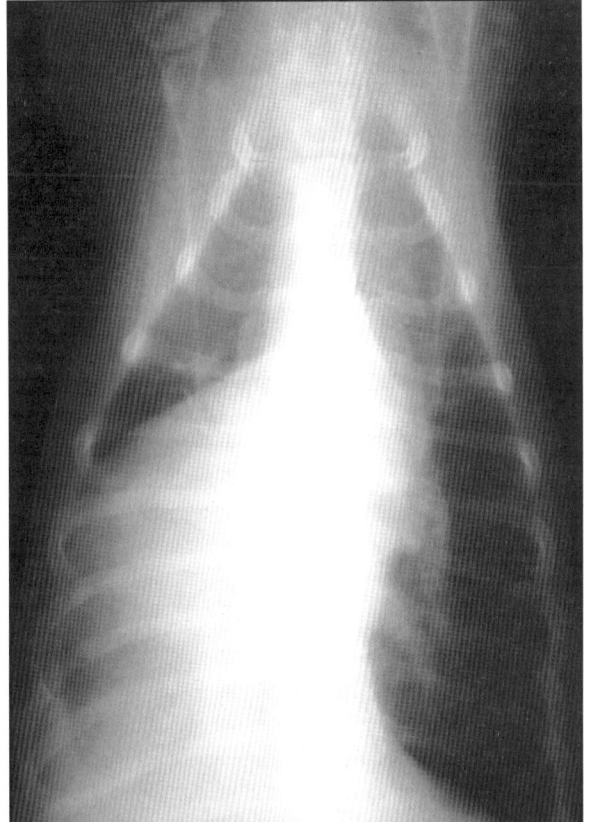
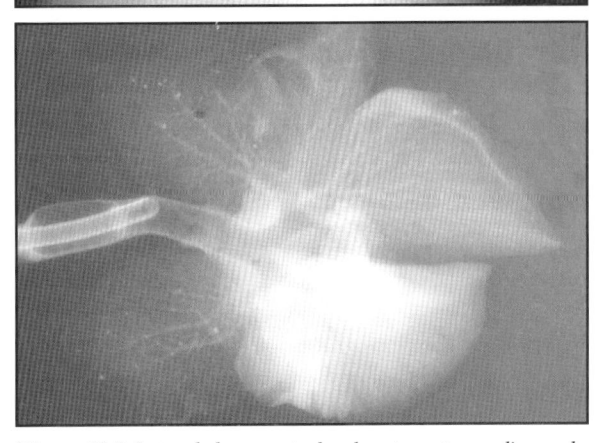

Figure 17.5: *Lateral, dorsoventral and post-mortem radiographs of a dog with a large right-sided lung mass. The right middle, caudal and accessory lobes are involved. The histological diagnosis was bronchogenic carcinoma with metastasis to the tracheobronchial lymph nodes and to the lungs.*

Courtesy of University of Wisconsin-Madison School of Veterinary Medicine Radiology Department.

Definitive diagnosis requires cytological or histological examination of neoplastic tissue. Occasionally, a diagnosis can be made from cytological examination of sputum or material obtained by transtracheal wash or bronchoscopy. More frequently, transthoracic needle biopsy or thoracotomy is required.

Management
Surgical excision of the tumour-bearing lung lobe(s) is the recommended form of therapy. Adjuvant systemic chemotherapy (for example, with cisplatin and vinblastine) may prove useful for patients with evidence of lymph node metastasis, or unresectable pulmonary involvement. Prognostic factors have not been thoroughly defined. Primary lung tumours tend to grow slowly, so that lobectomy may be followed by a prolonged period of good quality life, even in patients with incomplete resection of neoplastic tissue.

Metastatic neoplasia
Malignant tumours may metastasize to local draining lymph nodes, or to more distant sites. Haematogenous and lymphatic spread can occur. Distant metastasis to the lungs is very common, probably because the pulmonary capillary bed is the first one encountered by most tumour cells after release from the primary tumour. Tumour cells are prone to lodge in the first capillary bed encountered after release.

Although many different malignant tumours of small animals can metastasize to lung; *thyroid* and *mammary carcinomas, haemangiosarcomas* and *osteosarcomas* are particularly likely to do so.

Clinical signs
Patients with pulmonary metastatic neoplasia are usually presented for assessment of the primary tumour. Occasionally, the primary tumour is not evident and patients are presented for cough, increased respiratory rate and effort, or other signs similar to those found in primary lung neoplasia.

Diagnosis

Radiography: Assessment of the lungs for evidence of metastatic disease should be a routine practice in tumour-bearing patients. Radiographs may show multiple, discrete, round soft tissue pulmonary masses (so-called 'cannon balls') or a more miliary nodular pattern (see Figures 17.6 and 17.7). Metastatic mammary carcinoma in cats tends to produce a marked interstitial pattern without obvious nodules. Pleural effusion or (occasionally) pneumothorax may be present, secondary to metastatic disease. Unfortunately, physical examination and thoracic radiographs are relatively insensitive methods for detection of pulmonary metastases. The sensitivity of thoracic

radiography for the detection of pulmonary metastases can be improved somewhat by taking both left and right lateral recumbent views (Lang *et al.*, 1986). Nevertheless, tumour masses smaller than 5 mm in diameter are likely to be missed.

Diagnosis is usually presumptive, based upon the presence of a primary malignant tumour and compatible radiographic findings. Before a presumptive diagnosis is accepted, consideration should be given to other possible causes of nodular interstitial pulmonary disease. Fungal, mycobacterial, parasitic and non-infectious granulomatous diseases should be considered. Transtracheal wash and transthoracic fine needle aspiration may help to distinguish neoplastic from non-neoplastic disease.

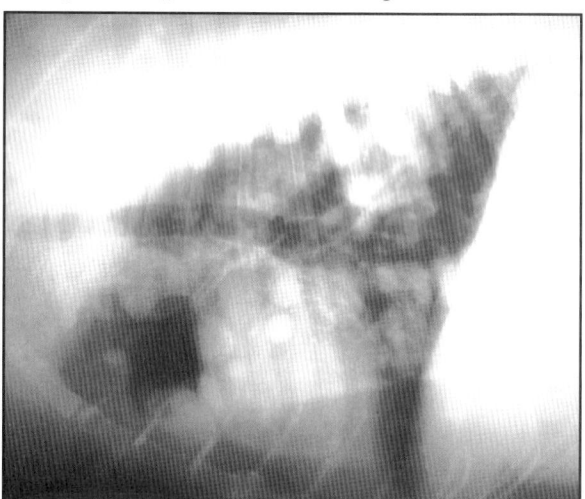

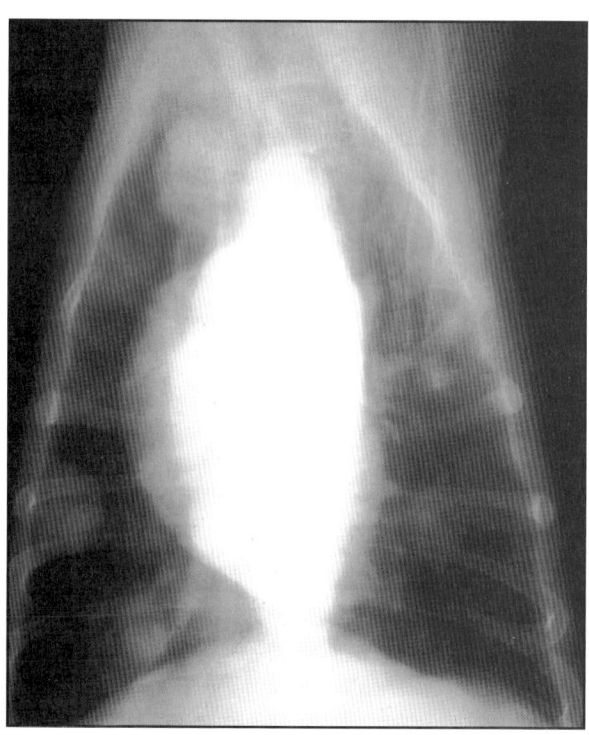

Figure 17.6: *Lateral and dorsoventral radiographs of the thorax of an 11-year-old, male neutered German Shorthaired Pointer showing metastatic prostatic carcinoma. Multiple 'cannonball' metastases are evident.*

Courtesy of University of Wisconsin-Madison School of Veterinary Medicine Radiology Department.

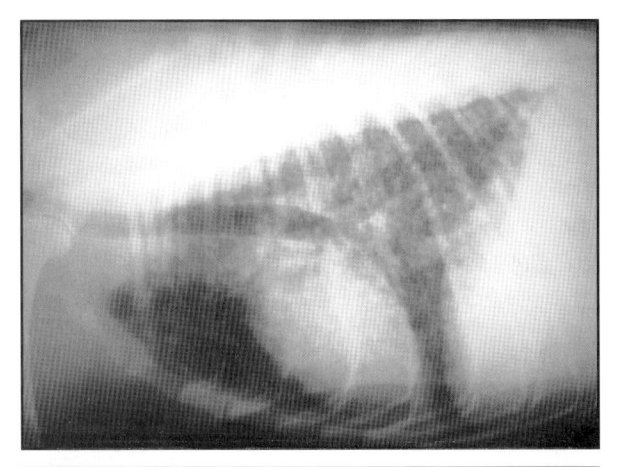

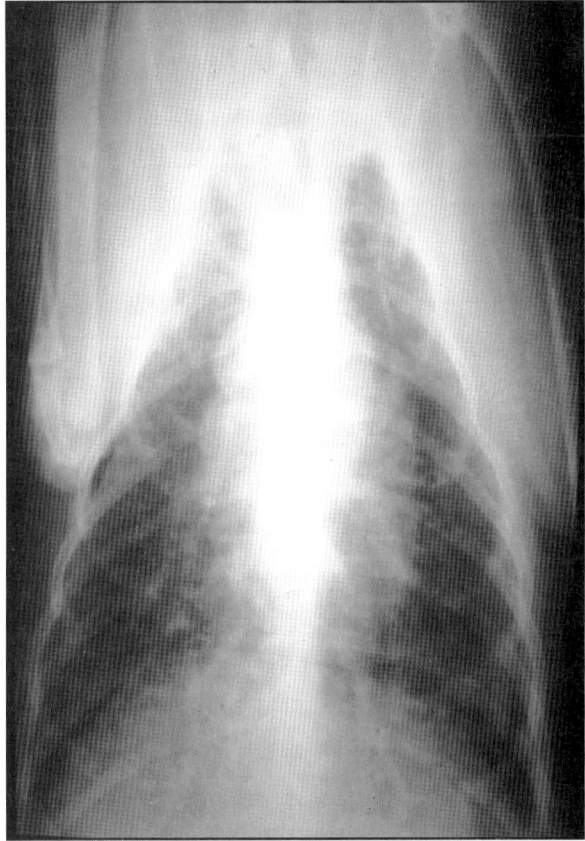

Figure 17.7*: Lateral and dorsoventral radiographs of the thorax of a 9-year-old female spayed Collie. The generalized, nodular interstitial pulmonary pattern was caused by metastatic haemangiosarcoma.*

Courtesy of University of Wisconsin-Madison School of Veterinary Medicine Radiology Department.

Management

Treatment of pulmonary metastatic neoplasia is usually difficult. Occasionally, when one or very few metastatic masses are found, surgical excision can be considered. This is rarely appropriate; but it may be the only therapeutic option if (for example) a tumour metastasis has eroded through the visceral pleura to cause pneumothorax. Several systemic chemotherapeutic protocols have been used for the management of pulmonary metastatic disease. The selection of drugs is usually based upon the sensitivity of the primary tumour. In general, results have been disappointing.

Multisystemic neoplasia

Malignant lymphoma (or lymphoma, lymphosarcoma) may involve the lung parenchyma. There is usually concurrent involvement of hilar, sternal and other mediastinal lymph nodes.

Clinical signs: These are highly variable and often non specific. The radiographic appearance of the lung parenchyma is also highly variable, with nodular, diffuse interstitial, alveolar and mixed patterns evident in various patients.

Diagnosis: The radiographic appearance may mimic that seen in several of the other diseases described in this chapter; in particular, some of the infectious diseases. Diagnosis of lymphoma can usually be made by cytological or histological examination of material obtained from affected lymph nodes. Although it may be tempting to assume that any pulmonary radiographic abnormalities are due to lymphoma, infectious disease should be ruled in or out (by transtracheal wash, cytology and culture).

Management: Treatment of lymphoma has been described elsewhere. If infectious bronchopneumonia is diagnosed, it should be treated aggressively, so as to avoid exacerbation when immunosuppressive anti-neoplastic therapy is started.

Other multisystemic neoplastic diseases such as mast cell tumour, various leukaemias, and multiple myeloma may occasionally involve the pulmonary parenchyma.

Non-cardiogenic pulmonary oedema

Although left heart failure is the major cause of pulmonary oedema in small animal patients, there are several other mechanisms that can lead to the accumulation of fluid in the pulmonary interstitium, alveoli and airways (see Figure 17.8). Some of the mechanisms that lead to pulmonary oedema are incompletely understood. Conditions that cause low plasma oncotic pressure predispose strongly to the development of pulmonary oedema. However, on their own, these conditions rarely cause oedema, unless there is concurrent increased intravascular hydrostatic pressure or increased vascular wall permeability. Lymphatic obstruction is an important cause of oedema elsewhere in the body, but rarely causes pulmonary oedema. Pulmonary oedema caused by increased vascular permeability is sometimes termed adult respiratory distress syndrome (ARDS; for a review see Frevert and Warner, 1992). ARDS is a term of dubious value, purloined from human medicine. In human medicine, the term is used to describe several different forms of acute, severe, non-cardiogenic pulmonary oedema, which require similar intensive therapy. Increased alveolar capillary permeability is a common feature of these disorders, although the cause of the increased permeability varies widely. In each case, the oedema fluid

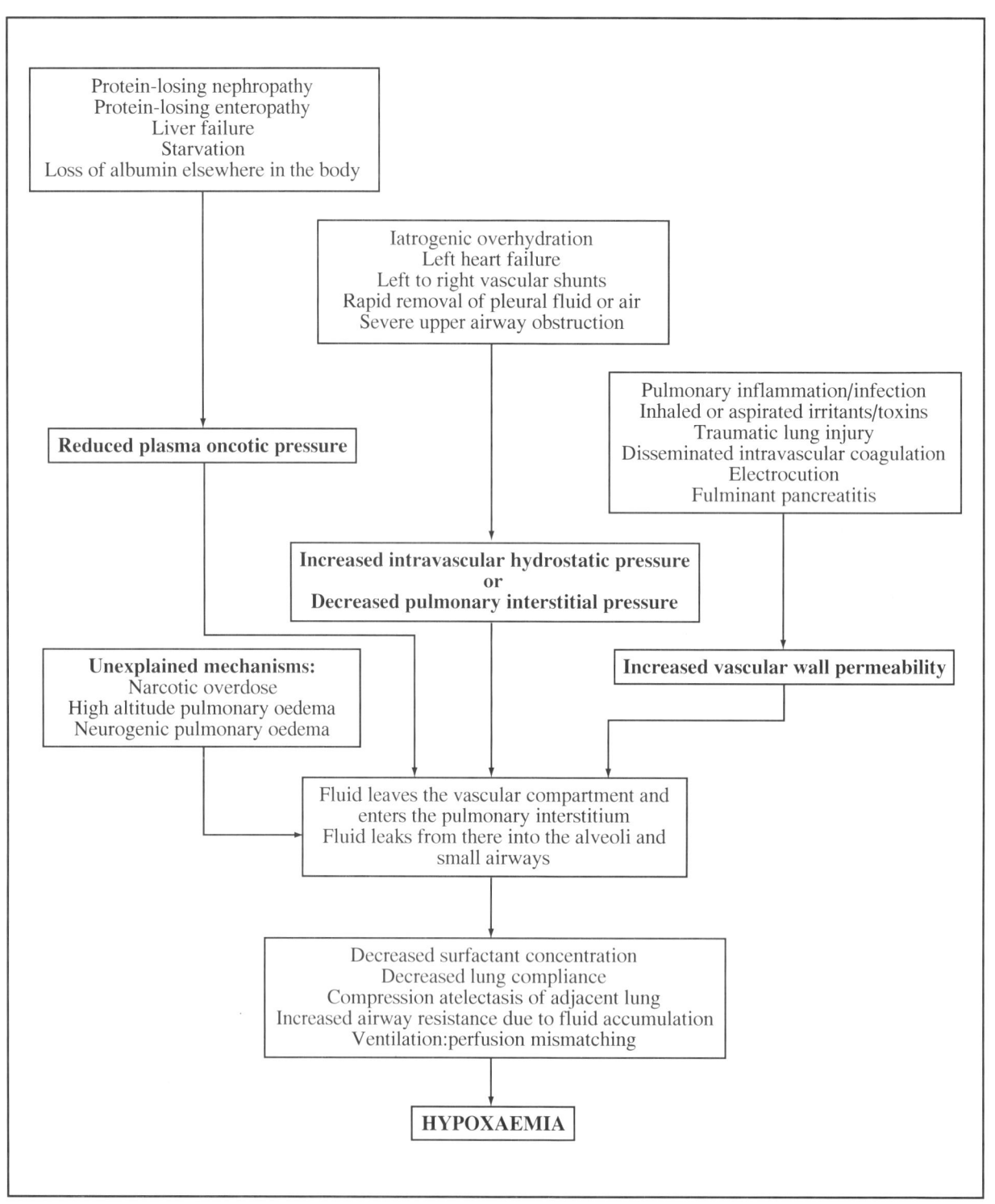

Figure 17.8: Major factors in the pathogenesis of pulmonary oedema.

has a high protein content and tends to accumulate despite normal or low pulmonary capillary hydrostatic pressure. The high protein content of the oedema fluid makes these conditions particularly difficult to treat.

Diagnosis

Diagnostic evaluation of patients with suspected non-cardiogenic pulmonary oedema should include history, physical examination, thoracic radiographs, routine haematological examination, serum chemistry profile and urine analysis. There may be a history of electrocution, head trauma, seizures or overzealous i.v. fluid therapy. Physical examination may reveal a cause for pulmonary oedema, or show evidence of oedema elsewhere in the body. Blood work may indicate low plasma oncotic pressure and suggest a cause for it. Urine analysis may show heavy proteinuria, an important cause of hypoalbuminaemia and low plasma oncotic pressure. Thoracic radiographs will help confirm the presence of interstitial and alveolar infiltrates.

The typical distribution of alveolar infiltrates differs between cardiogenic and non-cardiogenic pulmonary oedema. Non-cardiogenic pulmonary oedema typically causes dorsocaudal alveolar infiltrates, rather than the perihilar infiltrates seen in dogs and the diffuse, patchy infiltrates seen in cats with cardiogenic oedema.

Management

Non-cardiogenic pulmonary oedema of all kinds should be treated with cage rest, oxygen supplementation and avoidance of stress. Stressful medical procedures should be carried out with minimal restraint by technically proficient personnel; or should be delayed temporarily until oxygen supplementation and cage rest have produced some improvement. Aminophylline (10 mg/kg i.v. tid to qid) may be helpful in some cases. The loop diuretic frusemide (1–4 mg/kg i.v.) is very helpful in the management of pulmonary oedema due to increased intravascular hydrostatic pressure. It is less valuable in the management of increased vascular permeability and should not be used on its own in hypovolaemic patients. Patients with low plasma oncotic pressure should receive plasma volume expander therapy with stored plasma or colloidal gelatin. Patients with suspected neurogenic pulmonary oedema may benefit from mannitol (1.5 g/kg i.v. once). Treatment of increased permeability pulmonary oedema is challenging and varies somewhat, according to the inciting cause. Efforts should be made to identify and treat any underlying disorder. Bronchodilators, loop diuretics and shock doses of glucocorticoids may be of some benefit. Patients with ARDS are likely to require mechanical ventilatory support with PEEP because of hypoxaemic respiratory failure.

REFERENCES AND FURTHER READING

Berry CR, Moore PF, Thomas WP, Sisson D and Koblik PD (1990) Pulmonary lymphomatoid granulomatosis in seven dogs (1976-1987). *Journal of Veterinary Internal Medicine* **4**, 157

Cogan DC and Carpenter JL (1989) Diffuse alveolar injury in two dogs. *Journal of the American Veterinary Medical Association* **194**, 527

Darke PGG, Gibbs C, Kelly DF, Morgan AG and Pearson H (1977) Acute respiratory distress in the dog associated with paraquat poisoning. *Veterinary Record* **100**, 275

Dennis JS (1991) Clinical features of canine pulmonary thromboembolism. *Compendium of Continuing Education for the Practicing Veterinarian* **13**, 1811

Dennis JS (1993) The pathophysiologic sequelae of pulmonary thromboembolism. *Compendium of Continuing Education for the Practicing Veterinarian* **15**, 1595

Farrow CS (1983) Near-drowning (water inhalation). In: *Kirk's Current Veterinary Therapy 8th edn. Small Animal Practice*, ed. RW Kirk. W.B. Saunders Company, Philadelphia

Frevert CW and Warner AE (1992) Respiratory distress resulting from acute lung injury in the veterinary patient. *Journal of Veterinary Internal Medicine* **6**, 154

Hawkins EC, Ettinger SJ and Suter PF (1989) Diseases of the lower respiratory tract (lung) and pulmonary edema. In: *Textbook of Veterinary Internal Medicine, 3rd edn*, ed. SJ Ettinger. W.B. Saunders Company, Philadelphia

Herrtage ME and Clarke DD (1985) Congenital lobar emphysema in two dogs. *Journal of Small Animal Practice* **26**, 453

Lang J, Wortman JA, Glickman LT, Biery DN and Rhodes H (1986) Sensitivity of radiographic detection of lung metastases in the dog. *Veterinary Radiology* **27**, 74

O'Sullivan SP (1989) Paraquat poisoning in the dog. *Journal of Small Animal Practice* **30**, 361

Ogilvie GK, Haschek WM, Withrow SJ, Richardson RC, Harvey HJ, Henderson RA, Fowler JD, Norris AM, Tomlinson J, McCaw D, Klausner JS, Reschke RW and McKiernan BC (1989) Classification of primary lung tumors in dogs: 210 cases (1975-1985). *Journal of the American Veterinary Medical Association* **195**, 106

Roudebush P (1992) Infectious pneumonia. In: *Kirk's Current Veterinary Therapy 11th edn, Small Animal Practice*, ed. RW Kirk and JD Bonagura. W.B. Saunders Company, Philadelphia

Saxon WD and Kirby R (1992) Treatment of acute burn injury and smoke inhalation. In: *Kirk's Current Veterinary Therapy 11th edn, Small Animal Practice*. ed. RW Kirk and JD Bonagura. W.B. Saunders Company, Philadelphia

Tennant BJ and Haywood S (1987) Congenital bullous emphysema in a dog: a case report. *Journal of Small Animal Practice* **28**, 109

Pleural and Mediastinal Disease

Virginia Luis Fuentes

PLEURAL ANATOMY

The *parietal pleura* is a serous membrane lining the walls of the thoracic cavity, the diaphragm and the mediastinum. Its vascular supply comes from the intercostal, pericardial and diaphragmatic arteries (i.e. systemic circulation), so that the hydrostatic forces driving fluid out of the capillaries exceed the oncotic forces preventing fluid from leaving.

The *visceral* (or *pulmonary*) *pleura* adheres tightly to the surfaces of the lungs and follows all of their irregularities. It extends to the bronchi in all interlobar fissures, except between the cranial and caudal parts of the left cranial lung lobe. The pulmonary arteries supply blood to the visceral pleura, and drainage is into the pulmonary veins. The hydrostatic forces in the capillaries of the visceral pleura are therefore lower than in the parietal pleura, so that there is net uptake of fluid from the pleural space across the visceral pleura (Kinasewitz, 1998).

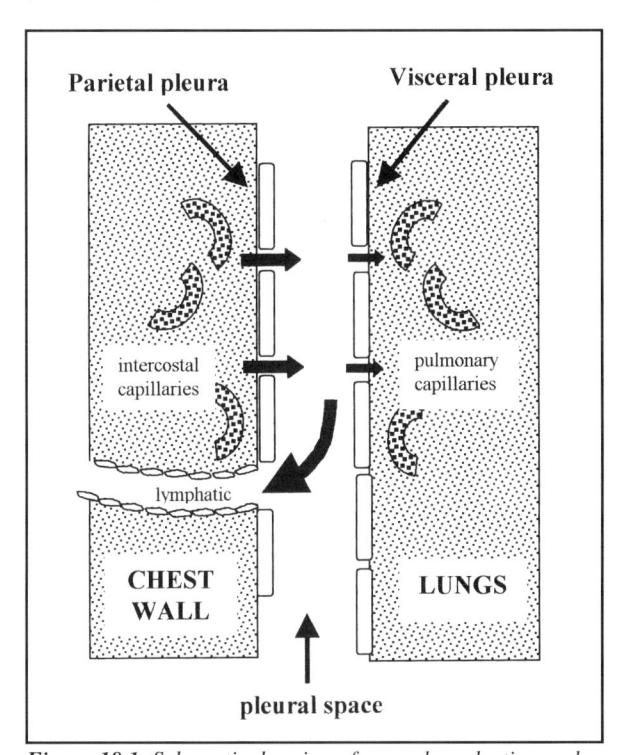

Figure 18.1: *Schematic drawing of normal production and drainage of pleural fluid.*

The pleural membranes contain an abundant lymphatic network. Large stomas in the parietal pleura connect with lymphatic collecting vessels, and ultimately empty into the thoracic duct. These lymphatics provide the main drainage route for the pleural space (Figure 18.1).

A small amount of fluid is normally present in the pleural space, which helps to lubricate the pleural surfaces and facilitate movement between the lungs and the thoracic wall during expansion.

PLEURAL DISEASE

Pleural disease is generally the result of an abnormal accumulation of fluid or air within the pleural space, termed *pleural effusion* and *pneumothorax*, respectively. A variety of aetiologies exist for both conditions (Table 18.1), although the net result is mechanical interference with ventilation, resulting in restriction of lung expansion. A general approach which includes thoracic drainage and adequate oxygenation is indicated in virtually all cases, but usually the underlying cause of the pleural disease must be addressed for satisfactory management.

PLEURAL EFFUSIONS

Pathophysiology

The parietal pleural membranes are leaky to fluid and protein. Fluid is drained from the pleural space predominantly by bulk flow rather than diffusion, and the parietal pleural stomas are large enough to accommodate intact erythrocytes. The parietal lymphatics have a large capacity for absorption, and can increase the rate of pleural drainage by up to 30 times the baseline rate (Broaddus and Light, 1994).

Pleural effusions are likely to develop if:

- The rate of pleural fluid production increases
- The rate of drainage decreases
- Both are affected.

	Type	Aetiology
Pleural fluids	True transudate	Hypoproteinaemia
	Modified transudate	Congestive heart failure Neoplasia Lung lobe torsion Diaphragmatic rupture
	Non-septic exudate	Feline infectious peritonitis Repeated thoracocentesis Reaction to thoracostomy tubes Neoplasia

	Septic exudate	Pyothorax:
		  extension of intra-thoracic infection
		  penetration of chest wall
		  haematogenous spread

	Chylous effusions	Congestive heart failure Neoplasia Trauma Congenital Thrombosis of cranial vena cava Lymphangiectasia Idiopathic
	Haemorrhagic effusions	Neoplasia Trauma Coagulopathy Lung lobe torsion
	Neoplastic	Lymphoma Mesothelioma Primary or secondary lung tumours Chemodectoma Metastatic pleural tumours
Pneumothorax	Open	Penetrating trauma Iatrogenic (thoracocentesis, biopsy procedures)
	Closed	Blunt trauma Foreign bodies Rupture of blebs, bullae, neoplasms, abscesses Spontaneous pneumothorax

Table 18.1: Pleural conditions.

Increase in fluid production

Changes in Starling's forces may arise with an increase in hydrostatic pressure (congestive heart failure) or from a decrease in colloid osmotic pressure (hypoalbuminaemia). These forces will result in a *transudate*, where the pleural membranes are not themselves abnormal. Alternatively, the pleural membranes may be affected by inflammation, infection or neoplasia and the resulting increased capillary permeability will lead to production of a protein- and cell-rich *exudate*. Pleural effusions may also arise directly from intra-thoracic lesions, such as haemorrhage following trauma or from a bleeding neoplasm.

Decrease in rate of drainage

The parietal lymphatics may be affected by obstruction of the stomata, intra-thoracic lymph node disease, or raised systemic venous pressures affecting the flow from the thoracic duct. Many disease processes may affect both the rate of fluid production and drainage.

Clinical signs

History

Although pleural effusions generally develop gradually, the onset of clinical signs may appear to be comparatively sudden to the owner (Davies and Forrester, 1996). The severity of clinical signs may vary according to the underlying cause, the rate of accumulation, and volume of fluid. Animals may be almost asymptomatic (slow accumulation, small volume) or they can be severely compromised (rapid accumulation and large volumes). Large volumes of fluid can be tolerated in non-stressed, unexercised animals, but these animals will decompensate rapidly and fatally if not handled with care. Owners may have noticed exercise intolerance, and a reluctance to lie down. There may also be a non-specific history of inappetence, weight loss, lethargy and dehydration. Occasionally, coughing may be reported if there is concurrent airway compression.

Physical examination

When clinical signs do develop, they usually manifest as dyspnoea with a prolonged inspiratory phase, sometimes with abdominal breathing. There is no associated upper respiratory tract noise (in contrast with upper airway obstruction, which also causes inspiratory effort). Physical examination often reveals decreased respiratory sounds and muffled heart sounds, which is particularly marked ventrally. Dullness on percussion of the ventral thorax may also be noted. Severe cases will be cyanotic and have a distended thoracic cage.

Diagnosis

With severely dyspnoeic patients, thoracocentesis should be carried out prior to radiography if a pleural effusion is suspected. This will not only provide useful diagnostic information about the nature of the fluid, but it will also make radiography less hazardous and more informative. Any minor risks of thoracocentesis are outweighed by the potential advantages.

Thoracocentesis can be performed by needle aspiration using a butterfly cannula (see Chapter 29). As much fluid as possible should be withdrawn using a three-way tap and syringe.

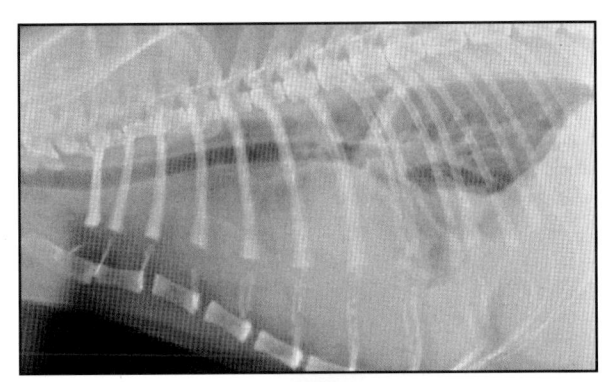
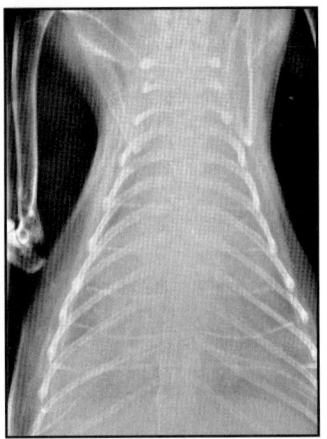

Figure 18.2: Lateral and dorsoventral radiographs of a 13-year-old cat with hyperthyroidism, showing leafing of the lung lobes, and an obscured cardiac silhouette.

Both sides of the chest should be drained to remove the maximum amount of fluid and ameliorate respiratory function. Aspirated fluid should be analysed grossly, microscopically and biochemically; samples should also be submitted for aerobic and anaerobic culture and sensitivity (Tyler and Cowell, 1989).

Careful *radiography* is used to detect the presence and amount of fluid, which may be evident as interlobar fissures and retraction or 'leafing' of lung lobe edges (Figure 18.2). It may also be possible to assess whether the fluid is free or encapsulated by adhesions. It may be possible to determine the underlying cause of the effusion with radiography, and thoracic radiographs should always be obtained post-thoracocentesis (see Chapter 5i). Contrast studies can prove useful in some pleural effusions (e.g. mesenteric lymphangiography for chylothorax, peritoneography for diaphragmatic ruptures).

Ultrasonography is used to evaluate cardiac and valvular function, the presence of pericardial effusion and mediastinal masses.

Types of pleural effusions

Effusions have been traditionally categorized in the laboratory as transudates, modified transudates or exudates, based on the amount of protein and cells (Table 18.2). This classification system can be useful as an initial diagnostic step, but there is considerable overlap between categories (Table 18.1). A cytological classification system can be used to divide the types of pleural effusions into categories according to the predominant cell type (Table 18.2). Protein levels and cell counts can provide further information.

True transudate

- Clear, colourless fluid with few cells, and low protein levels.

Hypoalbuminaemia is the principal cause of true transudates. Hypoalbuminaemia may result from protein-losing enteropathy, protein-losing nephropathy, or hepatic disease. Ascites or subcutaneous oedema may also be present.

Modified transudate

- Clear to moderately turbid, straw-coloured to amber or pink to red
- Low to moderate numbers of cells, moderate to high levels of protein
- Non-degenerate neutrophils, macrophages and mesothelial cells, small lymphocytes.

Many causes of pleural effusions result in modified transudates. Long-standing modified transudates may become more inflammatory in nature with time, so that they resemble exudates.

Type	Appearance	Fluid analysis	Cytology
True transudate	Clear, colourless or very pale yellow	Protein <25–30 g/l Cells <1.5 x 10⁹/l	Macrophages, lymphocytes, mesothelial cells
Modified transudate	Clear to moderately turbid; pale yellow/pink to straw-coloured/reddish	Protein <35 g/l Cells <1.0–7.0 x 10⁹/l	Macrophages, lymphocytes, mesothelial cells plus non-degenerate neutrophils
Non-septic exudate	Turbid, amber to reddish	Protein >30 g/l Cells >5.0 x 10⁹/l	Neutrophils, macrophages, lymphocytes
Septic exudate	Turbid or floccular, yellow/green/brown/red may be foul-smelling	Protein >30 g/l Cells 5.0–300 x 10⁹/l	Degenerate neutrophils, with phagocytosed bacteria
Chyle	White to milky pink/reddish	Protein >25 g/l Cells >0.4–20 x 10⁹/l	Small lymphocytes (few neutrophils); non-degenerate neutrophils, macrophages in long-standing effusions
Haemorrhage	Blood	Protein >30 g/l (nucleated) cells >3.0 x 10⁹/l (or >25% of peripheral blood values)	similar to peripheral blood
Neoplastic	Variable (see any of the above except true transudate)	Variable	Neoplastic cells may be present (e.g. lymphoma) or may not (haemangiosarcoma, chemodectoma)

Table 18.2: Cytological classification of pleural fluids.

Congestive heart failure

Pleural effusions are usually associated with right heart failure in dogs and cats, although small effusions can potentially develop with left-sided failure also. Signs of cardiac disease are usually present (e.g. murmurs, arrhythmias or gallop sounds) and distended jugular veins or ascites may be noted. Thoracocentesis may be used to relieve dyspnoea, but diuretics and specific cardiac treatment are used for long-term management.

Neoplasia

Neoplastic effusions may have enormously variable characteristics, and neoplastic cells will not always be evident on cytological examination, depending on the tumour type.

Lung lobe torsion

Lung lobe torsion may also be associated with haemorrhagic effusions and non-septic exudates. Lung lobe torsions may result in pleural effusions, and may occur spontaneously in narrow, deep-chested dogs. In other breeds of dog and cat, a pleural effusion may cause a lung lobe torsion. Reported predisposing causes include trauma, diaphragmatic hernia and thoracic surgery (Walter, 1987). The right middle lung lobe is most commonly affected. Torsions may be from 90 to more than 360°. Affected animals are frequently depressed, pyrexic and inappetent, in addition to being dyspnoeic.

Diagnosis of lung lobe torsions can be difficult; radiography may reveal atelectasis of the affected lobe, or abnormal orientation of lobar bronchi. Air bronchograms may also be present, or a bronchial lumen may terminate suddenly (Figure 18.3).

Management is as for other pleural effusions, but also includes lobectomy of the affected lobe.

Diaphragmatic hernia

Diaphragmatic hernia may also be associated with haemorrhagic effusions.

Entrapment of abdominal viscera in the chest following traumatic diaphragmatic hernia may lead to production of pleural fluid. Even partial herniation of hepatic tissue may result in significant effusions.

Diagnosis is made from plain radiographs or using

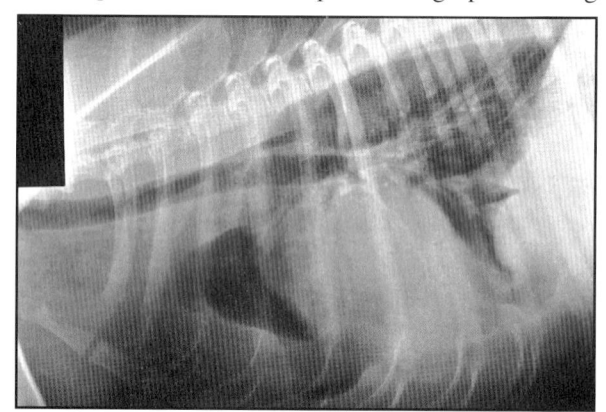

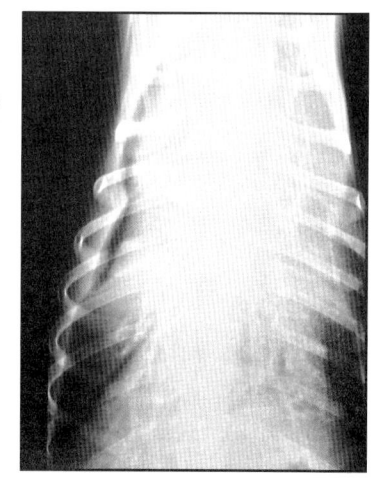

Figure 18.3: Lateral and dorsoventral radiographs of a 4-year-old Whippet with a pleural effusion and torsion of the right middle lung lobe.

barium studies to identify displacement of abdominal organs. Pneumoperitonography may also be used. Ultrasonography may be helpful in identifying diaphragmatic tears, particularly if there is minimal herniation.

Management requires repair of the hernia (see Chapter 30).

Non-septic inflammatory exudates

- Turbid, amber to reddish
- High protein levels and moderate to high levels of cells
- Hyper-segmented neutrophils, macrophages and lymphocytes.

In addition to specific conditions such as feline infectious peritonitis, non-septic exudates may develop from long-standing transudates or as a response to repeated thoracocentesis or to tube thoracostomies.

Feline infectious peritonitis (FIP)

The fluid associated with FIP may be very viscous with high protein levels (40–100 g/l). Ascites may sometimes be present, and serum globulins may also be high. Ocular changes may be present, such as anterior uveitis.

Septic exudate

- Turbid or floccular, yellow to green, brown or reddish and foul-smelling
- Very high cell counts (up to $300 \times 10^9/l$)
- Many degenerate neutrophils with intracellular and extracellular bacteria.

Pyothorax

The presence of infected, purulent fluid in the pleural cavity is termed pyothorax or empyema. The source of infection may be:

- Extension from structures within the chest (pneumonia, mediastinitis, oesophageal rupture)
- Introduction of infection through the chest wall (trauma, bite wounds, migration of foreign bodies or iatrogenic)
- Haematogenous spread.

Organisms commonly isolated include *Actinomyces, Nocardia, Bacteroides* spp, *Pasteurella* spp, and *Fusobacterium* spp. Anaerobic infections are particularly common in cats.

Affected animals are usually depressed and inappetent, with weight loss and dyspnoea. Most are pyrexic.

Radiography will reveal a pleural effusion that is sometimes unilateral or localized. Thoracocentesis yields a typical exudate with large numbers of degen-erate neutrophils on cytological examination. Gram stains should be made prior to receiving culture results; many organisms are difficult to grow and a positive Gram stain is invaluable if culture is negative. Pleural fluid samples must be submitted for aerobic and anaerobic culture. Anaerobic organisms are very common, and may be difficult to identify. Negative culture results do not rule out pyothorax, especially if previous therapy has included antimicrobials.

Management is based on effective thoracic drainage, and appropriate antimicrobial therapy. Thorough drainage requires placement of thoracostomy tubes and continuous suction. Intermittent drainage with indwelling chest tubes is less effective, but may still result in a successful outcome if drainage is carried out frequently. 'Stripping' of the tubes may be necessary to prevent the exudate from blocking the tubes. Repeated thoracocentesis will not result in adequate drainage, and will cause distress to the patient. As most infections are anaerobic, *ampicillin* is the first-line drug of choice. This should be given at high doses intravenously every 4–8 hours initially, then it can be given orally according to the animal's response. In cats, *clindamycin* (25 mg every 8 hours) should be given with ampicillin if *Bacteroides fragilis* is cultured (Bauer and Woodfield, 1995). The response to therapy can be assessed by the volume of exudate drained, and cytology and Gram stains of the fluid. If an adequate response is not obtained, cultures should be repeated. Once the volume of fluid recovered is less than 2 ml/kg per day, and cytology indicates non-degenerative neutrophils with no bacteria visible, then the chest tubes can be removed. Oral antibiotic therapy should be maintained for 6–12 weeks. Inadequate management may result in high mortality rates or chronic complications. With aggressive drainage, the prognosis is good (Turner and Breznock, 1988).

Chylous effusions

- White to pink or reddish
- Moderate to high numbers of cells, moderate to high levels of protein
- Predominantly small lymphocytes, with increasing numbers of neutrophils (especially in cats), macrophages, mesothelial cells and eosinophils with chronic effusions.

True rupture of the thoracic duct appears to be rare (Birchard *et al.*, 1988). Chylous effusions have been reported with thoracic neoplasia, right-sided cardiac failure, lymphangiectasia, trauma, cranial vena cava thrombosis associated with cannulation, and congenital or idiopathic causes (Birchard and Fossum, 1987). Afghan Hounds are over-represented in the literature (Fossum *et al.*, 1986). Oesophageal surgery, ligation of patent ductus arteriosus, or jugular catheterization procedures may result in iatrogenic chylothorax.

Diagnosis has traditionally been complicated by the requirement to distinguish 'true chyle' from 'pseudochylous' effusions. True chyle is derived from the fluid found in the thoracic duct and contains chylomicrons, whereas pseudochyle contains cholesterol or lecithin-globulin complexes that are responsible for the milky appearance. However, it is probably preferable to refer to 'chylous' or 'non-chylous' effusions, as pseudochylous effusions appear to be uncommon, and the fluid in the majority of chylous effusions in cats and dogs is probably true chyle. Chylous effusions are not always typically milky-appearing, and centrifugation can be helpful in demonstrating persistence of turbidity (in contrast with exudates, which will develop a clear supernatant on centrifugation). Other tests confirming a chylous effusion include comparing triglyceride levels in the effusion with serum. Chylous effusions will have triglyceride levels higher than serum levels.

Management can be very challenging. Even successful treatment of the underlying cause may not result in resolution of the chylothorax, and frequently the underlying cause is not readily corrected. Conservative management is usually attempted first, and consists of drainage of the fluid as necessary, with a low fat diet to reduce production of chyle. This is rarely successful. *Thoracic duct ligation* is effective in about 50% of cases, although it may be less effective in cats (see Chapter 30). Sometimes thoracic duct ligation will prevent accumulation of chyle, but production of a modified transudate persists. *Pleuroperitoneal shunts* have also been used to shunt chylous effusions from the chest to the abdomen (see Chapter 30). *Pleurodesis* has also been tried, where agents such as oxytetracycline hydrochloride are instilled into the (completely drained) pleural cavity in an attempt to create adhesions between the visceral and parietal pleura. Effective pleurodesis should limit the space into which chyle can accumulate. Unfortunately, it is often difficult to induce pleurodesis, and it can also be associated with considerable discomfort unless adequate analgesia is used.

Medical management has recently been attempted with use of *benzopyrones* or rutosides (Fossum, 1996).

Complications of chronic chylous effusions include *fibrosing pleuritis*, where the visceral pleura becomes grossly thickened and prevents re-expansion of the underlying atelectatic lung (Fossum *et al.*, 1992). Animals with severe fibrosing pleuritis may appear to have marked pleural effusions on radiography, but on drainage only a small volume of effusion is found to be present. The borders of the lung lobes may appear rounded with thickened edges. The prognosis is extremely guarded for affected animals, as surgical decortication often results in intractable pneumothorax.

Haemorrhagic effusions

- Sanguinous, non-clotting
- Erythrocytes, white cells, total protein >25% of serum values
- Differential white count similar to peripheral blood; no platelets and phagocytosis of erythrocytes in macrophages.

Thoracic trauma, bleeding neoplasms and coagulopathies may all cause haemothorax. Lung lobe torsions may also result in a haemorrhagic effusion. The history and evidence of trauma or bleeding at other sites may indicate the cause. Clotting tests may be indicated for coagulopathies, and radiography may be helpful for the diagnosis of tumours. Resorption of blood from the pleural cavity occurs rapidly via the parietal lymphatics; drainage of haemothorax following trauma is only indicated if dyspnoea is severe.

Neoplastic effusions

- Transudates, exudates, chylous and haemorrhagic effusions may all be produced by tumours
- Neoplastic cells may only be present with exfoliative tumours.

Both primary and metastatic tumours may produce pleural effusions. Mediastinal lymphomas will often result in the presence of lymphoblasts in pleural fluid. Adenocarcinomas may also exfoliate, and clumps of large, basophilic, pleomorphic cells may be seen. Metastatic carcinomas may also shed cells, and it may be possible to identify the tumour type with mast cell tumours or malignant melanomas. Sarcomas (such as haemangiosarcoma) do not tend to exfoliate. Activated mesothelial cells may be multi-nucleated, but should not be confused with neoplastic cells; air-dried smears should be submitted to a skilled cytopathologist. Malignant mesothelioma cells present a particular challenge, and pleural biopsy may be indicated. Biopsy procedures are also indicated for non-exfoliative intra-thoracic neoplasms.

PNEUMOTHORAX

Air may enter the pleural space via a breach in the chest wall ('open' pneumothorax), or via the lungs or mediastinum. *Open pneumothorax* may be the result of trauma, or may be iatrogenic. Potential iatrogenic causes include thoracocentesis and biopsy procedures, and inadequately sealed thoracostomy tubes. *Closed pneumothorax* may also be the result of trauma, as compression of the abdomen against a closed glottis can lead to rupture of a bronchus or the pulmonary parenchyma (Kramek and Caywood, 1987). *Sponta-*

neous pneumothorax occurs without a history of trauma, although pulmonary lesions are usually responsible (Holtsinger *et al.*, 1993). Rupture of pulmonary bullae or blebs, penetrating foreign bodies, or rupture of pulmonary cavitating neoplasms or abscesses may result in pneumothorax. True spontaneous pneumothorax has also been reported in dogs, where no underlying cause could be found.

Tension pneumothorax occurs when air can enter the pleural cavity, but the air cannot leave via the same entry point during expiration. Tears in the pulmonary parenchyma may act as a one-way valve.

Pathophysiology

The effects of a mild to moderate pneumothorax are similar to the effects of a pleural effusion. However, tension pneumothorax may lead to markedly increased intrapleural pressures. This leads to maximal chest expansion, so that the animal's ability to inspire is severely impeded. In addition, the raised intrapleural pressures interfere with venous return and thus reduce cardiac filling and cardiac output. As the lungs collapse, non-aerated areas of lung may be perfused, causing ventilation–perfusion mismatch. Tension pneumothorax is fatal unless treated rapidly.

History

Frequently there is a history of trauma, although signs with spontaneous pneumothorax may develop gradually.

Physical examination

The animal will usually be tachypnoeic, and in severe cases there will be cyanosis and pale mucous membranes. The chest may be distended with severe pneumothorax. The heart sounds may be muffled, and hyper-resonance may be detected on percussion.

Diagnosis

With suggestive clinical signs, the diagnosis may be confirmed by thoracocentesis. If the animal is sufficiently stable, radiographs should be taken. Classical findings of pneumothorax are retraction of lung lobes from the chest wall, with a radiolucent space free of vascular markings between the lungs and chest wall (Figure 18.4). The heart is frequently lifted off the sternum on lateral views. Where the pneumothorax is unilateral, the mediastinum may be markedly displaced to the opposite side. Underlying lesions may be evident on radiography, such as neoplasms or evidence of pneumonia. Blebs and bullae are often difficult to identify.

Management

If the pneumothorax is small and the animal is asymptomatic, then conservative management may be sufficient with close monitoring and cage rest only. With traumatic and iatrogenic pneumothorax, needle thoracocentesis may be adequate to drain the pleural cavity, although close monitoring should again be maintained. Spontaneous pneumothorax generally requires tube thoracostomy, and frequently requires surgical intervention to deal with the cause (Holtsinger *et al.*, 1993). Exploratory thoracotomy both allows detection of any underlying cause of spontaneous pneumothorax, and permits corrective lobectomy (e.g. for pulmonary bullae or blebs) (see Chapter 30).

DISORDERS OF THE DIAPHRAGM

Anatomy

The diaphragm is a musculo-tendinous sheet that separates the abdominal and pleural cavities. The central portion is tendinous, with muscular attachments radiating out to attach to the lumbar vertebrae, the ribs and the sternum. The aorta, the azygos and hemiazygos veins, and the thoracic duct pass through the diaphragm at the aortic hiatus; the oesophagus and vagal trunks pass through the oesophageal hiatus. The caudal vena cava crosses the diaphragm separately.

Diaphragmatic hernia

Any protrusion of abdominal contents into the thoracic cavity via the diaphragm may be termed a diaphragmatic hernia. Examples include congenital peritoneo–pericardial hernias (see Chapter 14), and hiatal hernias. The most common form, however, is traumatic diaphragmatic rupture. This is usually the result of blunt trauma (typically a road traffic accident) where compressive forces on the abdomen lead to rupture of the diaphragm and herniation of abdominal viscera into the thoracic cavity (Levine, 1987).

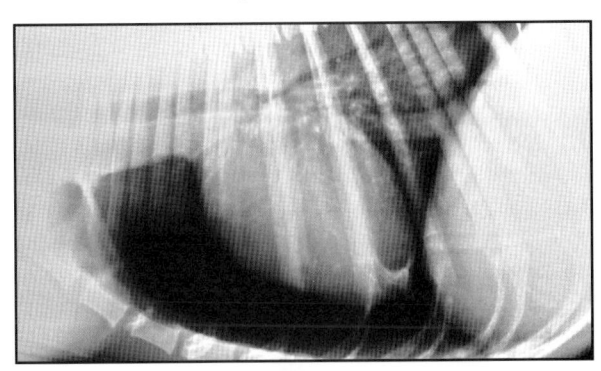
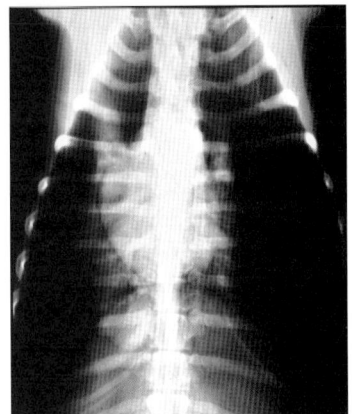

Figure 18.4: Lateral and dorsoventral radiographs of a severe tension pneumothorax in a Boxer, showing marked distension of the chest cavity and elevation of the heart from the sternum. The pneumothorax was caused by the sewing needle visible in the right caudal lobe overlying the diaphragm.

History

Animals may be presented immediately following a road traffic accident, and dyspnoea may be accompanied by signs of shock and other injuries, or respiratory signs may be minimal. Alternatively, animals may be presented a considerable period of time after the traumatic episode (even years later), and owners may need to be questioned closely. Acute exacerbations of chronic diaphragmatic rupture may occur following development of a pleural effusion, or dilation of a herniated stomach. Clinical signs may be restricted to signs of exercise intolerance in chronic cases, or gastrointestinal signs may be shown.

Physical examination

With acute and chronic diaphragmatic ruptures, affected animals may have muffled heart sounds, or a displaced apex beat. There may be evidence of a pleural effusion on percussion, or even increased resonance if there is a gas-filled abdominal viscus in the chest. If there is herniation of many abdominal organs, the abdomen may feel 'empty'.

Diagnosis

Radiography will frequently reveal evidence of diaphragmatic rupture (Figure 18.5), although pleural effusions may obscure abdominal organs and cause loss of the diaphragmatic outline. In addition, abdominal organs may move between the chest and the abdomen. Sometimes barium studies can be helpful in

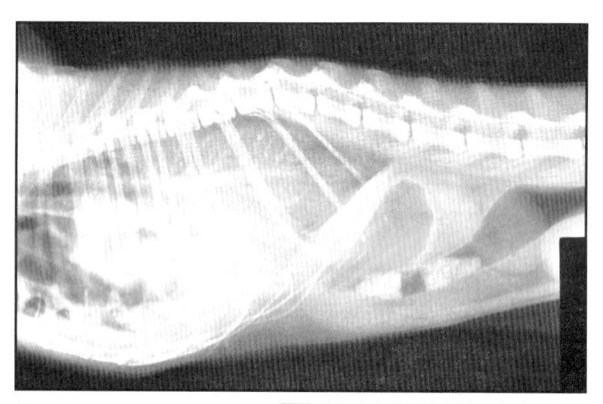

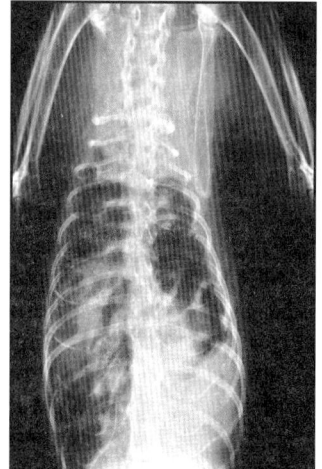

Figure 18.5: Lateral and dorsoventral radiographs of a 12-year-old cat with a diaphragmatic rupture caused by a road traffic accident as a kitten. Multiple intestinal loops are visible within the chest, with the stomach and colon the only parts of the gastrointestinal tract remaining within the abdomen.

outlining displacement of the gastrointestinal tract. Pneumoperitoneography and positive contrast peritoneography have been used to demonstrate small diaphragmatic tears. Ultrasonography is now used more commonly.

Management

Acutely presenting animals must be stabilized with treatment for shock and haemorrhage. Adequate oxygenation must be ensured, and any pleural effusions will usually need to be drained if not already carried out prior to diagnosis. However, the treatment for diaphragmatic rupture is *surgical repair*, and this should be carried out once the animal's condition is sufficiently stable (see Chapter 30). The prognosis is excellent with successful surgical repair.

Paralysis of the diaphragm

The diaphragm is innervated by the phrenic nerves, which arise from the cervical roots of C4–C7. Damage to the phrenic nerves may occur with cervical spinal trauma, space-occupying lesions in the chest, or with surgical procedures of the cranial mediastinum or pericardium. Unilateral damage to the phrenic nerves is rarely associated with significant clinical signs, but bilateral paralysis may cause dyspnoea associated with eating or recumbency. Confirmation of the diagnosis is obtained with fluoroscopy, which demonstrates minimal motion of the diaphragm with inspiration.

MEDIASTINAL DISEASE

Anatomy

The central extrapleural tissues of the chest form the mediastinum. The mediastinum is divided into three sections: the cranial, middle and caudal mediastinum; all covered by reflections of the parietal pleura.

The cranial mediastinum contains the heart, vessels to the head and neck, oesophagus, nerves and thymus. The middle mediastinum contains the heart and major vessels, tracheobronchial lymph nodes and oesophagus. The caudal mediastinum contains the oesophagus, aorta, caudal vena cava and phrenic nerves.

Mediastinal masses

Cranial mediastinal masses are common. Lymphoma is the most common cause (especially in cats). Other neoplasms affecting the cranial mediastinum include thymoma, thymic carcinoma and chemodectoma. Non-neoplastic masses include abscesses, haematomas and granulomas. Mediastinal masses may cause respiratory signs by production of pleural effusions, or by displacement of lung tissue if large. Compression of the oesophagus may lead to regurgitation (Figure 18.6); compression of the trachea and bronchi may cause coughing; and compression of the cranial vena cava may cause oedema of the ventral neck and head, and forelimbs.

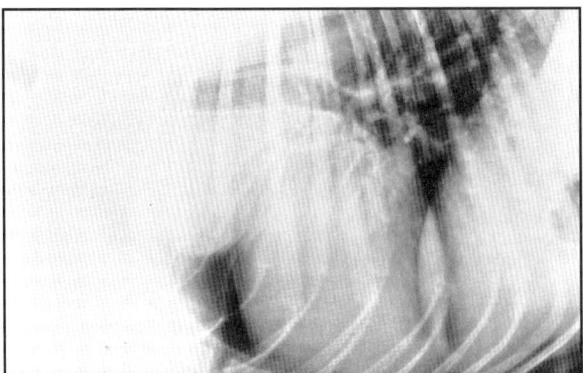

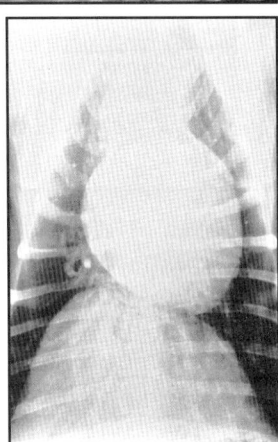

Figure 18.6: Lateral and dorsoventral radiographs of a Boxer with a cranial mediastinal mass, causing widening of the mediastinum on the dorsoventral view and dorsal displacement of the trachea on the lateral view. The mass was a chemodectoma.

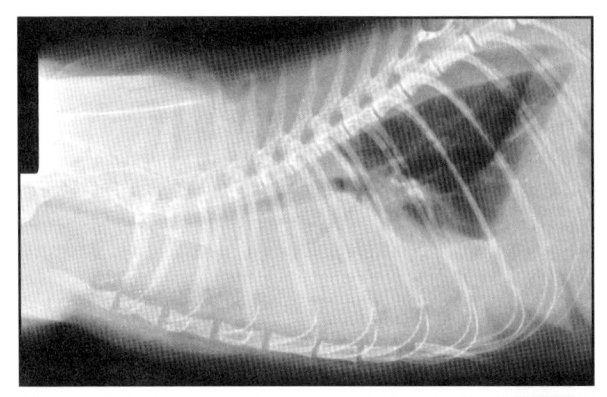

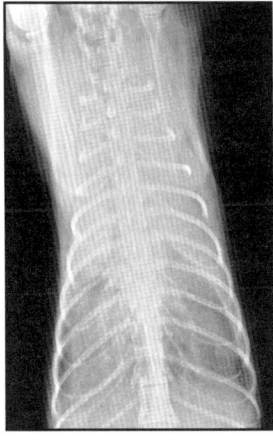

Figure 18.7: Lateral and dorsoventral radiographs of a 1-year-old cat with a thymic lymphoma, showing elevation of the trachea, a widened cranial mediastinum and an obscured cardiac silhouette.

Diagnosis

Clinical signs include incompressibility of the cranial chest – this is easier to detect in cats than dogs. Radiography will reveal a widened mediastinum, with displacement of the trachea and frequently, with neoplasia, pleural effusion (Figure 18.7). The heart and cranial lungs may be displaced caudally, although caution should be observed as large pleural effusions may sometimes mimic cranial mediastinal masses. Cytology of pleural fluid may suggest neoplasia (particularly with lymphoma), or a fine needle aspirate may be obtained from the mass. Ultrasound-guided biopsy of the mass may be helpful. If ultrasonography shows the lesion to be small, cystic, vascular, or close to major vessels or the heart, then biopsy material is better obtained at exploratory thoracotomy (see Chapter 30).

Management

Thymic lymphoma may respond to chemotherapy; surgical exploration of other masses is warranted to obtain biopsy material for a histopathological diagnosis. Excision of non-lymphomatous mediastinal masses may be attempted at the same time (see Chapter 30).

Pneumomediastinum

Pneumomediastinum is the presence of air within the mediastinum. This may occur as a result of pulmonary trauma or from wounds to the head and neck, so that air tracks between tissue planes. Pneumomediastinum is often accompanied by pneumothorax. Pneumomediastinum may also occur secondary to air-trapping with feline asthma.

Diagnosis

Affected animals may not show severe dyspnoea, unless there is significant concurrent pneumothorax. Subcutaneous emphysema may be present. Severe pneumomediastinum may impede venous return, and cause hypotension. Radiography shows mediastinal structures outlined by air, so that structures which are not generally seen may be clearly visible (e.g. the brachiocephalic trunk and azygos vein).

Management

Cage rest is often the only possible treatment for pneumomediastinum. Any associated pneumothorax, or underlying disease should obviously be treated.

Mediastinitis

Mediastinitis may be a sequel to oesophageal perforation, tracheal rupture or even stick injuries affecting the head and neck. Pneumothorax and pyothorax may be accompanying complications. Chronic mediastinitis may result in mediastinal granulomas. Tube thoracotomy may be necessary, and oesophageal and tracheal perforation will require surgical repair. Aerobic and anaerobic cultures should be carried out, and prolonged, aggressive antibiotic therapy is usually required.

Mediastinal lymphadenopathy

Enlargement of the mediastinal and sternal lymph nodes may be seen with lymphoma, metastatic neoplasia, pyothorax or mediastinitis, and tuberculosis.

REFERENCES

Bauer T and Woodfield JA (1995) Mediastinal, pleural, and extrapleural diseases. In: *Textbook of Veterinary Internal Medicine*, 4th edn, ed. SJ Ettinger and EC Feldman, pp 812–842. WB Saunders, Philadephia

Birchard SJ and Fossum TW (1987) Chylothorax in the dog and cat. *Veterinary Clinics of North America – Small Animal Practice* **17**, 271–283

Birchard SJ, Smeak DD and Fossum TW (1988) Results of thoracic duct ligation in dogs with chylothorax. *Journal of the American Veterinary Medical Association* **193**, 68–71

Broaddus VC and Light RW (1994) Disorders of the pleura. In: *Textbook of Respiratory Medicine*, 2nd edn, ed. JF Murray and JA Nadel, pp 2145–2163. WB Saunders, Philadelphia

Davies C and Forrester SD (1996) Pleural effusion in cats: 82 cases (1987 to 1995). *Journal of Small Animal Practice* **37**, 217–224

Fossum TW (1996) Feline chylothorax. *Proceedings of the American College of Veterinary Internal Medicine Forum*, Blacksburg, Virginia, pp 157–159

Fossum TW, Birchard SJ and Jacobs RM (1986) Chylothorax in 34 dogs. *Journal of the American Veterinary Medical Association* **188**, 1315–1318

Fossum TW, Evering WN, Miller MW, Forrester SD, Palmer DR, and Hodges CC (1992) Severe bilateral fibrosing pleuritis associated with chronic chylothorax in five cats and two dogs. *Journal of the American Veterinary Medical Association* **201**, 317–324

Holtsinger RH, Beale BS, Bellah JR and King RR (1993) Spontaneous pneumothorax in the dog – a retrospective analysis of 21 cases. *Journal of the American Animal Hospital Association* **29**, 195–210

Kinasewitz GT (1998) Pleural fluid dynamics and effusions. In: *Fishman's Pulmonary Diseases and Disorders*, 3rd edn, ed. AP Fishman, pp 1389–1409. McGraw-Hill, New York

Kramek BA and Caywood DD (1987) Pneumothorax. *Veterinary Clinics of North America – Small Animal Practice* **17**, 285–300

Levine SH (1987) Diaphragmatic hernia. *Veterinary Clinics of North America – Small Animal Practice* **17**, 411–430

Turner WD and Breznock EM (1988) Continuous suction drainage for management of canine pyothorax – a retrospective study. *Journal of the American Animal Hospital Association* **24**, 485–494

Tyler RD and Cowell RL (1989) Evaluation of pleural and peritoneal effusions. *Veterinary Clinics of North America – Small Animal Practice* **19**, 743–768

Walter PA (1987) Non-neoplastic surgical diseases of the lung and pleura. *Veterinary Clinics of North America – Small Animal Practice* **17**, 359–385

Specific Feline Cardiopulmonary Conditions

Rebecca L. Stepien

THE DYSPNOEIC CAT

Dyspnoeic cats present special problems to the veterinary practitioner. The usual pet feline lifestyle allows patients with substantial respiratory or cardiac disease to 'hide' this problem from the owner for long periods of time. If the disease is progressive, the patient will eventually be unable to hide the clinical signs. Unfortunately, recognition of clinical cardiopulmonary disease by the owner may occur only when the disease becomes an emergency situation.

Many serious cardiopulmonary diseases of cats result in non-specific clinical signs (e.g. lethargy and inappetence). The general nature of these presenting signs makes careful and thorough physical examination techniques mandatory.

DIFFERENTIAL DIAGNOSIS OF FELINE DYSPNOEA

Establishing a realistic differential diagnosis for dyspnoeic feline patients requires evaluation of the history, physical examination findings and results of any ancillary testing (see Chapter 7).

History

The owner of a dyspnoeic cat should be carefully queried as to the onset, recurrence pattern (if any) and physical description of the dyspnoeic episodes.

Onset

Although many clinical signs in ill cats appear to the owner to have occurred just prior to presentation, careful questioning may elicit recollection of prior similar episodes. Typical patterns relating to onset of dyspnoea are described in Table 19.1.

Nature of clinical signs

The physical characteristics of the dyspnoeic episodes are perhaps the most valuable aetiological clue in the history of the patient, and the owner should be asked about any progression or change since the onset of signs. The cat's dyspnoea may worsen with the stress and excitement of transport to the veterinary clinic, but occasionally, the transient episode may partially resolve by the time the patient arrives at the clinic.

Onset	*Recurrent dyspnoeic episodes ± cough over a period of years*	Chronic bronchitis; pulmonary fibrosis
	Recent onset and rapid progression	Pleural effusion; infectious diseases; allergic diseases
	Peracute onset (within 24 hours of presentation) Note: *slowly progressive causes of dyspnoea may appear to be peracute in onset if the patient decompensates rapidly*	Foreign body inhalation; pulmonary oedema (CHF); thoracic trauma; acute bronchoconstriction
Recurrence	*Recurrent dyspnoeic episodes that resolve without therapy*	Feline bronchial diseases
Response to therapy	*Frusemide*	CHF (pulmonary oedema or pleural effusion)
	Antibiotics	Recurrent infectious bronchitis; bronchopneumonia
	Corticosteroids	Inflammatory or allergic process
	Bronchodilators	Dynamic bronchoconstriction

Table 19.1: Historical findings in feline dyspnoea.

Severely dyspnoeic cats may assume characteristic postures to ease respiration (sternal recumbency with minimal movement, neck extension, elbows abducted). Panting in cats should be treated as an emergency until proven otherwise, especially if associated with cyanosis.

Cats with small airway or alveolar disease usually exhibit increased expiratory effort without inspiratory effort. Small airways collapse or constrict on expiration leading to air-trapping and progression of emphysema. Wheezing or bubbling sounds may be audible without a stethoscope. The combination of increased expiratory effort with wheezing is typical of cats with severe bronchial disease.

DIFFERENTIAL DIAGNOSIS OF FELINE COUGHING

Cats with cardiac disease or cardiac failure seldom cough unless they have heartworm disease, or their cardiac disease is complicated by pulmonary disease. Chronic and progressive coughing usually reflects pneumonic, neoplastic or advanced bronchial disease (Henik and Yeager, 1994), although cats with pyothorax may also cough. Diseases that involve the alveoli rarely cause coughing, unless the airways are also involved (however, many conditions involve both).

The presence a of cough may dictate the diagnostic plan. If pulmonary disease is suspected, tracheobronchial washes are helpful diagnostic tests. Bronchoalveolar lavage (BAL) and/or bronchoscopically guided lavage or brushings are recommended for diagnosis of respiratory disease not associated with coughing.

DIFFERENTIATING CARDIAC FROM PULMONARY DISEASE

Differentiation of primary pulmonary disease from cardiovascular disease is relatively straightforward in the majority of feline patients and is summarized in Table 19.2. History and physical examination are helpful to distinguish these causes of dyspnoea, but ancillary tests (thoracic radiographs, ECG) are often indispensable in the differentiation of cardiac versus pulmonary causes of dyspnoea (see individual conditions, later).

A finding of aortic thromboembolism in the presence of severe dyspnoea is pathognomonic for cardiac disease. Systemic signs associated with cardiac disease include hypothermia, weight loss, dehydration and an unkempt appearance. Prerenal azotaemia is common. Moderate to severe weight loss in an older patient with cardiac signs and a palpable cervical thyroid nodule suggests thyrotoxicosis as the underlying cause of cardiac abnormalities.

	Cardiac disease	Respiratory disease
Lethargy	+	±
Cough	–	+
Dyspnoea	+	+
Wheezing	–	+
Panting	+	+
Cyanosis	+	+
Pleural effusion	+	a
Heart murmur	+	±
Arrhythmia	+	b
Tachycardia	c	–

Table 19.2: *Differential diagnosis of clinical signs associated with feline cardiac or respiratory disease. + indicates sign is frequently associated with disease, – indicates sign is infrequently associated with disease. a: when seen in association with respiratory disease usually related to neoplastic disease, b: except respiratory sinus arrhythmia, c: occasional cats with congestive heart failure exhibit bradycardia.*

FELINE BRONCHIAL DISEASE

The terms 'feline bronchial disease', 'feline bronchopulmonary disease' and 'feline asthma' have been used to describe a disease syndrome in cats characterized by variable combinations of increased and sometimes profuse bronchial secretions, dynamic bronchoconstriction, and obstructive respiratory physiology. Although the subject of much laboratory and clinical investigation in recent years, the exact cause of this syndrome has not been well defined. As more information accumulates however, it has become apparent that the inflammatory bronchial disease recognized in the feline population is probably not a single entity, but may be several diseases with differing manifestations and responses to therapy (Table 19.3). Dye (1992) suggested that the diagnosis of feline bronchial disease is 'primarily a diagnosis of exclusion'. Diseases that can be directly treated (e.g. bacterial bronchitis) should be excluded before instituting chronic palliative care for inflammatory feline bronchial disease.

Incidence

Feline bronchial disease is often described as 'common', but it is unclear exactly what percentage of the feline veterinary population is affected by this set of disorders. In a retrospective study of 65 cases of feline bronchial disease diagnosed in the eastern United States, there was a predominantly female population affected, and Siamese cats were over-represented (Moise *et al*, 1989).

Classification of feline bronchial disease

Classification of feline bronchial disease is not straightforward. Previous descriptions of feline bron-

Disease	Age	Onset	Progression	Dyspnoea	Coughing	Wheezing	Therapy*	Typical therapeutic course	Comments
Bronchial asthma	Young middle-aged	Acute	Intermittent	Intermittent	Mild to moderate	Usually	Bronchodilators	Intermittent, dyspnoea may resolve spontaneously	Normal to overweight cats
Acute bronchitis	Middle-aged to old	Acute	Acute	Acute, variable severity	Productive	Usually	Corticosteroids Nebulization Antimicrobials, Anthelmintics	Once or intermittent	Often caused by infectious, or parasitic agents
Chronic bronchitis	Middle-aged to old	Chronic	Chronic	Less common	Intermittent or continuous	Some cases	Bronchodilators Corticosteroids Nebulization	Often lifelong	May have concurrent bronchial asthma (see below)
Chronic asthmatic bronchitis	Any	Acute intermittent bronchoconstriction with concurrent chronic bronchitis	Intermittent	Acute, severe	Chronic +/- productive	Acute/ chronic	Chronic phase: as chronic bronchitis Acute phase: as bronchial asthma	Chronic phase: lifelong Acute phase: intermittent	
Chronic bronchitis with emphysema	Middle-aged to old	Chronic	Chronic	Especially expiratory	Chronic, dry or productive	Usually	Bronchodilators Corticosteroids	Lifelong	Dyspnoea often severe at rest Air-trapping and bullae on radiographs

Table 19.3: Feline bronchial diseases.

*Note: in all cases, appropriate tests should be performed to rule out infectious or parasitic disease. If any of these conditions are diagnosed, initial therapy (other than emergency therapy) is directed to eliminating the underlying aetiology.

chial diseases tended to group animals with diverse signs as exhibiting various manifestations of essentially the same disease process (Bauer, 1989, Hawkins *et al.*, 1989), but it has become apparent that this population of sick animals may be divided based on clinical signs into categories that allow the use of specific therapies and more accurate prognostication. Dye and Moise (1992) suggested the division of feline bronchial disease patients into five categories: bronchial asthma, acute bronchitis, chronic bronchitis, chronic asthmatic bronchitis and chronic bronchitis with emphysema. This classification system is helpful in the clinical evaluation of individual patients because it is based on history, clinical signs and diagnostic test results rather than on histological findings, which are often not available in the clinical setting of pulmonary disease.

Aetiopathogenesis

The combination of problems underlying the clinical manifestations of bronchial disease include hyper-reactivity of the bronchiolar smooth muscle, and inflammation of the bronchial and bronchiolar linings. The hyperreactivity of the trachea and bronchi to irritating stimuli is similar to humans with asthma, and has led to application of the human terminology to cats. The hyperreactivity may reflect a true type I hypersensitivity response, autonomic imbalance, or mucociliary function abnormalities (Dye and Moise, 1992; Henik and Yeager, 1994). In some cases, signs of acute

bronchoconstriction are obviously temporally related to exposure to a 'triggering' substance or event, similar to findings in asthmatic people. This suggests imbalances between the bronchodilating non-adrenergic, non-cholinergic (NANC) system and bronchoconstricting cholinergic system (Dye and Moise 1992). Clinical signs of acute bronchoconstriction (expiratory effort, coughing, wheezing) are frequently seen in feline bronchial patients, but airway hypersensitivity is difficult to prove in the clinical setting.

Underlying inflammatory bronchial disease may lead to or help maintain acute bronchoconstriction through the release of bronchoconstrictive mediators from inflammatory cells that have migrated into the airway. Inflammatory mediators such as histamine and leukotrienes potentiate further inflammation and may in themselves cause bronchoconstriction (Dye and Moise, 1992). Inflammation may be acute or chronic, and is characterized by mucosal oedema and exudation; submucosal gland and goblet cell hyperplasia, and epithelial cell desquamation. If secondary bacterial infection is present, accumulations of mucus and pus may be present.

The final common pathway in feline bronchial disease is *airway obstruction* due to accumulations of mucus or mucopurulent exudates in airways already narrowed by bronchoconstriction. Chronically, expiratory obstruction to airflow leads to air trapping, and irreversible and progressive destruction of alveolar septa.

History and physical examination

Clinical subdivision of feline bronchial disease is based on history, clinical presentation and response to specific therapies (Table 19.3). Diagnostic testing is similar regardless of the classification. The findings on physical examination of feline bronchial disease vary with type and chronicity of disease. In general, dyspnoea, pulmonary crackles, wheezes and cyanosis are present in variable degrees. Heart rate may be decreased if respiratory effort is marked, and respiratory sinus arrhythmia may be present. The extent of the physical examination is strictly dictated by the level of distress exhibited by the patient, as intermittent supplemental oxygen and rest periods may be needed even during the initial examination.

Diagnosis

No definitive clinical diagnostic test for feline bronchoconstrictive disease exists; diagnosis is based on historical and clinical findings, compatible findings on ancillary testing, and exclusion of other causes of bronchial disease. Thorough initial work-up will definitively rule out other causes of bronchial disease, and the clinician can begin therapy with confidence. Initial therapies may need to be adjusted or changed if response is not adequate.

Minimum data base

A complete blood count, biochemistry and urinalysis allows exclusion of metabolic causes of dyspnoea, establishes a baseline to measure response to therapy and is vital if complications of therapy develop.

Haematological abnormalities reported to occur with feline bronchial diseases include circulating eosinophilia (18% of affected cats) and hyperproteinaemia (plasma protein > 75 g/l, 32% of cases). Circulating eosinophilia was not necessarily related to the predominant type of cell seen in bronchial lavage cytological samples (Moise *et al.*, 1989). In cases where circulating eosinophilia is observed, parasitic causes of pulmonary disease as well as feline heartworm disease (in endemic areas) should be ruled out using appropriate tests. Serum biochemical findings may reflect systemic changes such as mild dehydration. Urinalysis findings are normal unless systemic abnormalities are present.

Radiography

The radiographic changes in feline bronchial disease are summarized in Table 19.4. Thoracic radiographs are mandatory in the diagnosis and monitoring of feline bronchial disease. Early in the course of disease, changes may include minor accentuation of bronchial markings or development of mild interstitial infiltrates. If the cat's dyspnoeic events are intermittent, air-trapping (over-inflated lung fields, flattened diaphragm) may be noted during the event but later resolve. Bronchial wall thickening is evident

radiographically as 'doughnuts' when seen in cross-section and 'tram lines' (parallel lines) when seen in long-axis (Figure 19.1).

As the bronchial disease progresses or if complicated by secondary infection, the bronchial pattern may become more marked or more prominent interstitial patterns may develop. If bacterial pneumonia develops, alveolar infiltrates may be seen, especially in the ventral lung lobes. Although bronchial neoplasia cannot be completely ruled out on the basis of radiographic examination, 'typical' feline bronchial disease does not involve nodular or mass lesions or pleural effusion. Intrathoracic lymph nodes are normal in uncomplicated bronchial disease. Collapse of the right middle lung lobe is seen occasionally (approximately 10% of cases) and usually is thought to reflect chronicity of disease (Moise *et al.*, 1989).

When emphysema and signs of chronic obstructive pulmonary disease develop, thoracic radiographs may reflect permanent hyperinflation of lung fields. The cardiac silhouette may appear to be diminished in size and there is increased space between the cardiac silhouette and the diaphragm. The diaphragm is often flattened in appearance. In addition to signs of air-trapping, previous pulmonary patterns (bronchial, interstitial) are still present and the right middle lung lobe may be permanently consolidated (Figure 19.2).

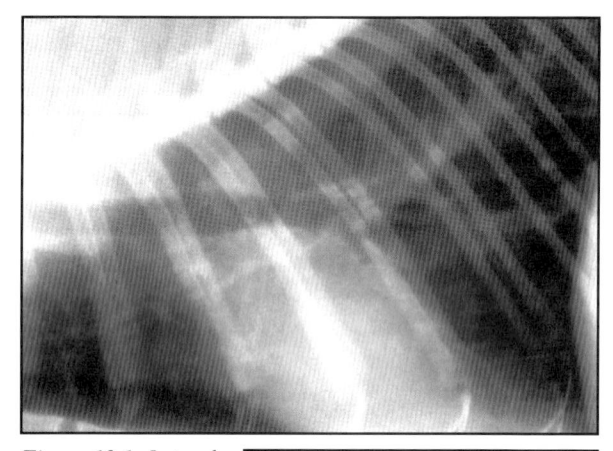

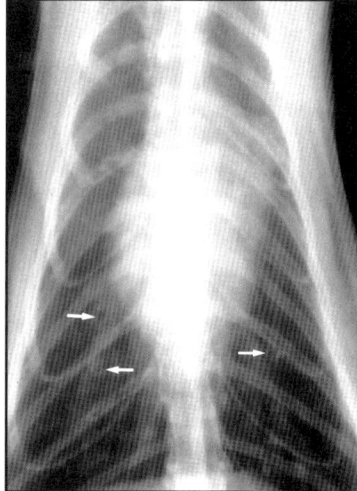

Figure 19.1: Lateral and dorsoventral radiographs from a 7.5-year-old MN domestic shorthaired cat with acute bronchitis. Although minimal changes are evident on the lateral exposure, bronchial thickening is evident as prominent 'doughnuts' (arrows) on the dorsoventral view, emphasizing the importance of taking two radiographic views in respiratory cases.

Early in disease course	• minor accentuation of bronchial markings • ± development of mild interstitial infiltrates • air-trapping during acute events • bronchial wall thickening (Figure 19.1)
Chronic bronchial disease, or if complicated by secondary infection	• bronchial pattern becomes more marked, interstitial patterns may develop • if bacterial pneumonia, alveolar infiltrates may be seen (especially ventral lung lobes) • collapse of the right middle lung lobe (approximately 10% of cases) (Moise *et al.*, 1989) • intrathoracic lymph nodes normal in uncomplicated bronchial disease
Emphysema and chronic obstructive pulmonary disease	• permanent hyperinflation of lung fields • cardiac silhouette may appear to be small • diaphragm flattened in appearance • previous pulmonary patterns (bronchial, interstitial) still present • right middle lung lobe may be permanently consolidated (Figure 19.2)

Table 19.4: *Radiographic findings in feline bronchial disease.*

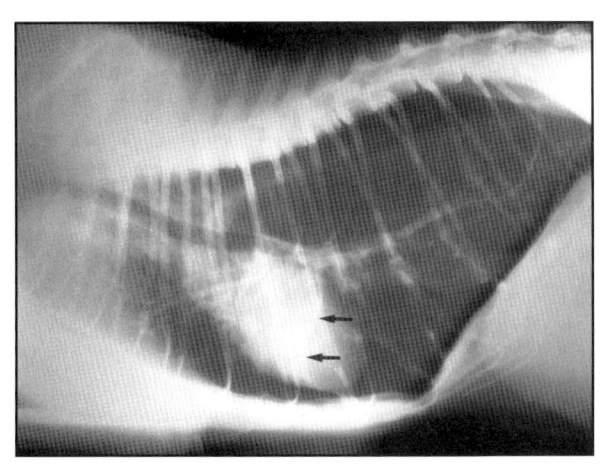

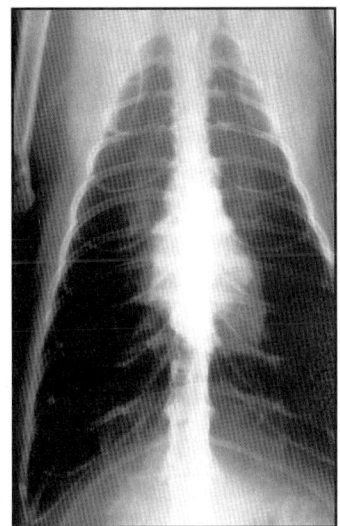

Figure 19.2: *Lateral and dorsoventral radiographs from an aged cat with chronic bronchitis and emphysema. Overinflation of the lung fields, a flattened diaphragm and increased space between the cardiac silhouette and the diaphragm are typical radiographic signs of air-trapping. In addition, a consolidated right middle lung lobe is indicated by the lobar sign evident on the lateral view (arrows).*
Courtesy of Dr Martha Moon.

Cytological examination

Cytological evaluation of the respiratory tract is important in the investigation of cats with suspected bronchial disease (see Chapter 5v). The choice of tracheal/bronchial wash versus bronchoalveolar lavage and bronchial brushings is based on the clinician's analysis of cost versus benefit. Typically, cats displaying dyspnoea without cough are chosen for bronchoscopic examination so that a 'deeper' sample can safely be retrieved from smaller airways. Bronchoscopic examination also allows direct observation of any bronchial obstruction or anatomical abnormality. Coughing cats, or cats showing both cough and dyspnoea can undergo bronchial lavage safely and effectively through the use of a sterile endotracheal tube and short-acting anaesthetics. In some cases, a non-bronchoscopic procedure is chosen because the presence of abundant mucus or the size of the patient's airway precludes bronchoscopic imaging. Supplemental oxygen should be administered before, during and after the procedure to minimise hypoxia, especially in animals with severe disease. Transthoracic lung aspirates are more useful in the diagnosis of parenchymal disease than bronchial disease.

Samples retrieved via bronchial brushings should be applied to a clean glass slide and submitted for cytological preparations. In some cases, Gram staining can be requested if bacteria are seen on the stained preparation. Bronchial lavage findings can be prepared by direct smear, but preparations often benefit by a concentration procedure (either table-top centrifugation or laboratory cytocentrifugation) prior to staining (Moise and Blue, 1983). An aliquot of the lavage fluid should be submitted for aerobic, anaerobic and *Mycoplasma* spp. culture.

Inflammatory lavage findings in cats with inflammatory bronchial disease are variable. Large proportions of any type of inflammatory cell (macrophages, neutrophils, eosinophils, mast cells) are abnormal. The cell type does not appear to be important in disease differentiation once other aetiological agents have been ruled out. Normal cats have been reported with up to 18% eosinophils in bronchial lavage specimens (Padrid *et al.*, 1991) and counts may vary over time in an individual cat (King and Fox, 1993). Hyperplastic goblet and epithelial cells may be present, and abundant mucus and coils of inspissated mucus indicative of small airway disease may be seen (Rebar *et al*, 1992, Greenlee and Roszel, 1984). Normal cats have minimal mucus, small numbers of macrophages and rare lymphocytes, neutrophils or ciliated columnar epithelial cells on bronchial lavage specimens.

Management options

Initial management of feline bronchial disease includes elimination of any underlying aetiologies and management of complicating secondary disease (e.g. bacterial infection). Long courses of antibiotics and in some cases intermittent therapy for bacterial bronchitis may be needed to control secondary infections.

A combination of medications is used in the chronic management of feline inflammatory bronchial disease; full resolution of chronic bronchial disease in cats is seldom permanently achieved. Respiratory emergencies are treated with oxygen and a variety of emergency drugs, but chronic respiratory signs are treated in a stepwise fashion, based on the clinical signs and ancillary testing results.

Respiratory emergencies

The most important components of emergency care of the patient with respiratory distress are oxygen and a low stress environment. Oxygen via nasal tube or face mask should be administered in a careful and relaxed manner. Oxygen chambers must be closely monitored for ambient temperature and humidity as well as adequate venting of carbon dioxide.

Adrenergic medications (adrenaline, isoprenaline, terbutaline) may be used in the acute respiratory emergency when severe bronchoconstriction limits respiration (Table 19.3). These medications promote bronchial smooth muscle relaxation by stimulating β_2 adrenoceptors. Adrenaline is useful in acute cases of reversible airway obstruction. It can be administered subcutaneously and usually requires one dose only. Side-effects include those resulting from alpha adrenoceptor stimulation: vasoconstriction, hypertension and arrhythmias. Terbutaline, a β_2 agonist, can be used as an emergency or maintenance bronchodilator (see Maintenance). Aminophylline, a methylxanthine bronchodilator, may be administered intravenously in acute respiratory emergencies, but should be injected very slowly to avoid adverse side-effects of hyperexcitability and worsening of signs.

Corticosteroids limit accumulations of exudate consisting of inflammatory cell debris, and limit hypersecretion of mucus mediated by inflammatory cells. Corticosteroids have a place in both emergency and maintenance care of bronchial disease. In cases of life-threatening respiratory distress, dexamethasone or prednisolone sodium succinate is administered parenterally, and the cat subsequently receives a tapering dose of oral corticosteroids (see Maintenance).

Anticholinergic medications are sometimes recommended to combat vagally mediated bronchoconstriction in acute emergencies (Dye and Moise, 1992), but their use may be accompanied by unwanted side-effects (Henik and Yeager, 1994).

Maintenance therapy

Maintenance therapy of cats with chronic bronchial disease consists of combinations of lifestyle changes, bronchodilators, corticosteroids and occasionally, antibiotics.

Avoidance of known triggering substances or events and weight loss may be all that is necessary to control mild cases of feline asthma. A hypoallergenic food trial may result in improvement in some cats (Henik and Yeager, 1994). As symptom severity or frequency increase, more pharmacological manipulation may be needed.

Bronchodilators are the next step in therapy for animals in whom lifestyle change is not effective. Bronchodilators for chronic use include terbutaline, theophylline and aminophylline.

Terbutaline mimics the bronchodilation normally induced by sympathetic nervous system stimulation. Recent studies have documented improvement in pulmonary function of some cats with bronchial disease after administration of terbutaline (Dye *et al*, 1992), but therapeutic plasma levels have not been reliably established. Side-effects of terbutaline include gastrointestinal upset or signs of hypotension (lethargy, depression, weakness).

Theophylline is the parent compound of several methylxanthine bronchodilators. Formulations of theophylline are dosed based on the amount of the parent compound (McKiernan, 1992). The pharmacokinetics of slow release preparations of theophylline in cats appear to be very product-specific; once daily dosing in the evening of Theo-Dur[R] tablets at 25 mg/kg appears to support accepted therapeutic plasma levels in the cat (Dye *et al*, 1992). Other preparations (e.g. 'sprinkle' preparations) may not be effective at this dosage (McKiernan, 1992). Aminophylline should be dosed according to its theophylline content (78%).

Chronic corticosteroid use is dictated by response to therapy without corticosteroids. Cats whose signs can be controlled by bronchodilator therapy may not need corticosteroids at all, or may only need them intermittently during 'flare-ups'. Mediators released by the inflammatory cells promote and perpetuate bronchoconstriction, and may contribute to long-term damage to the lung. With this in mind, aggressive corticosteroid therapy should be utilized if the animal is showing signs of severe airway inflammation. Initial dosage range of prednisolone is 0.5–2.2 mg/kg divided into 2 daily doses, using the higher end of the range for more severely affected animals. The dose is slowly reduced over 2–4 weeks to 0.5–1.0 mg/kg once daily according to the clinical progress of the patient. The ultimate goal is a dose of approximately 0.5 mg/kg every 2–3 days. Some animals may remain stable without any corticosteroid therapy until the next acute episode.

Antimicrobial therapy

Bronchial disease in cats may be complicated by secondary bacterial infections (Moise *et al.*, 1989; Ford, 1993). A wide range of isolates have been cultured from normal cats and cats with clinical bronchial disease (Henik and Yeager, 1994), but the presence of heavy growths of these organisms, anaerobic bacteria or *Mycoplasma* spp. should be considered abnormal. Ideally, antimicrobial therapy is based on identification of the organism and documentation of the sensitivity of the bacteria to specific antibiotics. A therapeutic trial of *doxycycline* (5 mg/kg PO twice daily for 3 weeks) has been recommended by some authors to treat presumptively for *Mycoplasma* spp. infections if culture for this organism is not available (Henik and Yeager, 1994).

Supportive measures for respiratory patients include rehydration and nebulization. Maintenance of hydration promotes liquefaction of airway mucus and allows mobilization of the mucus by the mucociliary apparatus. Chronically ill animals or those who are hospitalized and are inappetent quickly dehydrate, and require fluid therapy. The benefits of increased airway humidification via nebulization of 0.45% or 0.9% saline for 30–45 minutes every 4–12 hours have been reported, especially when the nebulization episodes are followed by coupage physiotherapy (Hawkins *et al*, 1989).

The following medications are generally contraindicated in animals with productive bronchial inflammatory disease: diuretics, anticholinergics, cough suppressants, beta-blocking medications (beta-blocking agents) and nonsteroidal anti-inflammatory agents.

FELINE CARDIOMYOPATHIES

Cardiomyopathy is defined as disease of the heart muscle. Most commonly, categorization of cardiomyopathy in cats includes dilated (DCM), hypertrophic (HCM), restrictive or intermediate (RCM) and 'undefined' cardiomyopathies. Although dilated cardiomyopathy is relatively easily recognizable in most cases, many cats do not easily fit into only one of the other categories and may have findings of more than one type of cardiomyopathy. It is unclear how these findings may affect success of therapy. 'Undefined' or 'intergrade' cardiomyopathies are described as those cardiomyopathies with some combination of hypertrophic, restrictive or dilated abnormalities. Other types of cardiomyopathy include infiltrative myocardial diseases, endomyocarditis (Bonagura, 1994; Bossbaly *et al.*, 1994) and an apparently congenital form of cardiomyopathy consisting of excessive moderator bands restricting the left ventricle (LV) (Liu *et al*, 1982).

Incidence

Cardiomyopathy is the most common acquired cardiac disease in the cat, and forms a major percentage of clinical feline cardiac cases.

History and clinical examination

The history and physical examination findings of many cardiomyopathic cats may be similar regardless of the type of cardiomyopathy, especially if congestive heart failure (CHF) is present. Typical physical findings of feline CHF are summarized in Table 19.5.

Mucous membrane colour variable	Normal, pale or cyanotic
Capillary refill time prolonged	
Systolic heart murmur	
Apex beat prominent	May be reduced if pleural or pericardial effusion is present
Heart rate usually elevated	May be normal or decreased if severe CHF is present
Arrhythmias	
Gallop rhythms	
Arterial pulse quality variable	Normal or weak, pulse deficits may be detected
Evidence of pulmonary oedema	Cyanosis and panting; crackles auscultated over localized or diffuse pulmonary fields, loudest at end-inspiration
Evidence of pleural effusion	Cyanosis and panting
	Pulmonary and cardiac sounds muffled or absent
Distended jugular veins	
Ascites (rare)	
Evidence of aortic thromboembolism (see later)	

Table 19.5: Physical examination findings in cats with congestive heart failure (CHF).

Cats with 'early' HCM or RCM may be diagnosed when asymptomatic if a heart murmur or gallop rhythm is detected on routine physical examination. Most cats with DCM are presented in CHF; central retinal degeneration is detected in approximately one-third of cats with taurine-deficient dilated cardiomyopathy. Undefined cardiomyopathies may have any combination of signs depending on the functional changes in the heart. Any type of cardiomyopathy may be complicated by peripheral thromboembolism.

Dilated cardiomyopathy

Aetiopathogenesis
Dilated cardiomyopathy is characterized by dilatation of cardiac chambers and poor systolic function in the absence of valvular, vascular or congenital disease. Three categories of dilated cardiomyopathy may be defined based on clinical testing:

- Taurine-deficient dilated cardiomyopathy (TDDCM)
- DCM due to unusual causes (e.g. toxic)
- Idiopathic dilated cardiomyopathy (IDCM).

Toxic causes of DCM appear to be rare; TDDCM and IDCM are the dilated cardiomyopathies most commonly seen in practice.

Taurine-deficient DCM
Prolonged and severe taurine deficiency was defined as the major cause of feline DCM in 1987 (Pion *et al.*, 1987). Since that time, changes in the formulation of most cat foods have resulted in a dramatic decrease in this type of cardiomyopathy. At present, animals at risk for taurine deficiency consist mainly of those animals on 'unusual' diets, i.e. research-related or home-cooked diets that are not properly balanced or supplemented.

Idiopathic DCM
IDCM is diagnosed when taurine deficiency and other known causes of DCM have been ruled out. The aetiology of this irreversible disorder is unclear, but IDCM may represent the end-stage of a myocarditis or endomyocarditis that was clinically silent until DCM developed.

Diagnosis
A diagnosis of feline DCM is based on the results of physical examination and ancillary cardiac testing, including radiography, electrocardiography, echocardiography and sometimes angiography.

Radiographic findings of DCM usually include severe cardiomegaly. With CHF, pulmonary venous and pulmonary arterial hypertension may be present, as well as localized or diffuse interstitial or alveolar

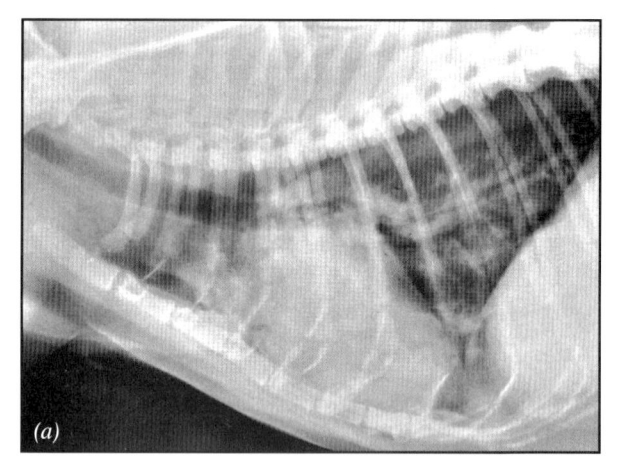
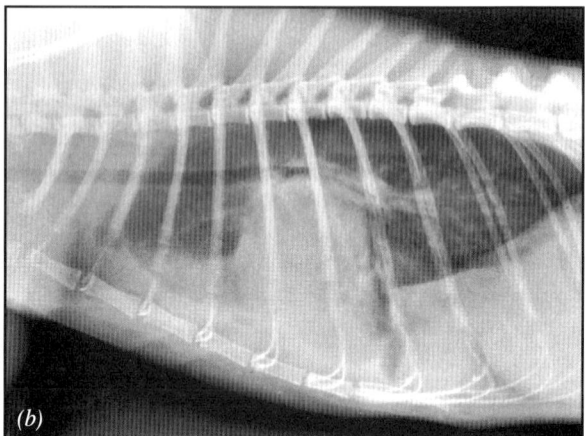
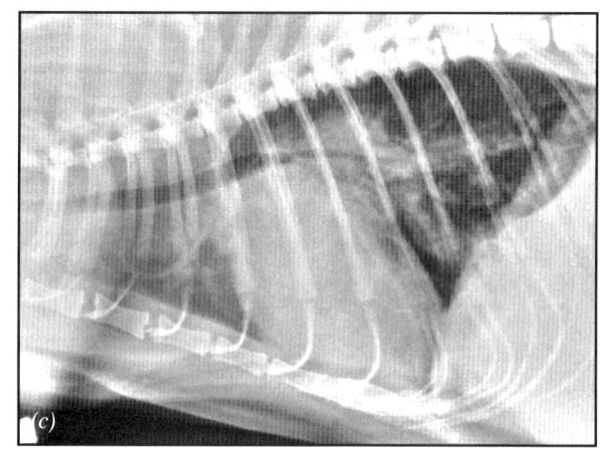

Figure 19.3: (a) *Lateral radiograph from a cat with taurine-deficient dilated cardiomyopathy and congestive heart failure. The cardiac silhouette is greatly enlarged, the caudal pulmonary arteries are enlarged and tortuous in appearance and there are diffuse alveolar infiltrates present.* (b) *Lateral radiograph from a cat with hypertrophic cardiomyopathy and congestive heart failure. The cardiac silhouette is enlarged, the caudal pulmonary arteries are enlarged and a moderate amount of pleural effusion is present.* (c) *Lateral radiograph from a cat with restrictive cardiomyopathy and congestive heart failure. There is generalized cardiomegaly with prominent left atrial enlargement; diffuse alveolar infiltrates and a small amount of pleural effusion are present. Comparison of these three radiographs emphasizes the 'overlap' of radiographic findings among the cardiomyopathies. It is usually not possible to diagnose the type of cardiomyopathy based on radiographic appearance alone.*

patterns (pulmonary oedema). Pleural effusion may obscure intrathoracic structures. Differentiation of various types of cardiomyopathy is often not possible based on thoracic radiography alone; all types of cardiomyopathy can lead to similar radiographic changes (Figure 19.3).

Electrocardiographic findings associated with DCM include changes in heart rate, conduction, complex size or rhythm, or the ECG may be normal. Any of these abnormalities is supportive evidence of cardiac disease and serious arrhythmias may require specific therapy.

Echocardiographic findings of DCM are specific. The LV is dilated (>18 mm at end-diastole) and fractional shortening is typically < 20% (and is often much lower). The left atrium is enlarged, leading to an increased left atrial:aortic ratio. The right atrium and right ventricle may also be enlarged, and small amounts of pericardial effusion may be present. On M-mode echocardiography, the E point to septal separation may be increased. Doppler examination may reveal mitral insufficiency.

A diagnosis of TDDCM involves recognition of typical cardiac and retinal changes and confirmation of low plasma taurine concentrations. Any cat with documented DCM should have plasma taurine concentrations measured; plasma taurine concentrations are normally approximately 50–120 nmol/l. Most cats with TDDCM have plasma taurine concentrations of 20 nmol/l or less.

Management strategies

Management of TDDCM includes therapy of CHF and supplementation with taurine. Success of therapy depends on successful management of CHF until tissue taurine concentrations are restored. Taurine supplementation begins while taurine concentrations are pending (Table 19.6). Taurine-deficient cats who survive CHF and receive appropriate supplementation usually show echocardiographic improvement in 3–6 weeks, and are usually successfully weaned off cardiac medications by 8–12 weeks.

Standard CHF therapy is used to manage TDDCM temporarily or as maintenance therapy in cases of IDCM, i.e. frusemide, digoxin and angiotensin converting enzyme (ACE) inhibitors. DCM is one of the rare instances in feline cardiac disease where acute inotropic support may be necessary. A dobutamine infusion may be used initially to support cardiac output if cardiogenic shock is present, and the patient is monitored for side-effects (e.g. seizures). If arrhythmias associated with myocardial disease are not life-threatening, specific therapy may not be required and the abnormalities may resolve with successful CHF therapy (Figure 19.4). Alternatively, supraventricular tachycardias may be successfully treated with digoxin and diltiazem, a calcium channel-blocking agent. Beta-blocking agents are generally avoided in animals in overt CHF due to negative inotropic effects, but may be used when CHF is resolved. Lignocaine is used with caution to treat sustained ventricular tachycardia.

Adrenaline	20 mg/kg SC every 30 minutes
Aminophylline	5 mg/kg IV slowly
Amlodipine besylate	0.625 mg/cat PO sid in the morning
Atenolol	6.25–12.5 mg/cat PO bid
Dexamethasone	0.2–2.2 mg/kg IV or IM
Digoxin	0.01 mg/kg PO every 48 hours
Diltiazem	1.5–2.5 mg/kg PO tid
Dobutamine	1–5 µg/kg/min, continuous infusion
Enalapril	0.25–0.5 mg/kg PO sid–bid
Esmolol	250–500 µg/kg IV slow bolus; 50–100 µg/kg/min continuous infusion
Frusemide	0.5–2.0 mg/kg PO, SC, IV or IM
Hydralazine	2.5 mg/cat PO sid–bid
Isoprenaline	0.1–0.2 ml of 1:5000 solution IM or SC
Lignocaine	0.25–0.75 mg/kg IV slowly
Nitro-glycerine ointment (2%)	5–10 mm of ointment applied cutaneously bid
Prednisolone sodium succinate	30 mg/kg IV
Prednisolone	*maintenance:* 0.25–1.1 mg/kg PO bid and taper (see text)
Propranolol	2.5–5.0 mg/cat PO tid, 0.05–0.1 mg/kg IV
Taurine	250–500 mg/cat PO bid
Terbutaline	*acutely:* 0.01 mg/kg SC or IV, repeat once if no effect in 5–10 minutes
	maintenance: 0.15 mg/kg PO bid, increase to 0.3 mg/kg PO bid if no effect and no adverse side-effects noted
Theophylline	4 mg/kg PO bid–tid (of theophylline salt)

Table 19.6: *Medications commonly used in the therapy of feline cardiorespiratory disorders. See text for specific indications. Note: Most of these medications are not approved for use in cats. IM: intramuscularly, IV: intravenously, PO: orally, SC: subcutaneously.*

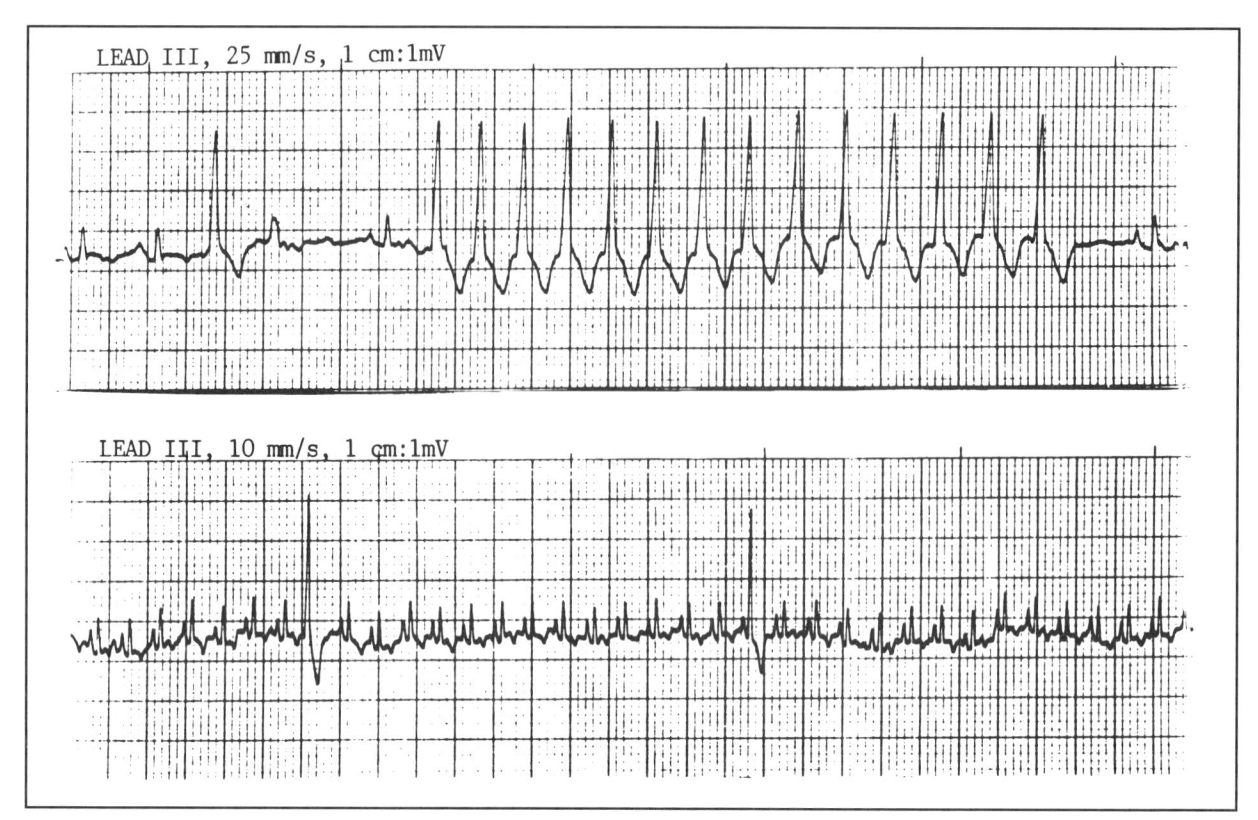

Figure 19.4: *Lead III electrocardiogram recorded from a cat with hypertrophic cardiomyopathy and congestive heart failure. Top: an underlying sinus rhythm (heart rate approximately 120 beats per minute) is complicated by single ventricular ectopics and paroxysms of ventricular tachycardia at 260 beats per minute (25 mm/s, 1 cm: 1 mV). Bottom: lead III electrocardiogram from the same cat after resolution of the congestive heart failure. Sinus rate is now 150 beats per minute with occasional single ventricular ectopic beats present. No anti-arrhythmic drugs were employed (10 mm/s, 1 cm: 1 mV).*

The prognosis for cats with IDCM controlled with medications is guarded to poor. Most cats with IDCM will survive 1-2 months with medical therapy, but occasional well-managed cats may live to 6 months.

Hypertrophic cardiomyopathy

Hypertrophic cardiomyopathy is a cardiac muscle disease characterized by variable thickening of the LV wall and interventricular septum (IVS). Dynamic aortic outflow obstruction may also be present. Non-cardiac diseases resulting in feline hypertrophic heart disease include aortic stenosis, systemic hypertension, hyperthyroidism and acromegaly (elevated growth hormone levels); these causes should be ruled out before idiopathic HCM may be diagnosed.

Incidence

HCM is a common diagnosis in the feline population and appears to be increasing in frequency. This increase may be due to a genuine increase in the prevalence of disease, or may reflect increased clinical awareness of the disease and increasing numbers of pet cats in the clinical population. The longest survival times are in asymptomatic cats with HCM; cats who are diagnosed in CHF at initial presentation have a much poorer prognosis (Atkins *et al.*, 1992).

Aetiopathogenesis

At present, HCM is considered to be idiopathic, but evidence suggests a genetic basis in some cats (Kittleson *et al.*, 1993). The primary dysfunction in the hypertrophic heart is diastolic, i.e. thickened, non-compliant ventricular walls limit functional diastole (ventricular filling). Reduced ventricular filling, limited luminal size and geometric changes in the ventricle (resulting in mitral valve distortion and mitral insufficiency) lead to decreases in cardiac output and eventually signs of CHF. Decreased myocardial perfusion secondary to hypertrophy leads to myocardial hypoxia and may form a substrate for arrhythmias. HCM may be complicated by LV outflow obstruction as the hypertrophied septum bulges into and obstructs the outflow tract during ejection (Figure 19.5). Systolic anterior mitral valve motion may further obstruct outflow and cause mitral insufficiency.

Diagnosis

Clinical examination and historical findings are similar in most respects to cats with other cardiomyopathies. If CHF is present, dyspnoea and tachycardia are the major clinical signs (see later for signs of thromboembolism). Many cases of HCM are 'clinically silent'; HCM should be included in the differential diagnosis for any murmur or gallop in an apparently healthy cat or a cat with signs of CHF.

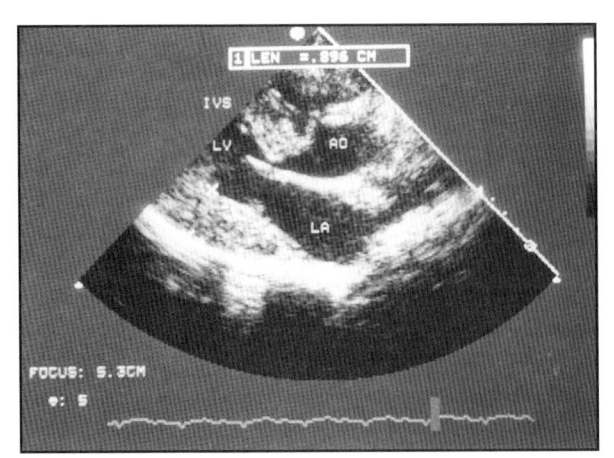

Figure 19.5: Two-dimensional echocardiograpm (right parasternal long axis view) from a 7-year-old MN domestic shorthaired cat with hypertrophic cardiomyopathy. The left ventricular free wall is thickened (8.9 mm) and the interventricular septum bulges into the left ventricular outflow tract in systole, leading to dynamic outflow obstruction. IVS, interventricular septum; LV, left ventricle; AO, aortic outflow tract; LA, left atrium.

Radiographic findings of HCM are variable. Sometimes a 'valentine-shaped' heart may be identified on the ventrodorsal radiograph; this appearance is due to left atrial enlargement and shifting of the cardiac apex to the right (Bonagura, 1994). Just as often, more generalized cardiomegaly may be present; the heart may appear globoid if pericardial effusion is present. On lateral views, the hypertrophic heart may appear elongated with a 'crease' present along the caudal border. Pulmonary oedema, pleural effusion or both may be present in cats with HCM.

Electrocardiographic findings frequently include sinus tachycardia, signs of LV hypertrophy (increased R wave amplitudes, left axis shift) and evidence of atrial enlargement (tall or wide P waves). Conduction disturbances are common; frequently, 'jagged' or irregular-looking QRS complexes of normal width indicate intraventricular conduction disturbances. Left cranial axis deviation is common and may be due to LV hypertrophy or left anterior fascicular block. Any arrhythmia may be seen, as well as a 'normal' ECG.

Two-dimensional echocardiography usually reveals LV hypertrophy involving the free wall and septum (diastolic LV free wall and septal thickness of >5.5 mm), large and sometimes hyperechoic papillary muscles, and left atrial enlargement. Thrombi may be present in the left atrial or LV lumen. Fractional shortening is normal to increased. Systolic anterior mitral valve motion may be documented on M-mode examination as movement of the anterior mitral valve leaflet towards the septum in systole. Doppler findings include mitral insufficiency and increased aortic outflow velocities if dynamic LV outflow obstruction is present.

Management strategies

Management of HCM depends on the clinical status of the patient. Current recommendations for asymptomatic HCM include beta-blockade or calcium channel-blocking agent therapy. There are no published reports to date evaluating the importance of early therapy of HCM; recommendations are based on clinical experience and studies of human HCM patients. At present, cats with HCM at the author's clinic are treated with *diltiazem* to promote diastolic relaxation and limit heart rate to < 200 bpm. If cats are asymptomatic but LV outflow obstruction or arrhythmias are present, a beta-blocking agent (*atenolol* or *propranolol*) is preferred. In cats with no clinical signs, the choice between beta-blocking and calcium channel-blocking agents is often based on ease of dosing and the owner's preference after discussion.

If CHF is present, *frusemide* and *glyceryl trinitrate* ointment are used to resolve pulmonary oedema and pleural effusion. Vasodilators (primarily ACE inhibitors) may be used with caution if no outflow obstruction is present. A recent study has indicated that clinical status of symptomatic cats with severe HCM improved greatly with diltiazem and frusemide therapy, and that in many cases frusemide could be discontinued after several days of therapy (Bright *et al.*, 1991). Although the number of cats studied was low and the cats had severe disease, cats treated with diltiazem showed improved clinical status. Diltiazem is presently the recommended therapy in the maintenance of cats with HCM. Beta-blocking agents have long been used in similar patients once CHF is resolved, especially those with sinus tachycardia or other arrhythmias. Clinical experience suggests that many cats do well with long-term maintenance beta-blocking agent therapy.

Restrictive cardiomyopathy

Aetiopathogenesis

Restrictive cardiomyopathy is characterized at postmortem examination by regional or global left ventricular myocardial fibrosis. Fibrotic tissue is thought to result in both systolic and diastolic dysfunction in the living animal. The underlying cause of RCM is unknown, but may be the result of previous myocarditis or eosinophilic infiltration, or be a previously undiagnosed case of HCM altered by chronic myocardial ischaemia and fibrosis. By the time damage is severe enough to lead to clinical diagnosis, the abnormalities appear to be irreversible.

Diagnosis

Historical and clinical findings of RCM are similar to HCM. Radiographs reveal moderate to severe cardiomegaly with evidence of severe atrial enlargement. Echocardiographic changes, as described by Bonagura (1994), encompass a constellation of two-dimensional, M-mode and Doppler findings, including:

- Normal to slightly decreased shortening fraction
- Left atrial enlargement inappropriate to the magnitude of hypertrophy, myocardial failure or mitral insufficiency
- Normal or thickened LV wall
- Mild or moderate dilation of the LV just below the mitral valve
- Decreased LV lumen size or narrowing in the mid-ventricle caused by fibrosis or fibrous bands
- Regional ventricular abnormalities including wall motion abnormalities
- Hyperechoic subendocardial foci, regional hypertrophy or moderator bands
- Mild or moderate right atrial and ventricular enlargement
- No or mild atrioventricular valve insufficiency
- Pericardial effusion of variable severity.

Any single cat may have any combination of these findings (Figure 19.6). Confusing combinations of findings of DCM, HCM and RCM commonly result in a diagnosis of 'undefined' cardiomyopathy, in which the description and therapy of the disorder is based on the exact combination of anatomical and functional abnormalities. A specific and presumably congenital type of RCM has been described in which thick, fibrous bands extend across the lumen or attach the papillary muscles to the free wall (Liu *et al.*, 1982); cats with CHF due to this abnormality are treated in much the same manner as those with other restrictive myocardial diseases.

Management strategies

Management of RCM is similar to that of DCM. *Digoxin*, *diuretics*, a *low salt diet* and *vasodilators* may be useful to control CHF. *Diltiazem* is used with caution in cats with a substantial hypertrophic compo-

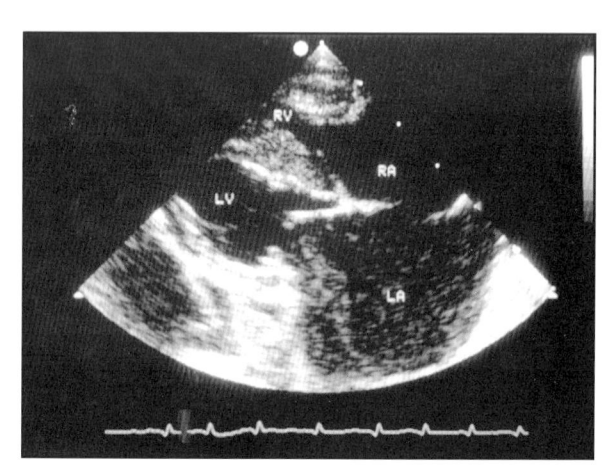

Figure 19.6: *Two-dimensional echocardiogram (right parasternal long axis view) from a MN domestic shorthaired cat with restrictive cardiomyopathy. The interventricular septum and right ventricular wall are mildly hypertrophied; there is severe enlargement of the right and left atria. RV, right ventricle; RA, right atrium; LV, left ventricle; LA, right atrium.*

nent, or in animals in which the primary dysfunction appears to be diastolic. Prognosis is guarded but some cats may live up to 1–2 years with careful therapy.

Aortic thromboembolism

Aortic thromboembolism (ATE) is a common and serious complication of the feline cardiomyopathies. Acute decompensation of cardiac disease due to the pain and stress of ATE or non-responsive paralysis after ATE may result in euthanasia of a previously stable cardiac patient.

Aetiopathogenesis

ATE in cats is most commonly associated with the primary cardiomyopathies. The coincidence of several mechanical and physiological abnormalities appear to be necessary components in the formation of a thrombus; all of these abnormalities may be present in animals with cardiomyopathy. *Damaged cardiac endothelium* provides a substrate for platelet adherence. A *hypercoagulable state* may be present, leading to abnormal platelet or clotting factor activation. Lastly, alteration of cardiac anatomy and function leads to *intracardiac blood stasis* and promotes clot formation.

When a thrombus leaves the heart and lodges in the peripheral vasculature, distal blood supply is disrupted. Thrombi release vasoactive substances (including serotonin and prostaglandins) that prevent effective collateral circulation. Ischaemia leads to necrosis of the affected muscle groups; if major organ vasculature is affected, bowel necrosis, acute renal failure or neurological abnormalities may result.

History and physical examination

The history of cats with ATE is typically acute in nature. Sudden onset of uni- or bilateral paresis of the hind limbs may occur when the cat is unsupervised or out-of-doors; the owner may suspect spinal trauma or fractured limbs. The cat may appear to be in pain, and may be tachypnoeic or have laboured breathing.

Physical examination findings are specific. Affected limbs are paretic or paralysed; there is pallor of the affected footpads or nailbeds and a lack of arterial pulse to the affected leg(s). The leg(s) are cool to the touch and may be stiff if contracture of major muscle groups is present. The cats often show evidence of pain by vocalization. Embolization of mesenteric vessels results in acute abdominal pain, and signs of acute renal failure may be present if renal arterial embolization has occurred. CHF is often present, and may have been present before embolization, or may be precipitated by the stress and pain of the ATE episode. Life-threatening CHF and arrhythmias are treated acutely, before management of ATE begins.

Diagnostic testing

Diagnosis of ATE or thromboembolism of other sites is based on physical examination, compatible history, physical evidence of cardiac disease (especially cardiomyopathy) and supportive testing. Angiography may delineate the obstruction but is rarely necessary and poses a significant anaesthetic risk to the patient. Echocardiographic examination may reveal thrombi within the atrium or ventricle.

Compatible biochemical findings include abnormalities reflecting organs affected. Severe muscle injury is evidenced by metabolic acidosis, elevations in LDH, CK, AST and ALT. Disseminated intravascular coagulation (DIC) may develop. Hyperkalaemia occasionally occurs, reflecting acidosis, muscle damage, acute renal failure or reperfusion phenomena.

Management strategies

Management of ATE begins with assuring the immediate survival of the patient; success of therapy for CHF (if present) will dictate the necessity of ATE therapy. Pretreatment neurological, muscular and vascular function is assessed; metabolic status is established via biochemical analysis and blood gas measurements. Over-diuresis is to be avoided; dehydration worsens peripheral perfusion.

Many ATE patients are humanely killed because of the severity of the signs, severity of concurrent heart disease or overall guarded prognosis for return to function. Patients who are or become systemically stable, often exhibit slow, steady progress towards function of the affected limbs. Some improvement in motor function may be seen as early as 3 days after ATE. Supportive care at home can result in gradual return to function over a period of weeks. Clinical experience indicates that if absolutely no improvement is seen in the first week, or if the limb itself deteriorates (cutaneous oedema formation, gas gangrene), recovery is unlikely. Limb amputation may result in a pain-free, functional pet, and is a reasonable option in an otherwise stable patient. Unfortunately, further episodes of ATE are common.

Immediate management of ATE consists of surgical removal of the thrombus, administration of thrombolytic drugs (tissue plasminogen activator (t-PA)), streptokinase, or supportive medical therapy.

Surgical embolectomy has long been considered to impose unacceptable risks for survival due to anaesthetic risk and possibility of precipitation of DIC. Recently, it has been suggested that surgery on stable animals may provide faster return to normal vascularity and should be re-evaluated (Bonagura, 1994). Surgery is contraindicated in patients in CHF.

Thrombolytic agents are commonly used in human beings for therapy of acute thromboembolism. *Tissue plasminogen activator* (t-PA) has been evaluated in a small number of cats and was reasonably successful (50% of cats showed improvement) at clot lysis; clinical use is limited by cost and a reported 50% mortality rate (Pion and Kittleson, 1989). Acute thrombolysis may result in reperfusion injury (characterized by hyperkalaemia and metabolic acidosis), and additional embolization if previously unidentified intracardiac thrombi are mobilized.

Streptokinase has been anecdotally reported (Bonagura, 1994) to be successful if administered within 8-12 hours of the onset of clinical signs (90 000 IU infused during first hour, then 45 000 IU/hour for up to 6 hours or until pulses return). However, mortality rates with streptokinase therapy may be no better than with t-PA.

The goals of medical therapy include alleviation of pain, prevention of further embolization and support of collateral circulation. Pain relief can be provided primarily through the use of opioid analgesics. The author most frequently uses buprenorphine (0.0075–0.01 mg/kg SC every 6 hours). Prevention of further clot formation is addressed through maintenance of hydration and administration of sodium heparin (200 IU/kg IV, then 200 IU SC three times a day for 2-3 days). Acepromazine (0.1 mg/kg SC three times per day, titrating to a maximum dose of 0.4 mg/kg until cat appears to be lightly sedated) may theoretically be used to promote vasodilation and collateral circulation. Acepromazine also increases sedation and may alleviate some patient stress. Controlled, comparative clinical trials of medical ATE therapy have not been reported.

Prophylaxis

Prevention of ATE is difficult. For many years, aspirin therapy (75 mg PO every 3 days) had been advocated to prevent thromboembolism in animals at risk. The effectiveness of this therapy has been questioned (Fox, 1991) and aspirin therapy is decreasing in popularity due to lack of documented efficacy. More recently, chronic oral warfarin therapy has been advocated to prevent feline ATE and results have been encouraging. Therapy with warfarin necessarily involves close monitoring of haemostasis parameters, and close owner supervision of the patient.

FELINE HYPERTENSION

Feline systemic hypertension has most frequently been associated with chronic renal disease or thyrotoxicosis. Other reported causes of hypertension are rare in the feline population (e.g. hypothyroidism, phaeochromocytoma, hyperadrenocorticism, primary aldosteronism) (Dukes, 1992). Feline hyperthyroidism is discussed elsewhere in this chapter; this section will concentrate on renal hypertension, thought to be the most frequent cause of hypertension in cats.

Incidence

Arterial hypertension is defined by most authors as a systolic and/or diastolic pressure of > 170/100 mmHg when measured by indirect Doppler-shift sphygmomanometry (Dukes, 1992; Littman, 1994). Studies suggest that between 60% and 75% of cats in renal failure have documentable elevations in arterial systolic pressure, diastolic pressure or both (Kobayashi *et al*, 1990, Lesser *et al*, 1992). The degree of renal insufficiency has not been related to the degree of hypertension in any study.

Aetiopathogenesis

Mechanisms of development of systemic hypertension in the setting of renal insufficiency include excessive sodium and therefore water retention by damaged kidneys, abnormal activity of the renin–angiotensin–aldosterone system (RAAS), autonomic dysfunction and alterations in locally vasoactive hormones in the vascular system (Ross, 1992). It is unclear which of these mechanisms is most important in the development of renal hypertension in cats, and multiple mechanisms may play a role. Published reports reveal variable results to multiple modes of therapy (Morgan, 1986; Littman *et al.*, 1988; Littman, 1994), suggesting that different medications may be effective in different animals, possibly based on the individual's mechanism of hypertension.

History and physical examination

Clinical signs relating to systemic hypertension relate to the underlying disease and to secondary organ damage. *Renal insufficiency* may be clinically apparent (dehydration, polyuria, polydipsia, small irregular kidneys, anaemia) or be subclinical in nature. *Hypertensive retinopathy* has been well described and consists of tortuosity of retinal blood vessels, retinal or vitreal haemorrhage, retinal detachment and blindness. The animal is often not noted to be abnormal until retinal detachment occurs and acute blindness is recognized by the owner. Successful therapy of hypertension may lead to retinal reattachment, but cats frequently remain functionally blind (Littman, 1994).

Cardiac manifestations of hypertension are due to ventricular hypertrophy secondary to the increased afterload of arterial hypertension. Concentric LV hypertrophy is accompanied by left atrial enlargement due to decreased LV compliance and/or mitral insufficiency. Heart rate may be elevated, and systolic murmurs, gallop rhythms and premature beats may be auscultated (Littman, 1994). Occasionally, diastolic murmurs typical of aortic insufficiency may be present (Morgan, 1986). Left-sided congestive heart failure may occur.

Diagnostic testing

Findings on diagnostic tests in cats with renal hypertension frequently reflect either the cause or the end-organ effects of the hypertension.

Haematology and *biochemistry* results may be normal or reflect findings consistent with chronic renal failure. *Urinalysis* usually reveals urine specific gravities that are inappropriately low and there may be evidence of proteinuria (Littman, 1994).

Thoracic radiographs may show cardiomegaly. Overt CHF is rare in uncomplicated hypertension.

ECG findings include tachycardias, and waveform changes consistent with LV or atrial enlargement.

Echocardiographic findings include concentric LV hypertrophy and left atrial enlargement. Doppler echocardiography may reveal mitral insufficiency and/or aortic insufficiency.

Abdominal radiography/ultrasonography may demonstrate small, irregular kidneys typical of chronic renal disease, or asymmetric adrenal glands indicative of neoplasia (i.e. phaeochromocytoma).

Blood pressure measurement

Definitive diagnosis of hypertension depends on measurement of arterial blood pressure. Several methods are available to measure blood pressure in cats, but the most dependable, repeatable and practical method appears to be through the use of Doppler-shift sphygmomanometry. This technique is simple, yields repeatable results, and is well-described elsewhere (Kobayashi *et al*, 1990; Lesser *et al*, 1992). Repeating measurements three to five times, and firm but gentle restraint of the patient increases accuracy and repeatability of measurements.

Management strategies

Attempts to control hypertension are aimed at preventing damage and minimizing progression of dysfunction in all affected organs. The clinician should approach therapy of hypertension in cats as a polysystemic disorder, and attempt to palliate the underlying disease (e.g. renal insufficiency) as well as controlling the dangerous side-effects of hypertension. Interestingly, successful management of hypertension did not appear to increase survival time in a recent review (Littman, 1994). However, in light of published data regarding the detrimental effects of chronic hypertension, and in the presence of anecdotal experience of improved quality of life in treated patients, control of hypertension appears to be desirable. A 20% reduction in or normalization of blood pressure measurements (Littman, 1994) is the desired goal of therapy.

Salt restriction has proven beneficial in the management of dogs with renal hypertension, especially when combined with other therapies (Cowgill and Kallet, 1986; Dukes, 1992), but has not been studied as a monotherapy in cats with hypertension.

Diuretics may be useful to reduce circulating volume in animals in whom inappropriate sodium excretion is the active mechanism for hypertension, but are not effective in all cases of renal failure-associated hypertension (Ross, 1992). Use of diuretics as monotherapy may lead to (further) activation of the RAAS, exacerbating sodium-retaining mechanisms and is not recommended.

Beta-receptor antagonists block adrenergically

mediated increases in cardiac output and renin secretion and have been advocated in therapy of hypertension in dogs and cats (Cowgill and Kallet, 1986; Snyder, 1991; Ross, 1992). Limited information regarding usc of these agents as monotherapy in hypertensive cats is available.

The two most common *vasodilating drugs* used in therapy of hypertension in cats are *hydralazine* and *enalapril* (or another angiotensin-converting enzyme inhibitor). Hydralazine hydrochloride lowers blood pressure by direct reduction of peripheral resistance. Disadvantages of hydralazine use for renal hypertension in cats include occurrence of reflex tachycardia and stimulation of the RAAS and fluid retention.

Angiotensin-converting enzyme inhibitors (ACE inhibitors) have been used to decrease blood pressure and limit proteinuria in people and animals with renal hypertension. ACE inhibitors reduce circulating volume, prevent further fluid retention and lower systemic blood pressure. Although no ACE inhibitors are approved for the treatment of renal hypertension in cats, enalapril (0.25–0.5 mg/kg once to twice daily) is frequently recommended.

Calcium channel-blocking agents are a diverse group of drugs that alter calcium kinetics at cell membranes, decreasing smooth muscle contraction, and may preferentially vasodilate the afferent renal arteriole (allowing maintenance of glomerular filtration rate, reduction of glomerulosclerosis and slowed progression of renal disease) (Ross, 1992). One recent uncontrolled study found *amlodipine besylate* to be effective as a monotherapy for renal hypertension in cats (Henik *et al.*, 1994).

Which combination of drugs is most appropriate for a given patient depends on the animal's response, the clinician's experience, other problems that may be present in the animal, cost and practicality of administration. In the author's experience, amlodipine besylate is successful in controlling hypertension in cats administered once daily. Alternatively, ACE inhibitors can be useful in some cats; beta-blocking agents may be added if ACE inhibition alone is not effective. Well-controlled, randomized, blinded clinical trials are clearly necessary to address this important clinical dilemma.

HYPERTHYROIDISM (THYROTOXICOSIS)

Hyperthyroidism is a common disease of middle-aged to older cats, and has significant cardiovascular consequences. In recent years, recognition of the prevalence of this disease has led to early diagnosis, and cardiovascular changes, though still documentable, result in congestive heart failure far less frequently (Broussard and Peterson, 1993; Fox *et al.*, 1993).

Incidence
Hyperthyroidism, usually diagnosed in animals greater than 10 years of age, is thought to be the most common feline endocrine disease. The polysystemic effects of thyrotoxicosis have been well described; an excellent review of thyroid disorders has recently been published (Ferguson, 1994).

Aetiopathogenesis
Feline hyperthyroidism results from adenomatous hyperplasia of the thyroid gland. These hyperplastic nodules are benign, but their growth and function do not appear to be controlled by normal feedback mechanisms. Excessive production of thyroxine (T4) and triiodothyronine (T3) leads to clinical signs of thyrotoxicosis (tachycardia, polyphagia, vomiting, diarrhoea, weight loss, polyuria and polydipsia).

Cardiovascular effects of thyrotoxicosis
Thyroid hormones have profound effects on the cardiovascular system, including increased heart rate, cardiac contractility and cardiac output, decreased systemic vascular resistance, arterial hypertension and direct stimulation of cardiac hypertrophy. These effects are partly due to the direct stimulatory effect of thyroid hormones on target tissues, and partially due to increased activity of and increased responsiveness to the sympathetic nervous system. In cats, therapy with beta-blocking agents reduces or eliminates some of the clinical signs associated with thyrotoxicosis, suggesting that the sympathetic nervous system plays a significant role in the pathogenesis of the feline disease. Interestingly, even though systemic vascular resistance is decreased, hyperthyroid cats are measurably hypertensive (Kobayashi *et al.*, 1990; Lesser *et al.*, 1992).

History and clinical examination
The systemic signs of hyperthyroidism have been well described (Peterson *et al.*, 1983; Jacobs *et al.*, 1986; Thoday and Mooney, 1992). Hyperthyroidism is considered a differential diagnosis for any acquired systolic heart murmur in older cats. The owner may not notice any signs directly referable to the cardiovascular system if CHF is not present. If CHF *is* present, the owner may notice that the cat is tachypnoeic or has laboured breathing, a 'pounding heart' and tachycardia.

Physical examination findings include weight loss, an unkempt appearance and sometimes an 'anxious' expression with hyperalert reactions and dilated pupils. There is often (but not invariably) a palpable thyroid nodule in the ventral cervical region. Heart rate is usually elevated and arrhythmias (including gallop rhythms) may be noted. Pulses may be hyperkinetic; pleural effusion may obscure a prominent left apical impulse or a right or left apical systolic murmur. Jugular distension may be present if the animal is in CHF. Pulmonary oedema may be suspected when crackles are auscultated over the pulmonary fields.

Diagnosis

Resting serum T3 and/or T4 levels usually establish a diagnosis of thyrotoxicosis. If these results are ambiguous, T4 levels should be repeated, or a T3 suppression test carried out. Assessment of the cardiac complications of thyrotoxicosis is as for other cardiac conditions:

- Thoracic radiographs may show cardiomegaly (Bond, 1986) or signs of CHF.
- ECG findings relate to the severity or chronicity of disease. Mildly affected animals may have a normal heart rate or sinus tachycardia. Severely thyrotoxic animals may have evidence of LV enlargement, tachyarrhythmias, or conduction defects.
- Echocardiographic findings vary from case to case. Values may be within normal range, yet qualitatively different from normal (Moise et al., 1986). LV hypertrophy or dilation, left atrial enlargement or aortic root enlargement may all be seen. The right side of the heart may also be enlarged. Fractional shortening may be increased (Figure 19.7). Echocardiographic abnormalities usually resolve with antithyroid therapy.

Systemic hypertension has been documented in cats with hyperthyroidism (Kobayashi et al., 1990; Lesser et al., 1992), but clinically evident hypertension appears to be rare in the population of hyperthyroid animals. Nonetheless, hyperthyroidism should be ruled out in cases of suspected or documented feline hypertension.

Management strategies

Definitive therapy of feline hyperthyroidism may involve chemotherapy (e.g. carbimazole), surgery or radioiodine therapy. Each modality has advantages and disadvantages and the interested reader is referred to a recently published review (Ferguson, 1994).

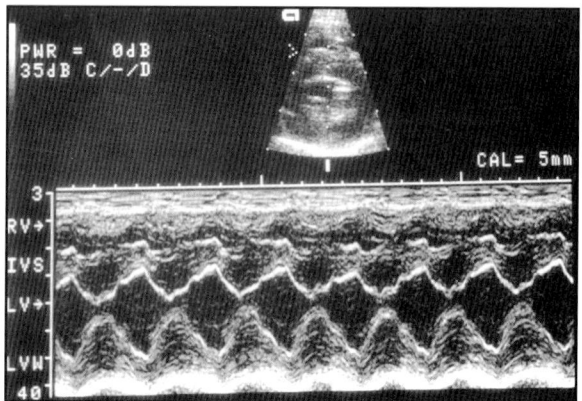

Figure 19.7: Left ventricular short axis M-mode echocardiogram from a 12-year-old MN domestic shorthaired hyperthyroid cat demonstrating typical findings of mild left ventricular and right ventricular dilatation, mild left ventricular and interventricular septal hypertrophy and increased contractile function.

Cardiovascular therapy

Recently, Bonagura (1994) suggested that therapy of thyrotoxic cats be based on classification into three clinical disease groups:

- Cats with CHF
- Cats with significant arrhythmias
- Cats who are free of clinical signs except for documented cardiomegaly or the presence of a murmur and/or gallop rhythm.

Therapy for cardiovascular abnormalities is initiated concurrently with antithyroid therapy.

Thyrotoxic cats with CHF are treated with typical CHF therapy and carbimazole therapy. Surgical thyroidectomy is contraindicated until CHF signs are resolved. Severe arrhythmias may resolve with resolution of CHF, but life-threatening arrhythmias should be treated immediately. Severe supraventricular arrhythmias in the presence of CHF may be treated with digoxin or diltiazem but beta-blocking agents should be avoided if possible until CHF is resolved.

Cats with tachyarrhythmias but no evidence of CHF are treated with beta-blocking agents and carbimazole. Propranolol is the beta-blocking agent of choice and is continued until the cat is euthyroid posttherapy, or the tachyarrhythmia resolves concurrent with clinical improvement. If surgery to resect the abnormal thyroid tissue is planned, this subset of patients receives beta-blocking agent with antithyroid chemotherapy until euthyroid. If cardiac status is stable, the cat can remain on beta-blocking agent therapy until recovered from surgery; the dose of beta-blocking agent can then be 'tapered' over a period of several days, then discontinued. Intraoperative arrhythmias may be treated with esmolol, an ultrashort-acting beta-blocking agent (IV, 50-100 µ/kg/min) or propranolol (IV, 0.05-0.1 mg slow bolus dose). Cats with no clinical signs of cardiovascular complications of thyrotoxicosis need not be treated with any cardiac medications and the chosen definitive therapy can be employed immediately.

REFERENCES

Atkins CE, Gallo AM, Kurzman ID and Cowen P (1992) Risk factors, clinical signs, and survival in cats with a clinical diagnosis of idiopathic hypertrophic cardiomyopathy: 74 cases (1985—1989). Journal of the American Veterinary Medical Association 201, 613

Bauer TG (1989) Pulmonary hypersensitivity disorders. In: Current Veterinary Therapy X, Small Animal Practice, ed.RW Kirk and JD Bonagura. WB Saunders, Philadelphia

Bonagura JD (1994) Cardiovascular diseases. In: The Cat, Diseases and Clinical Management 2nd edn, ed. RG Sherding. Churchill Livingstone, New York

Bond BR (1986) Hyperthyroid heart disease in cats. In: Current Veterinary Therapy IX, Small Animal Practice, ed. RW Kirk. WB Saunders, Philadelphia

Bossbaly MJ, Stalis I, Knight D and VanWinkle T (1994) Feline endomyocarditis: a clinical/pathological study of 44 cases. *Proceedings, 12th Annual ACVIM Forum* (abstract)

Bright JM, Golden AL, Gompf RE, Walker MA and Toal RL (1991) Evaluation of the calcium channel-blocking agents diltiazem and verapamil for treatment of feline hypertrophic cardiomyopathy. *Journal of Veterinary Internal Medicine* **5**, 272

Broussard JD and Peterson ME (1993) Changes in the clinical and laboratory findings in hyperthyroid cats from 1982-1992. *Proceedings, 11th Annual ACVIM Forum* (abstract)

Cowgill LD and Kallet AJ (1986) Systemic hypertension. In: *Current Veterinary Therapy XI, Small Animal Practice*, ed. RW Kirk. WB Saunders, Philadelphia

Dukes J (1992) Hypertension: a review of the mechanisms, manifestations and management. *Journal of Small Animal Practice* **33**, 119

Dye JA (1992) Feline bronchopulmonary disease. *The Veterinary Clinics of North America: Small Animal Practice* **22**, 1187

Dye JA and Moise NS (1992) Feline bronchial disease. In: *Current Veterinary Therapy XI, Small Animal Practice*, ed. RW Kirk and JD Bonagura. WB Saunders, Philadelphia

Dye JA, McKiernan BC and Rozanske EA (1992) Pulmonary function in cats with bronchopulmonary disease and acute response to IV bronchodilator challenge. *Proceedings, 10th Annual ACVIM Forum* (abstract)

Ferguson DC (ed.) (1994) Thyroid disorders. *The Veterinary Clinics of North America: Small Animal Practice* **24** (3)

Ford RB (1993) Role of infectious agents in respiratory disease. *The Veterinary Clinics of North America: Small Animal Practice* **23**, 17

Fox PR (1991) Evidence for or against efficacy of beta-blockers and aspirin for management of feline cardiomyopathies. *The Veterinary Clinics of North America: Small Animal Practice* **21**, 1011

Fox PR, Broussard JD and Peterson ME (1993) Electrocardiographic and radiographic changes in cats with hyperthyroidism: comparison of populations evaluated during 1979-1982 vs. 1992. *Proceedings, 11th Annual ACVIM Forum* (abstract)

Greenlee PG and Roszel JF (1984) Feline bronchial cytology: histologic/cytologic correlation in 22 cats. *Veterinary Pathology* **21**, 308

Hawkins EC, Ettinger SJ and Suter PF (1989) Diseases of the lower respiratory tract (lung) and pulmonary edema. In: *Textbook of Veterinary Internal Medicine* 3rd edn, ed. SJ Ettinger. WB Saunders, Philadelphia

Henik RA and Yeager AE (1994) Bronchopulmonary diseases. In: *The Cat, Diseases and Clinical Management* 2nd edn, ed. RG Sherding. Churchill Livingstone, New York

Henik RA, Snyder PS and Volk LM (1994) Amlodipine besylate therapy in cats with systemic arterial hypertension secondary to chronic renal disease. *Proceedings, 12th Annual ACVIM Forum* (abstract)

Jacobs G, Hutson C, Dougherty J and Kirmayer A (1986) Congestive heart failure associated with hyperthyroidism in cats. *Journal of the American Veterinary Medical Association* **188**, 52

King RR and Fox LE (1993) Eosinophil fluctuation in bronchoalveolar lavage fluid from normal cats. *Proceedings, 11th Annual ACVIM Forum* (abstract)

Kittleson MD, Pion PD and Meckhamer Y (1993) Hypertrophic cardiomyopathy in a group of highly interrelated Maine Coon cats. *Proceedings, 11th Annual ACVIM Forum* (abstract)

Kobayashi DL, Peterson ME, Graves TK, Lesser M and Nichols CE (1990) Hypertension in cats with chronic renal failure or hyperthyroidism. *Journal of Veterinary Internal Medicine* **4**, 58

Lesser M, Fox PR and Bond BR (1992) Assessment of hypertension in 40 cats with left ventricular hypertrophy by Doppler-shift sphygmomanometry. *Journal of Small Animal Practice* **33**, 55

Littman MP (1994) Spontaneous systemic hypertension in 24 cats. *Journal of Veterinary Internal Medicine* **8**, 79

Littman MP, Robertson JL and Bovee KC (1988) Spontaneous systemic hypertension in dogs: five cases (1981-1983). *Journal of the American Veterinary Medical Association* **193**, 486

Liu SK, Fox PR and Tilley LP (1982). Excessive moderator bands in the left ventricle of 21 cats. *Journal of the American Veterinary Medical Association* **180**, 1215

McKiernan BC (1992) Current uses and hazards of bronchodilator therapy. In: *Current Veterinary Therapy XI, Small Animal Practice*, ed. RW Kirk and JD Bonagura. WB Saunders, Philadelphia

Moise NS and Blue J (1983) Bronchial washings in the cat: procedure and cytologic evaluation. *The Compendium on Continuing Education for the Practicing Veterinarian.* **5**, 621

Moise NS and Dietze AE (1989) Bronchopulmonary diseases. In: *The Cat, Diseases and Clinical Management*, ed. RG Sherding. Churchill Livingstone, New York

Moise NS, Dietze AE, Mezza LE, Strickland D, Erb HN and Edwards NJ (1986) Echocardiography, electrocardiography, and radiography of cats with dilatation cardiomyopathy, hypertrophic cardiomyopathy, and hyperthyroidism. *American Journal of Veterinary Research* **47**, 1476

Moise NS, Weidenkeller D, Yeager AE, Blue JT and Scarlett J (1989) Clinical, radiographic, and bronchial cytologic features of cats with bronchial disease: 65 cases (1980-1986). *Journal of the American Veterinary Medical Association* **194**, 1467

Morgan RV (1986) Systemic hypertension in four cats: ocular and medical findings. *Journal of the American Animal Hospital Association* **22**, 65

Padrid PA, Feldman BF, Funk K, Samitz EM, Reil D and Cross CE (1991). Cytologic, microbiologic, and biochemical analysis of bronchoalveolar lavage fluid obtained from 24 healthy cats. *American Journal of Veterinary Research* **52**, 1300

Peterson ME, Kintzer PP, Cavanaugh PG, Fox PR, Ferguson DC, Johnson GF and Becker DV (1983) Feline hyperthyroidism: pretreatment clinical and laboratory evaluation of 131 cases. *Journal of the American Veterinary Medical Association* **183**, 103

Pion PD and Kittleson MD (1989) Therapy for aortic thromboembolism. In: *Current Veterinary Therapy X, Small Animal Practice*, ed. RW Kirk and JD Bonagura. WB Saunders, Philadelphia

Pion PD, Kittleson MD, Rogers QR and Morris JG (1987) Myocardial failure in cats associated with low plasma taurine: a reversible cardiomyopathy. *Science* **237**, 764

Rebar AH, Hawkins EC and DeNicola DB (1992) Cytologic evaluation of the respiratory tract. *The Veterinary Clinics of North America: Small Animal Practice* **22**, 1065

Ross LA (1992) Hypertension and chronic renal failure. *Seminars in Veterinary Medicine and Surgery (Small Animal)* **7**, 221

Snyder PS (1991) Canine hypertensive disease. *The Compendium on Continuing Education for the Practicing Veterinarian* **13**, 1785

Thoday KL and Mooney CT (1992) Historical, clinical and laboratory features of 126 hyperthyroid cats. *The Veterinary Record* **131**, 257

PART THREE

Therapy

Oxygen Therapy

Pamela J. Murison

INTRODUCTION

Oxygen is essential for life. Although some cells are capable of short-term anaerobic metabolism, inadequate oxygen delivery (DO_2) to tissues results in *tissue hypoxia*, and eventually results in cell death. Enriching inspired gas with oxygen increases the fractional concentration of inspired oxygen (FiO_2), and increases the diffusion gradient down the five elements of the oxygen cascade:

- Inspired gas
- Alveolar gas
- Arterial blood
- Capillary blood
- Mitochondria.

Oxygen therapy is also used to control pneumothorax, and as an adjunct in the treatment of carbon monoxide poisoning, clostridial infections and cancer chemotherapy.

TECHNIQUES

By cuffed endotracheal tube

In very depressed animals, an endotracheal tube provides a patent airway. An endotracheal tube in conjunction with a suitable breathing system provides an economical way to supply oxygen. Ventilation may also be assisted or controlled.

By tracheotomy tube

Oxygen may be delivered by a tube passed through a tracheal stoma. Attention must be paid to cleaning, and there is a considerable risk of tracheal irritation and infection with long-term use.

By mask

Masks are useful in emergencies because they are rapidly applied. However, poor fitting masks and low O_2 flows will cause rebreathing – the re-aspiration of expired CO_2. Some animals may resist the mask; struggling is counterproductive because it raises oxygen consumption. Constant attention is required to keep the mask in place and to ensure subjects do not inhale vomit or secretions.

Oxygen chamber/incubator

Oxygen chambers for small animals are commercially available, although ex-hospital human infant incubators are as effective and less expensive. In addition to raising FiO_2, these devices allow temperature and humidity to be controlled. Furthermore, the animal does not need restraint and long-term use is possible. However, the equipment may be expensive, occupy considerable space, and the technique is wasteful of oxygen. Examination requires that the cage be opened, which causes rapid falls in ambient oxygen levels. For these reasons, chambers are best used for small animals, e.g. cats.

Nasal catheter

Nasal catheters are tolerated by most animals and are suitable for long-term oxygen supplementation.. The nasal mucosa is first anaesthetized by instilling 1 ml of 2% lignocaine (dogs); or in cats, a few drops of proxymetacaine (Crisp, 1994). A soft rubber catheter is then measured against the head, from the nares to the medial canthus of the eye. The catheter should have multiple fenestrations at the tip to prevent jet lesions in the nasopharynx (Court, 1992). The tube is lubricated and inserted gently via the ventral meatus so that the tip comes to lie in the nasopharynx. Insertion is more difficult in very small puppies and kittens. The external portion of the catheter is passed over the dorsum of the nose, and between the eyes. Zinc oxide tape butterflies attached to the catheter are sutured, or glued to the skin. Approximately 50–100 ml/kg/min oxygen will maintain FiO_2 above 40% (Crisp, 1994).

Transtracheal insufflation

A large bore (14–16 gauge) over-the-needle intravenous catheter introduced into the lumen of the trachea between tracheal rings, or through the cricothyroid membrane, may be used to deliver oxygen. This option is useful in animals with facial injuries, when the introduction of a nasal catheter may cause further damage. Asepsis is important, and the catheter tip should be fenestrated in order to prevent jet lesions. Trans-tracheal oxygen pipes may be difficult to fix in position, especially in dogs with superfluous loose skin.

Hyperbaric oxygen therapy

A pressurized chamber can be used to deliver oxygen at a pressure greater than one atmosphere. The oxygen content of the blood is increased because oxygen is more soluble at higher pressures. Hyperbaric oxygen therapy is used mainly to facilitate wound healing. Direct access to the animal during treatment sessions is impossible, so the technique is unsuitable for distressed or unstable animals (Elkins, 1997).

PROBLEMS WITH OXYGEN THERAPY

Humidification

Oxygen from cylinders is dry and cold, and can damage respiratory mucous membranes (Nogushi *et al.*, 1973). When oxygen is to be administered for more than 2-3 hours, problems are reduced if inspired gases are humidified. There are several ways to achieve this:

- Heat-moisture exchangers
- Sterile saline (0.9%) instilled into the delivery tube or catheter (0.4 ml/kg/h)
- The gas is bubbled through sterile saline or water
- Nebulizers are used for 15 min/h (Hawkins, 1992).

Humidification is most important when the technique of oxygen supplementation bypasses the nasal or oral cavities, e.g. nasal catheters or transtracheal insufflation.

Toxicity

Oxygen toxicity is probably caused by free radicals which damage mucous membranes and invoke an inflammatory reaction. The results are hypertrophy of alveolar type II epithelial cells, injury to the pulmonary capillary endothelium and enhanced enzyme activity (Crapo *et al.*, 1980). Neonatal animals are less sensitive to toxicity, possibly because of antioxidant activity (Frank *et al.*, 1978). Clinical signs include tracheal irritation, cough, restlessness, anorexia, lethargy and dyspnoea. Toxicity occurs more rapidly when O_2 is administered under hyperbaric conditions. Despite this, 10-12 hours of 100% oxygen at normal pressure is unlikely to cause signs of toxicity in dogs (Paine *et al.*, 1941), especially if the animal is hypoxic when therapy started. Oxygen toxicity is slow to develop and initially reversible, whereas hypoxia can be rapidly lethal; fears of O_2

toxicity should not be used as a basis for withholding short-term O_2 therapy.

MONITORING RESPONSE TO OXYGEN THERAPY

The most useful sign of successful oxygen therapy is an amelioration of clinical signs. Cyanosis is the most obvious sign of low arterial oxygen tensions (PaO_2), and occurs when desaturated haemoglobin levels exceed 5 g/dl, irrespective of the oxygenated haemoglobin (HbO_2) levels. Therefore cyanosis may not be apparent in hypoxaemic animals with a low haematocrit, i.e. Hb <5 g/dl. Signs of cardiovascular hyperdynamism (tachycardia and hypertension) are often seen in the early stage of mild hypoxia. With time, the heart fails and terminal bradycardia with hypotension develops. Successful therapy results in lowered respiratory effort, a slowing of heart rate and an improvement in the animal's demeanour. The electrocardiogram shows characteristic changes when the myocardium becomes hypoxic; e.g. ST segment depression (ST elevation is less common); ST 'slurring'; and eventually ventricular ectopic activity. Changes in these signs may be used to gauge the effects of oxygen therapy on myocardial hypoxia. Pulse oximetry may also be useful, providing the probes are well sited, and are tolerated by the subject. However, the definitive diagnosis and assessment of effect depends on arterial blood gas analysis (see Chapter 6i).

REFERENCES AND FURTHER READING

Court MH (1992) Respiratory support of the critically ill small animal patient. In: *Veterinary Emergency and Critical Care Medicine*, ed. RJ Murtaugh and PM Kaplan, p. 575. Mosby, New York

Crapo JD, Barry BE, Foscue HA and Shelburne J (1980) Structural and biochemical changes in rat lungs occurring during exposure to lethal and adaptive doses of oxygen. *American Review of Respiratory Disease* **122**, 123-143

Crisp MS (1994) Critical care techniques. In: *Manual of Small Animal Practice*, ed. Sanders, p. 25. W.B. Saunders, Philadelphia

Elkins AD (1997) Hyperbaric oxygen therapy: potential veterinary applications. *Compendium of Continuing Education for the Practising Veterinarian* **19**, 607-612

Frank L, Bucher JR and Roberts RJ (1978) Oxygen toxicity in neonatal and adult animals of various species. *Applied Physiology* **45**, 699-704

Hawkins EC (1992) Ancillary therapy. Oxygen supplementation and ventilation. In: *Essentials of Small Animal Internal Medicine*, ed. RW Nelson and CG Couto, p. 247. Mosby-Year Book, New York

Nogushi H, Takumi Y and Aochi O (1973) A study of humidification in tracheostomized dogs. *British Journal of Anaesthesia* **45**, 844-848

Paine JR, Lynne D and Keys A (1941) Observations on the effects of prolonged administration of high oxygen concentrations in dogs. *Journal of Thoracic Surgery* **11**, 151

Medical Therapy of Cardiac Conditions

Janice McIntosh Bright

THERAPEUTIC STRATEGIES

The most appropriate method for treating a cardiovascular disorder is to identify and specifically remove the underlying cause, and numerous lesions affecting the heart and vasculature can, in fact, be definitively treated. However, when a specific aetiology cannot be identified or treated, non-specific (supportive) management is required. Moreover, some animals will benefit from supportive therapy given to stabilize their condition prior to a specific therapeutic intervention. This chapter addresses non-specific management of congestive heart failure and cardiac arrhythmias. Management of arterial thromboembolism, pulmonary thromboembolism, and systemic hypertension is discussed elsewhere (Flanders, 1986; Perry *et al.*, 1991; Dukes, 1992).

Management of congestive heart failure

Congestive heart failure (CHF) is a clinical syndrome characterized by inadequate cardiac output occurring in the presence of adequate venous return and circulatory congestion. Irrespective of the underlying cause or pathophysiological mechanism of the congestive failure, therapeutic goals include:

- Reducing ventricular filling pressures to alleviate signs of circulatory congestion (oedema)
- Improving cardiac performance (increasing forward stroke volume)
- Interrupting deleterious neural and hormonal compensatory mechanisms.

Rarely is a single therapeutic agent adequate, and combination therapy directed towards each of these goals is generally necessary for optimal patient management.

Reducing ventricular filling pressures

Although the pathophysiological mechanisms responsible for increased ventricular filling pressures (increased ventricular end-diastolic pressures) are variable in patients with CHF, *diuretics* should be used to normalize filling pressures, and thereby relieve oedema. Frusemide (furosemide) is considered

the diuretic of choice for management of patients with moderate to severe failure, because of its potency even in the presence of reduced renal blood flow, and because this diuretic potentiates the renal and pulmonary production of beneficial vasodilatory prostaglandins. In patients with mild or early heart failure, such as an asymptomatic animal with echocardiographic evidence of ventricular dysfunction, the use of diuretics may be counterproductive because the volume contraction they produce will increase plasma renin activity and minimize the stimulus for release of atrial natriuretic peptide. Patients with refractory oedema may benefit from the use of a second diuretic, such as a thiazide or an aldosterone antagonist, in combination with frusemide. Combined use of two diuretics which act at different sites in the nephron is often more effective than single agent therapy, particularly in patients with refractory right heart failure.

Diuretics should be dosed conservatively in animals that have CHF as a result of impaired diastolic function or mitral stenosis, for such patients require a greater than normal atrial pressure to achieve adequate ventricular filling.

Drugs with venodilating properties may be used in addition to diuretics for reduction of ventricular filling pressures and relief of congestion.

Improving cardiac performance

Whereas diuretics and venodilators are used to alleviate circulatory congestion regardless of the underlying cause of CHF, the most appropriate medical intervention(s) to increase cardiac output will vary depending upon the underlying pathophysiological mechanism. For example, stroke volume is likely to increase following administration of a positive inotropic agent to a patient with dilated cardiomyopathy, but such an agent is unlikely to improve cardiac output if administered to an animal with constrictive pericarditis. The only universally appropriate recommendation for increasing forward flow is to optimize heart rate and rhythm. Table 21.1 lists the common pathophysiological mechanisms of CHF and the most appropriate medical means of augmenting cardiac output for each mechanism.

Mechanism	Interventions

Haemodynamic overload
       Volume overload
 	
       Pressure overload
	Optimize heart rate and rhythm
	Surgical correction
	Arteriolar dilators (afterload reducers)
	Optimize heart rate and rhythm
	Surgical (or catheter) correction
	Treat hypertension if present

Myocardial systolic dysfunction *Impaired contractility*	Optimize heart rate and rhythm Positive inotropic agents Arteriolar dilators (afterload reducers)

Myocardial diastolic dysfunction
Impaired ventricular filling
       Hypertrophic cardiomyopathy
 	
       Restrictive cardiomyopathy
       Pericardial diseases
	Optimize heart rate* and rhythm
	Positive lusitropic agents
	Optimize heart rate and rhythm
	Optimize heart rate** and rhythm
	Pericardiocentesis and/or pericardectomy

Rhythm disturbances	Optimize heart rate and rhythm

†Diuretics and venodilators are used to relieve circulatory congestion in all patients with congestive failure regardless of the pathophysiological mechanism
*Sinus tachycardia is detrimental in patients with hypertrophic cardiomyopathy
**Sinus tachycardia is beneficial in patients with pericardial diseases

Table 21.1: *Pathophysiological mechanisms of congestive heart failure, with suggested interventions for increasing stroke volume†*

Interrupting deleterious compensatory mechanisms
Several neural and hormonal compensatory mechanisms become activated in patients with CHF in response to decline in cardiac performance. These compensatory mechanisms include:

- Generalized stimulation of the sympathetic nervous system
- Activation of the renin–angiotensin–aldosterone system
- Increase in secretion of arginine vasopressin (antidiuretic hormone).

Although activation of these neurohumoral systems is beneficial in situations of acute or mild failure, these peripheral compensatory mechanisms become detrimental in patients with chronic or more severe CHF. The vasoconstrictive and antidiuretic effects of compensatory neural and hormonal systems over-ride existing counter regulating mechanisms leading to increased congestion, greater impedance to blood flow, increased myocardial oxygen demand, reduced coronary perfusion, provocation of arrhythmias, deleterious deposition of myocardial collagen, decreased responsiveness of myocardial adrenergic receptors, and direct myocardial toxicity. Therefore, therapeutic interventions that interrupt deleterious neurohumoral pathways, and that stimulate endogenous vasodilating and natriuretic pathways, are likely to provide consist-

ent and sustained beneficial effects. It is known, for example, that *angiotensin converting enzyme inhibitors* provide more universal and more sustained beneficial effects than direct–acting vasodilators. *Frusemide*, in addition to its potent diuretic effects, stimulates the synthesis of beneficial vasodilating prostaglandins. Finally, *spironolactone*, a drug with weak diuretic properties, may provide significant benefits to patients with CHF when added to combination therapy with frusemide and angiotensin converting enzyme inhibitors (Weber *et al.*, 1992; van Vliet *et al.*, 1993; Zannad, 1993).

Management of impaired diastolic function
Hypertrophic cardiomyopathy, restrictive cardiomyopathy, and pericardial diseases are disorders characterized by diastolic dysfunction of the heart. When diastolic function is impaired, the ventricles cannot accept blood or fill adequately without a compensatory increase in atrial pressure. The impaired ventricular filling may result in congestive heart failure or in hypoperfusion without circulatory congestion manifested as weakness, syncope, or sudden death.

Animals with congestive heart failure as a result of impaired diastolic function should be given diuretics and venodilators to decrease the congestion and oedema. Frusemide is administered, either intramuscularly or intravenously, to those with life-threatening oedema. Large doses of diuretics should be avoided, however, because patients with abnormal diastolic function need a higher than normal atrial pressure to achieve adequate ventricular filling. Usually, positive inotropic agents are of little benefit because myocardial contractility is typically not impaired, and, administration of positive inotropic agents to patients with diastolic dysfunction may actually be deleterious because these agents increase the myocardial oxygen demand. Arteriolar dilation (afterload reduction) should also be avoided because animals with impaired ventricular filling are unlikely to have enough preload reserve to increase stroke volume in response to peripheral vasodilation.

In animals with hypertrophic cardiomyopathy, ventricular filling is reduced as a result of both reduced chamber compliance and a decreased rate and extent of active myocardial relaxation. Compliance is unlikely to increase in response to pharmacological interventions unless these interventions significantly reverse hypertrophy and fibrosis. Presently there are no drugs that consistently accomplish this. Impaired relaxation, however, can be reversed, at least in part, by administration of drugs that relieve myocardial ischaemia and alter myocyte calcium handling. Whereas *β-adrenergic antagonists* improve diastolic function indirectly by reducing heart rate and myocardial oxygen demand, these drugs impair active relaxation of the myocardium by reducing the intracellular concentration of cyclic AMP (cAMP). In contrast, the *calcium channel blocking agents* have a direct positive lusitropic effect. Improved left ventricular filling following treatment of patients with calcium channel antagonists comes about through a direct beneficial effect on abnormal calcium transients, through a decrease in regional asynchrony, and through improved myocardial perfusion.

Diltiazem is a calcium channel blocking agent that appears to be safe and effective in most cats with hypertrophic cardiomyopathy. Chronic administration of this drug has been shown to improve clinical signs as well as radiographic, echocardiographic, and laboratory indices of cardiac performance in affected cats (Bright *et al.*, 1991). Several sustained release preparations of this drug have recently been shown to provide therapeutic plasma concentrations when administered once or twice daily to normal cats (Atkins *et al.*, 1994; Baty, 1997).

Because myocardial relaxation is delayed and incomplete in patients with hypertrophic cardiomyopathy, tachycardia has an adverse effect on left ventricular filling and overall cardiac performance. The negative chronotropic properties of the beta-adrenergic antagonists and the calcium channel antagonists are useful, therefore, for slowing the sinus rate to prolong diastole and allow increased ventricular filling in affected animals. Similarly, ectopic rhythms that result in loss of a co-ordinated, sequential atrioventricular contraction pattern have an adverse effect upon ventricular filling, and should be suppressed if possible. Animals with persistent resting tachycardia, atrial fibrillation,

or paroxysmal tachyarrhythmias may require combination therapy with beta-adrenergic blockade and diltiazem to control heart rate and rhythm. However, patients receiving such combined therapy should be closely monitored for development of bradyarrhythmias and/or hypotension.

Restrictive cardiomyopathy occurs when ventricular compliance and, therefore, diastolic ventricular volume are impaired by endocardial, subendocardial, or myocardial replacement of myocytes with fibrosis or infiltrate. Contractile function is usually unimpaired, particularly in early stages of the disease. The medical management of restrictive cardiomyopathy is often unrewarding because without a means of reversing the infiltrative process, it is difficult, if not impossible, to improve ventricular compliance and filling. Treatment centres around preload reduction (diuretics and venodilators) and on anticoagulant drugs in an attempt to prevent systemic embolism. Unlike the situation in patients with hypertrophic cardiomyopathy, compensatory sinus tachycardia has a beneficial haemodynamic effect in patients with restrictive cardiomyopathy, because these patients have a rapid decline in ventricular pressure at the onset of diastole with peak filling occurring early in diastole. Thus, negative chronotropic agents such as digitalis, beta blocking agents and calcium channel blocking agents should not be used to suppress the sinoatrial node. However, by improving relaxation and dilating the coronary arteries, diltiazem may be of benefit to cats with a suspected ischaemic or hypertrophic component of the disease process. In addition, angiotensin converting enzyme inhibitors used at sub-hypotensive (non-vasodilating) doses and aldosterone antagonists may provide beneficial anti-fibrotic effects.

Pericardial disorders including pericardial effusions and constrictive pericarditis also impair diastolic filling. Pericardiocentesis or pericardiectomy are the only means of improving ventricular filling and cardiac performance in affected animals. As with all cardiac disorders, stroke volume will increase if the heart rate and rhythm are optimized. It should be noted that the haemodynamic features of patients with pericardial disease are similar to those of patients with restrictive cardiomyopathy; ventricular filling is limited to early diastole and, therefore, sinus tachycardia should not be suppressed. There is no haemodynamic advantage to slowing the sinus rate in order to prolong diastole.

MANAGEMENT OF ARRHYTHMIAS

Appropriate management of arrhythmias requires accurate electrocardiographic diagnosis (see Chapter 12). In addition, medical intervention must be justified by a favourable benefit to risk ratio. Cardiac arrhythmias are caused by a wide variety of cardiac and extracardiac disorders, many of which may be specifically treated (see Chapter 12). Therefore, an attempt should be made to identify and specifically treat precipitating or aggravating causes of the rhythm disturbance. Often overlooked in this regard is that many cardiovascular agents used for management of heart disease may be arrhythmogenic; particularly the cardiac glycosides, catecholamines, xanthine derivatives, and the antiarrhythmic agents themselves.

Medical management of bradyarrhythmias

Unless an underlying cause can be identified and specifically treated, an animal with a symptomatic bradyarrhythmia is likely to require implantation of an artificial cardiac pacemaker. *Parasympatholytic agents* are used to manage sinus bradycardia or conduction blocks that result from excessive vagal tone, but beneficial response to anticholinergic agents is less predictable in animals with drug-induced bradycardias. Similarly, parasympatholytic agents are usually ineffective in animals with diseases of the cardiac pacemaking and/or conduction system. By producing an increase in the rate of ventricular escape, *sympathomimetic agents* may be helpful for temporary management of bradycardia that is due to complete heart block.

Medical management of tachyarrhythmias

Non-specific medical management of pathological tachycardias requires distinguishing the arrhythmia as ventricular or supraventricular in origin. This differentiation is important because the efficacy of a selected antiarrhythmic agent is determined largely upon its ability to alter automaticity, conduction, or refractoriness in specific regions of the heart.

Many supraventricular tachyarrhythmias result from atrioventricular (AV) nodal re-entry of the cardiac impulses, and therefore, agents that slow AV nodal conduction, such as cardiac glycosides, β-blocking agents and calcium channel blocking agents, will often produce conversion to sinus rhythm. These same agents are also used for slowing the ventricular rate in patients with atrial fibrillation and atrial flutter. Drugs such as quinidine or procainamide that prolong the effective refractory period of the atrial myocardium are used to convert atrial fibrillation to sinus rhythm or to treat refractory supraventricular arrhythmias. Drugs such as lignocaine, procainamide, quinidine, or beta blocking agents often effectively reduce myocyte automaticity, decrease impulse conduction velocity, and prolong refractoriness such that ventricular arrhythmias are eliminated.

CARDIOVASCULAR THERAPEUTIC AGENTS

This discussion should be considered an introduction to the therapeutic agents most commonly used in the medical management of canine and feline cardiovascular disorders. The reader is encouraged to consult other texts (Bonagura and Muir, 1992) to obtain information on newer and less commonly used therapeutic agents, and also to obtain more detail regarding the pharmacological and pharmacokinetic properties of the individual drugs discussed. Table 21.2 contains a summary of current dose recommendations.

Diuretics

Thiazide diuretics

The thiazide diuretics produce an increase in sodium and water excretion by reducing sodium and chloride permeability of the distal convoluted tubules (Weiner, 1990; Pugh, 1991). These agents can increase renal sodium excretion five to eight fold and are, therefore, moderately potent diuretics. However, the thiazides become ineffective when renal blood flow is reduced, and are of little value as a single agent in patients with severe cardiac compromise. When used in combination with loop diuretics, they have a useful role in management of animals with severe congestive failure. Animals receiving a thiazide diuretic in combination with frusemide are particularly prone to electrolyte depletion.

Loop diuretics

The loop diuretics, including frusemide and bumetanide, have a rapid onset of action, a relatively short duration of effect, and a maximum diuresis significantly greater than other available diuretic agents. Because the loop diuretics impair the active transport of chloride and sodium in the ascending loop of Henle, their natriuretic capability exceeds by nearly ten times that of the thiazides. These drugs remain effective in the presence of reduced renal perfusion. Furthermore, renal dysfunction, unless extremely advanced, is not a contraindication for the use of these drugs (Pugh, 1991). However, the potency of the loop diuretics should be viewed as a 'double edged sword' in that these powerful diuretics can easily produce hypotension and electrolyte depletion, particularly in cats and inappetant dogs. Renal dysfunction may result from the concurrent administration of angiotensin converting enzyme inhibitors and large doses of loop diuretics.

Loop diuretics should be dosed to effect to control cardiogenic oedema. Parenteral administration (i.v. or i.m.) should be used in emergency situations. Parenteral administration may also be necessary in animals with severe right-sided failure because of intestinal malabsorption that develops in some of these patients.

Potassium sparing diuretics

Although several potassium sparing diuretic agents are available, spironolactone, acting by competitive antagonism of aldosterone in the renal tubules, is the only drug in this class that interrupts a deleterious compensatory mechanism. Because spironolactone has only mild diuretic properties, it has been traditionally used in patients

	Drug	Usual dose	Cautions and adverse effects
Diuretics	Hydrochlorothiazide	*Dog* 2–4 mg/kg q12–24 h *Cat* 1–2 mg/kg q12–24 h	Hypokalaemia, hyponatraemia, hypomagnesaemia, hypercalcaemia, and hypochloraemic alkalosis
	Frusemide	*Dog* 2–6 mg/kg q6–12 h i.v., i.m., s.c., p.o. *Cat* 1–4 mg/kg q12–24 h i.v., i.m., s.c., p.o.	Hypotension, dehydration, hyponatraemia, hypokalaemia, hypochloraemic alkalosis, and hyperglycaemia
	Spironolactone	*Dog* and *cat* 2–4 mg/kg q24 h p.o.	May cause hyperkalaemia when combined with ACE inhibitor therapy. May take 2–3 days to achieve peak effect
Cardiac glycosides	Digoxin	*Dog* 0.005–0.01 mg/kg q12 h p.o. (use lower dose in dogs >22 kg) 0.005–0.01 mg/kg q1 h i.v. to effect (Maximum total dose 0.02 mg/kg) *Cat* 0.01 mg/kg q48 h p.o. (avoid elixir in cats)	May cause lethal arrhythmias. May cause lethargy, anorexia, vomiting, diarrhoea, and depression. Hypokalaemia predisposes to toxicity. Renal dysfunction, hypoalbuminaemia, hypothyroidism, and use of quinidine or verapamil require dose reduction
	Digitoxin	*Dog* 0.02–0.03 mg/kg q8–12 h p.o.	May cause lethal arrhythmias. May cause lethargy, anorexia, depression, vomiting, and depression
Sympathomimetic drugs	Dopamine	*Dog* 2–7 µg/kg/min *Cat* 0.05–2 µg/kg/min	May cause sinus tachycardia and tachyarrhythmias (begin with lower dose and titrate upward)
	Dobutamine	*Dog* 5–20 µg/kg/min *Cat* 0.05–2 µg/kg/min	May produce sinus tachycardia and tachyarrhythmias. May produce seizures, vomiting or cardiac arrest in cats at higher doses
	Isoproterenol	*Dog and cat* 5 µg/kg i.v. 0.05–1 µg/kg/min	May produce profound sinus tachycardia and ventricular arrhythmias. Hypotensive
Phosphodiesterase inhibitors	Amrinone	*Dog and cat* 1–3 mg/kg i.v. followed by 30–100 µg/kg/min i.v.	May reduce blood pressure and produce reflex tachycardia at high doses
	Milrinone	*Dog and cat* 30–300 µg/kg i.v. followed by 1–10 µg/kg/min i.v.	May reduce blood pressure and produce reflex tachycardia at high doses. May exacerbate ventricular arrhythmias
Vasodilators	Glyceryl trinitrate ointment (2%)	*Dog* 5–15 mg q6–8 h transdermally	Caution owner to wear gloves when applying
	Nitroprusside	*Dog* 1–5 µg/kg/min initially increasing by 3–5 µg/kg/min increments	May cause severe hypotension and should not be used without blood pressure monitoring. Discontinue administration gradually
	Hydralazine	*Dog* 1–3 mg/kg q12 h p.o. (initial dose 0.5 mg/kg then titrate upward) *Cat* 2.5–10 mg q12 h p.o.	May cause sinus tachycardia, vomiting, weakness, depression. May cause a lupus-like syndrome
Angiotensin converting enzyme (ACE) inhibitors	Enalapril	*Dog and cat* 0.25–0.5 mg/kg q12–24 h p.o.	May cause a deterioration in renal function. May cause weakness, depression and hypotension. Use with caution in patients with renal dysfunction, hyponatraemia or dehydration
	Benazepril	*Dog* 0.25 mg/kg q12–24 h	May cause weakness, depression and hypotension. Use with caution in patients with renal dysfunction, hyponatraemia or dehydration
β-Adrenergic blocking agents	Propranolol	*Dog* 0.1–0.3 mg/kg i.v. 0.2–1.0 mg/kg q8 h p.o. *Cat* 0.002–0.06 mg/kg i.v. 0.2–1.0 mg/kg q8 h p.o.	May cause hypotension, weakness, bradycardia, and depression. May aggravate myocardial failure. May aggravate bronchoconstriction
	Atenolol	*Dog* 6.25–25 mg q12 h p.o. *Cat* 6.25–12.5 mg qd p.o.	(same as propranolol)
	Esmolol	*Dog and cat* 500 µg/kg slowly i.v. then 25–200 µg/kg/min	(same as propranolol)
Calcium channel blocking agents	Verapamil	*Dog and cat* 0.05–0.15 mg/kg i.v. *Dog* 1–3 mg/kg q8–12 h p.o.	May cause bradycardia, hypotension, AV block, and myocardial depression. Increases plasma digoxin concentration
	Diltiazem	*Dog and cat* 1.5–2.5 mg/kg q8 h p.o. (or for *cats* 10 mg/kg q12 h of Dilacor XR or 10 mg/kg q24 h of Cardizem CD) *Dog and cat* 0.1 mg/kg then 0.2 mg/kg/h i.v.	May cause bradycardia, hypotension, AV block, and myocardial depression
Antiarrhythmics	Lignocaine	*Dog* 2–6 mg/kg i.v. then 25–80 µg/kg/min i.v. *Cat* 0.25–0.75 mg/kg slowly i.v.	May cause tremors, nystagmus, restlessness, seizures, and vomiting. May cause AV nodal dysfunction in cats. May be proarrhythmic
	Tocainide	*Dog* 10–20 mg/kg q8 h p.o.	May cause same adverse effects as lidocaine.
	Mexiletine	*Dog* 5–10 mg/kg q12 h p.o.	May cause same adverse effects as lidocaine.
	Procainamide	*Dog* 2 mg/kg i.v. then 25–40 µg/kg/min i.v. 10–25 mg/kg q6 h p.o. , i.m. (sustained release q8 h p.o.) *Cat* 3–8 mg/kg q6–8 h p.o., i.m.	May be proarrhythmic. May cause AV block, hypotension, anorexia, vomiting, and a lupus-like syndrome. Negative inotrope
	Quinidine	*Dog* quinidine sulphate 5–20 mg/kg q6–8 h p.o. quinidine gluconate 5–20 mg/kg q6 h i.m.	May be proarrhythmic. May increase the ventricular rate in patients with atrial fibrillation. May cause hypotension, nausea, vomiting, diarrhoea, and depression. Negative inotrope
Anticholinergics	Atropine	*Dog and cat* 0.01–0.04 mg/kg i.v., i.m., s.c.	May cause miosis, emesis, sicca, diarrhoea, and tachycardia
	Glycopyrrolate	*Dog and cat* 0.005–0.01 mg/kg i.v., i.m. 0.01–0.02 mg/kg s.c.	(same as atropine)
	Isopropamide	*Dog* 2.5–5 mg q8–12 h	(same as atropine)
	Propantheline	*Dog* 3.75–7.5 mg q8–12 h	(same as atropine)

Table 21.2: Drugs used to treat cardiac conditions.

with heart failure in combination with more potent diuretics primarily for the purpose of reducing potassium loss. Recently, however, the vital role of aldosterone in sodium and water retention in patients with CHF has been recognized (Zannad, 1993), and preliminary data from human patients suggest that co-administration of spironolactone may be an effective means of managing CHF which has become refractory to combination therapy with loop diuretics and angiotensin converting enzyme inhibitors (van Vliet *et al.*, 1993).

Inotropic agents

Cardiac glycosides

Digitalis and various other cardiac glycosides have a relatively weak positive inotropic effect and a negative chronotropic effect that have been traditionally relied upon for chronic management of left ventricular systolic failure and for management of supraventricular tachycardias. Doubt exists, however, in regard to the sustained efficacy and safety of these agents in patients with sinus rhythm (Poole-Wilson and Robinson, 1989; Jaeschke *et al.*, 1990; Banerjee and Campbell, 1996). In humans, the indications for chronic digitalis therapy have recently been restricted to management of chronic supraventricular arrhythmias and management of systolic dysfunction in patients with severe left ventricular dilation, a third heart sound, and fluid retention (Bolognesi *et al.*, 1992).

Contraindications for use of the cardiac glycosides are numerous (Table 21.3).

| Digitalis intoxication |
| Cardiac diseases with predominant diastolic dysfunction |
| Advanced atrioventricular (AV) conduction block |
| Ventricular arrhythmias |
| Supraventricular arrhythmias in patients with ventricular pre-excitation |
| Acute myocardial infarction |
| Sick sinus syndrome |
| Acute myocarditis |

Table 21.3: Absolute and relative contraindications for cardiac glycosides.

The cardiac glycosides have direct effects on the electrical and mechanical activity of the heart and indirect effects mediated through the autonomic nervous system. Some of the therapeutic and most of the serious toxic effects are related to direct effects on the electrophysiological properties of the heart which include:

- Reducing the resting membrane potential, thereby slowing conduction velocity
- Reducing the action potential duration, resulting

in increased myocyte excitability
- Enhancement of automaticity, via an increase in the rate of spontaneous diastolic depolarization and creation of delayed afterdepolarizations.

However, when cardiac glycosides are administered to patients with CHF, the sinus rate usually decreases because of a drug-induced increase in vagal impulses and a reflexly mediated decrease in sympathetic tone (Hoffman and Bigger, 1990). The AV node is particularly sensitive to the indirect, vagomimetic effects of the glycosides producing a reduction in the rate at which atrial impulses can be conducted to the ventricles.

The most widely used digitalis preparations are *digoxin* and *digitoxin*. The pharmacokinetic properties and metabolism of these two drugs differ significantly. In addition, digoxin has a more pronounced vagally-mediated indirect effect than digitoxin. There is negligible hepatic metabolism of digoxin and, consequently, nearly all of the administered drug becomes available for distribution to the tissues. Moreover, only about 25% of digoxin in the plasma is bound to albumin. In contrast, digitoxin undergoes significant hepatic excretion and is more highly protein bound in the plasma (Hoffman and Bigger, 1990). Thus, digitoxin has a shorter plasma half-life than digoxin, and higher doses of digitoxin are needed to achieve therapeutic tissue concentrations (Table 21.2). Digoxin is primarily excreted in the urine. Therefore, renal dysfunction will reduce the rate of excretion of this drug increasing the plasma concentration. Frequent serum digoxin assays are required to establish and monitor dosage in azotaemic animals. Alternatively, digitoxin is excreted by the liver and can by used safely in dogs with renal dysfunction. However, digitoxin is not recommended for use in cats because of its long half-life (>100 hours) in this species. Many other factors such as age, presence of cachexia or ascites, hypoalbuminaemia, hypokalaemia, thyroid dysfunction, and interaction with other therapeutic agents will affect the availability, distribution, and elimination of the cardiac glycosides necessitating dosage modifications. In addition, the presence of myocardial failure or hypoxia increases myocardial sensitivity to the cardiac glycosides.

It is important, therefore, that patients be thoroughly screened prior to digitalis administration to identify factors that may require modification of the initial dosage. After glycoside therapy commences, the patient and the electrocardiogram should be monitored for signs of intoxication as well as for signs of improvement. A reduction in heart rate and reduced frequency of arrhythmia are desired effects in animals with tachyarrhythmias or ectopia. In other patients, signs of a beneficial response are less objective and include indirect evidence of improved tissue perfusion (improvement in strength, stamina, etc.). The glycoside dose should not be increased unless the patient is doing poorly *and* the serum digoxin concentration has been determined to be subtherapeutic. There is no reason to measure the serum digoxin concentration in patients that are doing well clinically and have no signs of possible toxicosis.

The clinical signs of digitalis intoxication vary from mild gastrointestinal upset to severe weight loss and life threatening arrhythmias. Anorexia and loose stools are very common side effects of digoxin administration that can complicate patient management by contributing to electrolyte depletion. Vomiting occasionally occurs without anorexia. The toxic effects of digitalis on the myocardium usually manifest as various cardiac arrhythmias which may be lethal. Ventricular ectopia such as isolated premature contractions, ventricular bigeminy or trigeminy, and ventricular tachycardia are common digitalis-induced arrhythmias. Atrial and junctional tachycardias, sinus bradycardia and arrest, second degree AV block, and junctional escape rhythms are also commonly observed. Whereas the adverse gastrointestinal effects of the cardiac glycosides may precede cardiac toxicity, this is not consistently true in animals with contractile failure.

Sympathomimetic agents
Among the various sympathomimetic agents only *dopamine* and *dobutamine*, because of their relative lack of vascular and positive chronotropic effects, are used for management of patients with CHF. These drugs are indicated for management of patients with severe, decompensated myocardial failure. In addition to stimulating the β_1-adrenergic receptors in the heart, dopamine stimulates the dopaminergic receptors of the renal and mesenteric vasculature, producing relaxation of the vascular smooth muscle and vasodilation in these areas. Thus, dopamine is likely to be a more useful therapeutic agent than dobutamine for patients with combined renal and cardiac disease. Dobutamine, however, is less arrhythmogenic. Both drugs must be given intravenously and, due to rapid development of β-receptor down regulation, are useful only for the first 24–48 hours of infusion. Patients with myocardial failure and atrial fibrillation should be given digoxin to prevent enhancement of AV conduction as a result of dopamine or dobutamine administration.

Isoprenaline (isoproterenol) is also a potent inotropic agent, but this agent has significant positive chronotropic and arrhythmogenic properties rendering it unsuitable for use in patients with heart failure.

However, by increasing the rate of ventricular escape, isoprenaline may be useful for the acute management of animals with complete heart block. *Adrenaline* (epinephrine) is a potent cardiac stimulant, but because of its positive chronotropic, arrhythmogenic, and vasoconstrictive properties, its usefulness in patients with cardiac disease is limited to cardiac resuscitative efforts.

Phosphodiesterase inhibitors
Amrinone, *milrinone* and *enoximone* are potent positive inotropic agents that produce their cardiotonic effects by inhibiting phosphodiesterase III, thereby increasing intracellular levels of cyclic AMP. These agents also relax vascular smooth muscle resulting in arteriolar dilation. Amrinone is available as an intravenous preparation in the USA, and both enoximone and milrinone are available for intravenous use in the UK. Milrinone is approximately 30–40 times more potent than amrinone. These positive inotropic agents are indicated for short-term management of severe myocardial failure, and may be efficacious in patients who have developed tachyphylaxis to the sympathomimetic inotropes. Whereas the catecholamines and cardiac glycosides are of questionable benefit in humans (Oakley, 1988) and in dogs (Bright, 1994) with failure of the right ventricular myocardium, the phosphodiesterase inhibitors have been shown to improve indices of right ventricular function in human patients (Konstam *et al.*, 1986). The drugs in this group have a large therapeutic index, but ventricular arrhythmias have been noted following administration in dogs. A beneficial effect of milrinone on clinical signs and ventricular performance has been reported in a group of dogs with naturally occurring CHF that were given the drug orally for a 4-week period (Keister *et al.*, 1990). However, data from human studies suggest that phosphodiesterase inhibitors are less effective and more arrhythmogenic than digoxin, and that milrinone has a deleterious effect on survival (Packer *et al.*, 1991a).

Vasodilating agents
Vasodilating agents are drugs used to relax vascular smooth muscle. These drugs are classified according to whether they act primarily on the capacitance vessels (venodilators), the resistance vessels (arteriolar dilators), or both (balanced vasodilators). They are further classified based upon mechanism of action (Table 21.4). In veterinary patients, vasodilators are

Venodilators	Nitrates (direct acting)	glyceryl trinitrate
Arteriolar dilators	Direct acting	hydralazine
	Calcium channel blocking agents	amlodipine
Balanced vasodilators	Direct acting	nitroprusside
	α_1-Adrenergic antagonists	prazosin
	Angiotensin converting enzyme (ACE) inhibitors	enalapril, captopril, benazepril

Table 21.4: Classification of vasodilators according to site and mechanism of action.

used to reduce preload and afterload in patients with CHF, and to reduce regurgitant flow and left atrial pressure in patients with mitral regurgitation. Less commonly, arteriolar dilators are used for management of systemic hypertension.

Venodilators increase venous capacitance, thereby decreasing ventricular diastolic pressures. *Arteriolar dilators* reduce vascular resistance with a subsequent increase in stroke volume and decrease in myocardial oxygen demand. In addition, some vasodilators, such as the calcium channel blocking agents, have direct coronary vasodilating properties.

Drugs with arteriolar dilating properties should not be used in patients with confirmed or suspected hypotension (animals with profound weakness, hypothermia, thready pulses, etc.). The condition of such patients should be stabilized with other agents prior to instituting afterload reduction. Arteriolar dilators are also contraindicated in animals with diastolic dysfunction and those with ventricular outflow obstruction.

Venodilators

Venodilators are used in combination with diuretics to relieve circulatory congestion. In dogs and cats, the nitrates are frequently used for venodilation, and although available in a wide variety of preparations for parenteral, sublingual, and transdermal administration, transdermal products are easiest to administer. Two percent *glyceryl trinitrate ointment* can be applied to a hairless area of the skin as a component of the initial therapy of patients with heart failure. Data indicate that some patients receiving transdermal nitrates develop tolerance to the drug with a reduced therapeutic effect. Also, it is unclear whether patients with CHF treated with a balanced vasodilator (e.g. enalapril, captopril, benazepril) will receive additional benefit from nitrate administration.

Arteriolar dilators

Some pharmacological agents have a relatively selective effect on the arterial smooth muscle. Such agents include the *calcium channel blocking agents* and the direct acting agent, *hydralazine*. Hydralazine has been used effectively in combination with diuretics for management of dogs with mitral regurgitation and in combination with diuretics and inotropic agents for treatment of myocardial failure. However, hydralazine administration often produces an undesirable increase in heart rate, as well as gastrointestinal upset. In addition, the beneficial effects of hydralazine may become attenuated by compensatory increases in sympathetic tone and renin secretion. The calcium channel blocking agents produce dilation of the arterioles and coronary vasculature and are frequently used for treating coronary artery disease and hypertension in people. Although these agents will reduce afterload, they are not generally recommended for patients with CHF because of their negative inotropic properties and

because of the adverse neurohumoral changes they induce (Packer, 1989). Recent data, however, indicate that *amlodipine*, a third generation calcium channel antagonist, may improve clinical signs, exercise tolerance, and left ventricular function in human heart failure patients (Packer *et al.*, 1991b).

Balanced vasodilators

Direct acting vasodilators: The direct acting agent, *nitroprusside*, and the angiotensin converting enzyme inhibitors have both arteriolar dilating and venodilating properties. Nitroprusside is an extremely potent intravenous agent which must be used with continuous monitoring of the arterial blood pressure. Its rapid onset of action, short half-life, and powerful vasodilating properties make it a useful drug for patients with acute, severe, life-threatening myocardial failure, mitral or aortic regurgitation, or systemic hypertension.

Angiotensin converting enzyme (ACE) inhibitors: The angiotensin converting enzyme inhibitors are a large family of drugs that produce vasodilation directly by blocking the formation of angiotensin II, and also indirectly by reducing sympathetic tone and reducing the degradation of kinins. The ACE inhibitors also have various other beneficial effects in patients with CHF (Table 21.5). At this time, ACE inhibitors are considered the vasodilators of choice for most dogs and cats with myocardial systolic dysfunction and volume overload. The deleterious effects on myocardial structure of locally produced angiotensin II have recently been recognized, and ACE inhibitors given at subhypotensive doses may prove to be an important component of therapy in patients with other types of CHF as well (Chatterjee, 1992; Zannad, 1993). Sustained beneficial haemodynamic effects of ACE inhibition have been documented in dogs with experimentally induced mitral regurgitation (Blackford *et al.*, 1990). ACE inhibition has also been shown to improve haemodynamics, clinical signs, and survival in dogs with naturally occurring heart failure resulting

Direct vasoconstriction
Aldosterone release
Vasopressin release
Facilitates noradrenaline release
Blocks neuronal uptake of noradrenaline
Adrenaline release
Augments pressor effects of vasopressin
Stimulates thirst
Stimulates central noradrenaline activity
Stimulates myocardial hypertrophy and fibrosis
Exacerbates arrhythmias

Table 21.5: Deleterious effects of angiotensin II in patients with congestive heart failure.

from mitral regurgitation and dilated cardiomyopathy (Co-operative Veterinary Enalapril Study Group, 1995).

Of the available ACE inhibitors, *captopril* and *enalapril* have been widely used in canine and feline patients, but enalapril has several advantages. Enalapril has a longer duration of action, produces less gastrointestinal upset, and is available in small tablet sizes suitable for cats and toy breed dogs.

The ACE inhibitors may have a deleterious effect on the renal status of patients with compromised renal function. Therefore, these drugs must be used cautiously or avoided in patients with significant renal impairment.

Calcium channel blocking agents

The calcium channel blocking agents are a heterogeneous group of drugs that reduce entry of calcium ions into the cells of various excitable tissues. Because calcium ions are vital to many processes including the activation of myocardial and vascular smooth muscle cells, these drugs are useful in a variety of cardiovascular disorders. As a general description of the calcium channel antagonists, these drugs have negative inotropic, positive lusitropic, and arteriolar dilating properties. In addition, they suppress sinoatrial automaticity and decrease AV nodal conduction velocity. However, specific agents vary significantly in their relative cardiodepressant, antiarrhythmic, vasodilator, and reflex sympathetic stimulating effects. Choice of a specific calcium channel antagonist must, therefore, be made after considering the nature of the disorder as well as the pharmacodynamic properties of the individual drugs.

Verapamil, nifedipine and *diltiazem* are the prototype or first generation calcium channel blocking agents. Of these, verapamil has the most potent effect on AV nodal conduction and is, therefore, a useful antiarrhythmic agent. Verapamil also has a more potent *in vivo* negative inotropic effect than either nifedipine or diltiazem and must be used extremely cautiously in patients with myocardial contractile failure. Verapamil tends to reduce the sinus rate and is a peripheral and coronary vasodilator.

Nifedipine has the least effect on AV conduction and the most potent peripheral vasodilating properties. This drug tends to cause a reflex sinus tachycardia making it an inappropriate choice for patients with hypertrophic cardiomyopathy.

The effects of diltiazem are somewhat intermediate between those of verapamil and nifedipine. This drug causes less peripheral vasodilation than nifedipine at equally potent coronary vasodilating doses. Diltiazem prolongs AV nodal conduction but not to the same degree as verapamil. Its negative inotropic effect is less than that of verapamil.

Several newer calcium channel blocking agents have been developed. These second generation calcium antagonists have more potent and selective coronary and peripheral vasodilating properties with less myocardial depression. They are used primarily for management of hypertension and ischaemic heart disease in people. These newer calcium antagonists, particularly amlodipine, may prove useful in the management of CHF as well.

Table 21.6 lists the uses and potential uses of the calcium channel blocking agents. Verapamil and diltiazem, by increasing the effective refractory period and delaying AV nodal conduction, are highly effective for converting re-entrant supraventricular tachycardia to sinus rhythm. Because the negative inotropic effects of diltiazem are less potent, it is a more appropriate antiarrhythmic agent than verapamil for patients with impaired systolic function. Verapamil and diltiazem may also be used to slow the ventricular response to atrial fibrillation and atrial flutter. The calcium channel blocking agents have little effect on intra-atrial and intraventricular excitability or conduction, and, therefore, these agents are usually ineffective for treatment of ventricular or atrial arrhythmias except those that occur because of myocardial ischaemia.

Diltiazem has been shown to reduce the severity of clinical signs, improve left ventricular filling, and enhance survival in many cats with hypertrophic cardiomyopathy (Bright *et al.*, 1991). The beneficial effects of diltiazem in this disorder are believed to result from a decrease in myocardial ischaemia, a reduction of sarcoplasmic calcium ion, and improved synchrony of ventricular relaxation.

Nifedipine is frequently used in people for acute and chronic management of systemic hypertension. Although available pharmacokinetic data would suggest that the half-life of this drug is too short to render it a useful antihypertensive agent in dogs, we have found it useful for management of systemic hypertension in some dogs, particularly those with renal failure.

Recent data indicate that *amlodipine*, a third generation agent, is a safe and effective drug for treatment of feline hypertension (Henik *et al.*, 1994). We have also used this drug successfully in hypertensive dogs and those with CHF that are intolerant of ACE inhibitors

Calcium gluconate or calcium chloride can be administered to antagonize the effects of calcium channel antagonists. Verapamil, if used in combination with digoxin will result in an increased plasma digoxin concentration.

Arrhythmias (supraventricular tachycardia, atrial fibrillation, atrial flutter)
Hypertrophic cardiomyopathy
Systemic hypertension
Pulmonary hypertension (?)
Congestive heart failure (?)
Myocardial protecting agents (cardiac surgery)

Table 21.6: *Uses and potential uses of calcium channel blocking agents in patients with cardiovascular diseases.*

β-Adrenergic blocking agents

The β-adrenergic blocking agents (β-blockers) competitively inhibit the binding of catecholamines to β-adrenergic receptors, thereby decreasing or inhibiting the effects of sympathetic stimulation. Most of these agents, such as *propranolol*, have a non-selective antagonistic effect on the β_1 and β_2 receptors; whereas others, such as *metoprolol* and *atenolol*, are relatively selective for the β_1 receptors of the heart. β-blocking agents may be used in the management of various cardiovascular disorders including supraventricular tachycardia and supraventricular ectopy, atrial flutter and atrial fibrillation, hypertrophic cardiomyopathy (to reduce heart rate, myocardial oxygen requirement, and intraventricular pressure gradients), ventricular ectopy, thyrotoxicosis, hypertension, and phaeochromocytoma. The response to therapy will reflect the dosage used as well as the underlying level of sympathetic tone. β-blocking agents may be combined with other antiarrhythmic agents, particularly for control of refractory ventricular arrhythmias. *Sotalol*, a potent non-cardioselective β-blocking agent, is the only β-adrenergic antagonist that prolongs the cardiac action potential duration, increases the refractory period, and lengthens the QT interval on the surface electrocardiogram. This drug, therefore, has direct antiarrhythmic and antifibrillatory properties, and has been widely and effectively used to control ventricular tachyarrhythmias in humans (Hohnloser and Woosley, 1994). However, little information is available regarding the clinical use of this β-blocking agent in veterinary patients.

Antagonism of sympathetic tone is potentially dangerous, especially in animals with myocardial failure. Therefore, low initial doses are used with gradual upward titration to achieve the desired effect (decrease in heart rate, reduction of blood pressure, etc.). β-blocking agents are usually administered orally, but esmolol and propranolol may be used intravenously for immediate control of supraventricular tachycardia. Contraindications for β-adrenergic blockade include bradycardia and impaired AV conduction, decompensating CHF, hypotension, bronchial asthma, and hypoglycaemia.

Cimetidine decreases the hepatic elimination of highly lipophilic β-blocking agents such as propranolol. Coadministration of β-blocking agents with calcium channel blocking agents may produce a profound reduction of heart rate, contractility and blood pressure.

Lignocaine, tocainide, and mexiletine

These antiarrhythmic agents have similar electrophysiological effects, and are used primarily for treatment of ventricular arrhythmias. These drugs exert their beneficial effects by decreasing automaticity and by prolonging the effective refractory period. They have little effect on conduction velocity and myocardial contractility. Lignocaine is administered intravenously using one or two initial boluses followed by constant infusion. It is the antiarrhythmic agent of choice for control of life-threatening ventricular arrhythmias. Mexiletine and tocainide are administered orally. All three agents may cause excitation of the central nervous system with nervousness, vomiting, twitching, and/or seizures. Diazepam should be used to control these adverse effects. Cats are very susceptible to the toxic effects of these drugs and may develop sinus node or AV nodal dysfunction in addition to the adverse neurologic signs.

Quinidine and procainamide

These drugs have similar electrophysiological and antiarrhythmic effects. Quinidine is used to treat atrial, junctional, and ventricular arrhythmias, and for the attempted conversion of atrial fibrillation to sinus rhythm. Procainamide is primarily used to treat ventricular arrhythmias. Whereas quinidine is used almost exclusively in dogs, procainamide is used in both dogs and cats. The antiarrhythmic effects of these drugs result from a drug induced reduction of automaticity and prolongation of the effective refractory period. Both drugs significantly depress conduction and have negative inotropic effects. Adverse gastrointestinal effects are common. Quinidine has a significant α-adrenergic blocking effect and may cause profound hypotension if administered by the intravenous route. Quinidine will increase the plasma digoxin concentration necessitating a reduction of the glycoside dosage.

Anticholinergic agents

Atropine and *glycopyrrolate* are anticholinergic agents that are administered parenterally for acute or short-term management of symptomatic sinus arrest, sinus bradycardia, sinus arrhythmia, and/or atrioventricular (AV) block associated with excessive vagal tone or with excessive doses of cholinergic drugs. Except in life-threatening emergencies, the intravenous route of atropine administration should be avoided otherwise temporary enhancement of sinus bradycardia or AV block may occur. *Isopropamide* or *propantheline bromide* are oral anticholinergic agents that are occasionally useful for management of animals with symptomatic sinus bradycardia and sinus arrest due to disease of the sinus node ('sick sinus syndrome'). However, clinical response to anticholinergic treatment of sinus node dysfunction is not usually sustained.

REFERENCES AND FURTHER READING

Atkins C, Johnson L, Keene B *et al.* (1994) Diltiazem pharmacokinetics and pharmacodynamics in cats. *Proceedings of the American College of Veterinary Internal Medicine* 12, 144

Banerjee AK and Campbell RW (1996) Digoxin therapy and survival in heart failure in sinus rhythm. *International Journal of Cardiology* 55, 9

Baty CJ (1997) Clinical update on feline hypertrophic cardiomyopathy. *Proceedings of the American College of Veterinary Internal Medicine* **15**, 149

Blackford LW, Golden AL, Bright JM *et al.* (1990) Captopril provides sustained hemodynamic benefit in dogs with experimentally induced mitral regurgitation. *Veterinary Surgery* **19**, 237

Bolognesi R, Tsialtas D and Manca C (1992) Digitalis and heart failure: does digitalis really produce beneficial effects through a positive inotropic action? *Cardiovascular Drugs and Therapeutics* **6**, 459

Bonagura JD and Muir WW (1992) Antiarrhythmic therapy. In: *Essentials of Canine and Feline Electrocardiography*, ed. LP Tilley. Lea and Febiger, Philadelphia

Bright JM (1994) Right ventricular function and right heart failure. *Proceedings of the American College of Veterinary Internal Medicine* **12**, 331

Bright JM, Golden AL, Gompf RE *et al.* (1991) Evaluation of the calcium channel-blocking agents diltiazem and verapamil for treatment of feline hypertrophic cardiomyopathy. *Journal of Veterinary Internal Medicine* **5**, 272

Chatterjee K (1992) Use of angiotensin converting enzyme inhibitors. *Heart Disease and Stroke* **1**, 128

Co-operative Veterinary Enalapril (COVE) Study Group (1995) Controlled clinical evaluation of enalapril in dogs with congestive heart failure. *Journal of Veterinary Internal Medicine* **9**, 243

Dukes J (1992) Hypertension: a review of the mechanisms, manifestations and management. *Journal of Small Animal Practice* **33**, 119.

Flanders JA (1986) Feline aortic thromboembolism. *Compendium on Continuing Education for the Practicing Veterinarian* **8**, 473

Henik RA, Snyder PS and Volk LM (1994) Amlodipine besylate therapy in cats with systemic hypertension secondary to chronic renal disease. *Proceedings of the American College of Veterinary Internal Medicine* **12**, 145

Hoffman BF and Bigger JT (1990) Digitalis and allied cardiac glycosides. In: *The Pharmacological Basis of Therapeutics* 8th edn, eds A Goodman Gillman, TW Rall, AS Nies and P Taylor. Pergamon Press, New York

Hohnloser SH and Woosley RL (1994) Sotalol. *New England Journal of Medicine* **331**, 31

Jaeschke R, Oxman AD and Guyatt GH (1990) To what extent do congestive heart failure patients in sinus rhythm benefit from digoxin therapy? *American Journal of Medicine* **88**, 279

Keister DM, Kittleson MD, Bonagura JD *et al.* (1990) Milrinone: a clinical trial in 29 dogs with moderate to severe congestive heart failure. *Journal of Veterinary Internal Medicine* **4**, 79

Konstam MD, Cohen SR, Salem DN *et al.* (1986) Effect of amrinone on right ventricular function: predominance of afterload reduction. *Circulation* **74**, 359

Oakley C (1988) Importance of right ventricular function in congestive heart failure. *American Journal of Cardiology* **62**, 14A

Packer M (1989) Pathophysiological mechanisms underlying the adverse effects of calcium channel-blocking drugs in patients with chronic heart failure. *Circulation* **80**, 59

Packer M, Carver JR, Rodeheffer RJ *et al.* (1991a) Effect of oral milrinone on mortality in severe chronic heart failure. *New England Journal of Medicine* **325**, 1468

Packer M, Nicod P, Khandheria BR *et al.* (1991b) Randomized, multicenter, double-blind, placebo-controlled evaluation of amlodipine in patients with mild-to-moderate heart failure. *Journal of the American College of Cardiology* **17**, 274

Perry LA, Dillon AR and Bowers TL (1991) Pulmonary hypertension. *Compendium on Continuing Education for the Practicing Veterinarian* **13**, 226

Poole-Wilson PA and Robinson K (1989) Digoxin – a redundant drug in congestive cardiac failure. *Cardiovascular Drugs and Therapeutics* **2**, 733

Pugh DM (1991) The urinary system. In: *Veterinary Applied Pharmacology and Therapeutics* 5th edn, eds GC Brander, DM Pugh, RJ Bywater and WL Jenkins. Bailliere Tindall, London

Van Vliet AA, Conker AJM, Nauta JJP *et al.* (1993) Spironolactone in congestive heart failure refractory to high-dose loop diuretic and low-dose angiotensin-converting enzyme inhibitor. *American Journal of Cardiology* **71**, 21A

Weber KT, Brilla CG, Campbell SE *et al.* (1992) Myocardial fibrosis and the concepts of cardioprotection and cardioreparation. *Journal of Hypertension* **10**, S87

Weiner IM (1990) Diuretics and other agents employed in the mobilization of edema fluid. In: *The Pharmacological Basis of Therapeutics* 8th edn, eds A Goodman Gillman, TW Rall, AS Nies and P Taylor. Pergamon Press, New York

Zannad F (1993) Angiotensin-converting enzyme inhibitor and spironolactone combination therapy: new objectives in heart failure treatment. *American Journal of Cardiology* **71**, 34A

Medical Therapy of Respiratory Conditions

Dawn Merton Boothe

Table 22.1 lists drugs used in the treatment of respiratory conditions.

ANTIMICROBIAL THERAPY

Bacterial infections

Infections of the lower respiratory tract are serious. Although generally less serious, infections of the tracheobronchial tree can contribute to more serious diseases such as asthma (Moise *et al.*, 1989). Important considerations to be made when selecting an antimicrobial for treatment or prevention of small animal respiratory infections include:

- The causative organism and its antimicrobial susceptibility
- Drug distribution to the respiratory tract
- The mechanism of action of the drug, particularly as it relates to bactericidal versus bacteriostatic effects
- Host toxicity
- Convenience of administration.

The routine use of antimicrobials for the treatment of chronic respiratory diseases is controversial. Distinction between infection and colonization should be made whenever possible. Selection of the antimicrobial is best based upon culture of the trachea or lower airways and susceptibility testing of the isolate. Although bactericidal drugs are preferred, no drug is bactericidal if adequate tissue concentrations are not achieved. In general, distribution to the lower airways is adequate to excellent for most drugs. However, the mucosa may represent a clinically important barrier to drug penetration and adjunct aerosol therapy may be indicated. Use of lipid soluble drugs may be preferred (i.e. quinolones) for upper airway infections.

Pasteurella sp. and *Moraxella* sp. (probably a non-pathogen) are the most common organisms isolated from the respiratory tract of cats with bronchial disease. In dogs, *Bordetella bronchiseptica* is the most common organism associated with tracheobronchial diseases, while *Bordetella* and *Streptococcus zooepidemicus* are common primary pathogens in pneumonia. Other pathogenic bacterial micro-organisms associated with respiratory disease in small animals include *E. coli*, *Pseudomonas* spp., *Klebsiella* spp., *Staphylococcus* spp. and α and β haemolytic streptococci (Amis, 1986; Conlon, 1990). Pulmonary abscessation may indicate infection by anaerobic bacteria (Boothe, 1990). The role of bacteria in chronic bronchial disease of dogs and cats is controversial (Padrid *et al.*, 1990).

Beta-lactam antibiotics are excellent first choice drugs for the treatment of most bacterial infections. The bactericidal aminopenicillin, *amoxicillin*, is well absorbed orally, is distributed to the lungs and is characterized by a broad spectrum of activity. The addition of the β−lactamase protectant, *clavulanic acid*, increases the efficacy of amoxicillin against both Gram negative (including *Pasteurella* sp. and *Bordetella*) and Gram positive anaerobes and aerobes. The combination drug is well tolerated in both dogs and cats. First generation cephalosporins (e.g. *cephalexin* and *cefaclor*) are also excellent choices for Gram negative organisms, although they may be less effective for the treatment of anaerobic infections. Third generation cephalosporins and extended spectrum penicillins (e.g. *ticarcillin* and *cefotaxime*) can be used for serious or life-threatening Gram negative infections.

The *fluorinated quinolones* (enrofloxacin) are very well distributed to the lungs and are bactericidal towards Gram negative aerobes (including *Pseudomonas* spp.) as well as *Mycoplasma* sp., an organism that may be associated with bronchial diseases (Moise *et al.*, 1989).

The *aminoglycosides* are also effective in life-threatening or complicated Gram negative infections. Their distribution to the lungs is adequate, although not as great as the quinolones. Aerosolization of aminoglycosides can enhance their therapeutic efficacy particularly for treatment of *Bordetella*-associated tracheobronchitis and *Pseudomonas* infections (Bemis and Appel, 1977). Absorption of *gentamicin* (up to 7.5 mg/kg in 3 ml saline) and *kanamycin* appears to be negligible in dogs following aerosolization by mask. While amikacin kinetics following aerosolization apparently have not been studied, it is unlikely that it will be systemically absorbed. Aerosolization of *polymyxin B* (3 mg/ml) is associated

Drug	Route	Dose (mg/kg)	Frequency (h)
Antimicrobials			
Amikacin	i.m., s.c.	7–10	12
Amoxicillin and			
clavulanic acid	p.o.	10–20	12
Gentamicin	i.v., i.m., s.c.	1–2	12–24
Cephalexin	i.m., s.c., p.o.	10–30	8–12
Chloramphenicol	p.o.	50	12
Enrofloxacin	p.o.	2.5	12
Bronchodilators			
β-Adrenoceptor agonists			
Adrenaline	i.m., i.v., s.c.	20 μg/kg of 0.01% solution	30 min (up to total dose of 0.5 ml)
	s.c.	0.1 ml/kg of 0.1% solution	
Clenbuterol	i.m., s.c., p.o.	0.8 μg/kg	12
Ephedrine	i.m., p.o.	*Dog* 5–15 mg (total)	
		Cat 2–5 mg (total)	
Isoprenaline	p.o.	0.44	6–12
	i.m., s.c., i.v.	0.1–0.2 mg total	6
	Aerosol	0.5 ml of 1:200 dilution	4 x 3
Orceprenaline	p.o.	0.5	6
	Aerosol		4 x 3
Albuterol	p.o.	5 μg/kg	8–12
	Aerosol	200 μg (human dose)	
Terbutaline	p.o.	1.25 mg total	12
Isoetharine	Aerosol	0.5–1.0 ml of 1:3 saline dilution	8
Methylxanthines			
Aminophylline	p.o.	*Dog* 10	6–8
		Cat 5–6	12
	i.v. infusion (emergencies)	2–5	8–12 over 30–60 min
Theophylline base	p.o.	*Dog* 5–10	6–8
		Cat 4 (based on 80% theophylline)	12
Theophylline anhydrous	p.o.	20 mg/kg	12 (dog)
base slow release			24 (cat)
Oxytriphylline	p.o.	10–15 (based on 65% theophylline)	8–12
Anticholinergic drugs			
Atropine	i.v., i.m., s.c.	0.02–0.04	as needed
Glycopyrrolate	i.v., i.m., s.c.	0.01–0.02	as needed
Glucocorticoids			
Prednisolone	p.o.	1–2	6–12
Prednisolone	i.v., i.m.*	2–4	4–6
sodium succinate			
Dexamethasone	i.v., i.m.*	0.2–2.2	
Triamcinolone	p.o.	0.25–0.5 mg total	24*
Beclomethasone			
dipropionate	Inhalant	200 μg (total human dose)	6–8
(*Taper doses to minimum effective dose)			
Antitussives			
Codeine	p.o.	1–2	8
Hydrocodone	p.o.	0.22	6–12
Butorphanol tartrate	s.c., i.m.	0.055–0.11	as needed
	p.o.	0.5–1.0	6–12
Dextromethorphan	p.o.	1–2	6–8
Morphine	i.m., s.c.	0.1	6–12
Mucolytics			
N-Acetylcysteine	p.o., i.m., i.v.	70–144	12
Bromhexine	i.m.	*Dog* 3–15	12
		Cat 3	24
	p.o.	*Dog* 2–2.5	12
		Cat 1	24

Table 22.1: Respiratory drug dosages.

with marked bronchoconstriction in human beings. Systemic antimicrobial therapy is indicated, in the author's opinion, in concert with aerosolization. If safe, the antimicrobial being aerosolized should be given systemically in order to generate bactericidal concentrations in the lung. Alternatively, a synergistic drug combination (e.g. aminoglycosides and penicillins) can be selected.

Although *sulphonamides* and *sulphonamide–trimethoprim* combinations are distributed well to respiratory tissues, the emergence of resistance by veterinary strains of several organisms decreases the utility of these drugs and the author seldom uses these drugs as first choice antimicrobials in complicated or serious infections (Conlon, 1990). *Clindamycin* can be useful for treatment of respiratory infections caused by Gram positive organisms. It accumulates in polymorphonuclear leucocytes and alveolar macrophages, and is indicated for treatment of lower respiratory tract infections caused by anaerobic organisms, *Staphylococcus aureus* and most *Streptococcus* spp. Diarrhoea may be a side-effect.

In the author's experience, the role of *tetracyclines* in the treatment of complicated infections is limited by the rapid development of resistance. However, they can be an excellent first choice for treatment, particularly for infections associated with *Pasteurella* and *Mycoplasma*. *Doxycycline* may be the preferred tetracycline because better solubility results in better bioavailability and enhanced cellular penetration.

Although chloramphenicol has been a good first choice antimicrobial for selected, uncomplicated respiratory tract infections, the drug is bacteriostatic and is not well tolerated in the cat. For public health reasons, it is generally recommended that chloramphenicol is only used where sensitivity testing indicates that no other antibiotic will be effective.

BRONCHODILATORS AND ANTI-INFLAMMATORY DRUGS

Chronic bronchial diseases are best treated by breaking the inflammatory cycle while immediately relieving bronchoconstriction. Anti-inflammatories and bronchodilators represent the cornerstone of therapy in most bronchial diseases. Because of a shared mechanism of action, most drugs which induce bronchodilation also reduce inflammation. Bronchodilators reverse airway smooth muscle contraction by increasing cAMP via β_2 adrenergic receptors; decreasing cGMP by inhibiting histaminergic or muscarinic receptors; or decreasing intracellular calcium ion concentrations. In addition, these drugs also decrease mucosal oedema and are anti-inflammatory because they decrease mediator release from inflammatory cells. Rapidly acting bronchodilators include β-adrenoreceptor agonists, methylxanthines and cholinergic antagonists.

β-Adrenoreceptor agonists

β-Receptor agonists are the most effective bronchodilators because they act as functional antagonists of airway constriction, regardless of the stimulus. They are most effective in states of bronchoconstriction. Large numbers of β_2 receptors are located on several cell types in the lung, including smooth muscle and inflammatory cells. Increased cAMP in smooth muscle cells causes relaxation. In the inflammatory cell, increased cAMP inhibits mediator release. β-Receptors also stimulate secretion of airway mucus, resulting in a less viscous secretion and enhanced ciliary activity.

Non-selective β-agonists such as *adrenaline*, *ephedrine* and *isoprenaline* (isoproterenol in the US) are the most important component of therapy of acute respiratory distress due to bronchoconstriction, e.g. in feline asthma. Adrenaline can be administered parenterally to achieve rapid effects. Drugs which have been given orally for chronic therapy include isoprenaline and ephedrine (Moise *et al.*, 1981). Both adrenaline and ephedrine cause α-adrenergic activity, which may cause vasoconstriction and systemic hypertension. Non-selective β-agonists may cause adverse cardiac effects due to β_1 receptor stimulation. These effects may be problematic in cats suffering from hypertrophic cardiomyopathy. Aerosolization reduces the adverse effects of non-selective β-adrenergic agonists by increasing β_2 specificity, since only these β receptors appear to line the airways.

At appropriate doses, β_2-selective agonists are not generally associated with the undesirable effects of β_1 adrenergic stimulation. However, few of these drugs have been used in small animal animals. *Clenbuterol*; *orciprenaline* (metaproterenol in the US - a derivative of isoprenaline), and its analogue, *terbutaline* (Bauer, 1986) have all been used in small animals. Rapid first pass metabolism of orciprenaline and terbutaline results in reduced systemic bioavailability following oral administration, thus oral doses are considerably higher than parenteral doses. Clenbuterol is excreted largely unchanged in the urine. All three drugs can cause β_1 side effects at high doses. *Albuterol* and *isoetherine* are examples of β_2 selective agonists which have been administered by aerosolization in small animals (Papich, 1986). Chronic use of β adrenergic agonists can result in refractoriness due to down-regulation (i.e. reduced numbers) of β receptors. This problem is largely avoided in people by using correct doses. Drugs which block β_2-receptors, such as propranolol and its congeners, are contraindicated in animals with bronchial disease.

Methylxanthines

Theophylline
The methylxanthine derivative, theophylline, has been the cornerstone of long-term bronchodilator therapy in small animals. Its mode of action was originally attributed to inhibition of phosphodiesterase (PDE), and increased concentrations of cAMP. However, this mechanism is controversial. Other possible mechanisms include antagonism of the bronchoconstricting neurotransmitter, adenosine, or interference of calcium mobilization.

As with β-agonists, theophylline is equally effective in large and small airways. Theophylline has other effects in the respiratory system which are important to its clinical efficacy. In addition to its bronchodilatory effects, it inhibits mast cell degranulation and thus mediator release, increases mucociliary clearance, and prevents microvascular leakage. A major advantage of theophylline compared with other bronchodilators, is increased strength of respiratory muscles and thus a decrease in the work associated with breathing. This may be important to animals with chronic bronchopulmonary disease.

Theophylline is one of the few drugs whose disposition has been studied in small animals. Regular aminophylline is well absorbed following oral administration in both dogs and cats.(McKiernan *et al.*, 1981; McKiernan, 1983). Elimination half-life is longer in cats compared with dogs, necessitating a smaller dose. In dogs, peak plasma drug concentrations of theophylline base occur 1.5 hours following oral administration (McKiernan *et al.*, 1981). Several sustained-release preparations have been studied in dogs. The rate of oral absorption of sustained-release products in dogs is apparently faster than in humans, although the extent of absorption varies with the preparation. The longer release time of theophylline from these products may allow twice-daily rather than thrice to four times daily dosing in dogs, and once-daily rather than twice-daily dosing in cats. Of the preparations studied, the anhydrous theophylline tablet is preferred in dogs. Sustained-release preparations appear to be better absorbed in cats when dosed in the evening (McKiernan *et al.*, 1989; Dye *et al.*, 1990). Therapeutic drug monitoring (TDM) may be useful in identifying the most appropriate dosing regimen. The range recommended in people (10–20 µg/ml) can be extrapolated to small animals until a more definitive range has been established in dogs and cats. Because theophylline is not water soluble, it can only be given orally. Salt preparations of theophylline are available for either oral or parenteral administration. Dosing of the various salt preparations must be based on the amount of active theophylline (theophylline base). *Aminophylline*, an ethylenediamine salt, is 80% theophylline, while *etamiphylline* (Millophyline-V), a camphorsulphonate, is 65% theophylline, and glycinate and salicylate salts are only 50% theophylline.

Theophylline causes a variety of adverse effects, including:

- Central nervous excitation (manifested as restlessness, tremors and seizures)
- Gastrointestinal upset (nausea and vomiting)
- Diuresis and cardiac stimulation (e.g. tachycardia).

Use of i.v. aminophylline is limited to patients who have not responded to β–agonist therapy. Rapid infusions or infusions of undiluted drug can cause cardiac arrhythmias, hypotension, nausea, tremors and acute respiratory failure. Compared to the salt preparations, theophylline is more irritating to the gastrointestinal tract than aminophylline. The side effects of theophylline are dose dependent and might be avoided to a large degree by appropriate dosing and therapeutic drug monitoring. Etamiphylline causes less diuresis than theophylline.

Anticholinergic drugs

Anticholinergic drugs compete with acetylcholine at muscarinic receptor sites. In the respiratory tract, they reduce the sensitivity of irritant receptors and antagonize vagally-mediated bronchoconstriction. Anticholinergic drugs have not proven clinically effective for the treatment of chronic bronchial disease in animals, and should generally be avoided because of their deleterious effects on respiratory secretions. The route by which anticholinergics are administered influences their bronchodilatory effects. Aerosolized *atropine*, a prototype anticholinergic drug, affects predominantly the central airways; whereas both central and peripheral airways are affected if the drug is administered i.v. Because atropine is highly specific for all muscarinic receptors, it causes a number of systemic side effects, including tachycardia, meiosis and altered gastrointestinal and urinary tract function. In the respiratory tract, atropine reduces ciliary beat frequency, mucus secretion and electrolyte and water flux into the trachea. The net effect is *decreased mucociliary clearance,* which is undesirable in patients with chronic lung disease. Aerosolization of atropine does not ameliorate adverse reactions. Because of these adverse effects of atropine, its role in the treatment of respiratory diseases is limited. Atropine should be reserved for facilitation of bronchodilation in acutely dyspnoeic animals. It is the treatment of choice for life-threatening respiratory distress induced by anticholinesterases. Combination of atropine with either β–adrenergic agonists or glucocorticoids will cause better bronchodilation than either drug alone.

Glycopyrrolate can also be used as a bronchodilator in small animals. Although its onset of action is slower than that of atropine, its half-life is 4–6 hours compared with 1–2 hours for atropine. Glycopyrrolate is twice as potent as atropine when aerosolized, although potency following systemic therapy has apparently not been compared between the two drugs. Systemic side-effects of glycopyrrolate are minimal.

Glucocorticoids

Glucocorticoids remain the most effective long-term therapy for inflammatory bronchial diseases such as feline bronchial asthma because they are both bronchodilatory and anti-inflammatory. Steroids have a 'permissive' effect on β_2-receptors. Receptor sensitivity to β–adrenergic drugs is increased and receptor density in the airways and affinity for β–adrenergic drugs may also be increased. Potentiation of β–adrenergic activity leads to bronchodilation as well as control of inflammation. Glucocorticoids prevent the formation of inflammatory mediators important in the pathophysiology of inflammatory bronchial diseases, including prostaglandins, leukotrienes and platelet activating factor. As a result, glucocorticoids decrease leukocyte accumulation, induce eosinopenia and lymphopenia, prevent and reverse increased vascular permeability, and reduce release of additional mediators. Glucocorticoids also alter macrophage function, modulate the immune system and inhibit fibroblast growth. Thus, glucocorticoids can modify all phases of inflammation important in bronchial disease.

The subcellular mechanisms by which glucocorticoids induce their effects result in a lag time before maximum anti-inflammatory effects are realized. The anti-inflammatory potency of the glucocorticoids varies with the drug. *Dexamethasone* is about 5–10 times more potent than *prednisolone* or *triamcinolone*. However, it is associated with more adverse reactions and takes longer to be effective. Dexamethasone phosphate can penetrate cells rapidly and has a faster onset of action. *Methylprednisolone* is also a rapidly acting glucocorticoid; however, its expense tends to limit its use to the preferred drug for prevention or reduction of oxygen radical formation following re-expansion of atelectatic lungs.

Glucocorticoids are given i.v. to achieve rapid effects in acute, life-threatening situations, or orally for long-term administration as maintenance drugs. Glucocorticoids are well absorbed following oral administration. The half-life of the various glucocorticoids ranges from about 1 hour (prednisolone) to 5 hours (dexamethasone). However, the duration of action (biological half-life) of the drugs is much longer. *Hydrocortisone* and other short-acting glucocorticoids are active for less than 12 hours. Intermediate drugs such as *prednisolone* and *triamcinolone* are active for 12–36 hours, while long-acting drugs such as betamethasone and dexamethasone are active for more than 48 hours. While twice-daily therapy should be used for the initial control of symptoms, particularly in patients that are seriously ill, alternate or every third day therapy at the lowest effective dose should be initiated as early as possible. Although cats appear to be less susceptible to the adverse effects commonly associated with long-term glucocorticoid therapy in dogs, alternate day dosing of short to medium acting drugs is recommended for both species. Administration for several months to life may be necessary in some animals. Despite their convenience, the use of depot or reposital forms of glucocorticoids is controversial because of their unpredictability in duration of efficacy. Glucocorticoids can also be administered by aerosol for rapid, local effects. Triamcinolone acetonide and beclomethasone dipropionate can be aerosolized although the benefit: risk ratio is greater for the latter. *Beclomethasone dipropionate* is a glucocorticoid whose anti-inflammatory effects are much greater following aerosolization because it is metabolized to a less active form as it passes through the liver after oral administration. As an aerosol (200 µg), it has proven useful for the control of asthma in human patients that respond poorly to other therapy or cannot tolerate systemic glucocorticoid therapy. Although studies have not proven the efficacy of aerosolization in small animals, this route may be indicated for treatment of acute exacerbations of disease or for animals intolerant to systemic maintenance glucocorticoid therapy.

Mast cell stabilizers

Although the mechanism of action of *sodium cromoglycate* is not certain, it appears to inhibit calcium influx into mast cells, thus preventing mast cell degranulation and the release of histamine and other inflammatory mediators. At high concentrations, cromoglycate inhibits IgE-triggered mediator release from mast cells. Some studies suggest that the activation of inflammatory cells other than the mast cells (e.g. macrophages, neutrophils and eosinophils) is also inhibited by cromoglycate. Cromoglycate is most useful as a preventative prior to activation of inflammatory cells. It is not significantly absorbed following oral administration and is characterized by a short half-life. Thus, effective therapy is dependent upon frequent aerosolization which limits its utility in the treatment of small animal diseases. Currently, cromoglycate is the safest drug used to manage asthma in people. It is associated with only minor side-effects and its discovery has revolutionized the management of bronchial asthma in people. Because of its wide therapeutic window, and its apparent efficacy in control of many inflammatory cells, its use in the control of small animal bronchial disease warrants further investigation.

Miscellaneous drugs

Several other drugs are currently being investigated for their use in the treatment of chronic inflammatory bronchial diseases. *Calcium channel blocking agents* may decrease mediator release, smooth muscle contraction, vagus nerve conduction, and infiltration of inflammatory cells. Although *non-steroidal anti-inflammatories* (NSAIDs) effectively block prostaglandins (PGs) through inhibition of cyclooxygenase, they do not appear to have any effect on lipooxygenase and therefore production of leukotrienes or other chemical mediators of inflammation. Additionally, NSAIDs non-selectively block all PGs, including those which provide some protection during periods of bronchoconstriction. Leukotriene production might be enhanced by NSAID therapy due to greater concentrations of substrate for leukotriene formation. Current efforts in NSAID research are oriented towards identifying drugs which successfully inhibit both arms of the arachidonic acid metabolic cascade or specific prostaglandin or leukotriene inhibitors. The recent development of drugs that inhibit leucotriene formation (zileuton, a lipoxygenase inhibitor) or block leucotriene receptors (zafirlukast) has proven an important advance in humans and may be helpful in animals. Neither *antiserotonins* nor *antihistaminergic drugs* have proven clinically useful in the control of small animal or human respiratory diseases (Zenoble, 1980). This reflects, in part, the lesser role that histamine and serotonin have in chronic bronchial diseases.

MANAGEMENT OF COUGHING

Antitussives
The goal of antitussive therapy is to decrease the frequency and severity of cough. Whenever possible, the underlying cause should be identified and treated. Cough suppressants should be used cautiously, and are contraindicated if the cough is productive. Irritant receptors, and perhaps chemo- and stretch receptors initiate the cough reflex (McKiernan, 1983; Slonim and Hamilton, 1987). Decreased bronchial diameter resulting in increased airflow velocity is probably the most important cause of irritant receptor stimulation. Diameter can be reduced by bronchoconstriction, or accumulation of mucus, other secretions, or inflammatory cells.

The cough reflex can be inhibited *centrally*

- At the cough centre in the medulla (Roudebush, 1982)

or it can be inhibited *peripherally*

- By removing the irritant or debris which is decreasing airway diameter
- By blocking peripheral receptors.

Centrally active antitussives
These are classified as narcotic and non-narcotic drugs. Narcotic antitussives depress the cough centre sensitivity to afferent stimuli. However, they can be associated with strong sedative properties, as well as constipation when administered chronically. *Morphine*, *codeine* and *hydrocodone* can be used for cough suppression in both dogs and cats. Hydrocodone is more potent than codeine and causes less respiratory depression. The narcotic agonist/antagonist, *butorphanol tartrate*, is a potent antitussive when given orally or parenterally in dogs and cats (Hosgood, 1990). An advantage of this drug is that it is not scheduled. *Dextromethorphan* is a non-narcotic opioid commonly found in over-the-counter cough preparations. It is used in small animals with minimal sedation and its antitussive efficacy is equal to codeine. It can be used safely in cats. Studies in humans have shown that the combination of dextromethorphan with a bronchodilator is superior to dextromethorphan alone.

Peripherally acting antitussives
Bronchodilators are powerful peripheral antitussives because of their effect on airflow velocity. *Ephedrine* peripherally induces bronchodilation and is a common constituent of over-the-counter preparations; *theophylline* and *isoprenaline* are also common ingredients. Other peripheral antitussives include mucokinetic agents and hydrating agents (Roudebush, 1982).

Mucokinetic drugs facilitate the removal of secretions from the respiratory tree.

Mucokinesis can be induced by

- Drugs which improve ciliary activity (e.g. β-receptor agonists and methylxanthines)
- Drugs which improve the mobility of bronchial secretions by changing viscosity (i.e. mucolytics).

Mucolytics
Viscosity of bronchial secretions can be decreased by

- Hydration (e.g. sterile or bacteriostatic water or saline)
- Increasing pH (e.g. sodium bicarbonate)
- Increasing ionic strength (sodium bicarbonate and saline)
- By rupture of sulphur (S-S) linkages in the mucus (e.g. acetylcysteine or iodine).

Hydrating agents can be administered parenterally (i.e. isotonic crystalloids) or by aerosolization. Home aerosolization can be easily achieved with a humidifier or steamed bathroom. The efficacy of aerosolization in liquefying airway secretions is controversial (Wanner and Rao *et al.*, 1980). The greatest benefit will occur in upper airways. It should be noted that bland aerosols such as water and saline can actually be detrimental to mucociliary function. The efficacy of ionic solutions or alkaline solutions compared with water in enhancing mucus mobility is controversial (Wanner and Rao, 1980).

N-Acetylcysteine is the most widely used mucolytic drug in humans (Ziment, 1988). While it appears to be efficacious following aerosolization, more recently, oral administration has become the preferred route. In Europe, the drug is available in solid and powder dosing forms. In humans, acetylcysteine is rapidly absorbed from the gastrointestinal tract and extensively distributed to the liver, kidneys and lungs, where it may accumulate. It is rapidly metabolized by the liver to cysteine and cystine.

The mechanism of acetylcysteine reflects destruction by the free sulphydryl group of the disulphide bonds of mucoprotein. Smaller molecules are less viscid and are unable to bind efficiently to inflammatory debris. In addition, *N*-acetylcysteine serves as a precursor to glutathione, a major scavenger of free oxygen radicals associated with inflammation. The drug also appears to induce respiratory tract secretions, probably via a gastro-pulmonary reflex. At higher oral doses, acetylcysteine will also induce vomiting. The indications for oral acetylcysteine therapy in people include toxic inhalants (including tobacco smoke), bronchitis, chronic obstructive pulmonary disease, cystic fibrosis, asthma, tuberculosis, pneumonia and emphysema and the adult respiratory distress syndrome. Acetylcysteine is often used in combination with aerosolized antimicrobials because it may improve antibacterial penetration of infected mucus, regardless of the route by which either drug is administered. Acetylcysteine therapy is associated with few adverse affects. In humans, doses as high as 500 mg/kg are well tolerated, although vomiting and anorexia can occur. Because it is metabolized to sulphur-containing products, it should be used cautiously in animals suffering from liver disease characterized by hepatic encephalopathy. Aerosolization of *N*-acetylcysteine can cause reflex bronchoconstriction due to irritant receptor stimulation, and should be preceded with bronchodilators.

Expectorants

Expectorants such as potassium iodide are common ingredients in over-the-counter cough preparations. They are not antitussives, but are often used as adjuvants for the management of cough by facilitating removal of the inciting cause. Expectorants increase the fluidity of respiratory secretions through several mechanisms. Bronchial secretions are increased by vagal reflex following gastric mucosa irritation (iodide salts, bromhexine); and directly by volatile oils or through sympathetic stimulation. While the combination of expectorants with antitussives may seem irrational, the antitussive drugs in these combination products do not appear to prevent stimulation of the cough reflex induced by liquefied secretions. The expectorant mechanism of action of *guaiphenesin*, a common ingredient of over-the-counter cough preparations, is unknown. It may be ineffective at the doses used in cough preparations. The clinical efficacy of expectorants has not been scientifically established, yet these drugs should be considered as potentially useful adjuvants to other medical therapy. *Bromhexine* is an expectorant that may also facilitate penetration of antimicrobials into the respiratory tract. Bromhexine should be used cautiously in patients with gastric ulceration or erosion.

Aerosolization as a route of drug administration

The primary indications for aerosolization are directly to deliver drugs to the respiratory tract, and to facilitate liquefaction and mobilization of respiratory secretions. The benefits of direct drug delivery include assurance that target tissues receive high concentrations while systemic exposure and potentially toxic reactions are avoided (e.g. aminoglycosides and anticholinergics). In addition, hepatic first pass metabolism following oral administration is circumvented, which serves to prolong the pharmacological effect of selected drugs (e.g. β-adrenergic agonists and beclomethasone).

Inhalation therapy in small animals has been reviewed (Court *et al.*, 1985). The success of patient response to aerosolized drugs is probably a reflection of adequate drug delivery rather than a function of drug efficacy. Predicting the amount of drug delivered to the target tissue is not possible in small animals. Factors which determine the amount of drug administered via aerosolization include:

- The aerosolizer used and the particle size it generates
- Technique of delivery (i.e. mask versus endotracheal tube and nose versus mouth)
- Flow rate of the delivery gas
- Patient factors (such as anatomy of the respiratory tract, and respiratory rate and pattern).

The optimum particle size for particle (and drug) deposition in the trachea is 2–10 µm, while that in peripheral airways is 0.5–5.0 µm. Reusable and disposable nebulizers that generate the correct particle size are commercially available (Figure 22.1). Less than 10–20% of aerosolized drug probably reaches the tracheobronchial tree, and even less will reach the peripheral airways. With progression of chronic disease, therapy may become less effective as the respiratory pattern of the patient becomes shallow and rapid: depth of aerosol penetration decreases and more drug is deposited in upper airways. Administration of an aerosol by mask or in an enclosed, treated environment (Figure 22.2) reduces drug delivery to the tracheobronchial tree because particles will be deposited in the nasal turbinates and oropharynx. The utility of aerosolization may be further limited because of stimulation of irritant receptors and reflex bronchoconstriction. Resistance by the animal to aerosolization may further exacerbate respiratory distress. Animals should preferentially be pre-treated with a β–adrenergic bronchodilator 10 minutes prior to aerosolization. Alternatively, a bronchodilator or theophylline should

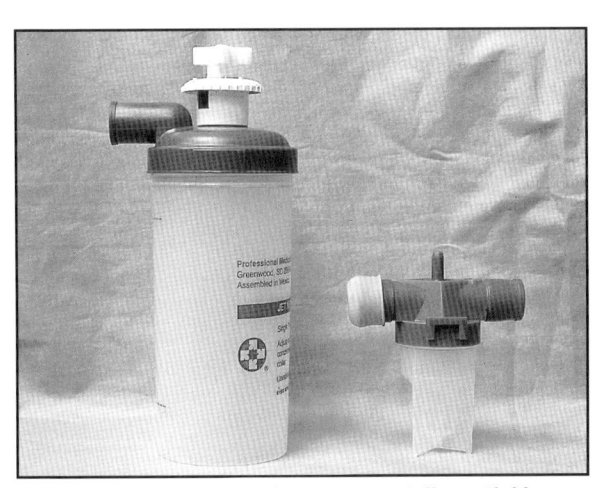

Figure 22.1: *An example of two commercially available aerosolizers that generate particles of the size appropriate for deposition in the respiratory tract. The larger aerosolizer fits directly to a large cage (see Figure 22.2a) while the smaller is used to aerosolize in a smaller, confined space (see Figure 22.2b).*

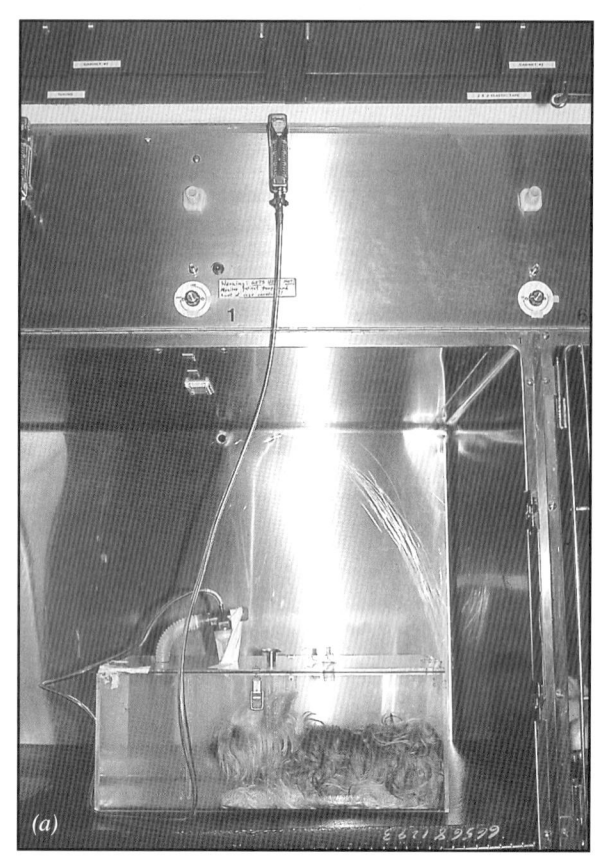

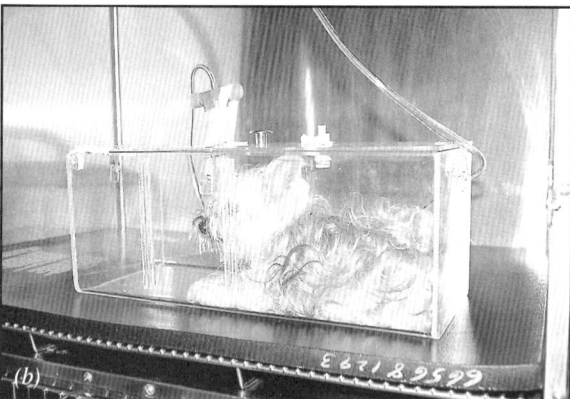

Figure 22.2: *Small patients can be aerosolized in a cat box. Oxygen (small tubing) is delivered to the aerosolizers where drug is added before it is delivered to the patient (larger tubing).*

be included in the aerosolized medicament (e.g. 100 mg aminophylline). Care should be taken not to overhydrate and flood the respiratory tract. Treatment of approximately 30–45 minutes should be repeated every 4–12 hours. In humans, aerosolization is a well established route of administration for bronchodilators and anti-inflammatories. In veterinary patients, aero-

solization is more commonly used for administration of antimicrobials and mucolytics. Indications include asthma, chronic bronchial diseases and infections of both lower and upper airways.

REFERENCES

Amis TC (1986) Chronic bronchitis in dogs. In: *Current Veterinary Therapy IX: Small Animal Practice*, ed. R.W. Kirk. WB Saunders, Philadelphia

Bauer T (1986) Pulmonary hypersensitivity disorders. In: *Current Veterinary Therapy IX: Small Animal Practice*, ed. R.W. Kirk. WB Saunders, Philadelphia

Bemis DA and Appel MJG (1977) Aerosol, parental, and oral treatment of *Bordetella bronchiseptica* infection in dogs. *Journal of the American Veterinary Association* 170, 1082

Boothe DM (1990) Anaerobic infections in small animals. *Problems in Veterinary Medicine* 2, 330

Conlon PD (1990) Antimicrobial drugs for respiratory tract infections. *Problems in Veterinary Medicine* 2, 362

Court MH, Dodman NH and Seeler DC (1985) Inhalation therapy. *Veterinary Clinics of North America: Small Animal Practice* 15, 1041

Dye JA, McKiernan BC, Neff-Davis CA and Koritz GD (1990) Chronopharmacokinetics of theophylline in the cat. *Journal of Veterinary Pharmacology and Therapeutics* 13, 278

Hosgood G (1990) Pharmacologic features of butorphanol in dogs and cats. *Journal of the American Veterinary Association* 196, 135

McKiernan BC (1983) Principles of respiratory therapy. In: *Current Veterinary Therapy VIII: Small Animal Practice*, ed. R.W. Kirk, p. 216. WB Saunders, Philadelphia

McKiernan BC, Davis CAN, Koritz GD, Davis LE and Pheris DR (1981) Pharmacokinetics studies of theophylline in dogs. *Journal of Veterinary Pharmacology and Therapeutics* 4, 103

McKiernan BC, Koritz GD and Davis LE (1983) Pharmacokinetic studies of theophylline in cats. *Journal of Veterinary Pharmacology and Therapeutics* 6, 99

McKiernan BC, Dye JA, Jones SD, Davis CAN and Koritz GD (1989) Sustained-release theophylline pharmacokinetics in the cat. *Journal of Veterinary Pharmacology and Therapeutics* 12, 133

Moise NS and Spaulding GL (1981) Feline bronchial asthma: pathogenesis, pathophysiology, diagnostics, and therapeutic considerations. *Compendium on Continuing Education for the Practicing Veterinarian* 3, 1091

Moise NS, Wiedenkeller D, Yeager AE, Blue JT and Scarlett J (1989) Clinical, radiographic, and bronchial cytologic features of cats with bronchial disease: 65 cases (1980-1986). *Journal of the American Veterinary Association* 194, 1467

Padrid PA, Hornof WJ, Kurpershoek CJ and Cross CE (1990) Canine chronic bronchitis: a pathophysiologic evaluation of 18 cases. *Journal of Veterinary Internal Medicine* 4, 172

Papich MG (1986) Bronchodilator therapy. In: *Current Veterinary Therapy IX: Small Animal Practice*, ed. R.W. Kirk, p. 278. WB Saunders, Philadephia

Roudebush P (1982) Antitussive therapy in small companion animals. *Journal of the American Veterinary Association* 180, 1105

Slonim NF and Hamilton LH (1987) Development and functional anatomy of the bronchopulmonary system. In: *Respiratory Physiology*, 5th edn, ed. D. Carson, p. 27. CV Mosby, St Louis.

Wanner A and Rao A (1980) Clinical indications for and effects of bland, mucolytic, and antimicrobial aerosols. *American Review of Respiratory Diseases* 122, 79

Zenoble RD (1980) Respiratory pharmacology and therapeutics. *Compendium on Continuing Education for the Practicing Veterinarian* 2, 139

Ziment I (1988) Acetylcysteine: a drug that is much more than a mucokinetic. *Biomedicine and Pharmacotherapy* 42, 513

PART FOUR

Surgical Techniques

Anaesthesia for Thoracic Surgery

R. Eddie Clutton

INTRODUCTION

Thoracic surgery makes specific demands on anaesthesia; opening the pleural cavity causes lung collapse and mandates the use of *positive pressure ventilation* (PPV). Improperly performed, PPV compromises cardiopulmonary function. Surgical manipulation also causes adverse physiological changes. Animals with cardiovascular and/or pulmonary disease undergoing thoracotomy are at increased risk; evaluation is often incomplete because haemodynamic and lung function testing is limited in companion animals.

Preoperative assessment and preparation

Little preparation beyond food deprivation is needed in cases with modest or no cardiopulmonary disease. The principal preoperative goal in animals with cardiac disease is to improve whole body oxygen delivery without increasing myocardial oxygen consumption and precipitating cardiac failure. Drugs used for this may affect the behaviour of anaesthetics agents, although withdrawing cardiac preparations usually creates more problems than it solves.

The broad goal of pulmonary preparations is to achieve a dry, 'clean', low-resistance airway using a combination of antibiotics, mucolytics, expectorants, corticosteroids and bronchodilators. Other readily correctable problems should be resolved before anaesthesia, e.g. pericardiocentesis for cardiac tamponade, pleural drainage for pneumothorax.

PRE-ANAESTHETIC MEDICATION

Pre-anaesthetic medication may be unnecessary in depressed, compromised animals, although avoiding stress is of paramount importance, especially in cases with 'air-hunger' or poorly controlled ventricular arrhythmias. Neuroleptanalgesic combinations are appropriate; low doses of acepromazine (12.5–25 µg/kg) combined with an opioid such as morphine or pethidine usually produce satisfactory sedation with mild haemodynamic effects. However, α_2-agonists (xylazine, medetomidine) should be avoided. In cases with respiratory disease, drugs depressing ventilation,

e.g. morphine, should be used at low doses, or withheld until the trachea is intubated, after which ventilation can be supported if necessary. In cardiac failure, all injectable drug doses are lower because drug volumes of distribution are reduced. Ill animals must be continuously observed after pre-anaesthetic medication is given, and a quiet environment (which improves drug effects) should be maintained. Oxygen delivery by mask for 2 minutes or so before induction eliminates pulmonary nitrogen and improves oxygen tension in anticipation of post-induction apnoea. However, 'pre-oxygenation' is unproductive if it excites the animal. Venous catheters should be placed before induction to anaesthesia.

INDUCTION

In debilitated cases, the particular drug used to induce anaesthesia is probably less important than the dose used. Appropriate doses are those that *just* provide sufficient jaw relaxation and suppression of laryngeal reflex activity for endotracheal intubation. Dose is based principally on the depressant effects of pre-anaesthetic medication and the medical condition. Inhalation techniques (mask or chamber) are satisfactory, providing excitement is not evoked. Chamber inductions are most suitable for cats. While atmospheric contamination with anaesthetic is inevitable, such techniques allow oxygen administration as consciousness is lost. The author uses a technique in which induction is attempted by mask, but completed with 'sleep' doses of injectable drug if the animal struggles. If arrhythmias are present, the electrocardiogram (ECG) is monitored during induction and anti-arrhythmic drugs like lignocaine (for ventricular arrhythmias) and atropine (for significant bradycardia or atrioventricular blockade) are made ready for injection. Nitrous oxide at inspired concentrations of 50–66% accelerates the induction rate with mask and chamber techniques. Its use lowers the inspired oxygen concentration, so N_2O should not be used in hypoxaemic animals. Because of its low blood gas solubility, nitrous oxide sequesters to gas-filled viscera and must not be used in cases of closed pneumothorax until these are opened by surgery.

This is not a problem in open pneumothorax when N_2O leaves through the thoracotomy incision or chest-wall defect.

MAINTENANCE

Drug selection

In high-risk cases, it is safer for anaesthetists to use drugs with which they are experienced, rather than to use unfamiliar agents which, in theory, may be more appropriate. A 'balanced' anaesthetic technique incorporating a sedative–hypnotic drug, an analgesic and a muscle relaxant is probably ideal. Drugs which maintain or increase cardiac output and blood pressure (e.g. ketamine-based combinations, isoflurane) seem attractive in 'high-risk cardiac' cases. However, these may increase myocardial work and myocardial oxygen consumption, and cause arrhythmias. Many anaesthetic agents, e.g. halothane, are especially arrhythmogenic in the presence of catecholamines. This does not preclude the use of such agents; rather it imposes a need to ensure minimum catecholamine levels. These are achieved by maintaining adequate 'levels' of anaesthesia and blood pressure, while avoiding hypoxia, hypercapnia and hypothermia.

Positive pressure ventilation

Opening the pleural cavity allows intrapleural and atmospheric pressures to equilibrate; lung on the opened side collapses under elastic recoil and surface tension forces and the mediastinum shifts to the non-disrupted side. Positive pressure ventilation (PPV) is necessary; there are at least five adverse consequences when patients with an open pneumothorax breathe spontaneously.

Spontaneous breathing; adverse effects during thoracotomy

Paradoxical respiration: When an animal with a unilateral pneumothorax breathes spontaneously, the lung on the 'opened' side paradoxically inflates on expiration and deflates on inspiration. The 'intact' side behaves normally.

Pendelluft: Air moves between right and left lungs without being expired. The volume of this 'pendulum air' or pendelluft depends on the relative size of chest wall defect and tidal volume. Pendelluft increases the work of breathing and anatomic dead space.

Mediastinal 'flap': In hemi-pneumothorax, the mediastinum moves towards the unaffected side during inspiration and limits lung inflation. This is particularly undesirable when animals are in lateral recumbency with the affected side uppermost, because mediastinal contents will further limit expansion of dependent lung. Mediastinal 'flap' restricts great vein filling and impedes venous return.

Reduced transmural venous pressure: Increased pleural pressure lowers venous transmural pressures, which in turn promotes venous collapse and limits venous return.

Atalectasis: In atalectatic (collapsed) lung, right-to-left intrapulmonary shunting (blood which is not exposed to ventilated alveoli) increases the volume of desaturated venous blood reaching the systemic circulation. This dilutes oxygenated arterial blood and lowers oxygen levels. Tendency to hypercapnia is offset by increased ventilation of uncollapsed lung.

During PPV, the inflation phase raises airway pressure above ambient. This prevents paradoxical ventilation and atalectasis, abolishes pendelluft and minimizes mediastinal 'flap'. Positive pressure ventilation also provides most of the energy required to ventilate the lungs and so 'whole body' oxygen consumption is lowered.

PPV technique

Airway: Positive pressure ventilation requires an airway which remains gas tight to the maximum inflation pressure (ideally about 20–25 cmH_2O). Tight-fitting masks are undesirable, as some gas inevitably enters the stomach and displaces the diaphragm cranially, reducing both the functional residual capacity and thoracic compliance. While the former predisposes to hypoxia, the latter increases the work of breathing and necessitates greater inflation pressures. Endotracheal intubation with a cuffed tube is almost mandatory.

Mode: Positive pressure ventilation can be performed manually or mechanically. The pros and cons of each mode are listed in Table 23.1.

Anaesthetic breathing systems for positive pressure ventilation: When manual ventilation is used, an appropriate anaesthetic breathing system with adequate fresh gas flows is required. The Magill, Lack and Parallel Lack systems are unsuitable for prolonged PPV unless uneconomically high flow rates and/or modified breathing patterns are imposed; they promote rebreathing and hypercapnia. With spontaneous breathing, circuit selection is usually based arbitrarily on body weight, and not on the animal's ability to overcome system resistance. These considerations are less important during PPV because the energy causing gas movement comes from the ventilator. However, breathing system resistance may be important before and after the period of controlled ventilation. The gas flow rates recommended during manual PPV in these systems are shown in Table 23.2.

	Advantages	Disadvantages
Mechanical ventilation	Accurate control of variables like tidal volume, respiratory rate, peak inspiratory pressure and inspiratory : expiratory ratio	Disconnection or cuff deflation may, if unnoticed, result in fatalities in 'paralysed' cases
	Constant variables create stable physiological conditions e.g. constant CO_2 promotes constant pH and K^+ levels	Mechanical failure can occur
	Constant rhythm depresses ventilation, provides narcosis and improves operating conditions	Barotrauma is more likely if inappropriate variables are set.
	Constant tidal volume (with constant flow generators) allows compliance to be quantified	Purchase and maintenance costs may be high
	Frees anaesthetist for other duties	
Manual ventilation	Circuit disconnections are appreciated immediately	Less accurate control of variables like tidal volume, respiratory rate, peak inspiratory pressure and inspiratory : expiratory ratio
	Mechanical failure cannot occur	Occupies full attention of anaesthetist
	Compliance changes are appreciated 'breath-by-breath'	Less rhythm i.e respiratory pattern, closer liaison between surgeon and anaesthetist required
	Barotrauma may be less likely	
	Inexpensive	

Table 23.1: *Advantages and disadvantages of manual and mechanical ventilation.*

Weight	Breathing system	Total flow ml/kg per min	O_2 flow ml/kg per min	N_2O flow ml/kg per min
			For 66% N_2O mixtures	*For 66% N_2O mixtures*
Up to 5 kg	Jackson-Rees modification of Ayre's T-piece	210–300	70–100	140–200
5–15 kg	Bain	300	100	200
>10 kg	Circle	90*	30	60
>10 kg	Horizontal To & Fro	90*	30	60

*If 100% oxygen is delivered in these systems total flow requirement is lower: 10–30 ml/kg/min are required.

Table 23.2: *Fresh gas flows for breathing systems during positive pressure ventilation.*

Monitoring positive pressure ventilation: In normal adult dogs a minute volume of 150–300 ml/kg per minute maintains normocapnia. A tidal volume of 15–20 ml/kg is delivered at a rate of 8–12 bpm. In cats, lower tidal volumes of 12–15 ml/kg are delivered at higher rates (10–15 bpm). (When PPV is imposed, the tidal volumes used are in excess of spontaneous breaths (normally 2.5–5 ml/kg). This is to compensate for elasticity in the ventilator and breathing system.)

The simplest way to assess ventilation is to observe chest wall movement, which should be perceptible, but not excessive. Minute volume can be quantified by respirometry, using a Wright's respirometer placed between the endotracheal tube connector and the patient end of the breathing system. If an in-circuit manometer is present, airway pressures of 20–25 cmH_2O are imposed. A useful way to monitor ventilation is based on the measurement of expired carbon dioxide (capnometry) although the definitive assessment relies on arterial blood gas analysis (specifically $PaCO_2$).

The inspiratory time should be about 1–1.5 seconds and the inspiratory:expiratory time ratio (I:E) should be in the order of 1:2 or 1:3. Temptation to maintain the lungs fully expanded at end-inspiration should be avoided; the lungs must return to end-expiratory position to permit venous return. During manual PPV, supranormal tidal excursions or 'sighs' should be imposed at 5-minute intervals.

Because of some potential adverse haemodynamic

effects of PPV (see below), the pulse rate and quality should be monitored during periods of controlled ventilation.

Suppressing respiratory activity

Positive pressure ventilation must 'over-ride' the animal's respiratory effort, as 'fighting the ventilator' raises mean intrathoracic pressure and makes precise surgery difficult. 'Fighting the ventilator' occurs because of inadequate ventilation (hypercapnia), acidaemia, hypoxaemia or inadequate anaesthesia in the face of surgical stimulation. Normal respiratory activity can be suppressed in several ways.

Hypocapnia: When metabolic rate is constant, pulmonary hyperventilation lowers $PaCO_2$ and removes the stimulus for inspiration. However, excessive hyperventilation is undesirable; respiratory alkalosis causes cerebral vasoconstriction and an adverse left-shift in the oxyhaemoglobin dissociation curve. Modest hyperventilation is the preferred means of suppressing spontaneous breathing in cats.

Neuromuscular blockade: Adequate doses of neuromuscular blocking agents totally suppress respiratory muscle activity, so their use requires a means for providing safe PPV for prolonged periods. The anaesthetist must also be able to identify inadequate anaesthesia (mydriasis, tachycardia, pallor, salivation, lacrimation, spasmodic facial and diaphragmatic twitching). Succinylcholine is uncommonly used in dogs and is too short-acting in cats to be useful. Neuromuscular blocking agents are useful in high risk cases because they relieve sedative–hypnotic drugs (which depress cardiovascular function) from the task of relaxing skeletal muscle; lower doses of the latter are needed thus preserving cardiovascular performance. Neuromuscular blockers are given by intravenous (i.v.) injection immediately after PPV is begun. Dose regimes for commonly used blockers are detailed in Table 23.3. Peripheral nerve stimulators facilitate dosing but are by no means vital.

Respiratory centre depression: Volatile anaesthetics and opioids reduce chemoreceptor sensitivity to CO_2. Opioids have only mild circulatory depressant effects, and so high doses can be used to suppress breathing. While morphine is satisfactory, short-acting agents like fentanyl and alfentanil, given by i.v. injection, are preferred (Table 23.4). Both drugs slow heart rate; if bradycardia becomes haemodynamically significant, atropine (40 µg/kg) should be given i.v.

Doses for opioids have not been established in cats, in which morphine (0.25 mg/kg slow i.v. or i.m.) is satisfactory. Pethidine may also be used (2–10 mg/kg i.m.) but the drug is unpredictable and relatively short acting.

Rhythmic lung inflation: Rhythmic lung inflation suppresses inspiratory drive even when $PaCO_2$ levels are normal or moderately raised.

Positive pressure ventilation; adverse effects

Positive pressure ventilation may reduce cardiac output, cause lung damage (barotrauma), augment ventilation/perfusion discrepancies in the lung and produce a variety of nebulous effects on other organs.

Drug	Loading i.v. dose (µg/kg)	Approx. duration (min)	Incremental i.v. dose (µg/kg)	Approx. duration (min)
Pancuronium bromide	100	30–85	33	20–30
Vecuronium bromide	100	25	45	15–21
	50	19	17	6–12
Atracurium besylate	500	40	200	10–22

Table 23.3: Dose regimes for commonly used neuromuscular blockers.

Opioid	Loading dose i.v. µg/kg	Increments i.v. µg/kg	Infusion µg/kg per min
Fentanyl	1–2.5	1–2.5 (every 25 min)	
Alfentanil	5–10	5 (every 5 min)	1–3

Table 23.4: Opioids used to induce respiratory centre depression.

Diminished cardiac output: During normal breathing, a decrease in pleural pressure is generated during inspiration which facilitates venous return and enhances cardiac output (the 'thoracolumbar pump'). Conversely, PPV raises intrathoracic pressure and impedes venous return, expelling blood from intrathoracic veins into the neck and abdomen. Diminished preload lowers cardiac output and hypotension may result.

Normally, compensatory increases in systemic vascular resistance (SVR) maintain blood pressure, but this response is obtunded by anaesthesia (see below). Fluid administration only partly restores preload. Mean intrathoracic pressure is the principal variable influencing cardiac output during PPV, consequently, problems are reduced (but not eliminated) on thoracotomy when intrapleural and ambient pressures equilibrate. Factors which raise mean intrathoracic pressure and reduce cardiac output during PPV and which, therefore, must be kept to a minimum by the anaesthetist include:

- Excessive inflation pressures (> 30 cmH$_2$O)
- 'Holding' peak inspiratory pressure
- Exerting positive end-expiratory pressure (PEEP)
- Using inspiratory: expiratory time ratios greater than 1:2.

When thoracic compliance is low, higher inflation pressures are needed to inflate the lungs (and maintain minute alveolar volume) and so mean intrathoracic pressure is raised. Thoracic compliance is relatively high in healthy small animals, therefore the effects of PPV are correspondingly mild.

Factors lowering thoracic compliance include:

- 'Fighting the ventilator'
- 'Closed' pneumothorax
- Obesity
- Pulmonary fibrosis
- Increased intraperitoneal pressure (or volume)
- Heavy draping (small animals)
- Misplaced surgical instruments (or hands).

The effects of PPV may become especially compromising in hypovolaemic animals, when cardiovascular disease is present or when compensatory mechanisms are suppressed by sympathetic block (general anaesthesia, extradural local anaesthesia, α_1-adrenoreceptor antagonism). Adverse effects are most likely when PPV is applied with the chest closed, i.e. before a closed pneumothorax is 'tapped' or at the end of thoracotomy.

Barotrauma: In dogs, a cough produces intrapulmonary pressures between 80 and 90 cmH$_2$O, while lungs supported by the thoracic cage and the abdominal musculature require bursting pressures between 80

and 140 cmH$_2$O (Soma, 1973). Pulmonary barotrauma (lung rupture) is very unlikely when PPV is conducted properly and in the absence of lung pathology, because normal inflation pressures used range from 15–25 cmH$_2$O.

Ventilation/perfusion discrepancy: Positive pressure ventilation alters normal *V/Q* relationships which may predispose to hypoxaemia. During spontaneous ventilation, inspired breath is distributed preferentially to lung in proximity to moving surfaces (i.e. peripheral lung fields) and to dependent lung. In PPV, gas distributes to peribronchial and perimediastinal areas, and for animals in lateral recumbency, the upper lung becomes preferentially inflated. Positive pressure ventilation increases anatomical dead-space (by increasing airway diameter) and alveolar dead-space (by hyperinflating alveoli in non-dependent lung).

Organ effects: Under certain circumstances, positive pressure ventilation has adverse effects on central nervous, renal and gastrohepatic function. For example, controlled ventilation may limit cerebral perfusion by raising cranial vena caval pressure and decreasing cerebral venous outflow, while ventilation-related reductions in cardiac output may lower cerebral blood flow. Positive pressure ventilation reduces urine output, glomerular filtration rate, sodium excretion and free water clearance. This partly results from reduced renal perfusion. In addition, PPV-related hypotension reduces aortic arch and carotid sinus baroreceptor activity. This increases renal sympathetic activity (producing antidiuresis and antinatriuresis), causes release of ADH and activates the renin–angiotensin system.

Patient monitoring during thoracotomy

Regular examination of vital signs (heart rate, rhythm, capillary refill time, pulse quality) is required to monitor adverse effects of PPV and surgery. Before thoracotomy, oesophageal stethoscopy provides information on cardiac rhythm, contractility and lung sounds. When the chest is open, lung expansion and venous return (distension of great veins) can be assessed by direct vision. The heart's rhythm and mechanical activity can be readily monitored, especially if the pericardium is open. Arterial blood pressure monitoring is useful during correction of anomalous conditions or when major haemorrhage is anticipated. In the latter, a central venous pressure line is useful for monitoring the adequacy of blood volume and provides a means for rapid fluid administration. Mucous membrane colour must be observed; pallor indicates hypoperfusion while cyanosis reflects hypoxaemia. Arterial blood pressure, urine output, simultaneous core versus peripheral temperature measurement and surgical oozing are useful indicators of perfusion. Arterial blood gas analysis is very useful, but unfortunately rarely available, to monitor adequacy of ventilation. Pulse oximetry monitors haemoglobin saturation and models equipped with bar plethysmographs simultaneously indicate pulsatile blood flow. Core temperature measurement using oesophageal thermistor probes are preferred to mercury-in-glass thermometers inserted *per rectum*. The adequacy of anaesthesia must be frequently appraised when neuromuscular blockers are used. Ventilators, equipment, endotracheal tube cuff pressures and breathing system integrity are frequently checked as disconnection or mechanical failure is rapidly fatal in paralysed animals.

Intraoperative analgesia

In cases with cardiovascular disease, the relatively high inspired concentrations of volatile anaesthetics required to produce adequate analgesia may compromise physiological function. In these, intraoperative analgesia is best achieved with opioids, preferably μ-agonists. While 'pre-emptive analgesia' has been difficult to demonstrate in humans, veterinary anaesthetists consider that opioids given before pain is generated (or perceived) produce more effective analgesia. Consequently, morphine (0.1–1.0 mg/kg i.m.) is probably best given as part of pre-anaesthetic medication, although in cats, it may be better to delay injection until the animal is unconscious (0.1–0.5 mg/kg i.m.). Alternatively, alfentanil or fentanyl can be used at the aforementioned doses.

Non-steroidal anti-inflammatory drugs can be used in conjunction with opioids as part of a 'polymodal analgesic' approach. These should be given *preoperatively* so that the drugs can prevent inflammatory cascades before they are initiated and 'leach' into inflammatory exudate. In dogs and cats, carprofen (4 mg/kg i.v.) or ketoprofen (2 mg/kg i.v., i.m. or s.c.) are options, with meloxicam for postoperative in-feed use.

Temperature management

Animals undergoing thoracotomy are likely to lose heat. Positive pressure hyperventilation with cold gases causes rapid 'core-cooling' by evaporation and conduction, while exposure of thoracic viscera for prolonged periods also promotes evaporative and convective heat losses. Hypothermia is common during correction of cardiac anomalies because patients are young (immature thermoregulatory mechanisms) and small (high surface area:volume ratio).

Intraoperative hypothermia is very undesirable, because it augments the central nervous depressant effects of anaesthetics, lowers myocardial contractility, predisposes to arrhythmias, causes left-shift in the oxyhaemoglobin dissociation curve and increases blood viscosity.

Heat loss is most easily limited by maintaining ambient temperatures and relative humidity at the highest levels consistent with comfortable working conditions. Applying topical heat (e.g. heater blankets), providing insulation (e.g. bubble wrap, aluminium foil) and eliminating draughts is also useful. Surgical preparation should not involve excessive clipping,

wetting, or the use of volatile disinfectants. During surgery, repeated flooding of the thorax with warmed irrigation fluid (38°C, by microwave) reduces evaporative and convective heat losses. Irrigant should not be allowed to dwell (and cool) '*in situ*' but be continuously removed by suction. Exposed serosal surfaces should be continuously moistened and covered. Ideally, inspired gases should be warmed and humidified. The depth of anaesthesia must not be excessive and surgery should be conducted as rapidly as possible.

Maintaining urine output

Several factors predispose to renal hypoperfusion and oliguria during thoracotomy. This may be important in animals with diminished renal function and/or those receiving potentially nephrotoxic drugs like some antibiotics or non-steroidal anti-inflammatory drugs.

Measuring urine output involves introducing catheters into the urinary bladder. The catheter is attached to a discarded fluid administration set and bag, and the latter rested on scales. One millilitre of urine weighs approximately 1 g, and an output of 1.0–1.5 ml/kg per hour is desirable during surgery. If this is not forthcoming, the level of anaesthesia and haemodynamic performance should be appraised because both inadequate anaesthesia and hypotension reduce renal perfusion. Fluid administration rate should be increased to improve effective circulating blood volume. If no response ensues within 30 minutes, frusemide 2–5 mg/kg i.v. is given, followed by a dopamine infusion 1–2.5 μg/kg per minute.

Anaesthetist–surgeon co-ordination

Anaesthetists and surgeons must co-ordinate their respective activities on at least five occasions during thoracotomy. Immediately *before* the pleural cavity is opened the anaesthetist must allow the lungs to deflate fully. Similarly, the lungs should be deflated whenever 'sharps' are within the thorax. If mechanical ventilation is used, surgeons must time their manipulation involving 'sharps', or otherwise request that ventilation be temporarily suspended. At the end of surgery, lung integrity is assessed by the anaesthetist imposing relatively high pressures (25–35 cmH$_2$O) while the lung is held under irrigation fluid. Lungs are also held in expansion before thoracic closure, when atelectatic lung is re-expanded. Finally, the lungs are fully inflated while the final sealing sutures are tied; this minimizes iatrogenic pneumothorax.

Management of adverse surgical effects

Surgery may produce unavoidable and undesirable physiological effects. Surgeons must be informed and be prepared to suspend surgery temporarily when these arise.

Occlusion of mediastinal structures

Great veins and atria may become twisted, compressed

or occluded when the heart is lifted and rotated. This reduces venous return and cardiac output. Liver retraction during diaphragmatic hernia repair may occlude the caudal vena cava, creating a similar effect. Rapid fluid administration is required when these unavoidable manoeuvres result in clinical signs like tachycardia and/or hypotension.

Vagal interference

Cardiac vagal fibres may be inadvertently stretched during surgery, e.g. tumour retraction, stapling procedures or whenever 'blind' traction is used, causing sudden bradycardia, bradyarrhythmias and even asystole. When these complications are seen, surgery must be suspended immediately and traction released. Atropine 40 µg/kg i.v. is then injected (if asystole is present, injection must be made into the left ventricular lumen). Surgery is resumed once heart rate increases or sinus rhythm is restored.

Reflex bradycardia is often encountered during correction of the patent ductus arteriosus (Bramham's sign) when the ductal ligature is tightened too rapidly. Loosening and re-applying the suture at a slower rate may avoid a repeated problem. If heart rate slows to significant levels, i.v. atropine may become necessary although often, pre-ligation rates return within 1–5 minutes of ligation.

Epicardial stimulation

Tactile stimulation of the epicardium with surgical instruments occasionally elicits arrhythmias. These are usually benign, although lignocaine (2–4 mg/kg) i.v. may become necessary if arrhythmias become more threatening or haemodynamically significant. If sustained stimulation is unavoidable, lignocaine infusion (25–75 µg/kg per minute) is preferred to repeat injections.

Haemorrhage

This is likely with operations upon vascular structures. Rapid fluid administration through several venous catheters may be required although outcome depends principally on surgical repair of the vessel wall.

Hypotension

Sudden hypotension results from arrhythmias, mechanical interference with venous return or acute depression of myocardial contractility caused, for example, by irrigating the heart with solutions which are cold, too concentrated, hyposmolar or radically different in ionic composition. The cause must be recognized and corrected immediately; fluid infusion and possibly inotropes, e.g. dobutamine (1–5 µg/kg per minute) may become necessary.

Cardiac arrest

Primary respiratory failure is highly unlikely when PPV is performed, and so during thoracotomy, cardiac arrest is nearly always iatrogenic or represents an end-stage event. Cardiac arrest is discussed in more detail later in this chapter.

RECOVERY

The goals of recovery are to restore full respiratory function while ensuring a comfortable, rapid convalescence.

Lung re-expansion

Before the thorax is closed, atelectatic lung is re-expanded to reduce postoperative venous admixture and to eliminate possible foci for bacterial growth. Inflation pressures of 30–40 cmH$_2$O may be necessary. These are not imposed 'acutely', but steadily increasing pressure is applied on successive breaths. Well-expanded lung may need manual depression at this time to divert inspired gas to non-expanded areas. Inflating lungs submerged under irrigation fluid allows a final 'leak-check'. At the point of chest wall closure (when either the final chest wall suture is tied or the chest drain is sealed) lungs are fully inflated to expel residual pneumothorax.

Re-expanding collapsed lung is not without hazard; hypotension occasionally occurs, possibly because previously compressed pulmonary vessels re-open, enlarging the vascular space. Fluids should be rapidly administered if tachycardia indicates hypotension is developing.

Widespread pulmonary oedema occasionally develops if chronically collapsed lung is re-expanded too rapidly. In cases like chronic diaphragmatic hernia, lungs should be expanded very slowly, ideally over 24 hours using continuous suction applied via tube thoracostomy.

Restoration of spontaneous ventilation

Anaesthetists should aim to restore spontaneous breathing as soon as the chest wall is closed. However, spontaneous breathing rarely follows the discontinuation of PPV because of one, or more commonly a combination, of the following:

* Hypocapnia
* Hypothermia
* Residual drug activity:
  neuromuscular blocking agents
  opioids
  volatile anaesthetics
  barbiturates.

Animals are 'weaned from the ventilator' by simultaneously increasing central nervous sensitivity to CO$_2$ (initiating recovery from anaesthesia), and raising plasma CO$_2$ tensions to a stimulant threshold. Breathing resumes with sub-normal $PaCO_2$ levels, although increasing CO_2 at weaning accelerates the onset of spontaneous effort. $PaCO_2$ is raised in several ways:

- By including 4% CO_2 in inspired gas (if the anaesthetic machine has this facility) this raises $PaCO_2$ by 30 mmHg
- By causing controlled re-breathing
    increasing mechanical dead-space
    reducing the fresh gas flow in non-re-breathing systems
    switching soda-lime canister 'out-of-circuit' in those systems which incorporate a switch
- Total ventilatory support may be withdrawn and the lungs inflated with 100% oxygen only when signs of de-saturation become apparent. Respiratory rates as low as 1 or 2 bpm may be required.

Neuromuscular blockade is antagonized when clinical signs of spontaneous recovery are evident (diaphragmatic twitching) or peripheral nerve stimulation indicates some degree of neuromuscular transmission. Antagonists include *either* edrophonium (500 µg/kg) and atropine (40 µg/kg) *or* neostigmine (50 µg/kg) and glycopyrrolate (10 µg/kg) mixtures. In both regimes, the anti-cholinesterase and anti-muscarinic components are mixed together in the same syringe and injected slowly over 30–60 seconds.

Antagonism of opioid drug activity using pure antagonists like naloxone is to be condemned as endogenous analgesic systems, as well as the effects of exogenous drug, will be reversed. The use of doxapram is only justified as a diagnostic step to distinguish central (brainstem depression) from peripheral (neuromuscular) causes of hypoventilation. Because it raises the level of consciousness and possibly, appreciation of surgical invasion, it has no role as a routine non-specific respiratory stimulant after thoracotomy.

Pain relief

The suppression of sympatho–adrenal responses is especially desirable in animals with cardiac disease because tachycardia and hypertension may cause arrhythmias and/or myocardial failure. Catecholamine-induced increases in renal vascular resistance may initiate renal failure when renal disease is present. Increased oxygen consumption, hyperglycaemia and an increased metabolic rate are other undesirable sympatho–adrenal changes. Analgesia restores ventilatory function and minimizes pulmonary complications in several ways: it allows normal respiratory patterns without 'splinting' and active expiration. 'Splinting' is the reflex contraction of expiratory muscles employed to prevent excess stretch, and therefore pain at the incision site. Active expiration reduces the time the chest wall is stretched and is therefore painful.

Analgesia allows normal minute ventilation volumes and large tidal volumes to be inspired. The latter are needed to re-expand atalectatic lung and for effective coughing, which aims to expel airway debris. 'Splinting', active expiration and pain-suppressed coughing promotes retention of airway secretions, airway closure and atelectasis. These in turn increase the work of breathing, and may result in hypoxia. Finally, effective analgesia allows animals to get up and walk, and to reposition themselves for optimum breathing comfort. It also improves their tolerance of pleural drains.

There are at least six ways to relieve post-thoracotomy pain, each technique having advantages and disadvantages. Choice is influenced by the nature of surgery (e.g. sternotomy versus intercostal thoracotomy). Usually, two or more techniques can be combined.

Systemic opioids

The use of systemically administered opioids was once unpopular because they cause some degree of hypoventilation. This drawback is now considered to be less relevant because respiratory depression can be avoided by using low doses or using a mixed agonist–antagonist drug. It is felt that systemic opioids may improve ventilatory performance when chest wall pain is present because they suppress splinting and by producing slow, deep breathing, increase minute alveolar ventilation.

In dogs, morphine (0.1–1.0 mg/kg) i.m., or slow (over 2 minutes) i.v. injection every 2–3 hours is suitable for post-sternotomy and post-thoracotomy pain. It can also be given at 0.1–0.25 mg/kg per hour as an infusion in a crystalloid solution. Higher doses are used when morphine is the only analgesic given; lower doses are appropriate for an opioid 'safety-net' when other analgesics are given. Doses also depend on the severity of surgery. In cats, loading doses of 0.1–0.5 mg/kg i.m. are suitable followed either by repeated doses (2- to 4-hour intervals) or i.v. infusion (0.05–0.1 mg/kg per hour). Other pure agonist opioids, e.g. methadone or pethidine, may be used (at equi-analgesic doses) but the quality of analgesia and comfort provided by morphine appears to be superior. Pethidine is short acting and often seems ineffectual in cats. Use of mixed agonist–antagonists like buprenorphine or butorphenol precludes the uncomplicated use of short-acting µ-agonists for intra-operative analgesia.

Repeated doses of analgesic are required when signs of discomfort are seen. There are no risks with 'addiction' (dependence) developing if analgesia is provided for the customary period of 24–72 hours. Continuous morphine (0.05–0.25 mg/kg per hour) is suitable in both species when pain is present.

Non-steroidal anti-inflammatory drugs

Carprofen (4 mg/kg) or ketoprofen (2 mg/kg) are

useful given preoperatively, along with systemic opioids as part of polymodal analgesic strategy.

Intercostal block

This technique is only feasible for intercostal thoracotomy. It is most easily performed before wound closure; approach is from the visceral side of the nerve with injections made at the caudal border of each rib (avoiding the intercostal artery and vein). Three, or preferably five segments cranial and caudal to the incision site are blocked. Catheters can be pre-placed for repeat injections but are readily dislodged. Bupivacaine 0.5 % with adrenaline, 0.5 ml per nerve, provides analgesia 12–20 minutes after injection which lasts 3–7 hours. The technique is poorly tolerated in animals which have recovered from anaesthesia, because injection is made externally and must pass through muscle, which reduces accuracy. Repeat injections are also required and the technique becomes time consuming.

Despite the apparent ease of nerve location, poor 'quality' block is the principal disadvantage of the technique; success may in part be due to paravertebral spread of injectate. With bupivacaine, overdose, or rapid systemic absorption can result in convulsions and arrhythmias. Paravertebral spread may result in widespread sympathetic blockade with segmental vasodilation and, through loss of local vascular resistance, hypotension. Flail segments may result from successful, multi-segmental block.

Interpleural local anaesthetic

Interpleural bupivacaine can be given through an interpleural catheter positioned in the sixth intercostal space. A dose of 1.5 mg/kg bupivacaine (0.5 % solution containing 1:100 000 adrenaline) is given when the animal appears to be in pain. Unfortunately, the technique relies on local anaesthetic suffusing the incision site which it reaches by gravity. Animals must therefore be positioned lying upon the surgical site.

Extradural opioids

In dogs, extradural morphine (0.1 mg/kg dissolved in 0.26 ml/kg sterile saline) injected at the lumbosacral junction produces analgesia without sympathetic nervous or motor blockade. Analgesia far outlasts systemic opioid administration (lasting about 24 hours), although the technique seems to rely in part on a systemic effect; animals appear to be sedated for 8–12 hours. In a recent experiment, extradural morphine (0.15 mg/kg) provided better analgesia than the same dose given i.v. (Popilskis *et al.*, 1993). Butorphanol (0.08 mg/kg diluted in a similar volume of saline) may be used instead of morphine. Doses are unavailable for cats.

Cryoanalgesia

This technique provides analgesia for 3–4 weeks in humans but has not been evaluated in companion animals. The intercostal nerve is dissected free and enveloped in an ice-ball generated by a cryoprobe. Structure and function is restored over 2–3 weeks without neuritis or neuromata formation.

TENS

Transcutaneous electrical nerve stimulation (TENS) uses a commercially available stimulating unit to deliver a low voltage high frequency (80 Hz) stimulus pattern to a spinal nerve. This is thought to excite myelinated dorsal horn A d fibres and suppress pain signals reaching the cord via small diameter unmyelinated c fibres. The technique is inexpensive, easy to apply and has no apparent side-effects. However, in many cases relief is incomplete or absent and so, in animals, the technique cannot be regarded as reliable.

Local infiltration/sternal fixation

After sternotomy, weight on the thoracic limbs creates painful abduction and shearing forces along the incision line. Breathing causes similar discomfort. This is limited if some sternebrae are left intact (unseparated) during the operation as this provides postoperative chest wall rigidity. Analgesia also results when bupivacaine-soaked swabs are placed on the retracted sections of sternebrae during surgery and before closure, when the incision line may be infiltrated with bupivacaine.

Pleural drainage

Residual pneumothorax, inflammatory exudate and blood can be removed from the interpleural space by reabsorption, intermittent aspiration, or with chest drains, in which suction is applied continuously or periodically. The technique used depends on the animal's size and the volume of exudate, blood or gas likely to be produced. Inspiring high concentrations of oxygen assists absorption of residual gas. Continuous suction via pleural drains also assists re-expansion of chronically atelectatic lung.

Endobronchial suction

Mucus and blood remaining in the airway after surgery predispose to distal airway collapse. They are unlikely to be cleared because animals are unlikely to cough effectively after thoracotomy. Also, the mucociliary carpet is 'paralysed' by anaesthesia. Foreign material must be aspirated by endobronchial suction before the endotracheal tube is removed. This must be judicious because distal airway collapse can also follow excessive vacuum. Suction is applied for 10-second periods only followed by three to five lung inflations using 100% O_2.

Oxygenation

Postoperative oxygen supplementation is desirable because it lowers the risk of tidal and alveolar hypoxia. It also evacuates residual pneumothorax by enlarging the arterio–venous gas tension difference, favouring gas transfer into pleural veins. Often, O_2 administration has to be continued beyond that time when chewing, 'gagging' and undesirable 'bucking' activity mandate the removal of the endotracheal tube. Delivery may be continued by:

- Oxygen cage
- Tracheostomy
- Nasotracheal catheter
- Mask
- Plastic bag.

The risk of oxygen toxicity is low in companion animals compared with human beings.

Positioning

Postoperative patient positioning is determined by the need to produce optimum oxygenation, to ensure patient comfort and to facilitate nursing. Sternal recumbency optimizes oxygenation but is poorly tolerated after sternotomy incision. Left lateral recumbency allows the larger right lung to remain uppermost and well expanded but may cause discomfort when surgery has been performed on this side.

Animals are usually allowed to recover with the affected side uppermost; this facilitates drain management, is less painful and promotes rapid re-expansion of affected lung. However, periodic re-positioning is useful because this allows bilateral lung expansion and causes interpleural gas 'pockets' to shift towards the drain and reduces the risk of decubital ulceration.

Assessing adequacy of ventilation after thoracotomy

After thoracotomy, breathing adequacy is assessed in several ways. Clinical signs should be observed, e.g. mucous membrane colour, chest wall excursion, respiratory rate and pattern (shallow, rapid breathing is less efficient than slow, deep breathing with spontaneous 'sighs'). Although the most informative test involves arterial blood gas analysis, this should reveal minimal $P(A-a)O_2$ values with low to normal $PaCO_2$ levels (36-40 mmHg; 4.32-4.78 kPa). A simple water manometer attached to the endotracheal tube before tracheal extubation can be used to measure peak negative inspiratory pressure generated during three successive inspirations (Table 23.5), although an aneroid manometer with a negative scale (calibrated in cmH_2O) is more convenient.

Re-warming

Postoperative hypothermia delays recovery, increases patient sensitivity to pain and through shivering, elevates whole body oxygen consumption at a time when ventilatory performance may be poor. Topical heat (infra-red lamps, hot-water bottles etc.) should be applied, the animal dried and insulation provided; this avoids further heat loss. Rectal or gastric lavage is a simple, effective technique to raise temperature. This involves introducing warm (40°C) water into the stomach or rectum by a funnel and siphon assembly; fluid is withdrawn (by lowering the funnel) after 3-6 minutes or so. Topical heat must be applied judiciously because poor cutaneous blood flow increases the likelihood of burns.

Although 'shivering' occurs in normothermic animals after halothane, and often indicates pain, it invariably elevates metabolic oxygen consumption and indicates the need for inspired air enrichment with O_2.

Urine output

Postoperative pain, hypotension and opioids may contribute to urine retention. Urine output should be maintained during recovery using infusions of crystalloids, periodic frusemide injections (2-5 mg/kg i.v. every 90 minutes or so) and/or dopamine infusion (about 1.0-2.5 µg/kg per minute).

Ongoing respiratory function

Clinical examination, thoracic radiography and arterial blood gas analysis may be used for the continued assessment of lung function.

Metabolic 'balance'

Postoperative calorific requirements are elevated and so animals should be encouraged to eat as soon as possible. Specialized techniques for feeding may be needed in anorexic animals. Postoperative fluid intake must be maintained by the parenteral route if necessary.

CARDIAC ARREST

For several reasons, cardiac arrest is relatively easy to manage during thoracotomy:

PINP (cmH_2O)	Comment
0 to -10	Adequate ventilation unlikely
-10 to -15	Adequate ventilation may just be possible
-15 to -20	Unable to overcome major airway resistance
-20 to -30	Able to cough and overcome major airway resistance

Table 23.5: Peak negative inspiratory pressure.

Drug	Use	Dose
Adrenaline	In asystole; to coarsen 'fine' fibrillation; to increase inotropy and systemic vascular resistance	100 µg/kg i.v.
Atropine	For vagally mediated asystole and critical atrioventricular blockade	40 mg/kg i.v.
Methoxamine	This α_1-agonist increases systemic resistance	500 µg/kg i.v.
Sodium bicarbonate	No longer recommended	
Calcium	No longer recommended during CPR *except* in hypocalcaemia, gross halothane overdose, or when HCO_3^- has been inadvertently given	
Methylprednisolone	Used for endotoxic and possibly 'vasculogenic' shock	30 mg/kg
Lignocaine	Used to control ventricular arrhythmias	Two boluses at 4 mg/kg, followed by infusion at 25–75 µg/kg per min
Dobutamine	Infusions maintain inotropy after cardiac activity is restored	1–5 µg/kg/min IV infusion

Table 23.6: *Drugs for use during cardiac arrest.*

- Internal cardiac compression can be used, which is considerably more effective than external compression
- Arrhythmias may be identified visually
- Accurate intravascular and/ or intracardiac injections are possible
- Aortic cross-clamping is possible
- Atrial and vena caval filling may be assessed; fluid and α_1 agonist administration can be adjusted accordingly
- Some assessment can be made of ventricular systolic function, allowing titration of inotropes
- Sub-normal cardiac temperatures can be easily corrected
- The adequacy of lung inflation can be established.

Internal cardiac compression: technique

- Open pericardium
- Use fingers or hands to 'milk' ventricles [the compression rate should be 80–120 per minute (dogs)]
- If atrial or venous filling is poor, use gravity, abdominal binding, fluids or α_1 agonists (e.g. methoxamine 0.1–0.5 mg/kg) to improve venous return

- Inflate lungs every third or fourth compression.

Drugs used to improve cardiac output should be injected into the left ventricular lumen (see Table 23.6). Injection must not be made into the left ventricular free wall or into branches of the coronary artery.

Electrical defibrillation

Electrolyte-soaked swabs are applied to the defibrillator paddles. The area of paddle in myocardial contact must be maximized. The defibrillator energy is set (0.1–0.5 J/kg). Personnel stand clear, oesophageal stethoscopes are disconnected, and the paddles are discharged (see Clutton 1993 and 1994).

REFERENCES

Clutton RE (1993) Management of peri-operative cardiac arrest in companion animals: part 1. *In Practice* **15**, 267–277

Clutton RE (1994) Management of peri-operative cardiac arrest in companion animals: part 2. *In Practice* **16**, 3–10

Popilskis S, Kohn DF, Laurent L and Danilo P (1993) Efficacy of epidural morphine versus intravenous morphine for post-thoracotomy pain in dogs. *Journal Of Veterinary Anaesthesia* **20**, 21

Soma L R (1973) *Controlled Ventilation of the Veterinary Patient.* Pitman-Moore, Inc., Washington.

Approaches to the Thorax

Barbara M. Kirby

CHOICE OF APPROACH

The most commonly used approaches to the thoracic cavity in dogs and cats include lateral thoracotomy, median sternotomy, and ventral midline coeliotomy with trans-diaphragmatic approach. Additional approaches include cranial thoracic wall flap, trans-sternal thoracotomy, and combined midline abdominal and thoracic approaches.

The most appropriate surgical approach to the thorax in an individual animal depends upon:

- The problem requiring surgical intervention
- The anatomical area of interest
- The degree of surgical exposure required
- The proposed surgical procedure
- Individual anatomical variations
- Personal preference or previous experience of the surgeon.

Critical assessment of a minimum of two radiographic views of the thorax is essential for operative planning for thoracotomy patients. Generally, ventrodorsal and right lateral thoracic radiographs are preferred, with the exposures made at peak inspiration. Additional radiographic views, as well as results of ultrasonography, echocardiography, angiography, lymphangiography and thoracocentesis, may provide valuable information to assist the surgeon's choice of approach in various circumstances.

Thoracic radiographs indicate the precise position of suspected intrathoracic lesions, and confirm the location of normal thoracic structures. These findings will then guide the choice of right versus left lateral thoracotomy, as well as the choice of the specific intercostal space. General guidelines for approaches to the thorax in dogs and cats for selected problems and procedures are given in Table 24.1. This is intended only as general guidance, with review of the individual animal's thoracic radiographs as the critical deciding factor.

THORACIC ANATOMY

The musculoskeletal anatomy of the thorax is obviously important in the chosen surgical approach, but will not be reviewed here. An internal thoracic artery and vein lie on each side of the sternum in the ventral thorax. These vessels can be encountered in both lateral intercostal thoracotomy and median sternotomy. Haemorrhage from transected internal thoracic arteries can be difficult to isolate and control. These vessels are best avoided. The intercostal artery, nerve and vein lie directly caudal to the corresponding rib on each side. Local anaesthetic infiltration of the intercostal nerves at the rib head for two or three intercostal spaces cranial and caudal to a lateral thoracotomy incision is a useful adjunct to systemic analgesics in thoracotomy patients. Haemorrhage from the intercostal arteries can be avoided during circumferential suture closure of the ribs by blunt passage of the swaged end of the needle around the ribs. Puncture of the intercostal artery in thoracocentesis is avoided by needle placement immediately cranial to the rib.

LATERAL THORACOTOMY TECHNIQUES

Lateral thoracotomy is the most commonly used approach to the thorax. Good exposure of the heart and lungs can be achieved. However, lateral thoracotomy provides good exposure of only those structures in the immediate vicinity of the thoracotomy, and only on the chosen side of the chest. Thus, it is critically important to choose the correct side and site for lateral thoracotomy, regardless of the specific technique chosen. Lateral thoracotomy does not provide adequate exposure of the entire thoracic cavity, as required for inspection of all pulmonary parenchyma in spontaneous pneumothorax, nor does it provide optimal exposure for most mediastinal masses. Median sternotomy is preferred in these instances.

Lateral thoracotomy can be performed on either the right or left sides of the thorax, anywhere from the third to tenth intercostal space or rib, depending on the reason for the thoracotomy. Cranial to the third rib and caudal to the tenth rib, little useful exposure of the thorax is obtained.

Lateral thoracotomy can be accomplished by a number of techniques, including standard and modified lateral intercostal thoracotomy, rib resection lateral thoracotomy, and rib pivot lateral thoracotomy.

Respiratory system

Thoracic structure	Procedure	Approach
Trachea	Tracheal collapse, stenosis	R3 or MS
	foreign body	R3-6
Lungs		L4-6 or R4-6 or MS
	L cranial lobectomy	L5
	L caudal lobectomy	L5 or L6
	R cranial lobectomy	R5
	R middle lobectomy	R5
	R caudal lobectomy	R5 or R6
	Accessory lobectomy	R6
	L hemipneumonectomy	L5 or L6 or MS
	R hemipneumonectomy	R5 or R6 or MS
Exploration	Pneumothorax	MS

Cardiovascular system

Site	Approach
PDA	L4
PRAA	L4
Pulmonic valve	L4 or MS
Aortic valve	MS
Tricuspid & mitral valves	MS (open heart techniques)
Subtotal pericardectomy	L5 or R5 or MS
Left atrium	L4 or MS
Right atrium	R4 or MS
Left ventricle	L5 or MS
Right ventricle	R5 or MS
VSD (pulmonary artery banding)	L4
Tetralogy of Fallot (Blalock or Potts)	L4
Heartworm removal	L4 or R5 or MS
Caudal vena cava	R7-9

Alimentary system and others

Site	Approach
Cranial oesophagus	R3-4 or MS
Caudal oesophagus	L7-9 or R7-9
Thoracic duct (dog)	R8-10
Thoracic duct (cat)	L8-10
Cranial mediastinum (masses)	MS or CTWF
Diaphragmatic hernia	CVMC

Table 24.1: Usual approach to the thorax for selected problems, procedures, or exposure of thoracic structures.

Key: *R (right), L (left): when followed by number indicates lateral thoracotomy at numbered intercostal space or rib number for rib resection or rib pivot procedures. MS, median sternotomy; CTWF, cranial thoracic wall flap; CVMC, cranial ventral midline coeliotomy; PDA, patent ductus arteriosus; PRAA, persistent right aortic arch; VSD, ventricular septal defect.*

Lateral intercostal thoracotomy

Lateral intercostal thoracotomy is the most common method of lateral thoracotomy. Access to the chest is gained by separation or transection of the muscles of the chest wall, layer by layer. The intercostal muscles are transected between adjacent ribs, and finally the parietal pleura is incised. Finnochetto or Haight self-retaining rib retractors are used to spread the ribs, with the chest wall beneath the retractors protected by moistened swabs In very small puppies and kittens, Wietlaner or Gelpi self-retaining retractors may be more useful than rib retractors, and have the advantage of being lighter in weight. They will, however, be less efficient in spreading the ribs. The ribs are more easily retracted cranially than caudally; thus if two adjacent spaces radiographically appear equally suitable for intercostal thoracotomy, it is usually better to choose the more caudal space.

The standard lateral intercostal thoracotomy involves transection of the latissimus dorsi muscle to gain access to the deeper musculature of the chest wall and intercostal space. A modification of this technique, sparing transection of the latissimus dorsi muscle, has recently been introduced (Dean and Pope, 1992). Use of the modified technique has been reported on either side at the fourth, fifth or sixth intercostal spaces in 16 dogs ranging from 2 months to 11 years of age. I have found the modified technique most useful in young, lightly muscled animals whose latissimus is elastic enough to be easily mobilized and retracted. To date, there has not been a comparative study between the two techniques published. In the experience of the author, there do not appear to be any major differences in postoperative morbidity between dogs with the modified technique in comparison to the standard technique, although those with the modified technique appear subjectively less lame on the affected forelimb in the early postoperative period.

The most commonly entered intercostal spaces are the fourth, fifth and sixth, as these provide access to most of the cardiopulmonary structures of surgical interest. A detailed description of the left fourth intercostal space thoracotomy is given below. The right third intercostal space thoracotomy provides good access to the intrathoracic trachea for application of extraluminal prostheses in tracheal collapse involving the thoracic trachea. It is usually combined with a ventral approach to the cervical trachea, as animals requiring thoracic tracheal support usually suffer cervical tracheal collapse also. The combined approach ensures good access to the thoracic inlet, often the site of the most severe collapse. Other specific sides and sites for lateral intercostal thoracotomy are given in Table 24.1.

The *left fourth intercostal space thoracotomy* is probably the single most commonly used approach to the thoracic cavity in dogs. It is the approach of choice for ligation of patent ductus arteriosus (PDA), one of the most common congenital heart defects in dogs. It is also the approach of choice for surgical repair of the most common variety of vascular ring anomaly in dogs, persistent right aortic arch (PRAA), where the oesophageal entrapment is relieved by double ligation and division of the ligamentum arteriosum. The left fourth intercostal space thoracotomy is also the approach for surgical relief of pulmonic stenosis by various techniques. It is sometimes used for access to the left cranial lung lobe, although the fifth intercostal space gives better exposure of the hilus of this lung lobe in most dogs.

The animal is positioned in right lateral recumbency. A small roll or sandbag under the chest may help to open up the intercostal space, and the forelimbs are pulled cranially and secured with leg ties. Hair is liberally clipped from the entire thorax, extending beyond the ventral and dorsal midlines, cranial to the caudal border of the scapula and including the axillary skin fold. The patient's skin and surgical team are routinely prepared for aseptic surgery, and the surgical field is routinely draped.

A vertical linear or curvilinear skin incision is made caudal to the scapula, and a scalpel incision is made through the subcutaneous tissue and cutaneous trunci muscle. Haemostasis should be meticulous, with ligation or electrocoagulation of bleeding vessels. Blunt dissection is used to isolate the ventral edge of the latissimus dorsi muscle.

In the standard technique, latissimus is transected from ventral to dorsal with Mayo scissors, and numerous muscular bleeding vessels are electrocoagulated or ligated.

In the modified technique, the ventral border of latissimus is incised with Metzenbaum scissors, and the incision is extended along ventral latissimus cranial and caudal for 4–8 cm; this cranial and caudal dissection is critical to allow retraction of latissimus. Latissimus is separated from underlying muscles with blunt finger dissection. The latissimus muscle is retracted dorsally by an assistant with hand-held retractors (or alternatively, a stay suture in the ventral border of the latissimus can be used to facilitate retraction of the muscle dorsally). The remainder of the procedure is identical to the standard technique.

The specific intercostal space is now identified by palpating cranially beneath latissimus to identify the first rib, and the ribs and intercostal spaces are counted caudally. The scalenus muscle normally inserts on the fifth rib (which helps to confirm the location of the fourth intercostal space) and is transected perpendicular to its fibres. The leaves of the serratus ventralis muscle are bluntly separated or transected, and the external and internal intercostal muscles are isolated and transected at the midpoint between adjacent ribs. The parietal pleura is pierced with the point of a scalpel blade at maximum expiration. Positive pressure manual or mechanical ventilation is required from this point. The parietal pleura is incised with Metzenbaum scissors.

The intrathoracic structures normally visible and accessible surgically from the left fourth intercostal space thoracotomy include:

- Ascending aorta
- Brachiocephalic trunk
- Left subclavian artery
- Descending aorta for several centimetres
- Main pulmonary artery
- Ductus arteriosus or ligamentum arteriosus
- Pulmonic valve
- Left auricular appendage
- Left phrenic nerve
- Vagus nerve.

Structures that are visible, but usually inaccessible surgically include:

- Thymus (in juveniles)
- Pericardium (usually fifth intercostal space for pericardectomy)
- Right ventricle
- Left ventricle.

Individual anatomical variations must always be kept in mind. Persistent left cranial vena cava is reported in up to 40% of puppies with PRAA, and in a small number of those with PDA. This anomaly is dramatically visible in the surgical field of a left fourth intercostal space thoracotomy, but is of no surgical importance other than that it should be recognized and reflected out of the way.

Closure of the lateral intercostal thoracotomy is begun by placement of circumferential sutures around the adjacent ribs. These sutures are intended only to bring the spread ribs back into their normal anatomical position. The ribs should not be overriding or tightly apposed. A water-tight and air-tight seal of the thoracic cavity is required. This seal is accomplished by meticulous layer-by-layer closure of the soft tissues. Simple continuous closure of each individual muscle layer is recommended. It is important that each layer of closure starts at the most dorsal aspect of the incision and is carried all the way to the most ventral aspect of the incision. When possible, depending on the size of the animal, the author uses a six- or seven-layer closure of the chest in lateral intercostal thoracotomy. The layers of closure, from deep to superficial are:

1. Simple interrupted circumcostal sutures.
2. Simple continuous apposition of transected intercostal muscles.
3. Simple continuous apposition of separated leaves of serratus ventralis muscle.
4. Simple continuous apposition of transected latissimus dorsi and scalenus muscles.
5. Simple continuous apposition of transected cutaneous trunci muscle.
6. Subcutaneous closure.
7. Skin closure.

Re-establishment of negative intrapleural pressure usually cannot be accomplished until after closure of the latissimus dorsi muscle layer, at the earliest. If a thoracostomy tube has been placed before closure of the chest, air can often be heard whistling through the open end of the chest tube with each ventilation when a good air-tight seal of the chest wall has been achieved. Bubbles of air or ballooning of the soft tissues between the ribs, most often seen at the ventral-most aspect of the incision, indicates inadequate soft tissue closure. An assistant can begin manually evacuating air and/or fluid from the pleural space once the latissimus is closed, when a chest tube is in place. This allows removal of the animal from assisted ventilation well before the end of the surgical procedure. When a chest tube is not indicated, negative intrapleural pressure is re-established with needle thoracocentesis at the end of the procedure.

Rib resection thoracotomy

Rib resection thoracotomy is indicated in circumstances where somewhat increased exposure than that gained by lateral intercostal thoracotomy is required. The lateral periosteum is sharply incised in the centre

of the rib to be resected. Using a blunt, curved periosteal elevator, the periosteum is circumferentially reflected from the rib. Using bone cutters, the rib is transected dorsally and ventrally and removed. With careful dissection, the periosteum on the medial side of the rib remains intact. This periosteum, with the parietal pleura attached, is sharply incised to gain access to the thorax. At closure, the periosteum on the medial and lateral sides of the rib are separately closed, leaving an intact periosteal tube for regeneration of the rib. In the author's experience, rib resection thoracotomy is rarely required. When the rib itself is involved in the disease process, such as in primary rib tumours, the periosteum is removed along with the rib. However, in most rib neoplasms, such as chondrosarcoma, *en bloc* resection of the mass requires removal of multiple ribs and thoracic wall reconstructive techniques.

Rib pivot thoracotomy

Rib pivot thoracotomy allows similar exposure to that gained by rib resection, while sparing the rib. It requires dorsal dissection to the level of the costovertebral articulation. The periosteum is incised and reflected as for rib resection. The rib is transected at the costochondral junction and rotated cranially using the costovertebral articulation as a hinge on which to pivot. At closure, the rib osteotomy is stabilized with orthopaedic wire placed in a hemicerclage fashion. Use of rib pivot thoracotomy was described in 11 dogs with primary pulmonary neoplasia involving a single lung lobe (Schulman and Lippincott, 1988). In these cases, lung lobectomy was performed with a mechanical stapling device. Stapling devices are sometimes difficult to manoeuvre into the proper position for lobectomy, with the exposure achieved with standard intercostal thoracotomy. Rib pivot thoracotomy provided excellent exposure in this case series, with neoplasms as large as 1300 cm^3 easily removed. Closure was simple and secure. Although the author has no personal experience with this procedure, its preservation of the rib seems preferable to discarding a normal structure, as in the rib resection thoracotomy.

MEDIAN STERNOTOMY

Exposure of the thoracic cavity by median sternotomy, or 'sternal split', allows thorough exploration of both hemithoraces. It is the approach of choice, in most instances, for masses in the mediastinum and for potentially bilateral pulmonary lesions, such as exploration for the cause of spontaneous pneumothorax. Lung lobectomy, however, is technically more difficult from this approach than lateral thoracotomy techniques. The structures of the heart base are relatively inaccessible by this approach. Subtotal pericardectomy can be performed by either median sternotomy or right or left lateral thoracotomy.

Technique

The animal is positioned in dorsal recumbency and supported by sandbags, a trough, or vacuum positioners, with the forelimbs pulled slightly cranially and secured. It is important that the animal is stable in this position, which can be difficult to accomplish in thin, deep-chested breeds of dog. The hair is liberally clipped, including adequate clip of the lateral chest walls for thoracostomy tube placement, if indicated. Skin preparation and draping are routinely performed. The ventral midline skin is incised from just cranial to the manubrium to just caudal to the xiphoid. Great care is taken to stay on the midline. The subcutaneous tissue is sharply incised. Meticulous haemostasis with electrocoagulation is required throughout the approach. The deep pectoral muscles are reflected for approximately 5 mm on either side of the midline of the sternebrae using periosteal elevation. The periosteum at the midline of the sternebrae is scored with a sharp scalpel blade or marked with electrocautery, to act as a guide for the sternal osteotomy. The sternebrae are divided using an oscillating saw, taking care to remain exactly on the midline through the entire thickness of the sternebrae to avoid damage to the internal thoracic arteries, lying just lateral to the midline on each side. The wound edges are protected with moistened swabs, and the sternotomy is spread with rib retractors.

The extent of median sternotomy required is variable. In complete median sternotomy, all sternebrae, including the manubrium and xiphoid process are sectioned. Complete median sternotomy gives the greatest exposure of the thoracic cavity, and in the author's opinion, is required for thorough exploration of the thorax as in spontaneous pneumothorax. Partial median sternotomy is sometimes indicated. Cranial median sternotomy, with the manubrium and first three or four sternebrae transected, may provide sufficient surgical exposure of the cranial mediastinum. Caudal median sternotomy, with the xiphoid and last three or four sternebrae transected is most often used in combination with cranial ventral midline coeliotomy for selected vascular, hepatic, and diaphragmatic herniation cases.

Closure technique

Closure of median sternotomy begins with reduction and internal fixation of the transected sternebrae. This is usually accomplished with orthopaedic wire in a figure-of-eight pattern. An air-tight and water-tight seal of the thoracic cavity is required, as in the lateral thoracotomy techniques, but is more difficult to achieve due to the paucity of muscle and soft tissue available on the ventral thorax. Careful reapposition of the elevated muscles and fascia with a simple continuous closure over the transected sternebrae and wire ends seals the thoracic cavity. Subcutaneous closure is with a simple continuous pattern and synthetic absorbable material. Skin closure is routine.

TRANS-DIAPHRAGMATIC THORACOTOMY

Diaphragmatic herniation is most often repaired from a cranioventral midline abdominal approach. Positive pressure ventilation in these cases must begin as soon as the *linea alba* is incised. Herniated viscera are retrieved from the thoracic cavity and returned to the abdominal cavity through the defect in the diaphragm. In congenital and chronic diaphragmatic hernias, where contraction and stenosis of the hernial ring may prevent reduction of the herniated organs, enlargement of the hernia by diaphragm myotomy may be required.

Surgical access to structures in the most caudodorsal thoracic cavity is occasionally gained by diaphragm myotomy, although lateral thoracotomy is more commonly used.

CRANIAL THORACIC WALL FLAP

Cranial thoracic wall flap combines cranial median sternotomy and unilateral intercostal thoracotomy. Ligation of the internal thoracic artery on the side of the intercostal approach is required. Exposure of the cranial mediastinum is improved with this technique, facilitating excision of some mediastinal masses.

TRANS-STERNAL THORACOTOMY

Trans-sternal thoracotomy involves bilateral intercostal thoracotomies made continuous by a transverse osteotomy of the sternum. Ligation of the internal thoracic artery on each side is required. Internal fixation of the transected sternum with cross-pins and a figure-of-eight wire is required for closure. Transsternal thoracotomy at the seventh intercostal space has been advocated for diaphragmatic hernia repair, although the indications for such an aggressive approach would be quite rare.

COMPLICATIONS

Complications associated with the thoracotomy itself, rather than the intrathoracic procedure or problem, are numerous and some are potentially life-threatening.

Haemothorax

Haemothorax in the immediate postoperative period may result from injury to one or both internal thoracic arteries or one or more intercostal arteries. Exploration of the wound and thoracic cavity may be required in animals with severe or persistent haemorrhage. Autotransfusion can be considered in animals with self-limiting haemothorax or preoperatively in those requiring exploration for the source of bleeding.

Pneumothorax

Pneumothorax occurring postoperatively in thoracotomy patients that have not had surgical insult to their lungs or airways may be the result of pulmonary injury by needle puncture during closure, entrapment of the periphery of a lung lobe in the closure or beneath the rib retractors, or overzealous thoracostomy tube aspiration resulting in injury to the lung parenchyma pulled into the chest tube. In most cases, intermittent or continuous aspiration of the chest tube will allow small air leaks to seal.

Subcutaneous emphysema

Subcutaneous emphysema is the result of inadequate closure of the overlying soft tissues, with escape of free air from the pleural space into the subcutaneous space. This is usually a minor, self-limiting problem. Broad spectrum systemic antibiotics are indicated for the prevention of septicaemia in severe subcutaneous emphysema. Exploration of the thorax and reclosure of the thoracotomy wound may also be required.

Rib fractures

Rib fractures or costovertebral luxations may result from excessive rib retraction. Specific therapy is not usually indicated, although supportive bandaging and prolonged analgesia may be required.

Wound complications

Wound complications are frequently encountered in all types of thoracotomies. Commonly encountered wound problems include oedema, wound swelling from fluid accumulation (seroma, haematoma, abscess), wound discharge, and dehiscence. Non-union of osteotomies of the sternebrae and ribs and osteomyelitis can be encountered in procedures requiring sectioning of bone. In one study, complication rates associated with median sternotomy were not statistically different from those associated with lateral thoracotomy, where wound complications were observed in four out of nine median sternotomies and 13 out of 36 lateral thoracotomies (Ringwald and Birchard, 1989). In a recent review of the complications of median sternotomy in 67 dogs and nine cats, no complications were reported in the cats, while the dogs had short-term and longer term complication rates of 19 and 22%, respectively (Burton and White, 1996). Four of the 37 dogs surviving more than 2 weeks after surgery developed radiographic evidence of sternal osteomyelitis. One dog suffered a sternal fracture and one suffered transient brachial plexus injury.

Lameness

Transient lameness of the ipsilateral forelimb in lateral thoracotomies is common.

REFERENCES

Burton CA and White RN (1996) Review of the technique and complications of median sternotomy in the dog and cat. *Journal of Small Animal Practice* **37**, 516–522

Dean PW and Pope ER (1992) Modified intercostal thoracotomy approach. *Journal of the American Animal Hospital Association* **28**, 87–91

Ringwald RJ and Birchard SJ (1989) Complications of median sternotomy in the dog and literature review. *Journal of the American Animal Hospital Association* **25**, 430–434

Schulman AJ and Lippincott CL (1988) Rib pivot thoracotomy. *Compendium of Continuing Education for the Practising Veterinarian* **10**, 927–931

Laryngeal Surgery

Richard A.S. White

LARYNGEAL PARALYSIS

Undoubtedly the most common indication for surgical intervention involving the larynx of small animals is the relief of laryngeal paralysis. Techniques for the management of laryngeal paralysis are intended to enlarge the rima permanently and ameliorate the restricted air flow. It should be emphasized that a variety of surgical procedures have been described for the treatment of this condition since it was first recognized (Cook, 1964), and there is ongoing controversy as to what are the most appropriate procedures. It is convenient to categorize these procedures according to whether or not the surgery disrupts the structures within the lumen of the larynx (Table 25.1).

Extralaryngeal	Intralaryngeal

Arytenoid lateralization
    unilateral
    bilateral
	Partial laryngectomy
	    ventriculocordectomy
	    partial arytenoidectomy

Re-innervation
    neuromuscular pedicle graft
    nerve anastomosis
	Castellated laryngofissure
	    conventional
	    modified

Table 25.1: Procedures for management of laryngeal paralysis.

Extralaryngeal procedures

Procedures which dilate the rima without disrupting the laryngeal mucosa have significant advantages and in the author's view are to be preferred. In particular, the following advantages are recognized:

- Gaseous anaesthesia can be maintained by routine endotracheal intubation throughout the surgery
- The risk of aspiration during surgery and the postoperative period is minimal
- The requirement for postoperative care, notably temporary tracheostomy management, is substantially reduced
- The incidence of intralaryngeal scarring is extremely low.

Arytenoid lateralization

Dilation of the rima by fixing the arytenoid(s) in abduction and attempting to mimic the function of the dorsal cricoarytenoid muscle has been described by various authors (Harvey and Venker-van Haagen, 1975; Lane, 1982; Rosin and Greenwood, 1982; LaHue, 1989; White, 1989; Burbidge *et al.*, 1993) and is now a well established technique. The procedure may be performed with a variety of modifications and the following is a description of the basic technique.

The unilateral procedure is performed with the patient in right lateral recumbency for a right-handed surgeon and vice-versa for a left-handed one. The neck is partially extended and supported on a pack. An incision is made at a point below the junction of the maxillary and linguofacial veins (Figure 25.1) and the fibres of the panniculus muscle split. The dorsal wing of the thyroid cartilage is palpated through the overlying soft tissue which is dissected bluntly to expose the thyropharyngeus muscle. This muscle is transected horizontally or its fibres split longitudinally to expose the dorsal wing of the thyroid cartilage. The thyroid cartilage can then be retracted laterally (Figure 25.2), allowing the fascial tissue lying between the thyroid and the cricoid to be broken down. At this point the firm cricothyroid articulation may be disrupted if required. Self-retaining retractors are used to retract the dorsal aspect of the thyroid laterally and the sharp prominence of the muscular process of the arytenoid cartilage overlying the rostrodorsal aspect of the cricoid cartilage is located by digital palpation. The fibres of the dorsal cricoarytenoid muscle fan out from this to the dorsal midline of the cricoid and are carefully transected to allow access to the cricoarytenoid articulation below. In cases of idiopathic paralysis, this muscle will be atrophied, but in cases of acute onset paralysis (e.g. trauma), the muscle remains substantial. It is very useful to leave part of the muscle attached to the muscular process to permit manipulation of the arytenoid during the procedure without tractioning the cartilage itself since it may prove to be friable in some cases. The arytenoid cartilage is now carefully separated with fine scissors from its underlying cricoarytenoid articulation without disrupting the laryngeal mucosa medially. The sesamoidean interarytenoid articulation is then cut which permits free movement of the cartilage.

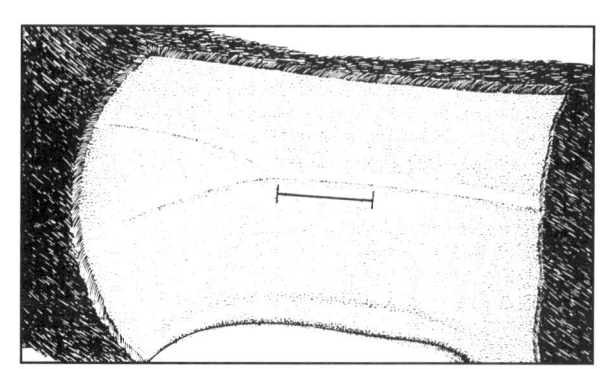

Figure 25.1: *Arytenoid lateralization: the incision is made below the bifurcation of the maxillary and linguofacial veins.* © *RAS White.*

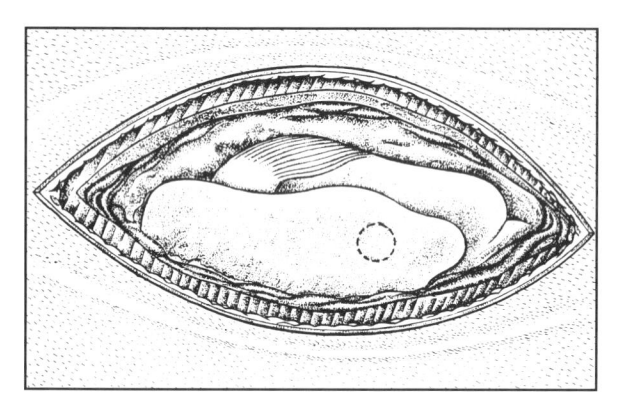

Figure 25.2: *Arytenoid lateralization: the thyropharyngeus muscle overlying the lateral aspect of the larynx is sectioned. The broken circle indicates cricothyroid articulation.* © *RAS White.*

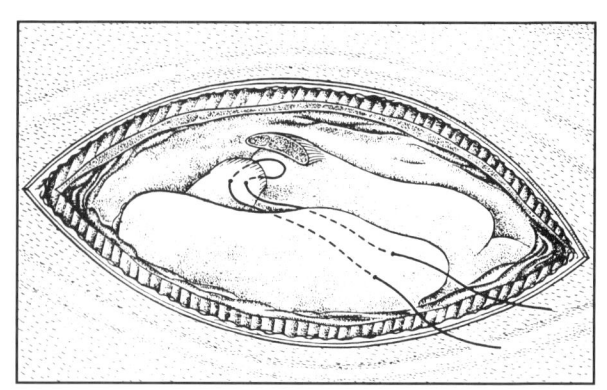

Figure 25.3: *Arytenoid lateralization: the arytenoid is separated from its articular attachments to the cricoid cartilage. The arytenoid is then anchored by means of a mattress pattern suture to the caudal cornu of the thyroid cartilage.* © *RAS White.*

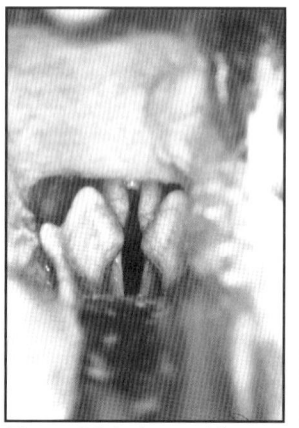
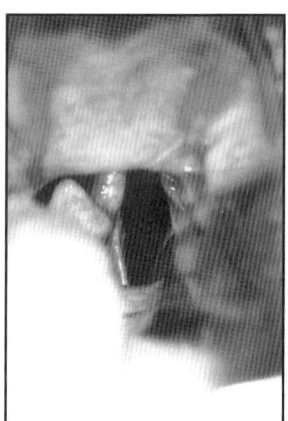

Figure 25.4: *Arytenoid lateralization: glottic inspection before surgery.*

Figure 25.5: *Arytenoid lateralization: glottic inspection after surgery.*

The arytenoid is now anchored in abduction by means of a suture prosthesis. A non-absorbable suture material is essential, since this will be required to retain the abducted arytenoid permanently. Materials such as polypropylene or monofilament nylon are most suitable, since stainless steel even when coated may tear through a more delicate cartilage. A swaged-on needle is used to introduce the suture through the thyroid cartilage immediately rostral to the caudal cornu. The needle is passed through the lateral aspect of the arytenoid, emerging in the centre of its articular face and is then passed back through this surface from a more medial point. The mattress pattern is completed by passing the suture through the medial face of the thyroid cartilage in the region of, but not immediately adjacent to, the original bite (Figure 25.3). The suture is now tied firmly but without overtensioning, since this may cause it to 'cheese wire' through the cartilages. The degree of arytenoid abduction can be inspected at this stage by temporarily removing the endotracheal tube. The thyropharyngeus muscle is closed routinely with absorbable sutures over the thyroid cartilage, and the potential dead space overlying the larynx is obliterated by meticulous closure of the various layers of overlying soft tissues. If not previously inspected, the larynx should be evaluated at this stage before the patient recovers consciousness to confirm that there is satisfac-

tory dilation of the rima (Figures 25.4 and 25.5). Any blood which may have accumulated in the laryngeal lumen, should the mucosa have been perforated during the procedure, should also be removed by suction.

Modifications of the above technique include the following:

- Bilateral arytenoid lateralization can be performed by repeating the above technique contralaterally with the patient in left-sided recumbency (Burbidge *et al.*, 1993). This has been recommended for younger, working dogs in which there may be a need for more glottic dilation to accommodate their greater exercise requirements (Rosin and Greenwood, 1982; Burbidge *et al.*, 1993). Bilateral surgery is reported to be associated with a higher incidence of postoperative dysphagia and aspiration
- A ventral approach has been described with the patient positioned in dorsal recumbency (Rosin and Greenwood, 1982) to permit bilateral surgery. Access to each arytenoid is achieved by rotating the larynx laterally about its longitudinal axis and is restricted compared with that achieved by the lateral approach

- Disarticulation of the cricothyroid junction is an optional step to allow further retraction of the thyroid cartilage and exposure of the cricoid and arytenoid cartilages. Some bleeding may occur from small vessels in the region of the articulation and it is important that this should be dealt with by careful diathermic cautery. Although omitting this step restricts access to the arytenoid cartilage, it shortens the operative time somewhat and may result in a more stable base to which the lateralizing prosthesis can be anchored. Bilateral disarticulation of the cricothyroid joint is reported to result in dorsoventral collapse of the rima (Lozier and Pope, 1992)
- Studies in post-mortem specimens (Lozier and Pope, 1992) suggest that sectioning the inter-arytenoid band with cricoarytenoid disarticulation allows greater dilation of the rima glottidis. The use of the cricoid rather than the thyroid cartilage for anchoring the prosthetic suture has been suggested as providing greater dilation of the rima (Lussier et al., 1996). It should be emphasized, however, that neither of these assertions has been supported by clinical studies.

Preoperative workup should include:

- Routine haematological and biochemical investigations, since almost all patients will be geriatric
- Thoracic radiographs to rule out co-existing pulmonary disease (e.g. primary neoplastic masses, aspiration pneumonia)
- Investigation of any dysphagic signs.

Postoperative care should include:

- A brief period of hospitalization to permit observation of the patient for any signs of respiratory distress. In most cases, this should be no more than 24 hours and patients should be discharged with instructions for limited exercise and permanent avoidance of collar use
- Perioperative antibiotic therapy, since there is potential for minor disruption of the laryngeal mucosa and perforation of the airway mucosa. Antibiotic therapy may be extended postoperatively if any risk of aspiration is perceived.

Complications of arytenoid lateralization include the following:

- Fragmentation of the arytenoid or thyroid may occur during the procedure if either cartilage is handled too vigorously or the prosthetic suture is repeatedly placed through the cartilage (Lane, 1982; White, 1989). In the event of this complication, the procedure should be repeated contralaterally
- Oedema may develop within the first 24–48 hours postoperatively in the perilaryngeal tissues causing obstruction of the rima and severe respiratory distress. Corticosteroids may be employed following a prolonged dissection to pre-empt this complication which may otherwise necessitate temporary tracheostomy intubation. The development of a seroma or haematoma is a similar possibility which may also necessitate airway bypass in severe cases
- Prosthetic avulsion is occasionally encountered in the immediate postoperative period and is normally due to the inclusion of an inadequate cartilage 'anchor' within the suture. Much less commonly, it may be seen as a chronic development several weeks or even months after surgery. A repeat, contralateral procedure is a feasible solution in cases in which a unilateral procedure has been performed
- Aspiration is in theory, at least, a complication of all procedures which leave the rima permanently dilated. Although this may appear as a potential problem after arytenoid lateralization, workers have reported no increase in the incidence of this problem after the unilateral procedure (White, 1989). There appears, however, to be more risk of dysphagia and aspiration following the bilateral surgery (Burbidge et al., 1993). Providing that the other glottic protection mechanisms (i.e. epiglottic movement, lateral food channels) remain functional after surgery the risk of aspiration after unilateral procedures should be acceptably low.

Prognosis
The long-term results of unilateral lateralization for older dogs with ILP are very favourable indeed, with rapid return to previous exercise function (Lane, 1982; Love et al., 1987; LaHue, 1989). In one long-term study of the results of unilateral lateralization, more than 90% of dogs were alive 1 year postoperatively and had little discernible stridor or exercise intolerance due to respiratory dysfunction (White, 1989). The technique can be applied to all sizes of dog and is also feasible in the cat (White et al., 1986; White, 1994).

Laryngeal re-innervation
Re-innervation of the larynx by both neuromuscular pedicle grafting (Greenfield et al., 1988) and nerve anastomosis (Rice, 1982) has been reported in dogs. Experimental studies with artificially created laryngeal paralysis have shown that the dorsal cricoarytenoid muscle can be re-innervated by transplanting a neuromuscular pedicle innervated by the first cervical

nerve (Rice, 1982). Dogs regained abductor function over periods of 9–11 months. The sternothyroid muscle was selected for the graft, since it is:

- Not innervated by the recurrent laryngeal nerve
- An inspiratory muscle and therefore provides synchronous abduction of the rima
- Has a nerve supply long enough to allow transplantation without undue tension on the graft.

A number of practical problems complicate this otherwise encouraging approach. Firstly, re-innervation has only been demonstrated in recently denervated (i.e. nerve-sectioned) muscle, and whilst this may be feasible for traumatic injuries of the laryngeal nerve, it may not be effective in chronic neuropathies such as ILP. Secondly, re-innervation of the intrinsic laryngeal muscles is indiscriminate such that simultaneous contraction of both abductors and adductors (synkinesis) may occur, resulting in uncoordinated movement of the arytenoids. Finally, the long interval between surgery and the clinical result represents an unacceptable delay in the management of the older dog with severe airway obstruction. Microsurgical repair of the caudal laryngeal nerve may be feasible in some instances, but this only has application for traumatic lesions (Rice, 1982).

Intralaryngeal procedures

Procedures which necessitate surgery within the lumen of the larynx are characterized by a number of significant intra- and postoperative considerations. These include the following:

- Endotracheal intubation is precluded during the procedure and hence maintenance of general anaesthesia dictates either placement of a temporary tracheostomy tube or continuous infusion of an intravenous agent
- Blood or tissue debris from the surgical site may be aspirated into the lower respiratory tract. The risk of aspiration during the procedure is further increased in the absence of endotracheal intubation
- The tracheostomy tube should be maintained *in situ* beyond the postoperative period to bypass any upper airway obstruction resulting from intralaryngeal oedema
- The surgical disruption or removal of the laryngeal mucosa is occasionally associated with intralaryngeal scarring or so-called 'webbing' which may severely stenose the airway at the level of the rima.

All of the above considerations should be examined carefully before selecting any intralaryngeal procedure. *It should be emphasized that a description of the* *intralaryngeal procedures is included here for the sake of completeness rather than the author's confidence in their suitability or efficacy in the management of laryngeal paralysis.*

Partial laryngectomy

Resection of the vocal folds, or ventriculocordectomy, is perhaps the oldest approach to creating a permanently enlarged rima (Harvey and Venker-van Haagen, 1975; Harvey and O'Brien, 1982). Several options exist, including resection of one or both folds, and combination of this with partial arytenoidectomy (i.e. removal of part of one or both arytenoid cartilages). Following the induction of anaesthesia, a mid-cervical, transverse tracheotomy is performed to permit gaseous anaesthesia via an endotracheal tube or cuffed tracheostomy tube (Harvey and Venker-van Haagen, 1975; Holt and Harvey, 1994a; Trout *et al.*, 1994). Conventional laryngeal intubation with intermittent withdrawal of the endotracheal tube from the anaesthetized patient to allow access to the surgical site is an alternative, but less desirable option for maintenance of anaesthesia. The dog is positioned in sternal recumbency with the mouth held open by means of a gag. The rima is visualized by simultaneous rostral retraction of the soft palate and ventral depression of the tongue and epiglottis.

Ventriculocordectomy

This is performed by grasping the vocal fold with long dissecting forceps and tensing it rostrally. Beginning at its attachment to the vocal process of the arytenoid the vocal fold and adjacent vocalis muscle are then resected (Figure 25.6) using either fine Metzenbaum scissors (Holt and Harvey, 1994a) or crocodile-action cup biting forceps (Harvey and O'Brien, 1982; Harvey, 1983a), the latter allowing for piecemeal removal of the fold. The procedure is repeated bilaterally. A small section of mucosa is left at the ventral commissure of the rima between the resected folds and is said to reduce the risk of postoperative intralaryngeal scarring (Harvey, 1983a).

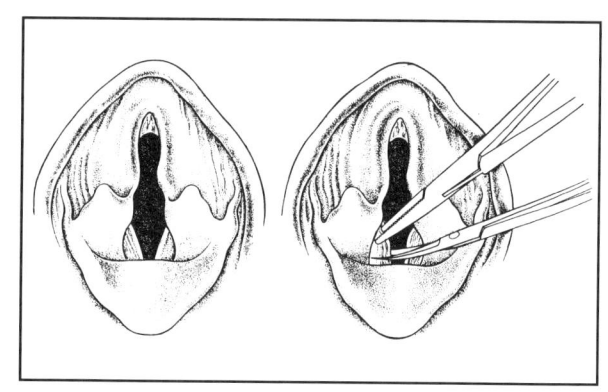

Figure 25.6: Ventriculocordectomy: the vocal folds are grasped and resected, leaving a small area of fold mucosa ventrally. © RAS White.

Partial arytenoidectomy

Arytenoid resection is performed in conjunction with ventriculocordectomy as described above. Cup forceps are then used to resect additional arytenoid cartilage (Harvey and Venker-van Haagen, 1975; Greenfield, 1987; Harvey, 1983a,b; Trout *et al.*, 1994). Opinion is divided as to how much of the cartilage should be removed in order to achieve the desired improvement in airway function. Previously, it has been customary to remove corniculate, cuneiform and vocal processes (Harvey and Venker-van Haagen, 1975; Harvey, 1983a,b), but more recent reports indicate that the incidence of postoperative complications, notably aspiration pneumonia, may be reduced by removal of only the corniculate process (Trout *et al.*, 1994). The procedure is performed unilaterally and the decision as to which side should be operated on is based on preoperative laryngoscopic examination in the case of unilateral paralysis.

Haemorrhage after partial laryngectomy procedures is controlled by direct pressure using a small dental sponge on the excision sites. Any blood clots or mucus which accumulate in the airway should be meticulously suctioned following the completion of surgery. The tracheostomy tube is maintained postoperatively and periodically occluded over the next 48 hours to ascertain at what point it may be safely removed. Antibiotic therapy should be maintained for several days after surgery to reduce the risk of pneumonia resulting from the aspiration of any debris (Harvey, 1983a; Holt and Harvey, 1994a; Trout *et al.*, 1994).

Complications of partial laryngectomy include the following:

- Aspiration pneumonia has been reported as a frequent and potentially fatal postoperative complication of vocal fold resection and partial arytenoidectomy (Harvey and O'Brien, 1982; Ross *et al.*, 1991). Recent reports suggest that bilateral vocal fold resection alone or alternatively, the use of an inflatable tracheostomy tube during surgery may result in a significant reduction in the incidence of this problem (Holt and Harvey, 1994a; Trout *et al.*, 1994)
- Glottic stenosis (Figure 25.7) may be encountered as a longer-term problem due to scarring ventrally of the site of the excised vocal folds (Harvey and Venker-van Haagen, 1975; Lane, 1982; Peterson *et al.*, 1991; Holt and Harvey, 1994a,b). The so-called 'webbing' granulation tissue may prove difficult to manage and may recur after resection (Matushek and Bjorling, 1988; Peterson *et al.*, 1992). Other techniques include lining the site with mucosal flaps (Matushek and Bjorling, 1988) or the use of a ventral silicone stent to dilate the rima (Peterson *et al.*, 1991). The tapering of doses of prednisolone following surgical resection has been reported as providing good results (Holt and Harvey, 1994b)

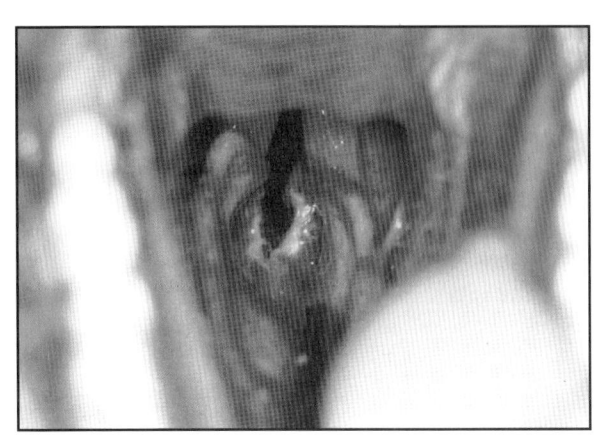

Figure 25.7: Glottic stenosis due to the development of scar tissue following ventriculocordectomy.

- Oedema may develop within the larynx at the resection sites (Greenfield and Dye, 1993), necessitating temporary tracheostomy. The perioperative use of dexamethasone sodium phosphate (0.25–1.0 mg/kg i.v.) or methylprednisolone sodium succinate (0.5–2.0 mg/kg i.v.) may reduce the incidence of this problem which otherwise prolongs the postoperative tracheostomy period.

Castellated laryngofissure

Ventral bisection and separation of the thyroid cartilage has been described as an alternative concept for glottic dilation (Gourley *et al.*, 1983). The technique as originally described for the dog was a modification of a procedure for the management of cricoid collapse in humans and involved the creation of a series of step-like incisions through the base of the thyroid cartilage (Figure 25.8a) following tracheotomy intubation. The castellated thyroid projections allow the two halves of the cartilage to be abducted ventrally thereby dilating the rima (Figure 25.8b). The basihyoid bone is then used to anchor the unstable thyroid fragments (Figure 25.8c). This technique is combined with bilateral ventriculocordectomy and consequently has many of the problems associated with intralaryngeal manipulation. There has been only one long-term study of the results of castellated laryngofissure (Gourley *et al.*, 1983).

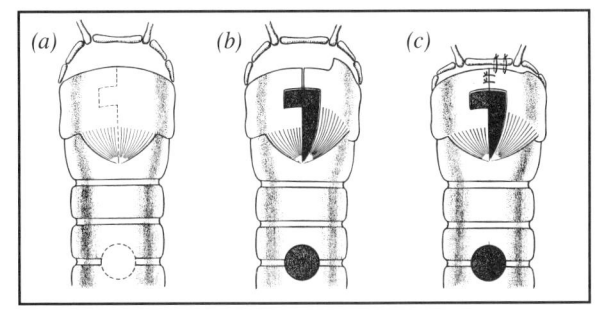

Figure 25.8: Castellated laryngofissure. (a) Step 1: a step-like incision is made through the ventral aspect of the thyroid cartilage and cricothyroid ligament. (b) Step 2: the hemithyroid is advanced unilaterally. (c) Step 3: the advanced hemithyroid is anchored to the basihyoid bone. © RAS White.

Modified castellated laryngofissure

The subsequent modification of the castellated laryngo-fissure procedure to include bilateral arytenoid lateralization (Smith *et al.*, 1986) underlined the unsatisfactory results achieved by the original procedure. There must be doubts too as to the rationale for the modified procedure, since it is clear that arytenoid lateralization alone is extremely successful in alleviating the signs of laryngeal paralysis (Lane, 1982; LaHue, 1989; White, 1989; Burbidge *et al.*, 1993) and there are few reports of the clinical use of modified castellated laryngofissure (Burbidge *et al.*, 1991).

LARYNGEAL EVERSION/COLLAPSE SYNDROME

Conservative management

In many dogs, laryngeal eversion/collapse is a progressive process and hence early detection and management of the underlying disease is essential to limit the ultimate extent of the condition. Upper airway obstruction in brachycephalic dogs should be relieved at an early age by lateralizing the nares, shortening the soft palate and resecting hyperplastic tonsils or redundant pharyngeal mucosal folds (Harvey, 1982a,b; Lane, 1982; Orsher, 1993). This may relieve the turbulence and abnormal airway pressures sufficiently to permit remission of the earliest changes within the larynx (i.e. mucosal oedema and eversion of the saccules) without additional management. For this reason, it is essential that every effort should be made to correct the underlying pathology before any surgical intervention involving the larynx itself is undertaken. The judicious use of steroidal, anti-inflammatory drugs may be helpful in promoting resolution of the laryngeal changes after upper airway surgery.

Resection of laryngeal saccules

In cases where the laryngeal changes are limited to chronic eversion of the saccules which does not respond to conservative management, resection of the everted tissue may be performed. The patient is prepared for surgery as for partial laryngectomy (see above) and positioned in sternal recumbency. The everted saccules are identified as small, red pea-like protrusions immediately behind the vocal folds and grasped with dissecting forceps. The saccules are resected through their base with fine scissors, and haemorrhage is controlled by direct pressure over the site (Harvey 1982a; Lane, 1982; Matushek and Bjorling, 1988; Lussier *et al.*, 1996) As is the case for laryngectomy procedures, the risk of postoperative aspiration may be reduced by temporary tracheostomy intubation.

Partial laryngectomy

Resection of the vocal folds and arytenoids has been used in the management of LECS (Harvey, 1982b;

Lane, 1982). The long-term results, however, are poor due to significant postoperative complications and the need for repeated surgeries to maintain the airway. Major intralaryngeal resection is therefore no longer recommended in the management of laryngeal collapse.

Permanent tracheostomy

Permanent tracheostomy is effective in the management of many advanced cases of laryngeal collapse, since not only does it provide immediate upper airway bypass, but it also relieves the abnormal airway pressures responsible for the degenerative changes involving the larynx. Permanent tracheostomies should be managed by careful cleaning during the initial 2–3 weeks when tenacious tracheal secretions may tend to occlude the opening. Thereafter, once-daily cleaning is sufficient to maintain its patency. Long-term problems include skin fold obstruction and stenosis of the stoma (Hedlund *et al.*, 1988).

Tracheostomy must be regarded as a salvage procedure and the long-term prognosis for dogs with advanced laryngeal collapse is very guarded. Techniques such as arytenoid lateralization, designed to alleviate the signs of laryngeal paralysis by enlarging the rima, are notoriously ineffective in the management of LECS, since the rigid cartilage 'chassis' essential for the success of the procedure is no longer present.

LARYNGEAL TRAUMA

Animals presented with airway obstruction due to laryngeal trauma frequently require prompt tracheostomy intubation to enable an airway to be maintained pending a more detailed evaluation of the larynx under general anaesthesia. Laryngeal trauma resulting from both compressive injuries and penetrating wounds is prone to perilaryngeal oedema and bruising. Early surgical intervention may exacerbate this and immediate management should, therefore, be limited to the control of any haemorrhage, debridement of non-viable tissue obstructing the airway and tracheostomy. In the case of penetrating wounds involving the perilaryngeal tissues, provision should be made for drainage and the removal of any residual foreign material (White and Lane, 1988). Anti-inflammatory and antibiotic therapy should be maintained with upper airway bypass until the oedema resolves, normally 3–5 days, at which time mucosal tears can be further debrided and repaired. Dislocations of the arytenoid cartilages or hyoid bones should also be corrected where possible at this time. Laryngeal function may be more meaningfully evaluated at this point, since laryngeal neuropraxia and paralysis are impossible to differentiate in the initial phases of the injury. In cases where laryngeal dysfunction is still evident, it is more practical to assume permanent paralysis and perform lateralizing surgery (see above) than to continue to manage the patient in the expectation of possible return of function. Injuries resulting in fibrosis around the arytenoid cartilages may result in the development of glottic stenosis in the longer term and management of this condition by lateralization may prove difficult. In such cases, there may be little alternative but to consider an intralaryngeal intervention or permanent tracheostomy.

Glottic stenosis due to intralaryngeal 'webbing' is a possible long-term complication of trauma and may be managed as previously described. The prognosis is guarded for return to normal laryngeal function in such cases.

LARYNGEAL NEOPLASIA

Few laryngeal tumours present as candidates for definitive surgical excision. The single exception to this is the oncocytoma (Figure 25.9), which is usually found as a discrete mass underlying the laryngeal mucosa (Wheeldon, 1982). The mass can often be removed by careful submucosal dissection from its position within the larynx, where it obstructs the rima.

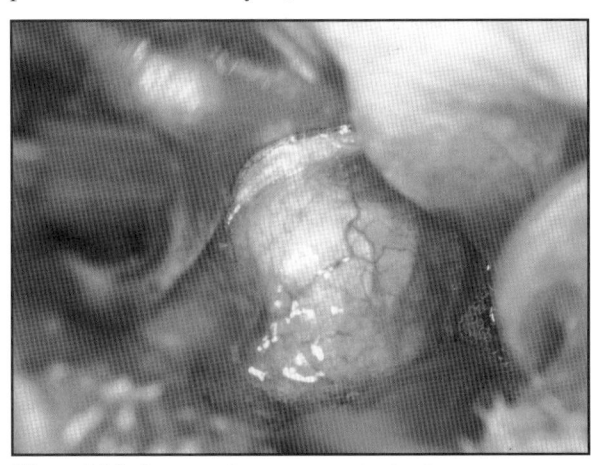

Figure 25.9: Laryngeal oncocytoma in the dog.

Ventral laryngotomy

Some benign tumours, and occasionally polyps, found within the larynx are less easily accessed via the rima and are better approached through a ventral laryngotomy wound. The patient is positioned in dorsal recumbency and the airway is maintained by either a narrow diameter endotracheal tube or temporary tracheostomy intubation during the procedure.

An incision is made through the cricothyroid ligament and continued forward through the ventral 'keel' of the thyroid cartilage. The two halves of the cartilage are separated by means of retractors to permit access to the mass and other intralaryngeal structures. The thyroid is repaired with simple interrupted sutures in its ventral aspect taking care to achieve accurate apposition and stability. The cricothryoid membrane is repaired in a continuous pattern to ensure an airtight seal.

Laryngectomy

Malignant laryngeal tumours (carcinomas, adenocarcinomas etc.) do not lend themselves to dissection from the larynx because of their tendency to local infiltration and their advanced stage at the time of detection. A variety of fanciful techniques for their management by partial laryngectomy have been described (Nelson, 1993), but are derived from human surgical literature and significantly, there are no long-term reports of their successful application in small animals. Laryngectomy combined with permanent total tracheostomy is, in theory, an option. The dearth of reports of the long-term results of its use in the management of canine tumours (Crowe *et al.*, 1986) should probably be regarded as an indication of its lack of success and suitability. Experience with this procedure in 10 dogs with malignant laryngeal tumours shows that the complication rate is high and few dogs go on to enjoy a normal quality of life for periods of more than 3 months after the surgery (White, RAS, unpublished data).

Megavoltage radiation therapy using twin oblique portals to spare the adjacent spinal tissue is commonly used in the treatment of laryngeal malignancy in humans. There are no reports in the veterinary literature of the routine use of radiation in this mode although it is certainly a viable possibility. Cytotoxic therapy is indicated in the management of lymphoma of the larynx in the cat and may achieve dramatic resolution of the clinical signs. The value of chemotherapy for other histological types is unknown.

The prognosis following surgical excision of the oncocytoma is guardedly good. Its growth is normally slow and does not appear to metastasize, although local recurrence over periods of many months or years is possible. Palliation of feline lymphomas is normally short-lived and the outlook for most malignant laryngeal tumours is poor. Since the overriding determinant is airway function, euthanasia is often sought by owners at an early stage in the disease.

REFERENCES AND FURTHER READING

Burbidge HM, Goulden BE and Jones BR (1991) An experimental evaluation of castellated laryngofissure and bilateral arytenoid lateralisation for the relief of laryngeal paralysis in dogs. *Australian Veterinary Journal* **68**, 268-272

Burbidge HM, Goulden BE and Jones BR (1993) Laryngeal paralysis in dogs: an evaluation of the bilateral arytenoid lateralisation procedure. *Journal of Small Animal Practice* **34**, 515-519

Cook WR (1964) Observations on the upper respiratory tract of the dog and cat. *Journal of Small Animal Practice* **5**, 309-329

Crowe DT *et al.* (1986) Total laryngectomy for laryngeal mast cell tumor in a dog. *Journal of the American Animal Hospital Association* **22**, 809-816

Gaber CE, Amis TC and LeCouteur A (1985) Laryngeal paralysis in dogs: a review of 23 cases. *Journal of the American Veterinary Medical Association* **186**, 377-380

Gourley VM, Paul M and Gregory C (1983) Castellated laryngofissure and vocal fold resection for the treatment of laryngeal paralysis in the dog. *Journal of the American Veterinary Medical Association* **182**, 1084-1086

Greenfield CL (1987) Canine laryngeal paralysis. *The Compendium of Continuing Education for the Practising Veterinarian* **9**, 1011-1020

Greenfield CL and Dye JA (1993) Laryngeal paralysis and collapse. In: *Disease Mechanisms in Small Animal Surgery*, ed. MJ Bojrab, pp. 371–375. Lea and Febiger, Philadelphia

Greenfield CL, Walshaw R, Kumber K *et al.* (1988) Neuromuscular pedicle graft for restoration of arytenoid abductor function in canine laryngeal hemiplegia. *American Journal of Veterinary Research* **49**, 1360–1366

Harvey CE (1982a) Upper airway obstruction. 3: Everted laryngeal saccule surgery in brachycephalic dogs. *Journal of the American Animal Hospital Association* **18**, 545–547

Harvey CE (1982b) Upper airway obstruction. 4: Partial laryngectomy in brachycephalic dogs. *Journal of the American Animal Hospital Association* **18**, 548–550

Harvey CE (1983a) Partial larygectomy in the dog. I. Healing and swallowing function in normal dogs. *Veterinary Surgery* **12**, 192–196

Harvey CE (1983b) Partial larygectomy in the dog. II. Immediate increase in glottic area obtained compared with other laryngeal procedures. *Veterinary Surgery* **12**, 197–201

Harvey CE and O'Brien JA (1982) Treatment of laryngeal paralysis in dogs by partial laryngectomy. *Journal of the American Animal Hospital Association* **18**, 551–556

Harvey CE and Venker-van Haagen AJ (1975) Surgical management of pharyngeal and laryngeal airway obstruction in the dog. *Veterinary Clinics of North America* **5**, 515–535

Hedlund CS, Tagner CH, Waldron DR and Hobson HP (1988) Permanent tracheostomy: perioperative and long-term data from 34 cases. *Journal of the American Animal Hospital Association* **24**, 585–591

Holt D and Harvey CE (1994a) Idiopathic laryngeal paralysis: results of treatment by bilateral vocal fold resection in 40 dogs. *Journal of the American Animal Hospital Association* **30**, 389–395

Holt D and Harvey CE (1994b) Glottic stenosis secondary to vocal fold resection: results of scar removal and corticosteroid treatment in nine dogs. *Journal of the American Animal Hospital Association* **30**, 396–400

LaHue TR (1989) Treatment of laryngeal paralysis in dogs by unilateral cricoarytenoid laryngoplasty. *Journal of the American Animal Hospital Association* **25**, 317–324

Lane JG (1982) Surgery of the conducting airways. In: *ENT and Oral Surgery of the Dog and Cat*, pp. 103–123. Wright PSG, Bristol

Love S, Waterman AE and Lane JG (1987) The assessment of corrective surgery for canine laryngeal paralysis by blood gas analysis: a review of thirty-five cases. *Journal of Small Animal Practice* **28**, 597–604

Lozier S and Pope E (1992) Effects of arytenoid abduction and modified castellated laryngofissure on the rima glottis in canine cadavers. *Veterinary Surgery* **21**, 195–200

Lussier B, Flanders JA and Erb HN (1996) The effect of unilateral arytenoid lateralization on rima glottidis area in canine cadaver larynges. *Veterinary Surgery* **25**, 121–126

Matushek KJ and Bjorling DE (1988) A mucosal flap technique for correction of laryngeal webbing. Results in four dogs. *Veterinary Surgery* **17**, 318–320

Nelson WA (1993) Upper respiratory system. In: *Textbook of Small Animal Surgery*, ed. D Slatter, pp. 773–776. WB Saunders, Philadelphia

Orsher RJ (1993) Brachycephalic airway disease. In: *Disease Mechanisms – Small Animal Surgery*, ed. MJ Bojrab, pp. 369–371. Lea and Febiger, Philadelphia

Peterson SW, Rosin E and Bjorling DE (1991) Surgical options for laryngeal paralysis in dogs: a consideration of partial laryngectomy. *Compendium of Continuing Education for the Practising Veterinarian* **13**, 1531–1539

Rice DH (1982) Laryngeal reinnervation. *Laryngoscope* **92**, 1049–1059

Rosin E and Greenwood K (1982) Bilateral arytenoid cartilage lateralisation for laryngeal paralysis in the dog. *Journal of the American Veterinary Association* **180**, 515–518

Ross JT, Matthiesen DT, Noone KE and Scavelli TA (1991) Complications and long-term results after partial laryngectomy for the treatment of idiopathic laryngeal paralysis in 45 dogs. *Veterinary Surgery* **20**, 169–173

Smith MM, Gourley IM, Kurpershoek CJ and Amis TC (1986) Evaluation of a modified castellated laryngofissure for alleviation of upper airway obstruction in dogs with laryngeal paralysis. *Journal of the American Veterinary Medical Association* **188**, 1279–1283

Trout NJ, Harpester NK, Berg J and Carpenter JC (1994) Long-term results of unilateral ventriculocordectomy and partial arytenoidectomy for the treatment of laryngeal paralysis in 60 dogs. *Journal of the American Animal Hospital Association* **30**, 401–407

Wheeldon ED (1982) Neoplasia of the larynx in the dog. *Journal of the American Veterinary Medical Association* **180**, 642–647

White RAS (1989) Unilateral arytenoid lateralisation: an assessment of technique and long term results in 62 dogs with laryngeal paralysis. *Journal of Small Animal Practice* **30**, 543–549

White RAS and Lane JG (1988) Pharyngeal stick penetration injuries in the dog. *Journal of Small Animal Practice* **28**, 13–25

White RAS, Littlewood JD, Herrtage ME *et al.* (1986) Outcome of surgery for laryngeal paralysis in four cats. *Veterinary Record* **118**, 103–104

White RN (1994) Unilateral arytenoid lateralisation for treatment of laryngeal paralysis in four cats. *Journal of Small Animal Practice* **35**, 455–458

Surgery of the Trachea and Bronchi

J. David Fowler

Surgery of the trachea and bronchi can be one of the most rewarding, or one of the most frustrating, endeavours taken on by the small animal surgeon. Numerous conditions, ranging from acute trauma, to degenerative diseases such as tracheal collapse, to foreign bodies and neoplasia may necessitate tracheal surgery.

The unique physiological function of the tracheobronchial tree poses challenges to the surgeon. It is obviously imperative that airway dynamics be maintained at all times, both during and following surgery. Thus surgery is quite often complicated by the presence of endotracheal tubes in the surgical field. Postoperative complications such as wound dehiscence, infection and wound contraction, which may be tolerated in other surgical settings, often pose a serious threat to the success of tracheal surgery. A knowledge of the specific anatomy and physiology of the trachea and bronchi is a prerequisite for a successful surgical outcome. The reader is referred to Chapter 1 for this information.

SURGICAL APPROACHES

Cervical trachea

The cervical trachea extends from the cricoid cartilage cranially to the thoracic inlet caudally. It is best approached through a ventral midline cervical incision with the animal in dorsal recumbency. Use of a bean bag or towel support dorsal to the neck will assist in exposure of the trachea.

Following incision of the skin and underlying platysma muscle extending from the larynx to the manubrium, the paired sternohyoideus and sternothyroideus muscles are separated. Caudal extension of the incision to the level of the manubrium requires sharp separation of the sternocephalicus muscles. Retraction of these muscles exposes the ventral aspect of the cervical trachea which is then easily dissected from surrounding loose connective tissue.

Several anatomical structures warrant consideration during surgical manipulation of the cervical trachea. The trachea receives a segmental blood supply which courses through paired lateral pedicles, and which originates from the cranial and caudal thyroid arteries. Complete disruption of the segmental vascular supply via dissection of both lateral pedicles has been associated with tracheal necrosis and should be avoided (Kirby *et al.*, 1991). More recent studies indicate that dissection of a single lateral pedicle does not result in transmural vascular disruption to the trachea (Coyne *et al.*, 1993).

The recurrent laryngeal nerves lie in close approximation to the trachea, and must be identified and avoided during surgical dissection. The left recurrent laryngeal nerve is variable in exact anatomical location, but is generally more closely associated with the trachea than is the right recurrent laryngeal nerve.

Other structures which pose fewer problems during tracheal mobilization, but which should be identified and avoided, include the paired thyroid glands, the oesophagus, the carotid arteries and vagosympathetic trunk.

Thoracic trachea and carina

The thoracic trachea and carina are approached through a right third intercostal thoracotomy. The animal is placed in left lateral recumbency, with the right foreleg tied forward. Skin and underlying cutaneous trunci muscle are incised from the costovertebral junction to the sternum. The latissimus dorsi muscle is dissected along its ventral border and retracted dorsally. Incision of the scalenus, serratus ventralis and intercostal muscles completes dissection of the thoracic wall.

Rib retractors are used to expose intrathoracic structures. The right cranial lung lobe is retracted dorsocaudally to remove it from the surgical field. The thoracic trachea is associated with the longus colli muscle dorsally, the oesophagus medially, and the cranial vena cava and vagosympathetic trunk ventrolaterally. The costocervical vein crosses the cranial thoracic trachea, whilst the azygos vein crosses the caudal thoracic trachea. Dissection and gentle retraction of these structures should allow adequate visualization of the thoracic trachea. Attention should be paid to the left recurrent laryngeal nerve, which is closely associated with the trachea, during medial dissection of the thoracic trachea. The costocervical vein may be ligated and transected if required for exposure of the cranial thoracic trachea, whilst the azygos vein may be ligated and transected for complete exposure of the tracheal bifurcation.

Tracheal wound healing

Ideal healing of a tracheal wound results in the re-establishment of normal tracheal mucociliary transport, tracheal flexibility and resistance to collapse, and minimal stenosis. Superficial wounds of tracheal mucosa which do not extend beyond the submucosal layer heal by migration, mitosis and differentiation of epithelial cells at the wound margin. Epithelium covers non-infected mucosal wounds within 24 hours of injury and differentiates into goblet and ciliated mucosal cells within 96 hours (Tangner and Hedlund, 1983). It is likely that many superficial mucosal wounds caused by endotracheal tube injury or tracheal foreign bodies are not clinically appreciated.

Deeper wounds which penetrate the submucosal layer heal by formation of granulation tissue and subsequent coverage by epithelium. The epithelium is often poorly differentiated, which may result in decreased mucociliary transport. Second intention healing invariably results in some degree of tracheal stenosis. In order to optimize wound healing and minimize stenosis, accurate apposition of tissue layers is critical. End-to-end anastomosis is generally recommended as the optimal method of tracheal reconstruction.

Excessive tension causes disruption of apposed tissues, scar formation and stenosis. It has been demonstrated that primary tracheal healing may occur in mature dogs, so long as tension on the suture line is not excessive. Stenosis is more likely to occur in puppies with moderate tension on the anastomosis. In practical terms, a greater amount of trachea may be safely resected in mature compared with immature dogs. The absolute number of tracheal rings which may be removed vary with the conformation of the dog and the elasticity of the trachea. Up to 60% of the trachea has been successfully resected in mature dogs (although this is certainly at the upper end of reasonable expectations), whilst the surgeon should not attempt resection of more than 25% of the trachea in puppies (Tangner and Hedlund, 1983).

Mucosal clearance is adversely affected by tracheal resection and anastomosis, especially in the absence of a normal cough reflex. Given successful primary healing of the tracheal defect, normal mucociliary clearance is expected to return within approximately 1 month of surgery.

GENERAL TECHNIQUES IN TRACHEAL SURGERY

Tracheal resection and anastomosis

Tracheal resection and anastomosis may be indicated for the management of congenital or acquired tracheal stenosis, trauma or neoplasia. During mobilization of the trachea, the surgeon should take care to dissect the lateral pedicles only over the area to be resected. This will ensure maintenance of an adequate segmental vascular supply to the cranial and caudal segments of the remaining trachea. Dissection of the lateral pedicles should be performed as close to the trachea as possible, taking care to preserve the recurrent laryngeal nerves.

Prior to resection of the diseased tracheal segment, retention sutures should be placed around the first cartilage ring, cranial and caudal to the segment to be resected. This prevents retraction of the tracheal segments and allows the surgeon to easily manipulate the tracheal ends. Three basic techniques of resection and anastomosis have been described (Lau *et al.*, 1980; Hedlund and Tangner, 1983) (see Figure 26.1). The

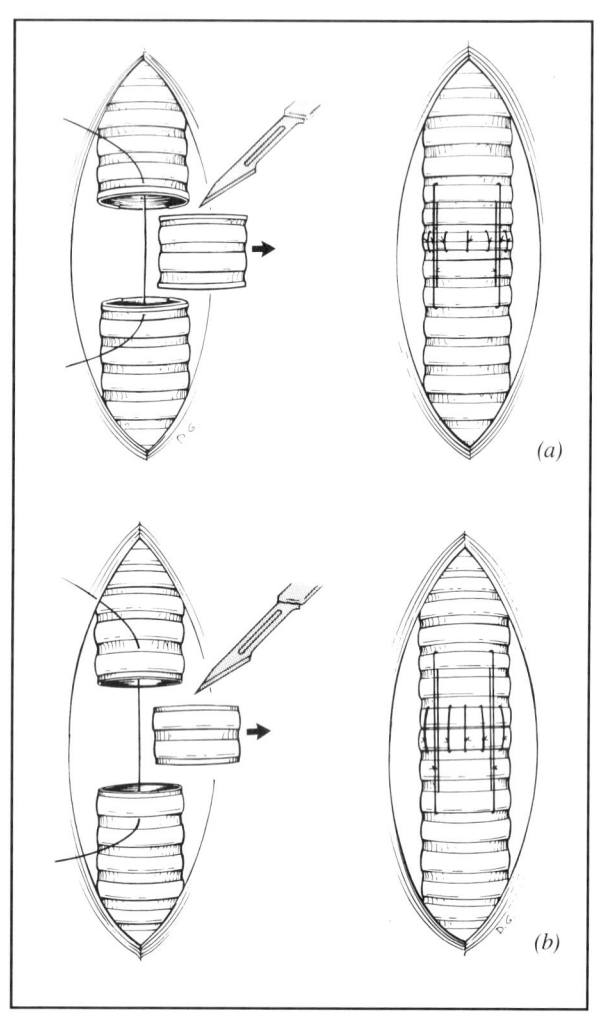

(a)

(b)

Figure 26.1: *(a) Diagrammatic representation of the split-cartilage technique for tracheal resection and anastomosis. Cartilage rings above and below the site of resection are split with a number 11 scalpel blade. Sutures are placed circumferentially around the split tracheal rings to provide apposition. Several retention sutures are placed around tracheal rings distant from the primary repair site to reduce tensile forces on the repair. (b) Diagrammatic representation of the annular ligament–cartilage technique. Division of the trachea is performed through the interannular ligament. Suture placement is identical to that described for the split-cartilage technique. Tissue apposition is less precise with this technique.*

specific technique to be used will depend largely on the preference of the surgeon and the size of the patient.

Simplified split-cartilage technique

A simplified split-cartilage technique is recommended in most situations. Following tracheal mobilization, the first cartilage ring above and below the segment to be resected is split with a number 11 scalpel blade. Tracheal repair is completed using simple interrupted, non-reactive monofilament sutures which encompass the split tracheal cartilages and penetrate mucosa; knots are tied extraluminally. Three to four retention sutures placed around the second tracheal ring above and below the anastomotic site are recommended to reduce tension on the repair site. The split tracheal cartilages heal via formation of fibrocartilage. This technique is generally accepted to result in less tracheal stenosis (0–24%) than other techniques of tracheal repair, but is not indicated in smaller animals, where the tracheal cartilages cannot be split without risk of fragmentation.

Annular ligament-cartilage technique

The annular ligament-cartilage technique is similar to the split-cartilage technique with the exception that initial tracheal resection is performed at the level of the interannular ligament. Subsequent suture placement is identical to that described for split-cartilage repair. Resultant tissue apposition is less accurate than in split-cartilage repair, with the cranial cartilage tending to override the caudal cartilage. Healing occurs by fibrous tissue formation. Stenosis may be more severe with the annular ligament-cartilage technique (0–45%). The annular ligament-cartilage technique is recommended for small dogs and cats.

Interannular technique

The interannular technique involves resection at the level of the interannular ligament. As much of the interannular ligament as possible is preserved in the resection. Repair is accomplished by placement of simple interrupted, non-reactive monofilament sutures through the preserved interannular ligament of the cranial and caudal tracheal segments. These sutures penetrate tracheal mucosa and knots are tied extraluminally. Retention sutures are utilized as described in previous techniques. Stenosis resulting from this technique has been reported in between 13 and 47% of cases. Tissue pull-out of sutures may be of more concern with this technique. Due to the increased technical difficulty of performing this technique, and very few reported advantages, the interannular ligament technique is not generally recommended for tracheal repair.

Following completion of tracheal anastomosis, the endotracheal tube should be withdrawn into the cranial segment. The trachea is then covered with sterile irrigating solution and the animal ventilated under moderate

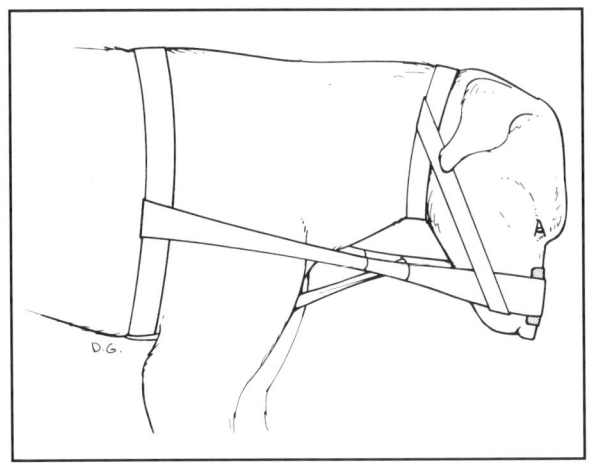

Figure 26.2: *A Martingale-type tape splint may be used for 2–3 weeks after tracheal repair to reduce movement and tension on the repair. This splint maintains the animal's head and neck in a flexed position.*

pressure. This will allow identification and repair of areas of air leakage. A Martingale-type tape splint may be applied postoperatively for 2–3 weeks to maintain the animal's neck in a flexed position and reduce tensile forces on the tracheal repair (see Figure 26.2).

Temporary tracheostomy

Temporary tracheostomies are indicated for short-term maintenance of a patent airway, usually in animals with significant airway obstruction at the level of the pharynx or larynx. In emergency situations, temporary tracheostomies may be performed under sedation and local anaesthesia, but general anaesthesia is recommended whenever possible.

Several types of temporary tracheostomy tubes are available for use. Most can be re-used following ethylene oxide sterilization. Tubes may be cuffed or non-cuffed. The tracheostomy tube should be flexible and minimally irritating to tissues. The author recommends the use of tubes containing an inner cannula which facilitates removal of tracheal secretions. The tracheostomy tube is maintained with the inner cannula in place. As tracheal secretions accumulate in the tube, the inner cannula is removed and cleansed (see Figure 26.3).

Temporary tracheostomy tubes are placed at the level of the second and third, third and fourth, or fourth and fifth tracheal rings. Numerous tracheal incision techniques have been described for tube placement, including U-shaped incisions, transverse interannular incisions, vertical incisions through two or more tracheal cartilages, or excision of portions of one or more tracheal cartilages. It appears that the specific incisional technique employed does not greatly affect postoperative tracheal stenosis. The author generally uses a transverse interannular incision between the third and fourth tracheal cartilages. The incision should extend less than 50% of the tracheal circumference in order to minimize postoperative stenosis. Placement of reten-

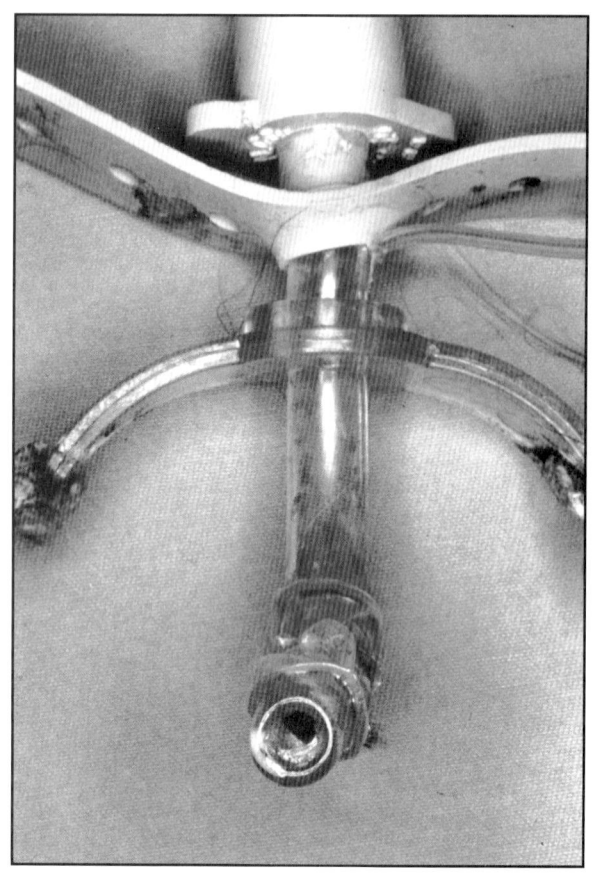

Figure 26.3: Tracheal secretions have accumulated in the end of this recently removed temporary tracheostomy tube. Frequent cleansing and suction of temporary tracheostomy tubes are required to prevent obstruction with tracheal secretions.

tion sutures around the tracheal cartilage above and below the tracheostomy site facilitates manipulation of the trachea and introduction of the tracheostomy tube.

The diameter of the temporary tracheostomy tube should be approximately 50-70% the diameter of the trachea. This will allow the animal to breathe around the tube if required. Following placement the tracheostomy tube is secured with sutures or gauze fixed to the tube and tied around the animal's neck.

Postoperative management of temporary tracheostomy tubes is critical. Obstruction of the tube with tracheal secretions may result in acute ventilatory compromise and death of the patient. Animals with tracheostomy tubes should therefore be monitored on a continuous basis. Management and removal of tracheal secretions is of paramount importance. Use of a cold water humidifier in the animal's cage helps to decrease the viscosity of tracheal secretions. The inner cannula of double cannulated tubes should be removed and cleansed initially every 15-30 minutes, and then at 1 hour intervals or as required during prolonged intubation. The trachea should be gently suctioned with a non-irritating suction catheter at this time. Instillation of 5-10 ml of sterile saline through the tracheostomy site several minutes prior to suctioning will help loosen tracheal secretions and facilitate their removal. Tra-

cheostomy tubes should be removed as soon as feasible. It is difficult to maintain temporary tracheostomy tubes for longer than a few days. Permanent tracheostomy techniques are indicated when longer periods of upper airway bypass are required.

Permanent tracheostomy

Permanent tracheostomy is indicated in instances where prolonged bypass of the upper airway is required. Laryngeal or upper cervical tracheal excision, pharyngeal or laryngeal radiation therapy and laryngeal collapse are examples.

Following retraction of the sternohyoideus muscles, an elliptical or rectangular segment is excised from the ventral trachea. The excised segment should be two to four tracheal rings in length, approximately one-third the diameter of the trachea and centred at the third to fifth tracheal ring. Although difficult to accomplish, it is advisable meticulously to incise through the tracheal cartilages preserving the integrity of the underlying mucosa. Blunt submucosal elevation of the segment to be excised may then be attempted.

The trachea is brought into apposition with the skin first, by suturing the sternohyoideus muscles dorsal to the trachea with several horizontal mattress sutures. A skin segment is excised to match the tracheal defect. Dermis is sutured to tracheal fascia surrounding the tracheostomy site using 2.0 or 1.5 non-reactive absorbable suture material. The tracheal mucosa is then incised and sutured to skin edges in a simple interrupted or simple continuous pattern (see Figure 26.4).

Animals with loose cervical skin folds may prove somewhat problematic. Fixation of the skin at the level of the stoma site often results in skin folds overlying the tracheostomy site once the animal recovers from anaesthesia and resumes an upright posture and movement of the head and neck. Excision of redundant skin folds is sometimes required as an adjunct procedure in these instances.

Management of the permanent tracheostomy site involves gentle cleansing with warm water or saline to remove accumulated tracheal secretions. The tracheostomy site may require cleaning as little as once daily or as often as hourly, depending on the amount of secretions present. Care should be taken not to disrupt the incision line while cleaning the stoma. Mucosal epithelium adapts rapidly to the decrease in humidity and temperature. After 2 weeks, the stoma generally requires minimal care.

It is important to warn owners that permanent tracheostomy may increase the possibility of aspiration of foreign bodies and water. Dogs with permanent tracheostomy must not be allowed to swim, and appropriate care should be taken during bathing to avoid submersion of the tracheostomy site. Animals with permanent tracheostomy may have an increased incidence of irritant tracheobronchial disease, but infec-

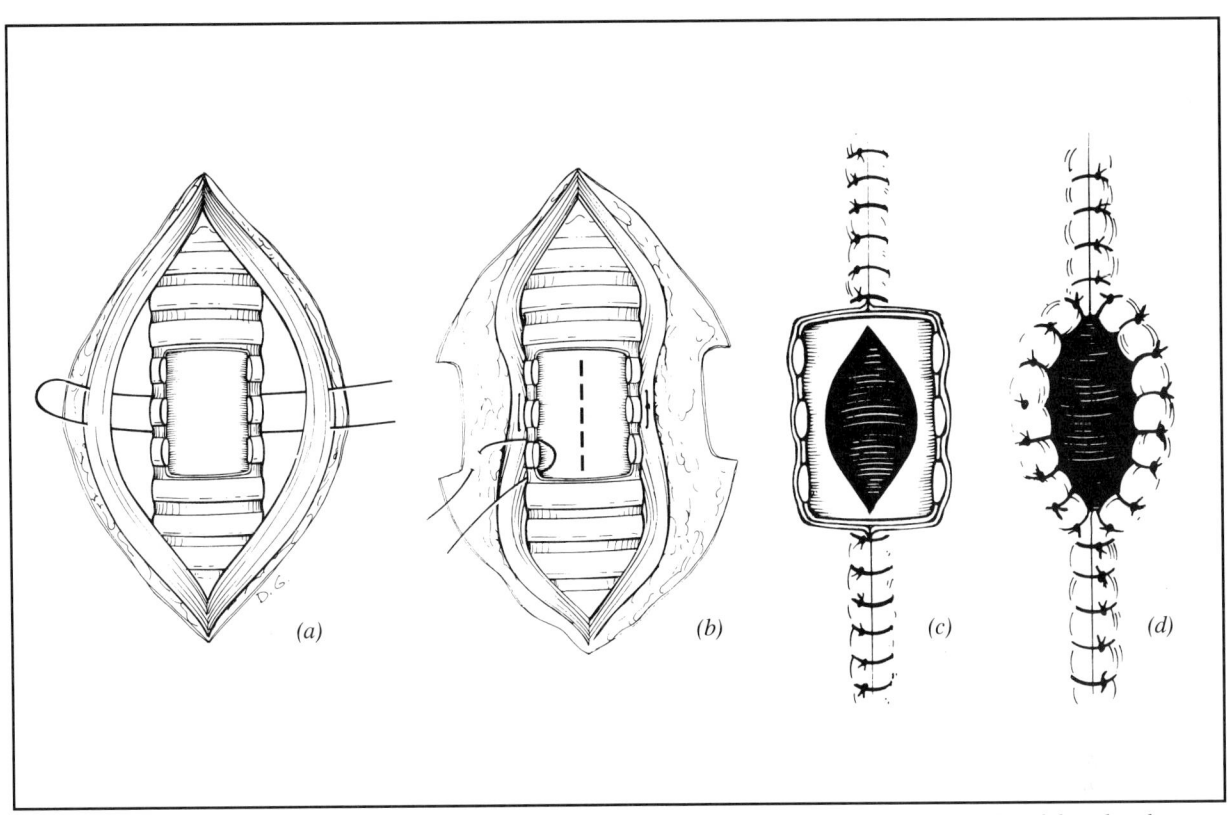

Figure 26.4: (a) Diagrammatic representation of permanent tracheostomy. A mattress suture has been placed dorsal to the trachea in the retracted sternohyoideus muscles. A rectangular resection of three tracheal cartilages has been performed, preserving the underlying tracheal mucosa. (b) A skin segment has been excised to match the tracheal defect. Trachea is sutured to overlying dermis to provide general apposition. (c) The tracheal mucosa has been incised longitudinally and skin edges have been apposed above and below the tracheostomy site. (d) Tracheal mucosa is sutured to skin edges using non-reactive 1.5 or 2.0 size suture.

tion of the respiratory tract has not been reported as a problem in normal dogs undergoing permanent tracheostomy.

Tracheal replacement

Techniques for total replacement of tracheal segments are largely experimental. A replacement technique with a suitably low complication rate remains to be defined. Several composite grafts consisting of biological and synthetic materials have been evaluated for tracheal replacement. One study utilized a prosthesis consisting of fine Marlex mesh with a continuous Teflon spiral which was covered with a graft of porcine collagen (Okumura *et al.*, 1993). This material was used for reconstruction of the cervical trachea. Although autogenous tissues were incorporated successfully into the graft, tracheal stenosis was a frequent complication. Autogenous skin or pericardium layered with hydroxyapatite rings and an omental pedicle flap were used for thoracic tracheal reconstruction in another study (Oizuma, 1993). Displacement of the hydroxyapatite rings, ventilatory insufficiency and tracheal stenosis were major complications. Microvascular transplantation of tracheal carinal allografts has recently been assessed (Ueda and Shirakusa, 1992). Although complications were frequent, successful outcomes were reported for up to 6 months with immunosuppressive therapy.

SPECIFIC SURGICAL DISEASES OF THE TRACHEA

Tracheal collapse

Tracheal collapse was first described in dogs in the 1940s. The reader is referred to Chapter 16 for descriptions of the pathophysiology and diagnosis of tracheal collapse in dogs.

Indications for surgical treatment

Indications and techniques for surgical treatment of tracheal collapse remain controversial. Advanced disease is often associated with a debilitated patient, and increased risk of anaesthetic and surgical complications. However, many animals with mild to moderate clinical signs may be adequately managed conservatively with cough suppressants, weight loss and environmental modifications. Dogs which suffer significant and persistent clinical signs despite conservative management, or which have life threatening compromise of ventilatory function should be considered candidates for surgical intervention.

Extent of tracheal collapse: The extent of tracheal collapse should be carefully assessed using radiography, fluoroscopy and endoscopy. Typically, collapse is most severe at the level of the thoracic inlet. The cervical and proximal thoracic trachea can be accessed through a ventral cervical approach. Collapse of the caudal portion of the intrathoracic trachea necessitates a right intercostal thoracotomy for adequate exposure. Collapse of the mainstem bronchi is a contraindication to surgical treatment for tracheal collapse.

Techniques

Early techniques for the surgical management of tracheal collapse revolved around attempts to reform the tracheal cartilages to a roughly spherical shape.

Chondrotomy of severely collapsed tracheal cartilages involved division of alternate tracheal cartilages on the ventral midline, resulting in the cartilage and dorsal tracheal membrane assuming a triangular, rather than a flattened, configuration. This technique met with minimal success since the redundant dorsal tracheal membrane could still prolapse into the tracheal lumen.

Plication of the dorsal tracheal membrane involved placement of horizontal mattress sutures in order to shorten the dorsal tracheal membrane. This procedure pulled the tracheal cartilages into a more spherical configuration, although decreasing luminal diameter. In the long term, tracheal rigidity is not adequate to maintain structural integrity with this technique.

Extraluminal techniques: In 1964, an extraluminal prosthesis for support of collapsed portions of the trachea was described (Schiller *et al.*, 1964). A cylindrical plastic tube with approximately 25% of its circumference removed, and with several holes for support of sutures, was used. The tube was secured to the trachea with 1.5 silk sutures. This prosthesis did serve to reconform the tracheal cartilages to a spherical configuration, but did not allow for tracheal flexibility. Support of long segments of trachea was difficult.

Hobson in 1976 described a modification of Schiller's technique involving the use of numerous 5 mm wide rings to support the trachea (see Figure 26.5). In this technique, the rings are formed from 3 ml syringe cases, and have several drill holes for suture placement. Multiple rings are placed at 5–10 mm intervals along the collapsed portion of the trachea. The open side of the prosthetic ring is positioned along the ventral aspect of the trachea and the tracheal cartilages and dorsal tracheal membrane are sutured to the ring using 2.0 or 1.5 non-absorbable suture material. Care must be taken to avoid incorporating the cuff of the endotracheal tube during suture placement. Moderate success has been associated with this technique. Complications include some loss of tracheal flexibility, inability to support the trachea between ring prostheses and potential erosion of the ring edge through the trachea.

Fingland in 1987 reported a further modification of the extraluminal prosthesis (see Figure 26.6). Spiral prostheses are formed from 3 ml syringe barrels or

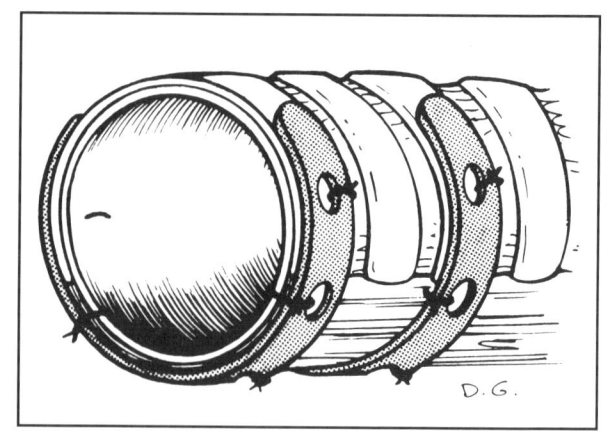

Figure 26.5: *Tracheal ring technique for repair of tracheal collapse as described by Hobson. Multiple incomplete rings with holes drilled for suture placement are formed from syringe casing. The rings are placed with the 'open' end overlying the ventral trachea. Sutures are placed to secure the tracheal cartilages and dorsal tracheal membrane to the ring.*

cases. The width of the prosthesis is 3 mm, with a distance of 6 mm between spirals. The spiral prosthesis is 'rotated' onto the collapsed segment of trachea and fixed circumferentially with non-absorbable suture material. The advantage of the spiral prosthesis over the total ring prosthesis is its ability to provide structural integrity along the entire length of the trachea. Initial descriptions of this technique involved complete dissection of both lateral pedicles, a procedure which was later found to be associated with a significant risk of transmural tracheal necrosis. A modified dissection procedure is now recommended wherein only the left lateral pedicle is dissected (Coyne *et al.*, 1993). The right lateral pedicle is left intact and small fenestrations are made to allow passage of the spiral prosthesis on each turn. This technique preserves the

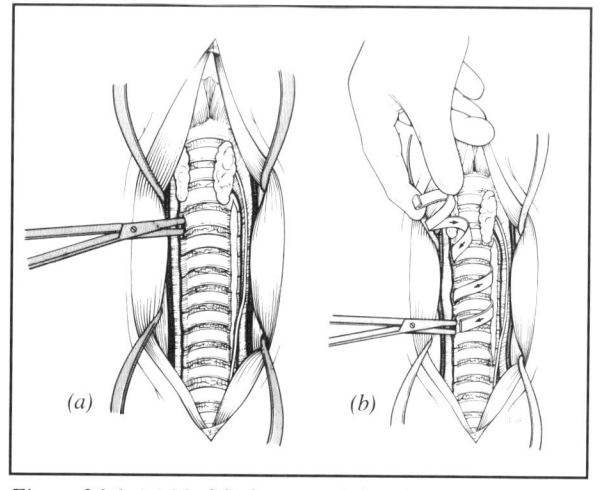

Figure 26.6: *(a) Modified approach for placement of the spiral ring prosthesis as described by Fingland. The left tracheal pedicle is completely dissected. The right tracheal pedicle is fenestrated between segmental vasculature in order to preserve the vascular integrity of the trachea. (b) The spiral ring is 'twisted' onto the trachea, taking care to feed the end of the spiral prosthesis through segmental perforations in the right tracheal pedicle.*

segmental vascular supply to the trachea along the right lateral pedicle and has not been associated with transmural necrosis. At present, use of the spiral ring prosthesis using the modified surgical approach preserving the right lateral tracheal pedicle appears to afford the best prognosis for long-term function.

Postoperative care

Postoperatively, dogs undergoing application of ring prostheses should be maintained in a non-stressful environment. Cough suppressants should be used in the immediate postoperative period and continued as required by the patient's response to treatment. Prophylactic broad spectrum, bactericidal antibiotics are recommended at the time of surgery. If preoperative tracheal wash indicates the presence of tracheobronchial infection, appropriate antibiotics based on culture and sensitivity results should be continued therapeutically. Sedation and analgesia may be required in the early postoperative period to reduce ventilatory stress. It is important to document normal laryngeal function at the time of anaesthetic recovery, as laryngeal paralysis is a potential complication. Owners should be made aware that surgery for tracheal collapse is an ameliorative, not a curative, procedure.

Various intraluminal prostheses have been evaluated, but have been associated with complications, including extrusion of the implant, erosion and granulation tissue formation, stricture and reduced mucociliary clearance (Sawada *et al.*, 1991). There is presently a resurgence of interest in defining an intraluminal prosthesis which can be applied endoscopically, provide tracheal support, and be incorporated into the tracheal lining with minimal inflammatory response.

Tracheal trauma

Tracheal trauma is often induced by altercations with other animals; penetrating injuries such as gunshots; blunt trauma, or inappropriate endotracheal intubation. Penetrating injury of the cervical trachea results in the formation of deep subcutaneous emphysema which may dissect extensively along the head, neck and trunk (see Figure 26.7). Intrathoracic tracheal trauma results in pneumomediastinum, which may extend to pneumothorax. Identification of the location and extent of tracheal trauma is required for successful management. Radiographic and endoscopic examinations are useful.

Small defects in the trachea occasionally may be managed conservatively. Cervical bandages may help in controlling air leakage from small defects in the cervical trachea. Thoracostomy drains may be required for management of air leakage resulting from intrathoracic tracheal trauma. Recovery from penetrating tracheal trauma is more predictable and rapid with surgical intervention. Debridement and direct suture repair of small defects may be adequate, whilst

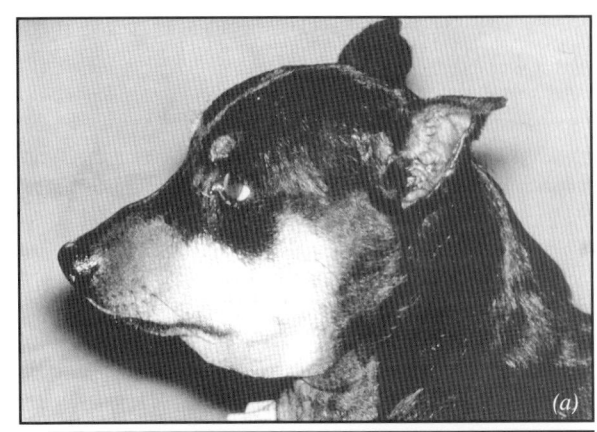

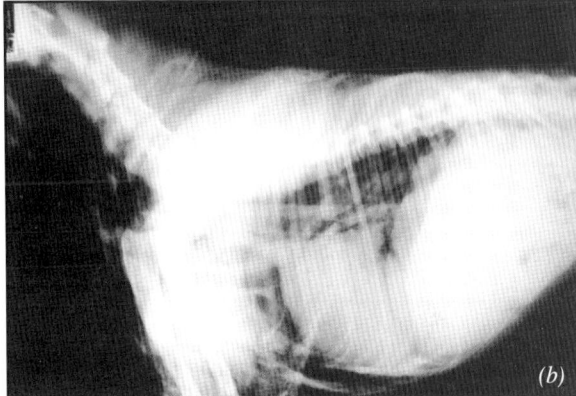

Figure 26.7: *(a) Photograph of a Miniature Pinscher presented after being attacked by a larger dog. The dog had suffered a tracheal laceration resulting in extensive subcutaneous emphysema. (b) Thoracic radiograph of the dog depicted in (a), showing superficial and deep subcutaneous and fascial emphysema consistent with tracheal laceration.*

resection and anastomosis may be required for larger defects. Local muscle flaps may be sutured over small tracheal defects in an attempt to control air leakage. Large defects should be managed by resection and anastomosis of the involved segment.

Tracheal and bronchial foreign bodies

Tracheal and bronchial foreign bodies most often affect sporting breeds and cats. Inhalation of foreign bodies into the trachea and bronchi is associated with an acute irritant tracheobronchitis, manifested as a sudden onset of coughing. Larger foreign bodies may result in impairment of air flow and respiratory compromise.

Surgery is not generally required for retrieval of tracheal and bronchial foreign bodies. Endoscopic visualization and retrieval using grasping or basket type forceps are usually successful. In instances where retrieval is not successful, or where endoscopic instrumentation is not available, surgery may be indicated. The approach is determined by the level at which the foreign body is lodged. Foreign bodies within the trachea or mainstem bronchi may be accessed by either a longitudinal or a transverse incision. Care should be taken to place the incision through a region of grossly normal trachea, since incision through an area of acute inflammation or infection increases the risk of dehiscence and stricture formation. A sterile endotracheal tube should be available for intraoperative intubation of the trachea or bronchus distal to the foreign body, if required. Following retrieval of the foreign body, the viability of tracheal/bronchial tissues is carefully assessed. The tracheal defect should be sutured with care and the incision checked under positive pressure ventilation for air leakage. A pleural or pericardial patch is sutured around the incision line to ensure an airtight closure (see Figure 26.8).

Broncho–oesophageal fistula

A broncho–oesophageal fistula is an abnormal communication between the oesophagus and a bronchus. Tracheo–oesophageal fistulae form between the trachea and oesophagus. Both are uncommonly reported in the dog, and are rare in the cat (Basher *et al.*, 1991). Broncho–oesophageal fistulae may be acquired secondary to trauma from oesophageal foreign bodies or,

less commonly, may be congenital. Animals present with clinical signs referable to the respiratory system. Coughing after eating and drinking, pyrexia, anorexia and weight loss are often observed. Regurgitation is a less frequent presenting complaint.

Treatment involves identification and obliteration of the fistula. Contrast oesophagrams and endoscopic examination will reveal the level of fistula formation. Dilute barium sulphate should be used for contrast examination, since oral iodinated contrast agents are hypertonic and can produce pulmonary oedema following entry into the lung. The majority of reported fistulae are associated with a traction diverticulum. The specific surgical approach depends on the level of the fistula. Following identification and dissection, the fistula is resected, and the involved bronchus and oesophagus are reconstructed. Stapling equipment is useful for rapid resection of the fistula.

The prognosis associated with broncho-oesophageal fistulae is good, unless secondary complications such as pneumonia or pulmonary abscesses are present. Significant associated lung pathology may necessitate pulmonary lobectomy following resection of the fistula.

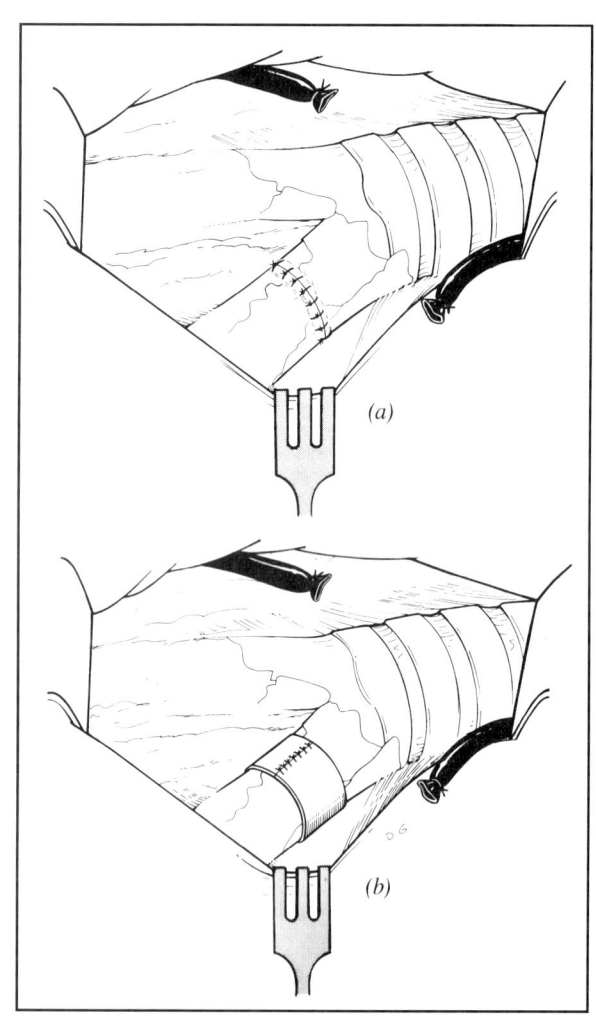

*Figure 26.8: (a) The carina is exposed through a right intercostal thoracotomy. Simple interrupted suture closure of the incised right mainstem bronchus has been achieved.
(b) A pleural or pericardial patch may be sutured around the bronchus to ensure an airtight closure.*

REFERENCES AND FURTHER READING

Basher AWP, Hogan PM, Hanna PE, Runyon CL and Shaw DH (1991) Surgical treatment of a congenital bronchoesophageal fistula in a dog. *Journal of the American Veterinary Medical Association* **199**, 479–482

Coyne BE, Fingland RB, Kennedy GA and Debowes RM (1993) Clinical and pathologic effects of a modified technique for application of spiral prostheses to the cervical trachea of dogs. *Veterinary Surgery* **22**, 269–275

Fingland RB, Dehoff WD and Birchard SJ (1987a) Surgical management of cervical and thoracic tracheal collapse in dogs using extraluminal spiral prostheses. *Journal of the American Animal Hospital Association* **23**, 163–172

Fingland RB, Dehoff WD and Birchard SJ (1987b). Surgical management of cervical and thoracic tracheal collapse in dogs using extraluminal spiral prostheses: results in seven cases. *Journal of the American Animal Hospital Association* **23**, 173–181

Fingland RB, Weisbrode SE and Dehoff WD (1989) Clinical and pathologic effects of spiral and total ring prostheses applied to the cervical and thoracic portions of the trachea of dogs. *American Journal of Veterinary Research* **50**, 2168–2175

Hauptman J, White JV and Slocombe RF (1985) Intrathoracic tracheal stricture management in a dog. *Journal of the American Animal Hospital Association* **21**, 505–510

Hedlund CS (1991) Tracheal resection and anastomosis. *Problems in Veterinary Medicine* **3**, 210–217

Hedlund CS and Tangner CH (1983) Tracheal surgery in the dog –part II. *The Compendium on Continuing Education* **5**, 738–748

Hobson HP (1976) Total ring prosthesis for the surgical correction of collapsed trachea. *Journal of the American Animal Hospital Association* **12**, 822–828

Kirby BM, Bjorling DE, Rankin JHG and Phernetton TM (1991) The effects of surgical isolation and application of polypropylene spiral prostheses on tracheal blood flow. *Veterinary Surgery* **20**, 49–54

Lau RE, Schwartz A and Buergelt CD (1980) Tracheal resection and anastomosis in dogs. *Journal of the American Veterinary Medical Association* **176**, 134–139

Oizuma H (1993) Experimental reconstruction of the mediastinal trachea with autogenous material – hydroxyapatite-omentum complex. *Nippon-Kyobu-Geka-Gakkai-Zasshi* **41**, 372–378

Okumura N, Nakamura T, Takimoto Y, Natsume T, Teramachi M, Tomihata K, Ikada Y and Shimizu Y (1993) A new tracheal prosthesis made from collagen grafted mesh. *ASAIO-J* **39**, M475–479

Park RD (1984) Bronchoesophageal fistula in the dog: literature survey, case presentations, and radiographic manifestations. *The Compendium on Continuing Education* **6**, 669–676

Rubin GJ, Neal TM and Bojrab MJ (1973) Surgical reconstruction for collapsed tracheal rings. *Journal of Small Animal Practice* **14**, 607–617

Sawada S, Tanabe Y, Fujiwara Y, Koyama T, Tanigawa N, Kobayashi M, Katsube Y and Nakamura H (1991) Endotracheal expandable metallic stent placement in dogs. *Acta Radiologica* **32**, 79–80

Schiller AG, Helper LC and Small E (1964) Treatment of tracheal collapse in the dog. *Journal of the American Veterinary Medical Association* **145**, 669–671

Tangner CH and Hedlund CS (1983) tracheal surgery in the dog – part

I. *The Compendium on Continuing Education* **5**, 599–606

Tangner CH and Hobson HP (1982) A retrospective study of 20 surgically managed cases of collapsed trachea. *Veterinary Surgery* **11**, 146–149

Ueda H and Shirakusa T (1992) Carinal transplantation. *Thorax* **47**, 968–970

Wang Z, Chi RC, Chen WX and Liu WZ (1991) Mucosal wound and cicatricial stricture formation in the dog trachea: an experimental study. *Journal of Laryngology and Otology* **105**, 207–209

Surgery of the Heart and Pericardium

Robert N. White

GENERAL CONSIDERATIONS

Before embarking on a surgical procedure within the thoracic cavity, it is imperative that the surgeon is well-versed in the anaesthetic techniques required. A high level of both surgical and anaesthetic skill and experience are required to carry out many of the procedures described. It is not acceptable to be able to complete the surgical exercise only to lose the patient for want of adequate anaesthetic and recovery facilities. It is essential that the surgeon is familiar with the pathophysiology of the cardiovascular disease for which the animal is to be treated and has a knowledge of the immediate effects of anaesthesia and surgery on the various conditions. Many of the procedures described require the use of specialized surgical instruments if they are to be treated successfully.

CONDITIONS OF THE PERICARDIUM AND PERICARDIAL CAVITY

The pericardium is a fibroserous covering of the heart. The fibrous pericardium is the connective tissue between the parietal serous pericardium and the adjacent pericardial mediastinal pleura. The serous pericardium is a closed sac that envelops most of the heart. The parietal layer adheres to the visceral layer, or epicardium, which tightly adheres to the heart.

PERICARDIOCENTESIS

Pericardiocentesis can be used as both a diagnostic and therapeutic procedure for cases of pericardial effusion. It involves the introduction of a needle or catheter into the pericardial sac. Sedation may be required for the procedure to be carried out safely, but in the majority of cases this is not necessary. An area is clipped on the right side from the sternum to the costochondral junction which encompasses the third to the seventh intercostal spaces. Pericardiocentesis is usually performed just below the costochondral junction at the right fourth, fifth or sixth intercostal

space. Penetration at this site will avoid lung tissue as the area overlies the cardiac notch. Other advantages of penetration of the pericardium at this site are associated with the cardiac anatomy; the site is ventral to the thin-walled right atrium, there are no coronary arteries located on the epicardium in this area, and the right ventricle is under relatively low pressure, so that penetration of the ventricular lumen is unlikely to result in catastrophic haemorrhage. The area is scrubbed and aseptically prepared. The ECG is continuously monitored so that any arrhythmias produced as a result of epicardial interference can be detected. The procedure may be performed with the animal standing or maintained in left lateral recumbency. The procedure should be undertaken in an aseptic manner. Local anaesthetic is infiltrated into the intercostal muscles at the proposed puncture site. A large bore (14–18 gauge), long (5–15 cm) over-the-needle catheter is inserted through a stab incision in the skin. Further fenestrations can be cut into the catheter prior to its insertion, but generally this is unnecessary. A syringe is attached to the needle and catheter/needle are advanced through the thoracic wall towards the heart. A slight negative pressure is placed on the syringe so that once the pericardial sac is entered, pericardial fluid will be aspirated. The catheter can then be advanced over the needle into the pericardial sac. If the catheter or needle contacts the epicardium, changes such as ventricular premature complexes will be seen on the ECG and the movement of the heart will be felt through the syringe. The arrhythmias usually cease when the catheter is retracted. Once the catheter is well placed in the pericardial sac, the needle can be completely removed and a three-way tap and extension set attached. As much pericardial fluid as possible is removed. Samples of the fluid are collected for laboratory analysis including cytology, culture and sensitivity. The fluid usually appears haemorrhagic or serosanguinous, and rarely clots. It is also possible to purchase catheters and catheter placement systems from veterinary catheter manufacturers that are specifically designed for pericardiocentesis in small animals. In general, these systems are placed with the aid of a guide wire using the Seldinger technique.

Pericardiectomy

Indications
The surgical removal of a portion of or the entire pericardium may be indicated for the following medically unresponsive conditions:

- Idiopathic pericardial effusion
- Constrictive pericarditis
- Heart base neoplasms
- Pericardial cysts
- Pericardial neoplasia.

It is usual that cases of idiopathic pericardial effusion will have been diagnosed and treated by pericardiocentesis. In some instances, this therapy will prove curative, but more commonly the effusion will reform. If the effusion recurs following two or three successful drainages, then a pericardiectomy should be considered. The surgical management of very long-standing cases with effusion can be difficult and less effective, since a restrictive epicarditis which is less amenable to treatment is commonly present. This epicarditis can be sufficient to produce continued clinical signs of right-sided heart failure. Therapeutic pericardiectomy should therefore be considered early in the management of this disease.

In individuals suffering from a heart base tumour which proves to be non-resectable, pericardiectomy may prove an effective palliative therapy. The clinical signs associated with the pericardial effusion will be resolved, and any effusion produced by the vascular neoplasm will be absorbed by the pleural surfaces of the thoracic cavity.

Technique
Pericardiectomy may be accomplished via a left or right fourth or fifth intercostal lateral thoracotomy, or by a median sternotomy. The choice of approach is governed to an extent by the underlying disease condition, although a median sternotomy is the only approach that will offer complete exposure of the entire pericardium up to the heart base (Figure 27.1). When performing a pericardiectomy, it is important to remove as much of the pericardium as possible. Removal of a small portion of pericardium (pericardial window) may effectively treat a pericardial effusion in the short term, but adhesions to the heart may seal the opening allowing an effusion to return. The phrenic nerves which run adjacent to the pericardium on either side of the thoracic cavity should be carefully dissected free and preserved. If dissection of these nerves proves impossible, a subtotal pericardiectomy can be performed to the level of each nerve on both sides. A portion of the resected pericardium should be submitted for histopathology and in some instances for culture.

In the diseased state, the pericardium becomes extremely thickened and vascular and great care should be taken to ensure adequate haemostasis during the resection. Electrocautery is very helpful, and may be considered mandatory when contemplating the procedure. It is essential that haemorrhage is controlled, and a thoracic drain is placed prior to thoracic closure. Should haemorrhage persist in the recovery period, it is possible that further surgery may be required to stop the bleeding.

Percutaneous balloon pericardiotomy
Recently, the technique of balloon pericardiotomy has been described for the treatment of recurrent pericardial effusion secondary to intrapericardial neoplasia (Cobb *et al.*, 1996). Under general anaesthesia and using image intensification, an over-the-needle catheter is introduced into the pericardium. The catheter is then used to introduce a guide wire into the pericardial sac. The guide wire is subsequently used to guide a balloon catheter across the pericardial wall. The balloon is then inflated the result of which is to tear a hole in the pericardial wall. This procedure represents a useful palliative procedure for patients with recurring pericardial effusion resulting from poor prognostic neoplasms (e.g. heamangiosarcoma) or in patients in which the financial constraints mean that a thoracotomy is not a management option.

Heart base tumours
Neoplasms which originate from the region of the ascending aorta are referred to as heart base tumours. The neoplasm most often encountered at this site is a chemodectoma of the aortic body (Figure 27.2). Chemodectomas tend to be locally invasive, but do not commonly metastasize. Invasive forms are often vascular, infiltrating the aortic, pulmonary artery and atrial walls, making surgical removal very difficult. Non-invasive forms are often discrete, well encapsulated with a smooth surface, and may be amenable to surgical resection. Clinical signs are related to pericardial effusion and right-sided heart failure.

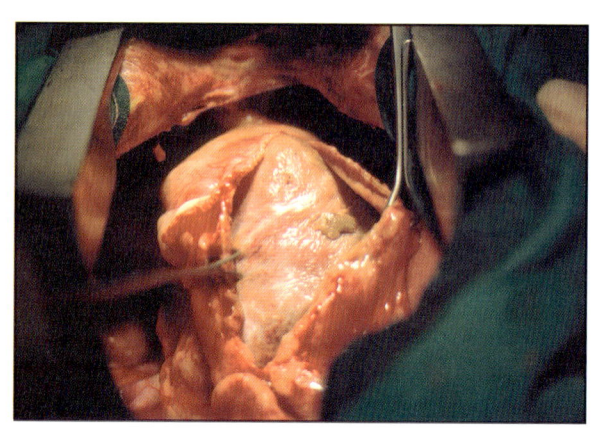

Figure 27.1: *Pericardiectomy being performed via a median sternotomy. Note the thickened and vascular pericardium and the presence of restrictive epicarditis.*

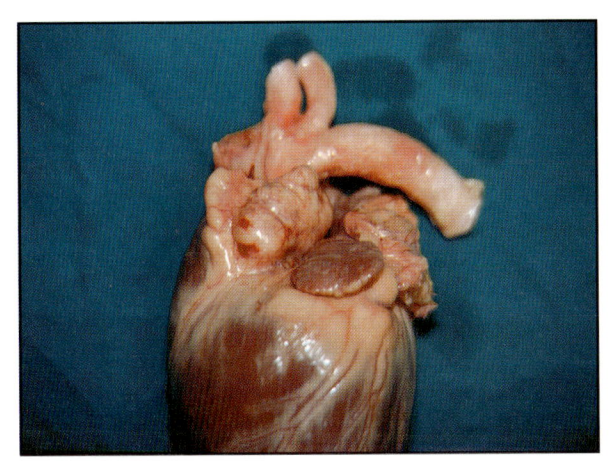

Figure 27.2: Cadaver specimen of a heart with a chemodectoma of the aortic body.

Technique

Surgical resection can be achieved via a left or right lateral fourth intercostal thoracotomy. Diagnostic investigations such as radiography and ultrasonography may indicate the preferred approach. Non-invasive forms may be carefully dissected off the aorta and pulmonary artery. This procedure must not be rushed, and is technically demanding. The surgeon should be familiar with the vascular surgical techniques required to repair tears in the pulmonary artery and/or aorta, should the need arise. Invasive and very large forms of the neoplasm will often be non-resectable. Individuals with non-resectable tumours in which the clinical signs were associated with pericardial effusion can be treated palliatively by performing a pericardiectomy. Tumour growth is often slow and long-term resolution of clinical signs can be achieved in some individuals (Thomas and Reed, 1986). The prognosis for individuals in which the neoplasm has infiltrated the myocardium is less favourable, and pericardiectomy may be of little benefit.

CONGENITAL CARDIAC CONDITIONS

Patent ductus arteriosus

Patent ductus arteriosus (PDA) results from a failure of the ductus to close after birth. If untreated, most individuals will only survive for the first years of life as the left-to-right shunting results in left-sided congestive heart failure. Early surgical ligation is the treatment of choice for left-to-right shunting PDAs. Surgery is not recommended for right-to-left shunting PDAs because ligating the ductus will generally result in a further increase in pulmonary artery pressure and pulmonary vascular resistance.

Technique

The ductus is accessible via a lateral left fourth intercostal thoracotomy. The cranial and caudal parts of the left cranial lung lobe are reflected caudally and

held reflected with a moistened swab. The ductus can usually be seen as a bulge between the dorsally positioned aorta and the ventrally placed main pulmonary artery. Systolic and diastolic fremitus will be felt at the site of the ductus.

Direct ligation: The ductus is approached either by opening the pericardium immediately ventral to the vagus nerve and reflecting the vagus nerve dorsally, or by opening the pleura adjacent to the ductus and reflecting the vagus nerve ventrally (Figure 27.3). In some dogs the dissection can be performed entirely extrapericardially; however, in dogs with a short ductus, it is usually necessary also to work intrapericardially. Right-angled forceps are used to bluntly open the fascia between the aorta and the main pulmonary artery both proximal and distal to the ductus. Care must be taken not to damage the left recurrent laryngeal nerve as it passes around the caudal aspect of the ductus. The right-angled forceps are passed gently, but firmly around the ductus from the distal fascia opening to the proximal fascia opening. This procedure requires great care and should not be rushed as rupture of the pulmonary artery or far

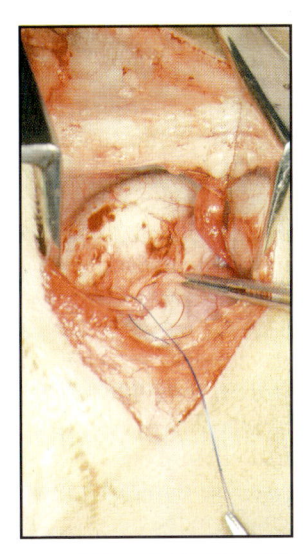
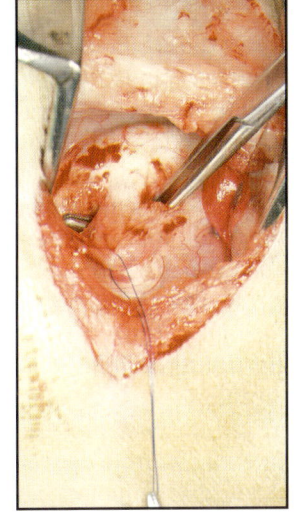
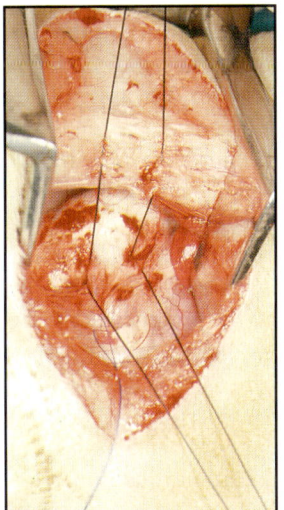

Figure 27.3: (a) Left lateral 4th intercostal thoracotomy in a dog with a patent ductus arteriosus. The vagus nerve has been reflected ventrally from the ductus with a polypropylene tie. An aortic bulge is present at the aortic ductus opening. (b) Right-angled forceps have been passed around the ductus. In this case, this dissection has been performed entirely extrapericardially. (c) Two silk ligatures have been placed around the ductus.

Reproduced from White (1994) with the permission of Veterinary International.

ductal wall may result. A loop of saline-soaked silk (0 to 2-0) is then placed in the jaws of the forceps and grasped. By using ligature-passing forceps it is impossible to inadvertently grasp the far wall of the ductus, thereby reducing the risk of accidental pulmonary artery or ductus rupture. The loop is then cut into two and positioned. The aortic (high pressure) side of the ductus should be tied first. Closure will result in an increased systemic blood flow which may lead to a rise in systemic vascular resistance. A marked vagally mediated reflex bradycardia (Branham's sign) may be seen in response to the pressure changes, and this can be so severe as to result in asystole. An anticholinergic drug such as atropine should be available at the time of ductus closure, and some surgeons feel it is prudent to close the ductus over at least a 5-minute period. A chest drain is placed and the thoracotomy closure is routine.

Indirect ligation (Jackson/Henderson technique):
The ductus is approached in a similar manner to that for direct closure (Jackson and Henderson, 1979). The mediastinum dorsal to the descending aorta is incised and further dissection to the medial aspect of the aorta is achieved bluntly with a finger. Blunt dissection in this manner should be continued until the aorta is completely mobilized on its medial aspect from the left subclavian artery to a region caudal to the ductus (often to the first intercostal arteries). A pair of narrow, blunt haemostats or a ligature forceps is passed around the aorta cranial to the ductus in a ventral to dorsal direction. Care is taken not to stretch the ductus excessively, and the tips of the forceps should be kept close to the aortic wall. A loop of saline-soaked silk (0 to 2-0) is then placed in the jaws of the forceps, grasped and passed around the medial wall of the aorta. The forceps are then passed around the aorta caudal to the ductus in a similar manner to that already described. The two free ends of the suture are grasped and passed around the medial wall of the aorta caudal to the ductus. The looped cranial suture is cut, and it is ensured that the two ligatures are not twisted around each other. The two ligatures can now be positioned and tied in a similar manner to that described for direct ligation.

This technique allows the placement of the ductal ligatures without direct dissection of the friable medial wall of the ductus and the pulmonary artery. Disadvantages of the technique include a longer surgical time; risk of iatrogenic damage to the thoracic duct which lies medial to the aorta; and the possibility of incomplete ductus attenuation due to the presence of mediastinal connective tissue snared within the ductal ligatures.

Ductal division: If the ductus arteriosus is found at surgery to be very wide and/or very short, or if iatrogenic trauma has resulted in a tear, the ductus must be divided and sutured.

This is a technically difficult procedure to perform, and requires the use of vascular occlusion clamps. The approach to the ductus is similar to that previously described. The mediastinum must be dissected off the lateral wall of the ductus, the main and left pulmonary arteries, and the aorta both cranial and caudal to the ductus. Care should be taken to visualize and preserve the left recurrent laryngeal nerve. It is important that both lateral and medial walls of the aorta are adequately exposed so that, should ductal rupture occur, the aorta can be cross-clamped both cranial and caudal to the ductus to minimize high pressure blood loss whilst repair is attempted. The ductus is cross-clamped with two pairs of vascular occlusion forceps which have fine teeth that are atraumatic and prevent slippage. The clamps are applied with the tips directly cranially and the aortic (high pressure) side should be applied first. It is important to keep close to the aortic wall so that when the second clamp is applied at least 2–3 mm of vessel lies between the forceps. The ductus can now be divided with a blade or scissors and the clamps gently rotated laterally to expose the cut edge of the ductus for suturing. The pulmonary artery end is then over-sewn with a double layer of continuous 5-0 polypropylene suture and the clamp removed. If there is any bleeding from the suture line, a swab can be placed over the suture line and retracted gently while the aortic end is closed. The aortic end is similarly closed with a double layer of 5-0 polypropylene and the clamp removed. Any haemorrhage from the aortic side will usually cease after a few minutes of gentle pressure with a swab.

Iatrogenic rupture of the ductus
Ductal surgery is generally relatively straightforward, although anyone contemplating performing surgery should be fully acquainted with emergency measures required to save the individual in which the ductus or main pulmonary artery ruptures on handling. In the event of severe haemorrhage, digital pressure should immediately be applied to the bleeding site. The spilt blood must be removed allowing visual assessment of the operative site, and this can only be achieved adequately with suction. If haemorrhage is severe, a blood transfusion may become necessary. A vascular occlusion clamp should be applied to cross-clamp the aorta cranial to the ductus and caudal to the brachycephalic and left subclavian arteries. This will allow the left ventricle to continue to eject blood, and will maintain perfusion to both the head and the heart. A second occlusion clamp should then be applied to the aorta caudal to the ductus to prevent retrograde aortic haemorrhage. Any haemorrhage will now be coming from blood flow in the pulmonary artery and will be dark blue. This is a low pressure system, making the haemorrhage less severe. Digital pressure will easily control this haemorrhage allowing the ductus to be divided. Good exposure of the pulmonary artery end

should now be achieved, and a partial occlusion clamp can often be used to achieve complete haemostasis and also allow pulmonary artery blood flow. The tear in the ductus and/or pulmonary artery can be closed with 5-0 polypropylene continuous sutures. The pulmonary artery end of the ductus can be closed as previously described, and the partial occlusion clamp removed. The aortic end of the ductus can be sutured and the caudal aortic cross-clamp removed. This can be followed by removal of the cranial aortic cross-clamp.

Outcome

The success rate of ductal surgery is probably greater than 95% in experienced hands. Individuals that are corrected early enough can be expected to live a normal life. However, approximately 1.5–2.0% of ductus ligations will recanalize (Eyster *et al.*, 1975). The cause of this is unknown, but if the recanalized blood shunting is substantial, the ductus should be divided.

There are a number of reports describing the occlusion of the ductus arteriosus using the transvenous catheter placement of an occlusion device such as a Raskind occluder or the Gianturco–Grifka occlusion device. These techniques require experience with intravenous catheterization techniques and image intensification equipment (fluoroscopy). Although these techniques are relatively non-invasive when compared with a thoracotomy, the cost of the devices and the variability of ductal anatomy seen in the dog may prevent these techniques from becoming widely available or accepted.

Vascular ring anomalies

Vascular ring anomalies are congenital malformations of the great vessels and associated structures which may lead to constriction of the thoracic oesophagus. Various ring anomalies have been reported in the dog and cat. The most common lesion reported in both the dog and the cat is the persistent right aortic arch (PRAA) which is readily amenable to surgical correction (Ellison, 1980). In general, the earlier surgical correction is performed, the greater the chance of a return to clinically normal oesophageal function.

Persistent right aortic arch (PRAA)

Animals with PRAA are frequently small, undernourished and immature, and anaesthetic management can be very challenging. The PRAA (Figure 27.4) can be approached via a left lateral fourth intercostal thoracotomy. The cranial and middle portions of the left cranial lung lobe are reflected caudally and maintained in position with a moistened swab. It is common to find an anomalous caval supply to the heart, and a persistent left cranial vena cava may be present. This, in general, should not be ligated unless the surgeon is sure that a normal right cranial vena cava is also present. A right hemiazygos branch may also be present. This often runs directly across the operative field and, if necessary, can be safely ligated and reflected ventrally. The great vessels of the heart should be further examined to ascertain the arterial anomalies present. In cases of PRAA, the ligamentum arteriosum is located as a fibrous ring between the proximal descending aorta and the pulmonary artery just cranial to the recurrent laryngeal nerve at the level of the oesophageal stricture. The ligament is bluntly dissected off the oesophagus. Great care should be taken not to perforate the thin oesophageal wall of the pouch cranial to the stricture. In a number of cases, a patent ductus arteriosus is present (Figure 27.5). There is often no blood flow

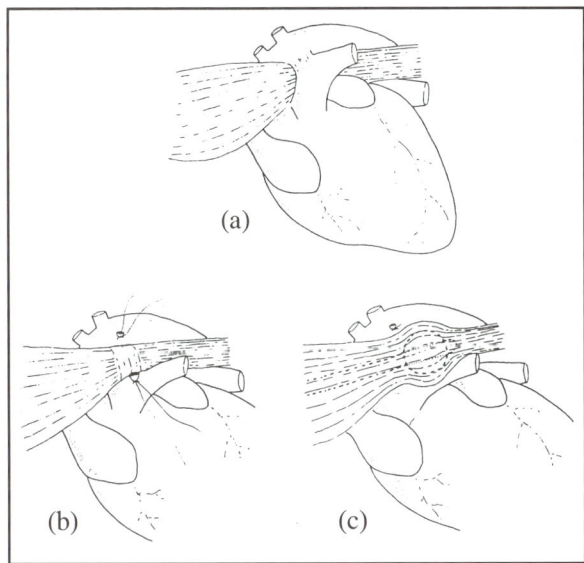

Figure 27.4: *Persistent right aortic arch. (a) The aorta can be seen running on the right side of the oesophagus. (b) The ligamentum arteriosum is double ligated and transected. Remaining fibrous bands are freed from the surface of the oesophagus. (c) This procedure can be achieved more readily if a Foley catheter with an inflated balloon is used to distend the oesophagus at the site of the entrapment.*

Reproduced from White (1994) with the permission of Veterinary International.

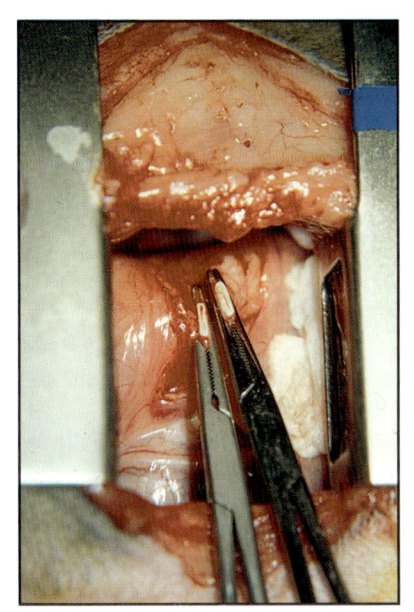

Figure 27.5: *An intraoperative photograph demonstrating a persistent right aortic arch in which a patent ductus arteriosus was present. Cardiac auscultation of this dog prior to surgery had never demonstrated any form of murmur.*

across the ductus because of the presence of the entrapped oesophagus, and it may have a similar appearance to that of a non-patent ligamentum. It may only become apparent that the ductus is patent at the time of division. For this reason, it is advisable to ligate the ligamentum both close to the aorta and also close to the pulmonary artery with surgical silk. The structure can then be divided. The oesophagus should be carefully dissected free from the aorta and pulmonary artery. Any remaining constricting, fibrous bands are freed from the oesophagus. This procedure can be achieved more readily if a Foley catheter with an inflated balloon is passed per os to distend the oesophagus at the site of the entrapment. Plication or resection of the redundant cranial oesophageal pouch is not recommended, because it only inverts redundant tissue and will not restore normal oesophageal peristalsis. Closure of the thoracotomy is routine after the placement of a thoracic drain.

Other vascular ring anomalies

Anomalous retro-oesophageal left/right subclavian artery: If a retro-oesophageal left or right subclavian artery is anomalous and producing oesophageal constriction, it must be elevated from the oesophagus, ligated and transected. Collateral circulation is sufficient to compensate for its ligation. An aberrant left subclavian artery may be seen in conjunction with a PRAA. Careful assessment of the oesophagus for a further constriction cranial to the ligamentum arteriosum may reveal the aberrant vessel. An aberrant right subclavian artery may be seen in conjunction with a normal left aortic arch (Hurley *et al.*, 1993). A left lateral thoracotomy may fail to determine the cause of the constriction with this anomaly. Therefore, selective angiography and oesophageal endoscopy may be required to confirm the diagnosis.

Double aortic arch: This is a well recognized although very rare form of vascular ring anomaly. Surgery for this is technically difficult and consists of division of the smaller of the two arches at its distal end, just proximal to the junction with the larger of the two arches. This can usually be achieved via a left lateral thoracotomy, since the smaller of the two arches is usually on the left side. The ligamentum should also be ligated and divided.

Outcome
It is rare for the oesophagus to attain normal function following surgery, and follow-up oesophageal motility studies frequently show persistent marked dilatation of the oesophagus. The placement of a gastrostomy tube at the time of vascular ring surgery may be considered. All food and water should be administered via this route for a 4–6 week period post-surgery. This nil-by-mouth regime may allow some reversal of the oesophageal dilatation during the rapid growth of the individual which occurs during this time. In some individuals, in addition to surgical management, continued dietary control such as feeding from a height may be required. The prognosis for cases of persistent right aortic arch following surgery ranges from good to poor depending on the severity of oesophageal dilatation and the delay in undertaking the corrective procedure. The high incidence of post-surgical complications and the possible need for prolonged dietary management should be fully explained to the owner of an animal suffering from a vascular ring anomaly prior to undertaking any surgical intervention.

Pulmonic stenosis
Pulmonic stenosis is an obstruction of blood flow from the right ventricle into the pulmonary artery, and the stenosis may occur at the valvular, subvalvular, infundibular or supravalvular location.

Valvular stenosis is considered to be most common and results from thickening or fusion of the free edge of the three pulmonic valve leaflets. Commissures are commonly well defined but adherent to the pulmonary artery wall. The pulmonary artery valve annulus is often stenotic.

Subvalvular stenosis is caused by a fibrous membrane just proximal to the pulmonic valve. When this lesion occurs very close to the pulmonic valve, differentiation of the condition from valvular stenosis may be difficult and this form of lesion has been described as pulmonic valve dysplasia.

Supravalvular stenosis as an isolated lesion is very rare, and presents as a stricture of the main pulmonary artery.

Infundibular muscular hypertrophy of the right ventricular outflow tract is generally caused by concentric muscular hypertrophy of the right ventricle as a result of long-standing pulmonic valve stenosis.

The severity of the stenotic lesion can be quantified by direct or indirect measurement of the pressures within the right ventricle and pulmonary artery to determine the pressure gradient across the lesion. Pressure gradients have been classified as mild (less than 50 mmHg), moderate (50–100 mmHg) and severe (greater than 100 mmHg). The treatment of choice for moderate and severe pulmonic stenosis is surgical correction.

There are many surgical procedures that have been advocated for the treatment of pulmonic stenosis and these include:

- Bistoury technique, for valvular and discrete subvalvular stenosis
- Modified Brock procedure, for subvalvular lesions
- Valvulotome valvotomy, for dysplastic pulmonic valve obstructions
- Inflow occlusion and pulmonary arteriotomy (Swan procedure), for valvular, discrete subvalvular and dysplastic valve lesions

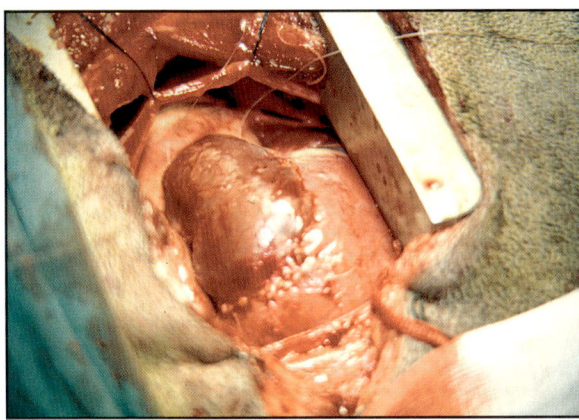

Figure 27.6: *Pericardial trans-annular patch-graft: final appearance of blood-filled patch following the cutting of the stenotic lesion and right ventricular outflow tract.*

Reproduced from White (1994) with the permission of Veterinary International.

- Patch-graft technique (closed or open trans-arterial valvulotomy), which is effective for all forms of stenosis including muscular infundibular hypertrophy
- Conduit repair, for bypassing the stenotic lesion
- Open trans-arterial valvulotomy with cardiopulmonary bypass
- Trans-cutaneous balloon valvuloplasty, for valvular, discrete subvalvular and dysplastic valve lesions.

Balloon valvuloplasty

Balloon valvuloplasty is a relatively safe procedure to perform and should be considered as the simplest and safest technique for the initial treatment of pulmonic stenosis (Brownlie *et al.*, 1991; Martin *et al.*, 1992). Balloon valvuloplasty is most effective for the treatment of valve stenosis caused by fusion of the valve leaflet commissures. It appears to be less effective when used to treat cases with a marked muscular infundibular hypertrophic component to the stenosis and, although the procedure may produce an improvement in these patients, they are likely to require further surgery.

Closed patch-graft technique

Of the other procedures described, excluding those requiring cardiopulmonary bypass, the most effective is probably the patch-graft technique (Figure 27.6) as it can be used to treat all forms of pulmonic stenosis (Breznock and Wood, 1976; Orton *et al.*, 1990). This procedure can be performed via a left lateral fourth or fifth intercostal thoracotomy. An autograft of pericardium or a synthetic material such as polytetrafluoroethylene (PTFE) is generally used for the graft material. The pericardium is harvested by careful mobilization of the left phrenic nerve from the pericardial surface. It is important that the pericardium is not punctured during this procedure. A large rectangular window of pericardium is then resected and

cleaned of any pericardial fat. Once the pericardium is opened it is important to assess the coronary vasculature of the heart for evidence of an anomalous left coronary artery passing across the right ventricular outflow tract (Buchanan, 1990). Although this vessel is a rare finding, its presence would mean abandoning the patch-graft procedure for another surgical method since the graft cannot be adequately placed without the severance of the anomalous coronary artery. Assuming normal coronary anatomy, a 2-0 multifilament stainless steel wire is passed into the right ventricular outflow tract below the stenosis and exits above the stenosis through the lateral wall of the main pulmonary artery. It is important that the wire passes across the stenosis within the vascular lumen. The passage of the wire may be guided by initially passing a catheter and stylet across the stenosis. The cutting wire can then be passed through the catheter and the catheter withdrawn. Small (5-0) polypropylene purse-string sutures may be placed around the entry and exit sites if any substantial haemorrhage occurs. The two ends of the wire are reflected ventrally and 5-0 polypropylene sutures are then placed at the four corners of the patch site. The graft is then sutured in place using a continuous suture pattern from each of the four corner sutures. A small portion of the ventral border of the graft is left unclosed so that the cutting wire can be removed by 'sawing' through the obstructed outflow tract. Care should be taken not to damage the patch in this process. The remaining ventral border sutures are now placed. The procedure opens the obstructed area of pulmonic stenosis and a portion of the right outflow tract into the patch, thus effectively turning a stenosis into an incompetence. A chest drain is placed and thoracotomy closure is routine.

Inflow occlusion and open patch-graft technique

Open graft valvuloplasty is accomplished using inflow occlusion and mild hypothermia. Inflow occlusion involves the complete interruption of venous flow to the heart. This in turn will dramatically reduce the cardiac output and is considered to result in complete cardiac arrest. In normothermic patients, the circulatory arrest period should be kept to a minimum (ideally less than 2 minutes, but certainly no more than 4 minutes). When mild whole body hypothermia (30–34°C) is employed, the cardiac arrest time may be extended to 6 minutes. Mild hypothermia may easily be achieved in small animals by simply avoiding measures usually employed to maintain body temperature during the anaesthetic period. An ability to re-warm the individual following the surgical procedure is essential if this procedure is to be undertaken.

Inflow occlusion can be achieved from either left or right lateral thoracotomies or via a median sternotomy. Snares are placed around the cranial and caudal venae cavae and the azygos vein (Figure 27.7). The cranial

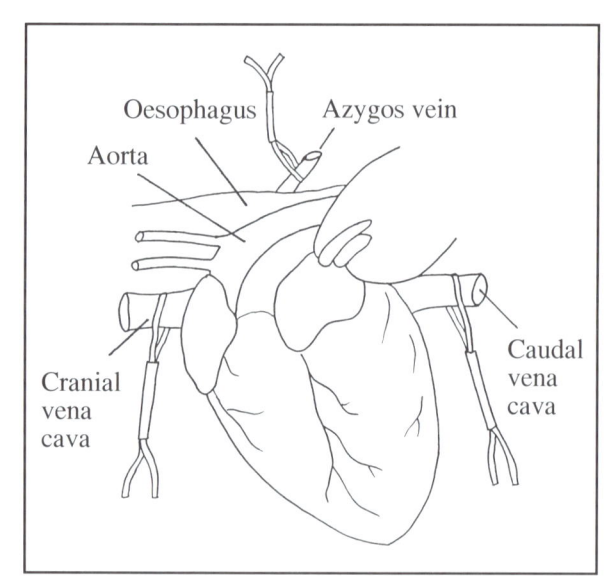

Figure 27.7: The position of the venous occlusion snares during inflow occlusion on the left side.

vena cava is located in the mediastinum, cranial to the heart and ventral to the brachycephalic artery. The caudal vena cava is located in the caudal mediastinum in the plica vena cava. When a left fourth or fifth thoracotomy in undertaken, some difficulty may be experienced in trying to snare the caudal vena cava especially if some degree of cardiomegaly is present. Gentle cranial rotation of the heart will generally allow access to the vessel, but may induce a greatly diminished cardiac output during cardiac rotation. The azygos vein can be snared by locating its insertion into the cranial vena cava as it joins the right atrium (right-sided approach) or by dissecting dorsal to the oesophagus and aorta (left-sided approach). The animal is well ventilated and the venous snares snugged up. The right side of the heart will take about 15 seconds to empty.

Open patch-graft valvuloplasty is generally accomplished via a left fifth intercostal thoracotomy. Orton *et al.* (1990) describe making a partial thickness incision in the right ventricular outflow tract. An autogenous pericardial or synthetic PTFE patch is then sutured to the ventriculotomy incision and the cranial aspect of the pulmonary artery. Venous inflow occlusion is then initiated and the pulmonary artery and right ventricle are incised full thickness. Suction will be required to remove any residual blood within the right heart and also to remove blood entering the right heart from the coronary sinus. Dysplastic pulmonic valve leaflets are incised or excised as necessary. Suturing of the pulmonary artery to the patch graft is completed and inflow occlusion is discontinued. The heart is resuscitated as necessary. In the author's opinion, the partial ventriculotomy incision will tend to bleed producing a blood clot which must be removed prior to making the full thickness incision. If the clot is not removed, it may enter the pulmonary artery producing an embolus.

Inflow occlusion and pulmonary arteriotomy

Pulmonary arteriotomy during inflow occlusion is an effective surgical treatment for all forms of pulmonic stenosis, excluding those accompanied by significant muscular infundibular stenosis (Malik *et al.*, 1993). This procedure (Figure 27.8) offers little advantage over closed valve dilation for simple pulmonic stenosis and, therefore, is probably rarely indicated in small animals with pulmonic stenosis. The surgical approach for the technique is via a left lateral fourth or fifth intercostal thoracotomy. Inflow occlusion is performed in a manner as described above. The right side of the heart will take about 15 seconds to empty depending on the degree of pulmonic stenosis. Once this is seen to have occurred, the pulmonary artery is cross-clamped distal to the proposed incision site. Polypropylene stay sutures can be placed in the main pulmonary artery prior to the inflow occlusion to make its handling easier during the procedure. The main pulmonary artery can then be opened. During the procedure, venous drainage from the coronary supply to the heart will continue to drain into the right atrium and right ventricle making the use of suction mandatory. A narrow suction probe is often useful, so that it can be passed across the valvular stenosis to lie within the right ventricle. The valve is exposed and the leaflets are untethered from the pulmonary artery wall and the commissures are sharply incised so that a maximum orifice is obtained. Subvalvular tissue which requires removal can also be resected through this approach. Once the corrective surgery is completed, a partial vascular occlusion clamp can be applied to the pulmonary artery across the incision site. The circulation is re-established by releasing the snares and removing the pulmonary artery cross-clamp. The pulmonary artery incision is closed with continuous 5-0 polypropylene sutures. As with all inflow occlusion techniques, total occlusion time should be kept to a minimum.

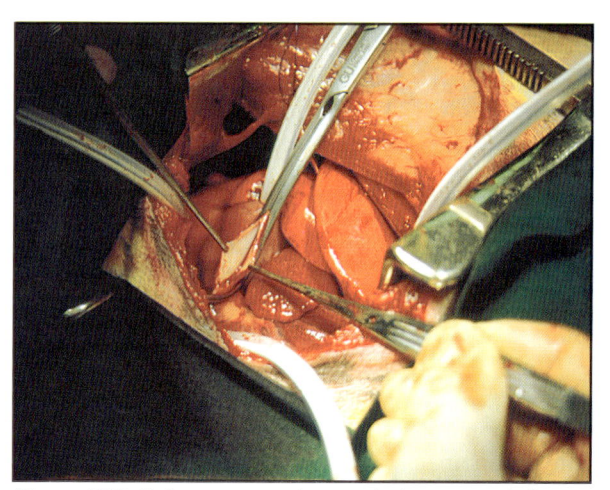

Figure 27.8: Pulmonary arteriotomy during venous inflow occlusion in a dog with valvular pulmonic stenosis.

Reproduced from White (1994) with the permission of Veterinary International.

There are few long-term studies available regarding the prognosis following surgical intervention for pulmonic stenosis, but it appears that surgical correction in individuals not in right-sided failure carries a very favourable outlook. All forms of pulmonic stenosis surgery should be considered technically very demanding, and should not be undertaken without careful planning, the relevant surgical expertise and adequate surgical instrumentation.

Aortic stenosis

The three broad forms of aortic stenosis recognized in small animals are supravalvular, valvular and subvalvular. The subvalvular form is the commonest recognized in the dog. Subvalvular aortic stenosis (SAS) can be categorized further into fixed and dynamic forms (Sisson, 1992). Both forms of the stenosis can be accompanied by other congenital cardiac defects including mitral valve dysplasia. Surgical therapeutic options for SAS in the dog include balloon catheter dilation, closed trans-ventricular dilation (Dhokarikar *et al.*, 1995) and open surgical resection (Monnet *et al.*, 1996).

Surgical intervention in dogs with valvular or subvalvular aortic stenosis should be considered for dogs with substantial ventricular hypertrophy and systolic gradients across the stenosis above 75 mmHg. Both forms of valve dilation may be performed without cardiac bypass. Cardiac catheterization with a balloon catheter is usually performed via one of the carotid arteries and requires radiographic image intensification (fluoroscopy). Transventricular dilation of the aortic valve may be accomplished via either a median stenotomy or a left fifth lateral thoracotomy. A

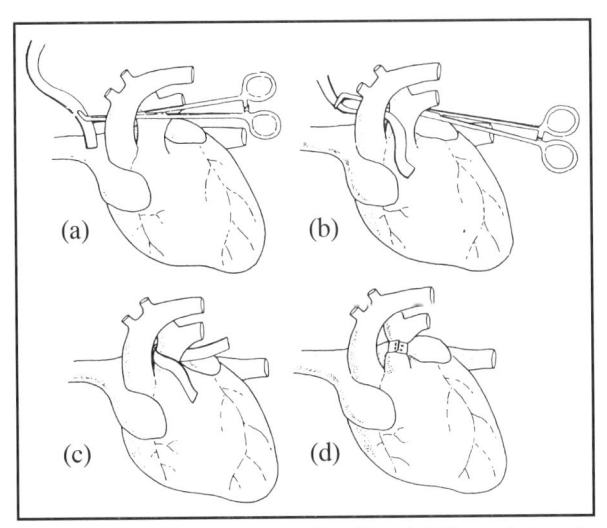

Figure 27.9: *Pulmonary artery banding. (a) The technique is illustrated with a right-angle clamp passed around the aorta to enable an umbilical tape to be placed between the aorta and the pulmonary artery. (b,c) The clamp is passed through the transverse sinus, which delivers the band around the pulmonary artery. (d) The band is tightened to reduce pulmonary flow.*

Reproduced from White (1994) with the permission of Veterinary International.

buttressed mattress suture tourniquet (2-0 to 0 polypropylene) is placed in the left ventricular apex. The relevant sized valve dilator is passed through a ventricular stab incision. The dilator is positioned across the stenosis by palpation of the tip of the instrument in the ascending aorta. The valve dilator is opened to dilate the subvalvular ring or split fused commissures of the valve cusps. It is suggested that, although both dilatory procedures carry a low mortality, neither results in long-term reduction to the systolic pressure gradient.

With the advent of cardiopulmonary bypass in small animals, techniques involving the open resection of SAS lesions appear to hold the most promise for the treatment of this condition in the dog. Correction is performed via an aortotomy performed through a right fourth intercostal thoracotomy. Aortic leaflets are gently retracted revealing the subvalvular fibrous ridge which is sharply excised. Care must be taken not to damage the anterior leaflet of the mitral valve or the conduction tissues located in the septum.

Ventricular septal defects

Most isolated ventricular septal defects (VSDs) in the dog and the cat occur in the membranous region of the interventricular septum below the aortic valve on the left side, and are covered by the cranial (anterior) aspect of the tricuspid septal leaflet on the right side (infracrista ventricularis lesion) (Weirich and Blevins, 1978). Lesions rarely occur below the pulmonic valve (supracrista ventricularis lesion) or in the muscular region of the interventricular septum.

Surgical therapy for VSDs involves either the palliative procedure of pulmonary artery banding to reduce pulmonary blood flow, or closure of the defect during an open heart procedure. Surgical intervention should be considered for a large, haemodynamically significant VSD. Definitive patch closure of a VSD can be accomplished during cardiopulmonary bypass in dogs over 15 kg in body weight. A perimembranous (infracrista ventricularis) lesion may be corrected from the left side via a right ventriculotomy approach.

If the primary repair of the lesion is not technically feasible, palliative pulmonary artery banding should be considered (Figure 27.9) (Eyster *et al.*, 1977). The procedure can be performed via a left lateral fourth intercostal thoracotomy. The pericardium is opened and dissection between the aorta and pulmonary artery reveals a plane for passage of right-angled forceps between the great vessels. The blades are first passed around the aorta, and the banding tape (umbilical tape) is pulled through between the aorta and pulmonary artery. The forceps are then passed in a cranial direction through the transverse sinus, a recess between the anterior surface of the atrial chambers and the posterior surface of the great arteries. The end of the tape is passed through the sinus so that it now surrounds the pulmonary artery. This technique avoids direct dissection around the delicate pulmonary artery. The band can now be tightened with the aim of reducing the pressure in the pulmonary artery to half or just less than half the systemic pressure, so that a balance is achieved between pulmonary and aortic blood flow (Figure 27.10). The exact degree of narrowing of the pulmonary artery can be difficult to judge, and requires the measurement of the pressure in the pulmonary artery distal to the band. This pressure is compared with the systemic pressure measured via a direct arterial pressure line. Once the appropriate pressure in the distal pulmonary artery has been achieved the two strands of the band are sutured together to maintain the required diameter before it is tied with multiple square knots. If the band is tied too tightly, hypoxaemia will result; pulse oximetry can be used during the ligation procedure to assess arterial oxygen saturation. Thoracotomy closure, after the placement of a thoracic drain, is routine.

If the technique is performed on very immature animals, subsequent growth and maturation may produce a relative narrowing of the pulmonary artery at the banding site. This may produce excessive constriction of the pulmonary artery and pulmonary hypoperfusion. Few long-term follow-up studies following surgical therapy for VSDs are available, but primary closure should be curative, while the results of pulmonary artery banding depend on the adequate reduction in pulmonary blood flow. If the right and left side of the heart become balanced the long-term prognosis should be favourable (Eyster *et al.*, 1977).

Mitral valve disease

Although mitral valve disease is commonly recognized in the dog, there have until recently been few reports describing surgical therapies for the management of valvular disorders. With the availability of safe cardiopulmonary bypass techniques, open correction for mitral valve disease has become a therapeutic possibility. Therapeutic options include valvuloplasty, annuloplasty and valve replacement. The valve is exposed via a left atriotomy. Valvuloplasty techniques attempt to reconstruct a damaged, regurgitant valve to one which is competent and of normal diameter. Annuloplasty techniques generally attempt to narrow the dilated valve annulus thus narrowing the mitral valve ring to the correct size, allowing the cusps to meet and making the valve competent.

Valve prostheses fall into two categories; tissue and mechanical valves. There is no perfect valve substitute but porcine bioprosthetic valves, unlike mechanical valves, generally do not require lifetime anticoagulation minimizing the risks of anticoagulant-related bleeding (Figure 27.11). Valve replacement relies on the availability of these valves from the human field. There is also a question regarding the lifespan of such devices in the dog, although recent reports suggest long-term successful outcomes are possible (White *et al.*, 1995, 1997).

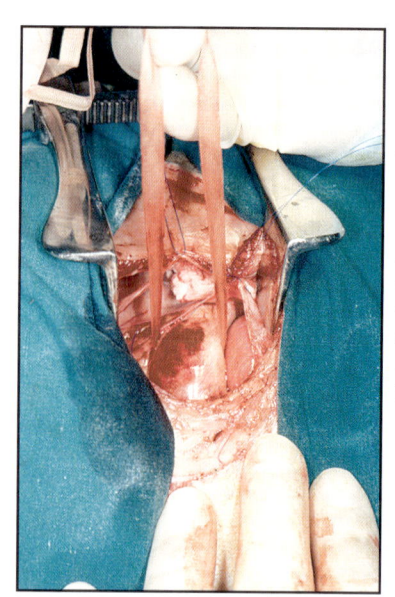

Figure 27.10: A length of umbilical tape has been passed around the main pulmonary artery. The band can now be tightened to reduce the pressure in the pulmonary artery to half or just less than half the systemic pressure.

Reproduced from White (1994) with the permission of Veterinary International.

Tetralogy of Fallot

The condition of tetralogy of Fallot comprises a combination of pulmonary outflow tract obstruction, ventricular septal defect (VSD), overriding of the aorta and right ventricular hypertrophy. The haemodynamically most important abnormalities are the large VSD situated just below the non-coronary and right coronary cusps of the aortic valve, and the pulmonary outflow tract obstruction which results in a decrease in pulmonary blood flow (Ringwald and Bonagura, 1988). The combination of a VSD and pulmonic stenosis alone may produce clinical signs which are indistinct from those seen when all four components of the tetralogy are present.

The primary surgical repair requires cardiopulmonary bypass and consists of closing the VSD, relieving the pulmonary outflow tract obstruction by resection of the excessive infundibular muscle, and enlargement of the valve annulus by ventriculotomy/pulmonary arteriotomy and insertion of a transannular patch-graft.

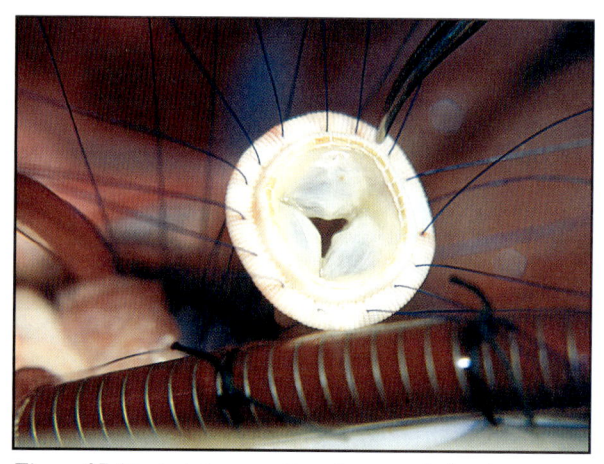

Figure 27.11: An intraoperative photograph showing a porcine bioprosthetic valve being sutured to the mitral valve annulus via a left atriotomy.

Palliative surgical corrections for the disorder attempt to increase pulmonary blood flow and consist of creating a left-to-right vascular shunt between a systemic artery and the pulmonary artery. The easiest of these procedures to perform is a modified Blalock/Taussig anastomosis. The approach is via a left lateral fourth intercostal thoracotomy. The left subclavian artery is identified running in the cranial mediastinum dorsal to the brachycephalic artery. It is dissected along its length as far cranially as possible. It is then ligated and divided as far distally as possible. A bulldog clamp is placed on the proximal end of the divided artery to prevent haemorrhage. The artery is swung towards the pulmonary artery. It is important that it does not become kinked by this procedure, as this will reduce blood flow along its length. An end-to-side anastomosis can then be performed between the free end of the subclavian artery and the main pulmonary artery. A vascular partial occlusion clamp can be used on the pulmonary artery while the anastomosis is completed, to allow the procedure to be undertaken with a beating heart. The left internal thoracic artery may be considered as an alternative to the left subclavian artery in cases where subclavian artery kinking is likely (Holmberg *et al.*, 1985). Kinking can also be prevented by harvesting an autogenous arterial graft by ligation and division of the proximal left subclavian artery. Vascular clamps are placed on the pulmonary artery and ascending aorta. Incisions are made in each vessel and an end-to-side anastomosis is performed to each vessel using 5-0 polypropylene suture. The diameter of the subclavian artery limits the systemic flow of blood to the lungs so that they do not become overperfused. Another advantage of the technique is that the subclavian artery grows with the patient so that the flow to the lungs increases to compensate for the growth of the individual. Closure is routine following the placement of a thoracic drain.

Cor triatrium dexter

Subdivision of the right atrium into cranial and caudal chambers by an anomalous membrane is referred to as cor triatrium dexter. The dividing membrane arises as a result of persistence of the embryological right sinus venosus valve. The most common clinical presentation is abdominal distention caused by ascites and systemic venous congestion of the caudal half of the body. Jugular distension is absent. The clinical signs are usually seen at a very young age. Diagnosis may be confirmed with echocardiography and selective angiography. Successful surgical management has been achieved by splitting or cutting the dividing membrane (septectomy) via a right atriotomy under inflow occlusion.

Miscellaneous

Many of the other congenital cardiac conditions can be treated surgically, but most require the use of cardio-pulmonary bypass. Continued advancements in the techniques of cardiopulmonary bypass will allow this condition, and many of the other defects such as atrial septal defects, persistent truncus arteriosus, transposition of the great arteries and common atrioventricular canal, to become amenable to surgical correction.

CARDIOPULMONARY BYPASS

The essential purpose of cardiopulmonary bypass (CPB) is to provide a stilled, bloodless heart with blood flow temporarily diverted to an extracorporeal circuit that functionally replaces the heart and lungs. Modern CPB will provide respiratory, circulatory and thermoregulatory functions. Respiratory function supports adequate and controllable carbon dioxide elimination in accordance with carbon dioxide production, to maintain the arterial carbon dioxide concentration in a desired range for the temperature of the blood. It also will provide oxygen transport to the blood which matches body oxygen consumption. Circulatory function of CPB maintains a desired perfusion pressure and flow while minimizing trauma to the formed elements of the blood. The thermoregulatory functions of CPB are complex, but essentially it will allow body temperature to be decreased, which in turn lowers body metabolism. Hypothermia will also permit the use of lower blood flows, thereby decreasing blood trauma. Profound hypothermic levels will reduce metabolism to the point where the body will tolerate total circulatory arrest for extended periods of time without demonstrable cellular destruction. CPB may also provide flaccid hyperkalaemic myocardial arrest and hypothermic myocardial preservation by actively cooling the heart with cold cardioplegic solutions. The last thermoregulatory function of CPB is to restore the individual to normothermia prior to termination of the procedure.

The essential elements of the CPB machine and circuit are shown in Figure 27.12. Desaturated blood exits the patient's vena cava through the venous cannula(e) and is drained by gravity through a large bore polyvinyl chloride tubing into a venous blood reservoir. The blood is drawn from this reservoir by the roller pump and then passes through the membrane oxygenator. One or more cardiotomy sucker lines will allow heparinized blood to be removed from the operative field and returned to the venous reservoir. The oxygenated blood then flows through an arterial filter and back through the arterial cannula to either the femoral artery or the aorta. The circuit is generally primed with a non-blood solution (lactated Ringer's) which is fully heparinized. During CPB any drugs required by the patient are added to the venous reservoir of the bypass circuit. In preparation for CPB the patient must be fully heparinized so that blood coagulation within the CPB circuit does not occur. At the end

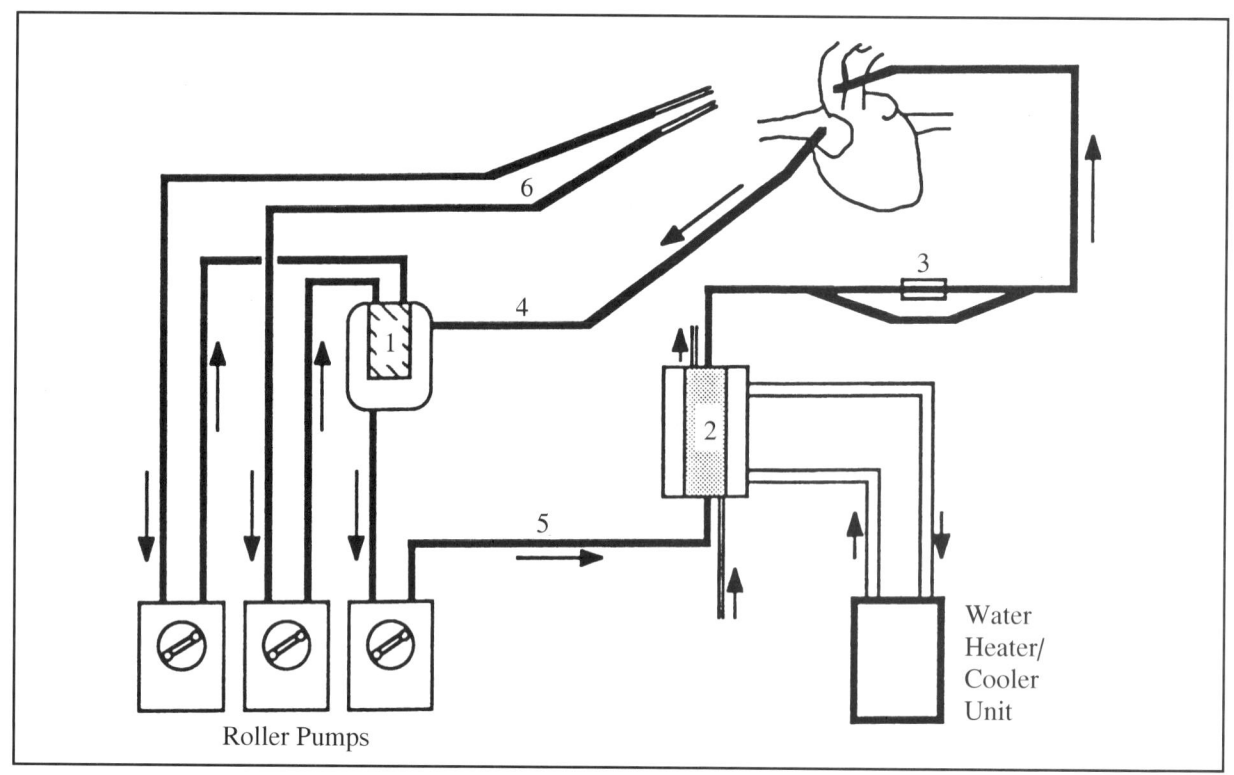

Figure 27.12: The essential elements of a CPB circuit. (1) Venous reservoir. (2) Membrane oxygenator which incorporates a heat exchange unit. (3) Arterial line blood filter and bubble trap. (4) Venous line siphoning blood from the right atrium/vena cava to the venous reservoir. (5) Main pump line taking blood from the venous reservoir and pumping it through the oxygenator before returning it to the patient via the arterial line and the aortic cannulation site. (6) Cardiotomy sucker lines returning free blood from the operative field to the venous reservoir.

Reproduced from White (1994) with the permission of Veterinary International.

of the bypass procedure, once all the cannulae have been removed, the anticoagulation is reversed with protamine sulphate.

All of the intracardiac surgical repairs can be technically better performed on a stilled heart which can be opened. Once all the technical problems of placing an animal on cardiopulmonary bypass have been overcome, it is likely that the most effective intracardiac repairs will be achieved in this way.

PACEMAKER IMPLANTATION

The implantation of an artificial pacemaker for the heart is indicated in both dogs and cats suffering from the following conditions which are medically unresponsive and for which no primary disease can be identified.

- High grade second degree atrioventricular (AV) block
- Complete AV block
- Persistent atrial standstill
- Sinus bradycardia
- Sinus arrest
- Sinoatrial (SA) block
- Bradycardia–tachycardia syndrome
- 'sick sinus syndrome'.

The artificial pacemaker has two major components; the pulse generator which contains the micro-circuitry and the battery, and the lead which delivers the electrical impulse to the myocardium. Pulse generators are manufactured to perform different functions. These functions are letter coded on the external surface of the pacemaker casing. Generally, in the veterinary field, pulse generators with ventricle pace and ventricle sense are used. These are usually fixed rate, although some have certain functions such as the discharge rate which can be programmed.

The leads can be divided into those with either epicardial or endocardial placement electrodes.

- Epicardial electrode leads are implanted with the electrode placed into the myocardium on the surface of the heart
- Endocardial electrode leads are implanted within the right ventricle.

The leads can be further classified into either unipolar or bipolar configurations.

- The unipolar system has the cathode (–) electrode at the tip of the lead and the anode (+) electrode as the pulse generator casing. In this configuration the pacing current has to pass through the body tissues to complete the circuit

- The bipolar system has both the anode and cathode electrodes near the tip of the pacemaker lead. In this configuration the pacing current only has to travel a very short distance to complete the circuit.

These configurations affect the electrical characteristics of the lead systems. The bipolar system has a high resistance to electromagnetic interference, whereas the unipolar system has superior sensing characteristics.

An external pacemaker is considered essential if the procedure of pacemaker implantation is to be carried out safely. In conjunction with an endocardial lead placed into the right ventricle via an external jugular vein, it will allow the heart to be temporarily paced during the anaesthetic and surgical procedure. This should be considered mandatory for the implantation of epicardial leads. An electrocardiogram (ECG) should be monitored throughout the implantation procedure and cardiac resuscitative drugs should be available in the event of an emergency. Successful pacing will generate a pulse rate equal to that set by the pulse generator and a characteristic ECG which includes pacing spikes.

Epicardial lead placement

Epicardial lead placement requires the implantation of the electrode into the apex of the left ventricle. Three basic approaches are described:

- Lateral fifth intercostal thoracotomy (right or left)
- Cranial midline laparotomy and partial caudal midline sternotomy
- Cranial midline laparotomy and transdiaphragmatic approach.

All three methods require the exposure of the apex of the left ventricle. An avascular insertion site on the ventricular wall is chosen and the corkscrew tip of the epicardial lead is implanted into the myocardium. Epicardial leads are usually packaged with an insertion tool which allows firm and proper placement. The pulse generator is sited in a superficial site so that it can be easily replaced should it malfunction in the future. The site of placement is also governed by which approach to the heart is performed. The generator is commonly placed subcutaneously behind the last rib following a lateral thoracotomy (Yoshioka *et al.*, 1981), whereas it may be placed within the cranial abdomen following both the transdiaphragmatic and median sternotomy approaches (Fox *et al.*, 1986). Sufficient slack lead should be left in the thorax to prevent any tension being placed on the epicardial insertion site. For all systems, the unipolar system is activated when the circuit is completed by placing the generator

against the internal body tissues. The bipolar system becomes active when the lead is connected to the pulse generator and, unlike the unipolar system, this process is unaffected by the position of the pulse generator.

Endocardial lead placement

Endocardial lead placement requires the transvenous implantation of the electrode in the chamber of the right ventricle (Darke *et al.*, 1989; Sisson *et al.*, 1991). The procedure can be carried out under heavy sedation and with local anaesthesia. Venous access is usually gained via either the left or right external jugular vein. The neck of the individual is clipped on the proposed side and aseptically prepared. Local anaesthetic is infiltrated at the level of the external jugular vein and dorsally for the placement of the pulse generator. A small skin incision is made over the external jugular vein and the vein is exposed by a combination of sharp and blunt dissection. A 5-0 polypropylene purse-string suture is placed in the lateral wall of the vein. A stab incision is made into the vein within the purse-string and the lead is inserted caudal into the vein lumen. The lead is directed into the apex of the right ventricle under fluoroscopic guidance. A wire stylet passed down a central lumen of the lead will aid this procedure. The lead can be connected to a temporary external pacemaker while a subcutaneous pocket is created for the pulse generator via a second dorsally placed incision. The lead is secured within the right ventricle by suturing it to the cutaneous tissues surrounding its entrance site to the external jugular vein. The portion of lead that is outside the vein can then be passed through a subcutaneous tunnel to the pulse generator pouch. The lead is then attached to the pulse generator which is placed within its pocket. The pocket and the vein incision site are closed with non-absorbable suture. The neck should be bandaged for 5–7 days to prevent the animal from interfering with the surgical site, and to minimize the formation of a seroma within the pulse generator pocket. This procedure is simple and quick to perform and when performed carefully, lead dislodgement from the ventricle is rare. In most cases the lead placement can be undertaken under sedation, and should anaesthesia be required for the surgical formation of the pocket, this can safely be achieved once the animal is temporarily externally paced.

Ideally, for all systems of implantation, the pacing and sensing thresholds of the patient should be measured during the implantation procedure. A pacing systems analyser is required to perform this procedure and the information can be used to assess whether the electrode has been sited optimally. Some external pacemaker units can also be used to estimate the patient threshold at the time of temporary pacing during the implantation procedure.

REFERENCES AND FURTHER READING

Breznock EM and Wood GL (1976) A patch-graft technique for correction of pulmonic stenosis in dogs. *Journal of the American Veterinary Medical Association* **169**, 1090-1094

Brownlie SE, Cobb MA, Chambers J, Jackson G and Thomas S (1991) Percutaneous balloon valvuloplasty in four dogs with pulmonic stenosis. *Journal of Small Animal Practice* **32**, 165-169

Buchanan JW (1990) Pulmonic stenosis caused by single coronary artery in dogs: four cases (1965-1984). *Journal of the American Veterinary Medical Association* **196**, 115-120

Cobb MA, Boswood A, Griffin GM and McEvoy FJ (1996) Percutaneous balloon pericardiotomy for the management of malignant pericardial effusion in two dogs. *Journal of Small Animal Practice* **37**, 549-551

Darke PGG, McAreavey D and Been M (1989) Transvenous cardiac pacing in 19 dogs and one cat. *Journal of Small Animal Practice* **30**, 491-499

Dhokarikar P, Caywood DD, Ogburn PN, Stobie D and Burtnick NL (1995) Closed aortic valvotomy: a retrospective study in 15 dogs. *Journal of the American Animal Hospital Association* **31**, 402-410

Ellison GW (1980) Vascular ring anomalies in the dog and cat. *Compendium of Continuing Education for the Practising Veterinarian* **2**, 693-705

Eyster GE, Whipple RD, Evans AT, Hough JD and Anderson LK (1975) Recanalised patent ductus arteriosus in the dog. *Journal of Small Animal Practice* **16**, 743-749

Eyster GE, Whipple RD, Anderson LK, Evans AT and O'Handley P (1977) Pulmonary artery banding for ventricular septal defect in dogs and cats. *Journal of the American Veterinary Medical Association* **170**, 434-438

Fox PR, Matthiesen DT, Purse D and Brown NO (1986) Ventral abdominal, transdiaphragmatic approach for implantation of cardiac pacemakers in the dog. *Journal of the American Veterinary Medical Association* **189**, 1303-1308

Holmberg DL, Bowen V, Pharr JW and Kruth S (1985) Microsurgical management of tetralogy of Fallot in a cat. *Journal of the American Veterinary Medical Association* **186**, 708-709

Hurley K, Miller MW, Willard MD and Boothe HW (1993) Left aortic arch and right ligamentum arteriosum causing esophageal obstruction in a dog. *Journal of the American Veterinary Medical Association* **203**, 410-412

Jackson WF and Henderson RA (1979). Ligature placement in closure of patent ductus arteriosus. *Journal of the American Animal Hospital Association* **15**, 55-58

Komtebedde J, Ilkiw JE, Follette DM, Breznock EM and Tobias AH (1993) Resection of subvalvular aortic stenosis - surgical and perioperative management in seven dogs. *Veterinary Surgery* **22**, 419-430

Malik R, Church DB and Hunt GB (1993) Valvular pulmonic stenosis in bullmastiffs. *Journal of Small Animal Practice* **34**, 288-292

Martin MWS, Godman M, Luis Fuentes V, Clutton RE, Haigh A and Darke PGG (1992) Assessment of balloon pulmonary valvuloplasty in six dogs. *Journal of Small Animal Practice* **33**, 443-449

Monnet E, Orton E, Gaynor JS, Boon J, Wagner A, Linn K, Eddleman LA and Brevard S (1996) Open resection for subvalvular aortic stenosis in dogs. *Journal of the American Veterinary Medical Association* **209**, 1255-1261

Orton EC, Bruecker KA and McCracken TO (1990) An open patch-graft technique for correction of pulmonic stenosis in the dog. *Veterinary Surgery* **19**, 148-154

Ringwald RJ and Bonagura JD (1988) Tetralogy of Fallot in the dog: clinical findings in 13 cases. *Journal of the American Animal Hospital Association* **24**, 33-43

Sisson D (1992) Fixed and dynamic subvalvular aortic stenosis in dogs. In: *Current Veterinary Therapy XI*, ed. RW Kirk and JD Bonagura, pp 760-766, WB Saunders, Philadelphia

Sisson D, Thomas WP, Woodfield J, Pion PD, Luethy M and Delellis LA (1991) Permanent transvenous pacemaker implantation in forty dogs. *Journal of Veterinary Internal Medicine* **5**, 322-331

Thomas WP and Reed JR (1986) Pericardial disease. In: *Current Veterinary Therapy IX*, ed. RW Kirk. WB Saunders, Philadelphia

Weirich WE and Blevins WE (1978) Ventricular septal defect repair. *Veterinary Surgery* **7**, 2-7

White RN (1994) Cardiac surgery in companion animals. *Veterinary International* **6**, 3-24

White RN, Boswood A, Garden OA and Hammond RA (1997) Surgical management of subvalvular aortic stenosis and congenital mitral dysplasia in a golden retriever. *Journal of Small Animal Practice* **38**, 251-255

White RN, Stepien RL, Hammond RA, Holden DJ, Torrington AM, Milner HR, Cobb MA and Hellens SJ (1995) Mitral valve replacement for the treatment of congenital mitral valve dysplasia in a bull terrier. *Journal of Small Animal Practice* **36**, 407-410

Yoshioka MM, Tilley LP, Harvey HJ, Wayne ES, Lombard CW and Schollmeyer M (1981) Permanent pacemaker implantation in the dog. *Journal of the American Animal Hospital Association* **17**, 746-750

Pulmonary Surgery

Martin Sullivan

INTRODUCTION

Regardless of the disease that has necessitated the need for surgery to the lungs, the surgical techniques available all follow very similar general principles. To avoid repetition when dealing with individual conditions, it is simpler to describe the broad approach and focus on specific variations when dealing with individual diseases.

ANATOMY

The bronchial tree commences at the bifurcation of the trachea dorsal to the heart. The bifurcation is located beneath the fifth intercostal space from a surgical point of view. At the hilus of the lung, each bronchus is accompanied by a pulmonary artery and vein, with a smaller but significant bronchial artery. The pulmonary veins lie ventro-medially, the left arteries dorso-caudally, and the right arteries ventro-lateral relative to the bronchi (Figure 28.1). The bronchial arteries are usually single, but in a significant number of cases (10%), there may be double bronchial arteries. Lung parenchyma is spongy, and provides poor grip for suture material.

Site and approach

As pulmonary surgery is not an everyday practice for most veterinary surgeons, it is essential to identify the location of the lesion as far as side and lobe are concerned. Failure to do so will thwart good surgery and may even be embarrassing. The lesion should be identified with the aid of pre- and post-drainage radiographs where appropriate. As a general rule, the lungs are best approached via the fifth intercostal space, since the hilus is located beneath this intercostal space:

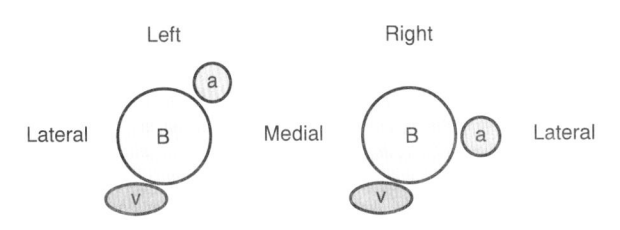

Figure 28.1: Anatomy of the bronchial vessels.

where adhesions are suspected caudally, then the sixth intercostal space will provide more room for manoeuvre. The instruments and detailed approach are given elsewhere (see Chapter 24).

Stapling devices
Stapling devices are expensive, but they significantly reduce surgery time, because there is reduced dissection and no need to place ligatures. The most appropriate device is a linear stapler.

Partial lobectomy

Indications
The main indications for partial lobectomy are lesions located in the middle and distal thirds of lung lobes:

- Cyst/bullae
- Small abscess
- Small tumour
- Laceration
- Biopsy of discrete and diffuse lung disease.

Option 1
The affected lobe is exteriorized, and the area to be resected is isolated from the rest of the lobe by placing one or two crushing forceps across normal lung. A continuous horizontal mattress of 1.5–2 m polyglactin 910 is placed 0.5 cm proximal to the crushing forceps. Once placed, the portion of lung is resected by cutting close to and proximal to the forceps. This leaves an edge of lung tissue that has not been damaged; and is finely oversewn with 1–1.5 m polyglactin 910 (Figure 28.2).

Option 2
Alternatively, if a linear stapler is available, it may be used to resect and close the lung. The area of lung to be resected is isolated from the rest of the lung by the stapler, which is then screwed down to crush the tissue, bringing the staples and anvil into line. A single cartridge of staples is fired to produce two staple lines and the lung is cut distal to the stapler.

After the lung tissue has been removed, the pleural cavity is flooded with enough sterile saline to check for

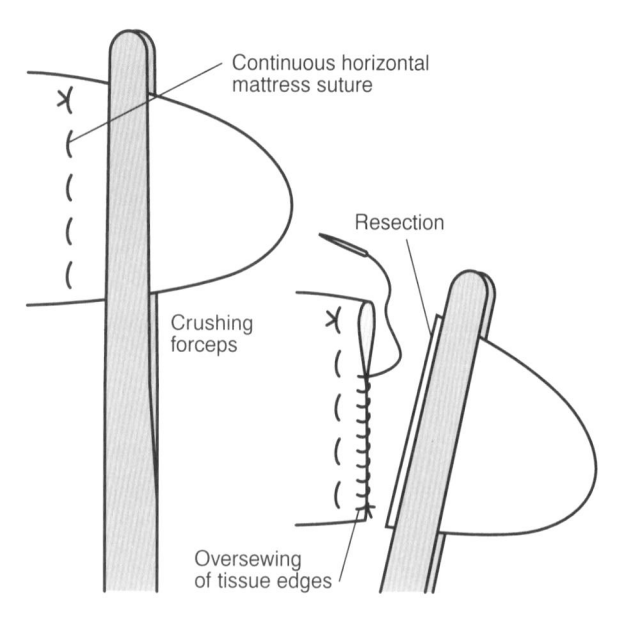

Figure 28.2: Partial lobectomy: use of sutures.

leakage from the now submerged suture line. Minor leaks can be ignored, but larger leaks should be stopped with additional sutures. Residual fluid is aspirated from the chest, a drain placed and the thorax closed.

Complete lobectomy

Indications

- Large emphysematous bullae
- Tumour
- Abscess
- Bronchiectasis
- Bronchial foreign body
- Lobe torsion.

A standard fifth intercostal approach is used to reach the hilus. Normal lobes are packed off with soaked swabs.

Option 1
The pleura and perihilar connective tissue are dissected dorsally to clear a path to the lobar artery, which should be ligated first to quench blood flow to the lobe. Dissection down onto the artery should be cautious, and fine Metzenbaum scissors or haemostats are suggested. The artery is not crushed with forceps, but a double loop of ligating material (2–2.5 m absorbable suture material) is passed between the vessel and the bronchus. The loop is cut and the artery is double ligated, with care taken to place the sutures without dragging on the artery. A third transfixing suture is then placed through the artery between these two ligatures, but close to the proximal suture. The artery may then be transected. The lobe is retracted dorsally to expose the medial aspect of the lung and the pulmonary vein. As the pulmonary vein is fairly fragile

and easily lacerated, extreme care must be taken dissecting around the vessel to allow ligature placement. The bronchus is cleared of any residual connective tissue and crushed with two forceps. The bronchus is sectioned between the two forceps and the lung lobe removed. To close the bronchus, it is first necessary to collapse the annular lumen of the bronchus. This is achieved by placing 2–2.5 m monofilament nylon horizontal mattress sutures through the cartilage of a bronchial ring proximal to the clamp. Enough space should be left to permit a further more distal row of sutures to be placed in the membranous portion of the bronchus between the clamp and the suture line. The bronchus is transected close to the clamp on the proximal aspect. The free membranous edge, which has not been damaged by the clamp, is now oversewn with a simple continuous layer of 1.5–2 m polyglactin 910 (Figure 28.3). Residual debris is removed from the chest and the suture line tested for leaks by covering the stump with saline. If any occur, then additional sutures are placed. Once all but minor leaks have been stopped, the pleura and connective tissue at the hilus are brought together to cover the stump. This helps to reduce postoperative air leakage and also reduces postoperative adhesions.

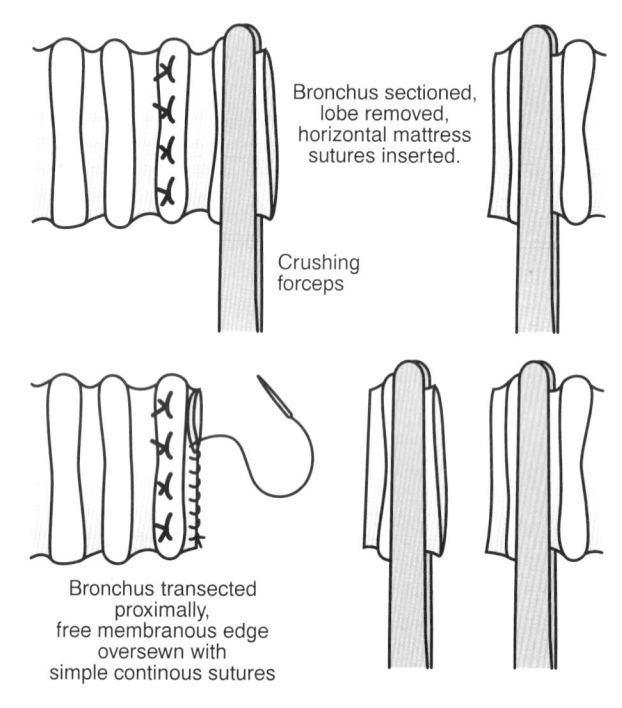

Figure 28.3: Complete lobectomy.

Lung abscess and bronchiectasis
Care must be taken to mop any spillage from the cut bronchus with a moistened swab to prevent contamination of the pleural cavity.

Neoplastic lung lobes
To overcome the difficulty of manipulating the bulky mass of the lobe in the chest, the lung lobe is clamped above the hilus, sectioned and removed to give better

exposure of the pedicle. Lobectomy for lung lobe torsion is also best dealt with by the same type of removal (see Chapter 30). Once the lobe is removed, the more distal clamp is removed and the connective tissue is dissected clear to expose the pedicle. The vessels are then ligated and the closure of the bronchus carried out as already described.

Option 2

A much more satisfying alternative is to use a linear stapler. This avoids the necessity to dissect around the hilus to isolate and clamp the blood vessels and the need to ablate the bronchial lumen and oversew the edges. The stapler is slid alongside the lobe to be removed and turned so that the pedicle lies within the jaws of the stapler. The guard is pushed forwards to prevent tissue escaping and the arm is screwed down to crush the tissue against the anvil and bring the staple cartridge into position. The gun is fired and a double row of staples is placed across the bronchus. The bronchus is sectioned distal to the gun and the lung removed. The staple gun is then removed and the staple line checked for leaks. Whilst the stapling devices are expensive, the time that is saved more than warrants their use.

Pneumonectomy

Pneumonectomy is indicated when a lesion affects one side of the lungs, leaving the contralateral side essentially unaffected. The surgical procedure is the same as for lobectomy, with the exception that the pulmonary artery is meticulously oversewn as well as ligated. This is best done with 1–1.5 m prolene or similar as a simple continuous suture. However, the indications for pneumonectomy are exceedingly rare in veterinary practice.

Thoracic Drainage

Martin Sullivan

INTRODUCTION

The pleural cavity requires drainage in those disease states where it is no longer a potential space. Either air or fluid may become interposed between the visceral and parietal pleura in such volumes as to compromise respiratory function significantly.

The need to drain the pleural cavity in small animals is not an everyday occurrence; furthermore, in many situations the ideal equipment is not to hand and compromises have to be made. The result is that the sort of drain chosen and the manner in which it is maintained may depend largely on available equipment and personnel, on the perceived need and, to a certain extent, on personal preference. Thus three forms of drainage may be considered: single episode drainage, temporary drainage, persistent drainage.

Indications

- Sample acquisition
- Simple pneumothorax
- Recurrent pneumothorax
- Hydrothorax
- Pyothorax
- Chylothorax
- Haemothorax
- Post-thoracotomy drainage to expand lungs
- Pleurodesis.

Types of chest drain

- Wide bore needle
- Large plastic intravenous catheter
- Proprietary trocarred chest cannula
- Intravenous tubing.

All of the above need some form of connector such as a three-way tap, Heimlich valve or multiple bore tube connector, and a means of suction, such as a 50 ml syringe or suction pump.

CLOSED CHEST INSERTION

Thoracocentesis

Single episode drainage is needed once a diagnosis of pleural effusion has been made and the nature of the effusion needs to be determined. Closed chest drainage is done where there is no indication for a thoracotomy to implant the drain, as inspection of the pleural space or thoracic organs is not warranted. In addition, this method may be used where the chest is to be drained on a single occasion towards the end of a thoracotomy. The most frequent indication for closed drainage is where a diagnosis of pleural effusion has been reached and a simple drainage alleviates the respiratory compromise and permits sample acquisition for evaluation of the nature of the effusion.

The animal should be prepared by infiltrating the site of the proposed drain with local anaesthesia. The site will depend on the material to be aspirated and the position of the animal during aspiration (Table 29.1).

Local anaesthetic is infiltrated into the skin directly over the proposed intercostal space, or one and a half intercostal spaces caudally if a large bore drain is going to be used. Local infiltration should also include the intercostal muscles, taking care not to hit the periosteum of the rib, which is very painful for the animal.

Where a single tap is being done with an intravenous needle, care must be taken to avoid laceration of the lung which all too easily occurs as the lung expands with air and rubs along the sharp edge of the needle. In this situation, the needle should penetrate

Positioning	Site for air aspiration		Site for fluid aspiration	
	Space	Location	Space	Location
Lateral recumbency	7th	mid-third	not applicable	not applicable
Sternal recumbency or standing	7th	dorsal third	4th or 7th	ventral third

Table 29.1: Sites for pleural drainage.

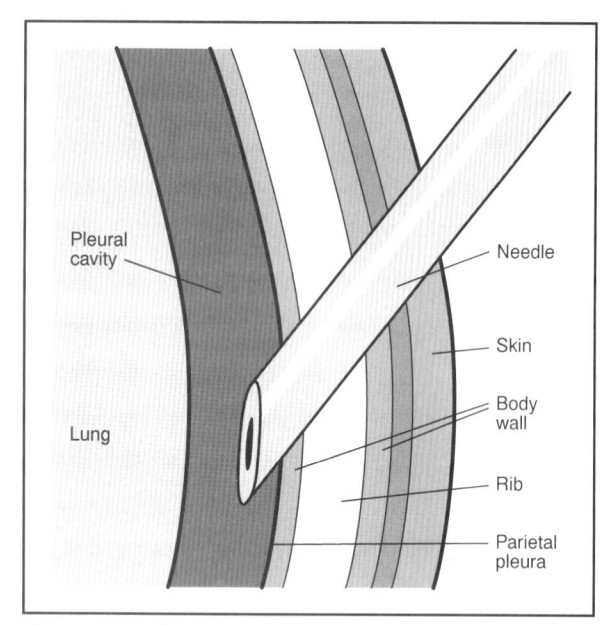

***Figure 29.1:** The needle is orientated so that the bevelled end is parallel to the rib cage.*

the pleural cavity and then be re-directed so that the needle lies somewhat parallel to the ribcage with the bevel facing the lung (Figure 29.1).

This positioning is not possible with a plastic intravenous catheter, which inevitably kinks at the hub. To reduce the risk of lung laceration further, a piece of plastic extension tubing interposed between the syringe and the needle allows manipulation of the three-way tap and syringe without excessive movement being transmitted to the needle. Using a butterfly catheter achieves the same result without having to cobble the extension tubing together.

Tube thoracostomy

A second method, particularly when the fluid is reactive or temporary drainage is required, is to use a commercial thoracic cannula with a trocar, or *thoracostomy tube*. These come in a variety of sizes, but most are designed for use in humans, and an adult cannula can easily be 30 cm in length, which is often too long. Thoracostomy tubes are available in sizes ranging from 14 to 40 French gauge, and the tube diameter should approximate the width of the mainstem bronchus (unless the pleural effusion is very viscous). Smaller cannulae are available. The hubs of these cannulae are generally quite bulky, and great care must be taken to protect these from patient interference, since they are going to be present for a number of days. These cannulae come with a steel luminal trocar, which allows them to be forced into the thorax in very heavily sedated or anaesthetized patients.

Technique

The skin is clipped and prepared for aseptic surgery; in addition, sterile gloves should be worn. A small nick is made in the skin, one and a half to two intercostal

spaces caudal to the eventual point of entry into the chest. The cannula is inserted through the incision and is used to drag the skin forward so that the point of the cannula lies perpendicular to the chosen intercostal space. The cannula should be held loosely in a fist 3–4 cm beneath the hub, so that when the top of the cannula is hit positively with the palm of the other hand, the trocar and cannula will only be driven far enough forward to ensure the parietal pleura is breached (Figure 29.2).

The trocar is then withdrawn enough to allow the point to be sheathed by the cannula, and both are advanced into the chest. The trocar may need to be withdrawn completely to allow the cannula to be pushed cranially and ventrally to lie on the floor of the thorax.

Where these cannulae are not available, a piece of drip tubing can be pressed into service. Five or six small holes are made in the distal end. These can be made by bending the tube back on itself and removing the corner of the fold with scissors to create a hole; this is repeated to fenestrate the tube. The tip of the tube is grasped in medium-sized curved artery forceps and driven through, forwards and into the pleural cavity from a skin incision two intercostal spaces caudal to the entry point into the chest.

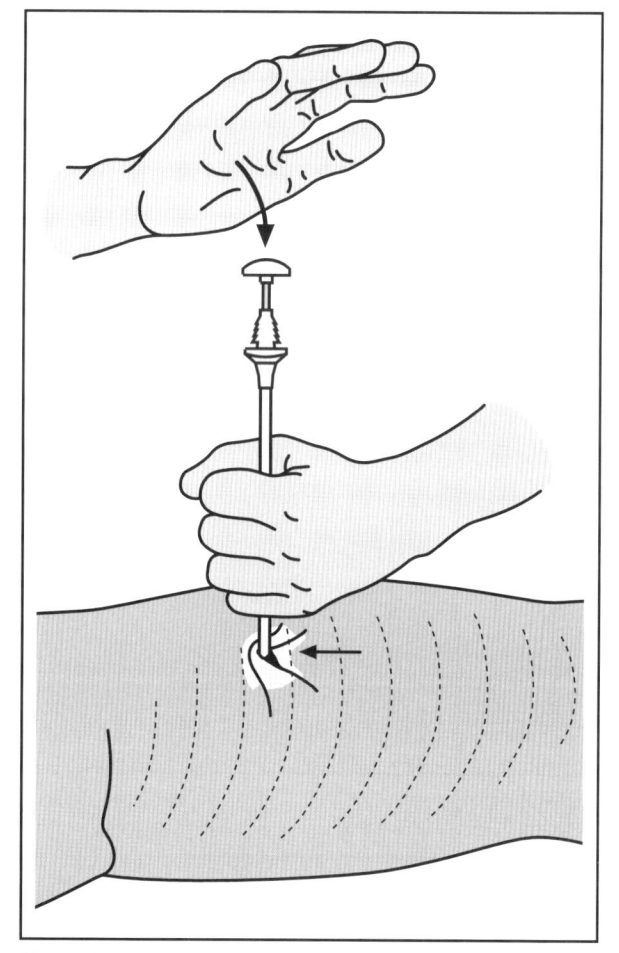

***Figure 29.2:** Tube thoracostomy.*

OPEN CHEST INSERTION

Animals that have had thoracotomies should have residual air and fluid removed towards the end of the surgery once the chest wall has been closed.

Maintenance of chest drains
The type of maintenance necessary will depend on the length of time for which it is anticipated that the tube will be required. For sample acquisition, there is no need for maintenance, since the drain is removed immediately the sample has been obtained. In those animals that have had a thoracotomy, many cases do not need to have the drain left *in situ* and the tube can be removed after drainage. To some ears this might sound heretical, but active animals often dislike 'bits protruding', and are frequently keen to dislodge them. Situations where there is little need to leave a drain are those thoracotomies where the lungs have not been breached, or where there has been little or no pleural effusion before surgery and little produced during surgery.

The keys to successful chest drainage are security of the tube, protection from animal interference, and a method that permits trouble-free drainage. Securing the drain is very important, and best achieved with a Chinese snare (or 'finger-trap') suture to anchor the tube to the skin. Using tape in the form of a butterfly cannot be relied on if the tape becomes wet.

Intermittent drainage
The seal between the suction apparatus and the drain is important. Heimlich valves are very bulky and not very successful in small animals. Three-way taps are very useful, but many prefer to add a clip proximal to the tap to ensure complete occlusion of the tube so that a pneumothorax will not occur if the tap is dislodged. The hub of the drain and the connecting apparatus is best protected by being hidden beneath a soft flexible bandage and layer of cotton wool. An Elizabethan collar is advisable, and the animal should be closely monitored to prevent interference with the tube. The amount of fluid or air aspirated at each occasion should be recorded, and this will guide the frequency of aspiration.

Continuous drainage
Underwater seals are bulky, difficult to manage, and require continuous observation of the animal to prevent the drain being dislodged from the underwater seals. They are thus only suitable for recumbent or inactive animals. Commercial systems are also available for continuous drainage, but still require constant monitoring. Negative pressures of $10-20$ cmH$_2$O are usually adequate for most pleural effusions, although higher pressures may be necessary for pyothorax. Aspiration pressures should not exceed 20 cmH$_2$O

Tube removal
The timing of tube removal depends on the quantity and rate of fluid accumulation. This is usually delayed until less than 4 ml/kg is aspirated per day. The long term presence of a chest drain may initiate an inflammatory response which may actually encourage fluid production. The Chinese snare suture is removed, and the tube is rapidly withdrawn; this may cause some discomfort. The wound should be sutured if necessary, and covered with a dressing for 48 hours.

Complications
The most important complication of the placement of chest drains is pneumothorax, if the end of the tube becomes open to the atmosphere. This can be rapidly fatal. Seroma formation and infection are other possible complications.

Surgery of Pleural and Mediastinal Disease

Claire J.A. Spackman

SURGICAL MANAGEMENT OF PLEURAL DISEASE

Pleural effusion is surgically treated in three ways: by removal of the effusion via tube thoracostomy; by transferring the effusion into the peritoneal cavity or the circulation by pleuroperitoneal or pleurovenous shunting; or by obliteration of the pleural space by pleurodesis.

In some types of pleural effusion, more specific surgical treatment is possible, for example, thoracic duct ligation for idiopathic chylothorax, lung lobectomy for lung lobe torsion and spontaneous pneumothorax, and surgical repair of diaphragmatic hernias.

Tube thoracostomy
Tube thoracostomy is covered in Chapter 25.

Pleuroperitoneal and pleurovenous shunting
Active and passive pleuroperitoneal shunting are used to treat intractable pleural effusions in dogs and cats. This procedure relieves dyspnoea by transferring pleural fluid to the peritoneal cavity, where the greater surface area of the peritoneal membrane allows more complete reabsorption. Analysis of the pleural fluid is a vital first step in using this procedure. Pleuroperitoneal shunting is contraindicated for septic pleural effusion, but may be indicated as a palliative measure with neoplastic effusion and incurable cancer.

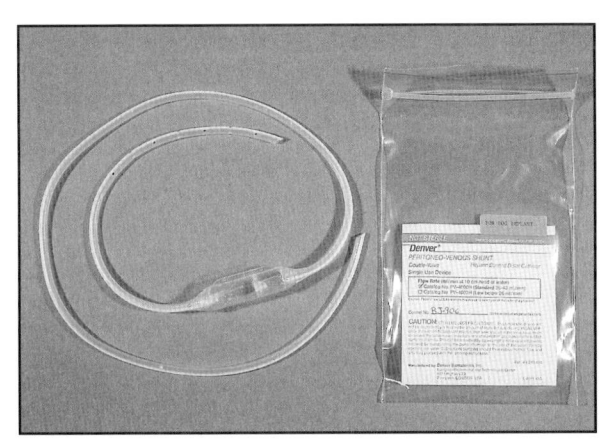

Figure 30.1: The double-valve Denver peritoneal–venous catheter may be used for active pleuroperitoneal shunting.

Active pleuroperitoneal shunting
Double-valve Denver peritoneal–venous catheters (Figure 30.1) have been used successfully in dogs for active pleuroperitoneal shunting. In small dogs and cats, Hakim–Cordis ventricular–peritoneal catheters have been used. Both of these devices are costly. Additional fenestrations are added to the venous portion of the catheter, which is then implanted into the thorax. The catheter is tunnelled subcutaneously under the external abdominal oblique muscle and positioned so that the pump chamber lies over the ninth rib. The peritoneal end is then tunnelled further caudally and placed into the peritoneal cavity through a stab incision or a grid laparotomy. The pump is sutured securely around the rib with non-absorbable suture. External compression of the pump is begun immediately, and is well tolerated by most dogs and cats after the immediate postoperative discomfort has passed. The pump is compressed repeatedly twice a day, each time until it becomes non-compressible. Ascites may be evident for 1–2 weeks postoperatively but does not require treatment.

Active pleuroperitoneal shunting has been used to treat persistent chylothorax. In human neonates, cases treated with shunts resolved within 3 months. Resolution has also been reported in cats (Donner, 1989). One dog treated for persistent non-chylous effusion after ligation of the thoracic duct was well and active 5 years later (Brumm and Smeak, 1992).

Pleurovenous shunting
This technique has also been used successfully in dogs with chylothorax (Willauer and Breznock, 1987). In this procedure, the venous portion of the catheter, which is not fenestrated, is implanted through a pursestring suture into the thoracic vena cava or the azygos vein and advanced to the level of the right atrium. This is technically more demanding surgery than pleuroperitoneal implantation, and may be complicated by fatal haemorrhage or thrombosis.

Passive pleuroperitoneal shunting
This is accomplished by implanting transdiaphragmatic Silastic catheters or by placing fenestrated Silastic sheeting in a defect created in the diaphragm. Pleural

fluid diffuses through these openings, aided by changes in respiratory pressures. This technique has been used in two cats (Peterson *et al.*, 1989), but long-term results in another study were not encouraging. Failure of drainage as a result of adherence of liver or omentum to the mesh was common.

Complications

Reported complications of pleuroperitoneal shunting include clotting of the pump valve, which necessitated replacement of the device; pleural compartmentalization, which was alleviated by placement of a second device on the contralateral side of the chest; and post-caval thrombosis, which was resolved rapidly with systemic anticoagulation. Transient abdominal distension occurs commonly. In very small patients, passive drainage is less technically demanding and less expensive. In addition, active drainage requires daily effort from the animal's owner, whereas passive drainage does not.

Pleurodesis

Pleurodesis (also called pleural sclerosis or pleural symphysis) is a method of treating pleural effusion, either fluid or air, by inducing adhesions between the parietal and visceral pleurae and thus obliterating the pleural space. Pleurodesis is used as a last resort, when other medical and surgical treatments have failed. Both chemical and mechanical methods of pleurodesis have been used.

Chemical pleurodesis is performed by instilling an irritant into the pleural space. Tetracycline is the recommended agent. The suggested procedure is:

- Completely drain the pleural cavity with thoracostomy tube(s) – verify that drainage is complete by radiography
- Instil 35–40 mg/kg of tetracycline diluted in up to 75 ml of sterile H_2O
- Follow with up to 200 ml of air to ensure contact of the tetracycline solution with all pleural spaces
- Rotate the animal to distribute the solution
- Drain the pleural cavity 2 hours later
- Maintain the chest tube until drainage is less than 4 mg/kg per 24 hours.

This procedure is based on that used in human patients, because few successful cases of pleurodesis have been reported in dogs and cats. General anaesthesia has been suggested, and also adding lignocaine, to a concentration of 0.25%, to the tetracycline solution. Pleural drainage is important to allow pleural surfaces to form adhesions and may be needed for 10 days or more. Analgesics may be needed throughout this period. The use of talc to induce adhesions is popular in human medicine and has recently been reported to be safe and effective in dogs.

Mechanical pleurodesis is performed by abrading the pleural surfaces with a dry surgical swab. Median sternotomy is necessary to reach all pleural surfaces. This procedure may cause haemorrhage and air leaks from the lung surfaces. Mechanical pleurodesis may be combined with tetracycline infusion.

Pleurectomy (excision of the parietal pleura) is not recommended, because the resulting haemorrhage and air leaks are severe.

Thoracic duct ligation for chylothorax

Thoracic duct ligation is usually recommended for treatment of idiopathic chylothorax in both dogs and cats. Idiopathic chylothorax is often associated with lymphangiectasia, which can be diagnosed by lymphangiography. If chylothorax is caused by trauma, medical therapy plus tube thoracostomy and drainage of the pleural space is suggested, because a ruptured thoracic duct may heal spontaneously. Continuous pleural drainage is preferred in chylothorax, to speed healing and reduce the risk of fibrosing or constrictive pleuritis (see Chapter 18). Successful treatment of chylothorax associated with thoracic neoplasia or cardiac disease requires correction of the primary disease, and possibly thoracic duct ligation with or without pleuroperitoneal shunting. In all cases, chylothorax must be given a guarded prognosis.

Lymphangiography is carried out by cannulating an abdominal lymphatic vessel. In order to improve visualization of these lymphatics which may be very small, especially in cats, food is withheld for 12 hours before surgery. Starting about three hours before induction of anaesthesia, the patient is fed either corn oil or cream, 2ml/kg, at hourly intervals. Either a paracostal or ventral midline coeliotomy is done, the caecum is exteriorized and a lymph vessel between the caecocolic lymph nodes and the cisterna chyli is isolated by placing 2-0 or 3-0 silk ligatures around it. A 22-gauge catheter is secured with the ligatures and extension tubing attached to it. The abdominal incision is closed around the tubing, which may also be sutured to the body wall for security. A three-way stopcock is attached to the tubing and an aqueous contrast medium (1 ml/kg diluted in 0.5 ml/kg saline) injected. A lateral thoracic radiograph is taken as the injection is completed. A lymphangiogram is used to diagnose lymphangiectasia and ruptures of the thoracic duct, and also to identify branches of the duct which may require ligation. Dogs vary greatly in branching of the thoracic duct.

Technique

Thoracic duct ligation is done through a right lateral thoracotomy at the 10th intercostal space in dogs. In cats, the approach is through a left lateral thoracotomy, at the 10th space, or through an incision in the left diaphragm. Methylene blue (1%) injected into the lymphangiography catheter will improve visualization of the duct but is not recommended if a leak is present, because the dye will spread over the pleural surfaces and make identification of the duct more difficult. The thoracic duct is located dorsolateral to the aorta and ventrolateral to the azygos vein. Haemoclips or silk ligatures are used to ligate the duct and its branches. Haemoclips are preferred because of ease of application and because they may serve as markers if further lymphangiograms are needed. An alternative method is *en bloc* ligation of all structures in the caudal mediastinum dorsal to the aorta, including the azygos vein. This approach should eliminate development of lymphatic anastomoses around the ligated duct, but no success rate for this technique has been reported. Occlusion of the thoracic duct by transcatheter embolization with cyano-acrylate has been successful in experimental work, but the few clinical cases reported had no better rate of success than reported with ligation.

After thoracic duct ligation, lymphangiography is repeated to ensure that ligation is complete. The catheter is removed by removing the body wall suture, if any, and pulling gently on the exteriorized tubing. Following thoracic duct ligation, a thoracostomy tube is kept in the patient. Pleural effusion, either chylous or non-chylous, may persist for some time postoperatively. Drainage of this fluid is important to prevent the very grave complication of fibrosing pleuritis. If thoracic duct ligation is successful, chylous effusion will stop within 1 week after surgery. If fluid production continues and no unligated branches or new anastomoses of the thoracic duct can be identified on repeated lymphangiography, then a shunting procedure or pleurodesis may be done. Alternatively, a pleuroperitoneal or pleurovenous shunt or Silastic transdiaphragmatic tubing or mesh is installed at the same time as thoracic duct ligation.

Complications

The most common complication of thoracic duct ligation is failure to resolve chylothorax. Subcutaneous and peritoneal accumulation of chyle may occur after thoracic duct ligation or occlusion. Other complications are those common to thoracotomy and to thoracostomy tubes. A serious complication of chylothorax is fibrosing or constrictive pleuritis. This condition has been treated by decortication, a surgical technique in which the dense fibrous peel covering the pleura is removed by sharp and blunt dissection. If this technique is done soon after the peel forms, it may be useful; although some degree of pneumothorax will be present postoperatively. With time, however, blood vessels will form which extend from the peel deep into the lung parenchyma. At this stage, decortication is a high-risk technique which may result in severe haemorrhage as well as pneumothorax. Decortication may also be used to treat constrictive pleuritis secondary to haemothorax and pyothorax.

Lung lobectomy for lung lobe torsion

Treatment of lung lobe torsion is by thoracocentesis and lobectomy of the affected lobe. A thoracostomy tube is used to drain the pleural cavity before general anaesthesia and maintained postoperatively. The affected lobe(s) is determined by radiography after the chest has been drained. Lateral thoracotomy is the best approach and should be used unless bilateral torsions are present. Lobectomy can be done from a median sternotomy approach, but isolation of the hilar structures is more difficult. Instead of individually ligating the pulmonary artery, vein and bronchus, in lung lobe torsion the entire twisted pedicle is clamped with large non-crushing forceps and the lobe is excised. The stump is then divided into its anatomical components and ligated, using monofilament suture. This technique minimizes the risk of releasing toxins from the often necrotic lung tissue into the circulatory system, which may happen if the torsion is reduced before lobectomy.

Complications

Complications of lobectomy for lung lobe torsion include pneumothorax, haemothorax, and occurrence of torsion in another lobe. The thoracostomy tube is kept in place until pleural effusion has ceased. Any developing haemothorax or pneumothorax will be easily detected. If pleural effusion persists or redevelops, the chest must be drained completely and the patient radiographed again. If a second lobe has twisted, a second lobectomy is performed, but the prognosis is much worse. Afghan Hounds may be more prone to develop torsion of a second lung lobe and should perhaps be given a more guarded prognosis. Dogs can tolerate acute resection of approximately 50% of the total lung mass.

Partial lobectomy is often used for an isolated pulmonary bulla, which is one cause of spontaneous pneumothorax. If a bulla is located in the proximal one-third of a lung lobe, removal of the entire lobe is indicated. If multiple small bullae (sometimes called pulmonary blebs, and sometimes numbering in the hundreds) are scattered over the surface of several lobes, pleurodesis is the only surgical option. Median sternotomy is the best approach for exploration in cases of spontaneous pneumothorax, because all of the lung can be assessed and pleurodesis, if needed, may be done at the same surgery.

Correction of diaphragmatic hernia

Surgical correction of traumatic diaphragmatic hernia is performed as soon as the patient is stable. Hernia repair done within 24 hours of trauma has a high mortality rate. The only indication for emergency repair is the presence of the stomach in the pleural cavity, because gastric distension causes rapidly fatal lung compression. In these cases, the dilated stomach is decompressed by inserting a hypodermic needle through the left thoracic wall, and surgery follows as quickly as possible. In other cases the animal is treated for shock, given supplemental oxygen if needed, and closely monitored until ready for surgery.

Technique

Midline ventral coeliotomy, starting at the xiphoid and continuing caudally beyond the umbilicus, is the preferred approach. If the hernia is long-standing and adhesions are present within the thorax, the incision is extended by partial median sternotomy of the most caudal sternebrae. The entire diaphragm should be examined, because occasionally multiple hernias are found. Herniated viscera are gently retracted into the abdomen. The hernia may need to be enlarged if herniated liver or spleen is too large to pass through the defect. If the hernia is of more than 2 weeks duration, any adhesions are divided by sharp dissection under direct visualization, because mature adhesions have an excellent blood supply. Early fibrinous adhesions are simply peeled apart. After the liver and spleen are returned to the abdomen, careful examination is made for areas of necrosis; partial resection or lobectomy may be indicated. The liver must be positioned anatomically in the abdomen – accidental twisting of a lobe is easily done.

Hernia repair has been done with many different suture materials and in several different suture patterns. Monofilament non-absorbable suture, such as polypropylene or monofilament nylon, works well. Sizes from 0 to 3-0 metric are appropriate. Simple continuous or continuous locking patterns or simple interrupted sutures are frequently used. Suturing of vertical tears begins at the most dorsal part of the hernia and continues ventrally, with care being taken not to reduce the size of the caval hiatus. In circumcostal tears, which are more common in cats, the torn edge of the diaphragm is brought back to its lateral and ventral position by passing sutures through the diaphragm and around the rib. In all cases a substantial bite of tissue is taken at each pass of the needle.

In fresh hernias and in many chronic hernias, the diaphragm can be closed primarily. If the edges of the hernia cannot be apposed, an abdominal flap graft may be developed from the peritoneum and the transverse abdominal muscle caudal to the diaphragm. Synthetic mesh has often been used, but is associated with a higher rate of complications.

Fluid in the chest should be aspirated before the hernia is closed, and a thoracostomy tube positioned if one is not already in place. Before and during tightening of the last suture in the hernia, the anaesthetist inflates the lungs fully to evacuate as much air as possible from the pleural space. Postoperatively, the thoracostomy tube is kept in place until pleural effusion ceases. If effusion is profuse, re-herniation should be suspected.

Complications

Complications of repair of diaphragmatic hernias are numerous but all are rare, if the patient survives the surgery. Death during or shortly after surgery may be caused by re-perfusion injury of the liver or other viscera. Re-herniation is associated with excessive tension on the suture line, or suture that is too small or that loses strength too quickly. If synthetic mesh is used, chronic inflammation and persistent infection may occur if the mesh is contaminated or if it is not sutured so as to prevent movement against the diaphragm. Hiatal hernia has recently been reported as a postoperative complication of chronic diaphragmatic herniation and also in association with a pleuroperitoneal hernia.

Peritoneo–pericardial diaphragmatic hernias in dogs and cats are congenital defects. Repair in many cases can be done without separating the diaphragm from the pericardium, simply by plicating the diaphragmatic edges from an abdominal approach after reducing the hernia contents. The edges are debrided and closed with a single or double continuous layer of suture. The chest is not opened. With this technique, a pocket of pericardium is formed. If this pocket is large, the air trapped in it is aspirated through the diaphragm with a hypodermic needle. If the hernia is very large, it may be impossible to appose the edges. In this case, the pericardial sac is used, either as a free graft or a flap, to close the defect in the diaphragm. No attempt is made to close the pericardium. This procedure opens the pleural cavity and controlled ventilation must be used.

Complications of repair are rare. Associated congenital defects of the sternum and abdominal wall are corrected during closure of the coeliotomy incision.

Diaphragmatic paralysis

One cause of the dyspnoea seen in bilateral diaphragmatic paralysis is paradoxical cranial displacement of the flaccid diaphragm during inspiration. Surgical tightening of the diaphragm by plication of the central tendinous portion, using interrupted inverting polypropylene sutures, has been suggested to eliminate this movement. A patient in which this technique was used had improved arterial blood gas values (Greene *et al.*, 1988). Plication is even more effective for unilateral paralysis, possibly acting by improving the kinetics of the normal side.

SURGICAL MANAGEMENT OF MEDIASTINAL DISEASE

Surgical exploration of the cranial mediastinum is indicated for biopsy of masses or for surgical removal of neoplasms. Thymoma is the mediastinal neoplasm most commonly treated by surgical resection. Biopsy procedures are performed through a 3rd or 4th intercostal lateral thoracotomy.

Thymectomy

For thymectomy, median sternotomy is the preferred approach, because the entire thoracic cavity is exposed, although a lateral approach is also possible, especially in cats.

The procedure is more easily and successfully done in cats, which often have encapsulated tumours. Thymoma in the dog is more often invasive and may require resection of pleural, pericardial, or lung tissue. A mediastinal lymph node should be removed with the thymoma for staging of the tumour.

Complications

The most common complication of thymectomy is haemorrhage. Careful dissection is required, especially at the craniodorsal margin of the thymus which is adjacent to the cranial vena cava. The phrenic, vagus and recurrent laryngeal nerves and the terminal thoracic duct are also in the cranial mediastinum, as are the oesophagus, trachea, and major arteries. A thoracic drain is placed at surgery; if no haemorrhage or pneumothorax develops, the drain is removed 24 hours later.

REFERENCES AND FURTHER READING

Aronsohn MG, Schunk KL, Carpenter JL and King NW (1984) Clinical and pathological features of thymoma in 15 dogs. *Journal of the American Veterinary Medical Association* **184**, 1355-1362

Auger JM and Riley SM (1997) Combined and pleuroperitoneal hernia in a shar-pei. *Canadian Veterinary Journal* **38**, 640-642

Birchard SJ and Fossum TW (1987) Chylothorax in the dog and cat. *Veterinary Clinics of North America: Small Animal Practice* **17**, 271-283

Birchard SJ and Gallagher L (1988) Use of pleurodesis in treating selected pleural diseases. *Compendium of Continuing Education* **10**, 826-833

Birchard SJ, Smeak DD and Fossum TW (1988) Results of thoracic duct ligation in dogs with chylothorax. *Journal of the American Veterinary Medical Association* **193**, 68-71

Birchard SJ, Smeak DD and McLoughlin MA (1998) Treatment of idiopathic chylothorax in dogs and cats. *Journal of the American Veterinary Medical Association* **212**, 652-657

Bonath KH (1996) Diaphragmatic surgery. In: *Complications in Small Animal Surgery*, 1st edn, ed. AJ Lipowitz, DD Caywood, CD Newton and A Schwartz, pp 245-263. Williams & Wilkins, Baltimore

Bonath KH (1996) Thoracostomy and thoracocentesis. In: *Complications in Small Animal Surgery*, 1st edn, ed. AJ Lipowitz, DD Caywood, CD Newton and A Schwartz, pp 239-243. Williams & Wilkins, Baltimore

Boudrieau RJ and Muir WW (1987) Pathophysiology of traumatic diaphragmatic hernia in dogs. *Compendium of Continuing Education* **9**, 379-385

Breznock EM (1988) Chylothorax: innovative surgical manipulations to a difficult surgical problem. *Veterinary Surgery* **17**, 30-34

Brumm FR and Smeak DD (1992) Pleural compartmentalization in a dog with a pleuroperitoneal shunt. *Veterinary Surgery* **21**, 205-207

Caywood DD (1996) Chylothorax. In: *Complications in Small Animal Surgery*, 1st edn, ed. AJ Lipowitz, DD Caywood, CD Newton and A Schwartz, pp 201-203. Williams & Wilkins, Baltimore

Colt HG, Russack V, Chiu Y, Konopka RG, Chiles PG, Pedersen CA and Kapelanski D (1997) A comparison of thoracoscopic talc insufflation, slurry, and mechanical abrasion pleurodesis. *Chest* **111**, 442-448

Donner GS (1989) Use of the pleuroperitoneal shunt for the management of persistent chylothorax in a cat. *Journal of the American Veterinary Medical Association* **25**, 619-622

Farnsworth R and Birchard SJ (1996) Subcutaneous accumulation of chyle after thoracic duct ligation in a dog. *Journal of the American Veterinary Medical Association* **208**, 2016-2019

Fossum TW (1993) Feline chylothorax. *Compendium of Continuing Education* **15**, 549-565

Fossum TW, Birchard SJ and Jacobs RM (1986) Chylothorax in thirty-four dogs: a retrospective study. *Journal of the American Veterinary Medical Association* **188**, 1315-1317

Fossum TW, Forrester SD, Swenson CL, Miller MW, Cohen ND, Boothe HW and Birchard SJ (1991) Chylothorax in cats: 37 cases (1969-1989). *Journal of the American Veterinary Medical Association* **198**, 672-678

Fossum TW, Evering WN, Miller MW, Forrester SD, Palmer DR and Hodges CC (1992) Severe bilateral fibrosing pleuritis associated with chronic chylothorax in five cats and two dogs. *Journal of the American Veterinary Medical Association* **201**, 317-324

Glennon JC, Flanders JA, Rothwell JT and Shelly S (1987) Constrictive pleuritis with chylothorax in a cat: a case report. *Journal of the American Animal Hospital Association* **23**, 539-543

Gores BR, Berg J, Carpenter JL and Aronsohn MG (1994) Surgical treatment of thymoma in cats: 12 cases (1987-1992). *Journal of the American Veterinary Medical Association* **204**, 1782-1785

Greene CE, Basinger R and Whitfield JB (1988) Surgical management of bilateral diaphragmatic paralysis in a dog. *Journal of the American Veterinary Medical Association* **193**, 1542-1544

Helphrey ML (1982) Abdominal flap graft for repair of chronic diaphragmatic hernia in the dog. *Journal of the American Veterinary Medical Association* **181**, 791-793

Hodges CC, Fossum TW and Evering W (1993) Evaluation of thoracic duct healing after experimental laceration and transection. *Veterinary Surgery* **22**, 431-435

Johnson KA (1993) Diaphragmatic, pericardial, and hiatal hernia. In: *Textbook of Small Animal Surgery*, 2nd edn, ed. DH Slatter, pp 455-470. WB Saunders, Philadelphia

Johnston GR, Feeney DA, O'Brien TD, Klausner JS, Polzin DJ, Lipowitz AJ, Levine SH, Hamilton HB and Haynes JS (1984) Recurring lung lobe torsion in three Afghan Hounds. *Journal of the American Veterinary Medical Association* **184**, 842-845

Kagan KG and Breznock EM (1979) Variations in the canine thoracic duct system and the effects of surgical occlusion demonstrated by rapid aqueous lymphography, using an intestinal lymphatic trunk. *American Journal of Veterinary Research* **40**, 948-958

Kerpsack SJ, McLoughlin MA, Birchard SJ, Smeak DD and Biller DS (1994) Evaluation of mesenteric lymphangiography and thoracic duct ligation in cats with chylothorax: 19 cases (1987-1992). *Journal of the American Veterinary Medical Association* **205**, 711-715

Klebanow ER (1992) Thymoma and acquired myasthenia gravis in the dog: a case report and review of 13 additional cases. *Journal of the American Animal Hospital Association* **28**, 63-69

Laing EJ and Norris AM (1986) Pleurodesis as a treatment for pleural effusion in the dog. *Journal of the American Animal Hospital Association* **22**, 193-196

Martin RA, Richards DLS, Barber DL, Cordes DO and Sufit E (1988) Transdiaphragmatic approach to thoracic duct ligation in the cat. *Veterinary Surgery* **17**, 22-26

Nelson AW (1993) Lower respiratory system. In: *Textbook of Small Animal Surgery*, 2nd edn, ed. DH Slatter, pp 777-804. WB Saunders, Philadelphia

Orton EC (1993) Pleura and pleural space. In: *Textbook of Small Animal Surgery*, 2nd edn, ed. DH Slatter, pp 386-399. WB Saunders, Philadelphia

Pardo AD, Bright RM, Walker MA and Patton CS (1989) Transcatheter thoracic duct embolization in the dog: an experimental study. *Veterinary Surgery* **18**, 279-285

Peterson SL (1996) Postcaval thrombosis and delayed shunt migration after pleuro-peritoneal venous shunting for concurrent chylothorax and chylous ascites in a dog. *Veterinary Surgery* **25**, 228-230

Peterson SL, Pion PD and Breznock EM (1989) Passive pleuroperitoneal drainage for management of chylothorax in two cats. *Journal of the American Animal Hospital Association* **25**, 569-572

Pratschke KM, Hughes JM, Skelly C and Bellenger CR (1998) Hiatal hernia as a complication of chronic diaphragmatic herniation. *Journal of Small Animal Practice* **39**, 33-38

Read RA (1981) Successful treatment of organising hemothorax by decortication in a dog - a case report. *Journal of the American Animal Hospital Association* **17**, 176

Schwartz A (1996) Thymectomy. In: *Complications in Small Animal Surgery*, 1st edn, ed. AJ Lipowitz, DD Caywood, CD Newton and A Schwartz, pp 323-328. Williams & Wilkins, Baltimore

Smeak DD, Gallagher L, Birchard SJ and Fossum TW (1987) Management of intractable pleural effusion in a dog with a pleuroperitoneal shunt. *Veterinary Surgery* **16**, 212-216

Suess RP, Flanders JA, Beck KA and Earnest-Koons K (1994) Constrictive pleuritis in cats with chylothorax: 10 cases (1983-1991). *Journal of the American Animal Hospital Association* **30**, 70-77

Takeda S, Nakahara K, Fujii Y, Matsumura A, Minami M and Matsuda H (1995) Effects of diaphragmatic plication on respiratory mechanics in dogs with unilateral and bilateral phrenic nerve paralysis. *Chest* **107**, 798-804

Wallace J, Mullen HS and Lesser MB (1992). A technique for surgical correction of peritoneal pericardial diaphragmatic hernia in dogs and cats. *Journal of the American Animal Hospital Association* **28**, 503-510

Wingfield WE, Bliven MT and Quirk PE (1985) Use of continuous chest drainage in dogs and cats. *Journal of the American Animal Hospital Association* **21**, 29—32

Willauer CC and Breznock EM (1987) Pleurovenous shunting technique for treatment of chylothorax in three dogs. *Journal of the American Veterinary Medical Association* **191**, 1106—1109

Thoracic Cage Defects

J. David Fowler

Injuries to the thoracic wall arising from trauma, infection and neoplasia are common in small animals, and functional reconstruction of the chest wall must be considered when planning therapy for these conditions. In minor cases involving contusion or non-displaced rib fractures, management may be as simple as providing analgesia to improve ventilatory function. Complex problems arising from ablative cancer surgery or severe trauma may require more advanced reconstructive techniques.

The chest wall is, by nature of its compliance, a resilient structure. Any injury to the chest wall should therefore draw the attention of the clinician to the possibility of considerable injury to underlying thoracic and abdominal organs. Chest wall injury is often associated with pneumothorax, haemothorax or cardio-pulmonary contusion which may further embarrass ventilatory or cardiac function. The chest wall must provide a closed pleural space, resist paradoxical motion during respiration, and protect underlying internal organs. Loss of any of these functions necessitates intervention to restore chest wall integrity.

This chapter focuses on the aetiology of chest wall injury and reconstructive options to restore anatomical and functional integrity of the chest wall. The reader is referred to earlier sections of the manual for discussion of recognition and management of parenchymal injuries which often accompany chest wall trauma.

CHEST WALL TRAUMA

Contusion

Contusion of the chest wall is frequently seen in animals suffering any form of blunt trauma. Contusion in itself does not compromise the functional integrity of the chest wall. Resultant pain, however, may diminish ventilatory effort. This is rarely problematic except in the instance of associated pleural or pulmonary disease. Provision of analgesia, along with treatment of any associated internal thoracic injury, are usually sufficient in the management of chest wall contusion. Analgesic agents with limited respiratory depressant effects, such as butorphanol, are recommended.

Fractured ribs

Fractured ribs most commonly occur secondary to severe blunt trauma, such as in motor traffic accidents. Rib fractures may be single, but often involve multiple ribs. Less commonly, segmental fractures in multiple ribs occur. The significance of rib fractures depends upon their number, displacement and the presence or absence of intrathoracic injury.

Non-displaced rib fractures are most commonly treated by provision of analgesia and rest. Chest bandages may provide support and reduce pain associated with rib fractures, but should be used cautiously, since they may further compromise ventilatory effort. Rib fractures may be associated with laceration of intercostal vessels. Haematoma formation and haemothorax may result. With drainage of the haemothorax, haemorrhage is generally self limiting. Continued accumulation of blood in the pleural space necessitates exploratory surgery and ligation of the lacerated vessels, following appropriate cardiovascular stabilization.

Rib fractures displaced into the pleural space may lacerate underlying lung lobes, and should be reduced and surgically stabilized. Life-threatening concomitant injuries should be addressed prior to surgery. In instances where stabilization is not possible due to the severity of thoracic wall injury, surgery should not be delayed. Intramedullary K-wires, cerclage wires, or spinal plates are recommended for reduction and stabilization of rib fractures (see Figure 31.1). Further stability may be attained through debridement and repair of traumatized soft tissues.

Flail chest

Flail chest is caused by segmental fractures involving multiple adjacent ribs, resulting in a free floating segment of thoracic wall. The loss of structural integrity results in paradoxical movement of the chest wall during respiration. Paradoxical chest wall motion not only compromises the dynamics of chest wall expansion, but more importantly causes continued contusion to underlying pulmonary parenchyma. Ventilation-perfusion mismatch caused by developing lung contusions results in further hypoxaemia. The unstable chest wall segment must be stabilized to prevent ongoing pulmonary trauma.

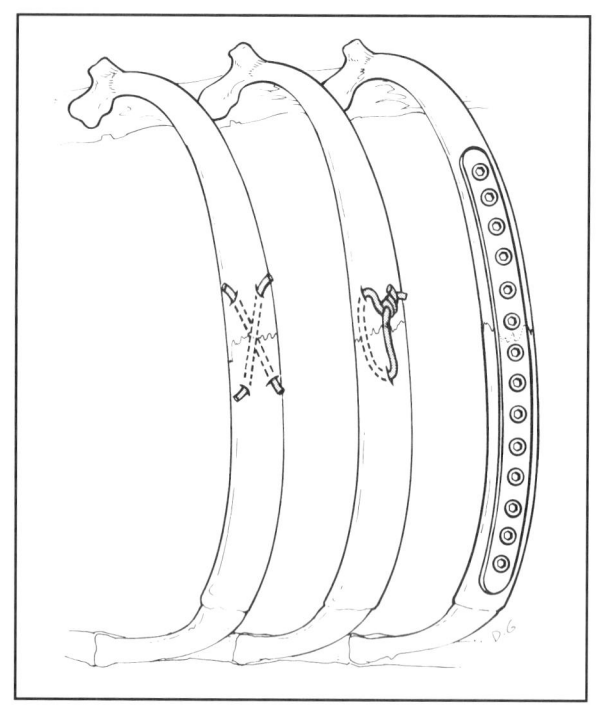

Figure 31.1: *Multiple methods are available for the stabilization of displaced rib fractures, including cross pinning with intramedullary wires, cerclage wiring and application of bone or spinal plates.*

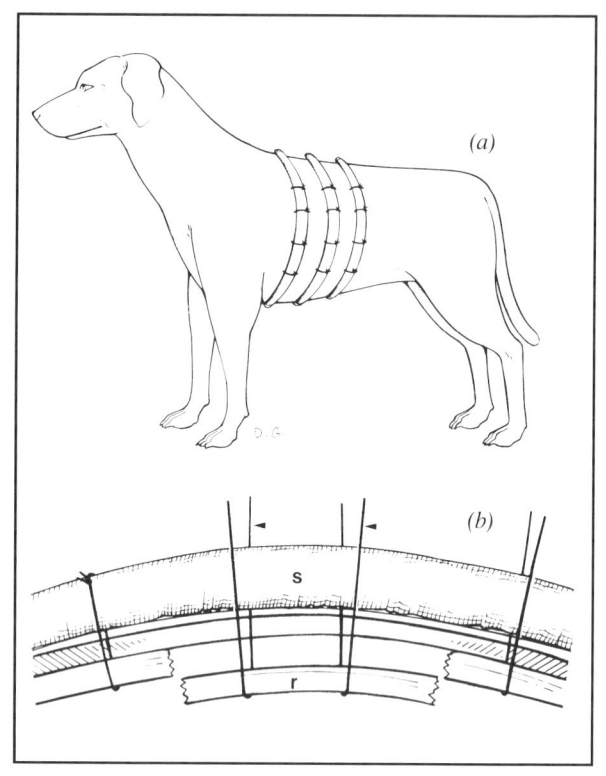

Figure 31.2: (a) *Flail chest may be stabilized by application of splint material moulded to the normal thoracic wall contour. The splint is laid over the flail segment in such a manner that it spans the defect and overlies intact rib above and below. Encircling sutures are placed percutaneously to surround the underlying rib. The sutures are tied around the splint, thereby fixing the unstable segment to the splint. Splints may be maintained for several weeks.* (b) *The splint is shown in profile with the underlying segmental rib fracture.* (r) *rib,* (s) *splint,* (arrow) *encircling suture.*

Flail chest is best managed by external splinting techniques. An external aluminium rod frame onto which the flail segment is sutured has been described (Kolata, 1981). Aluminium rods or thermoplastic splint material contoured to the shape of an intact rib may also be used (see Figure 31.2). The splint is placed to overlie one of the fractured ribs. Multiple monofilament non-absorbable sutures are placed using a large half-circle needle such that they encircle the rib and splint. Care must be taken to avoid trauma to underlying pulmonary parenchyma. Enough sutures are placed to incorporate the unstable segment of rib along with stable portions of the rib above and below the segmental fractures. One splint may be applied to each involved rib to achieve maximal stability of the flail chest. A loosely applied bandage protects the splints from disruption. Although general anaesthesia is advantageous, splint application may be accomplished using local anaesthesia in compromised patients.

External splints for flail chest may be used for temporary support during patient stabilization, or may be used for definitive repair. In the case of temporary splinting, internal fixation of rib fractures and associated soft tissues is accomplished following stabilization of the animal. External splints used for definitive repair should be maintained for 3-4 weeks to allow traumatized soft tissues to heal and provide support to the chest wall.

Open chest wounds

Penetrating injuries from bite wounds, gunshots or projectiles may result in open chest wounds. The clinician must consider several factors in deciding how best to manage such injuries. First and foremost is the animal's cardiopulmonary status. If pneumothorax is present, the pleural space must be evacuated. Continued accumulation of air in the pleural space signifies air leakage through tracts caused by the penetrating injury, or damage to pulmonary parenchyma. Continued air leakage through the penetrating wound should be managed by gentle cleansing of the surrounding area followed by application of petroleum jelly and a gauze bandage to the wound.

Sharp penetrating injuries cause minimal soft tissue disruption. Bandaging alone, or early surgical exploration and direct repair of soft tissues is indicated in these instances. Unfortunately, open chest wounds in small animals more often result from altercations with other animals (McKiernan *et al.*, 1984). The resulting wounds are a combination of laceration, crush and avulsion injury and should be considered heavily contaminated. Broad spectrum bactericidal antibiotic therapy is indicated. Surgical exploration and aggressive debridement of traumatized and contaminated tissues should be performed as soon as possible following cardiopulmonary stabilization. Soft tissues must be reconstructed after debridement to ensure maintenance of chest wall integrity.

NEOPLASIA OF THE THORACIC WALL

Primary tumours of the chest wall most frequently arise from the ribs or sternebrae. Osteosarcoma and chondrosarcoma are reported most frequently, with haemangiosarcoma and fibrosarcoma being relatively less common. In a recent retrospective study of 26 primary tumours of the thoracic wall, osteosarcoma accounted for approximately 60%, while chondrosarcoma accounted for 34% of all tumours (Veterinary Co-operative Oncology Group, 1993).

Animals with chest wall neoplasia most often present due to the presence of a noticeable mass. Occasionally thoracic wall tumours are associated with pleural effusion and affected animals are presented with signs of ventilatory insufficiency. The costochondral junction is most frequently involved, and large dogs are more prone to osseous tumours of the chest wall. There appears to be no predilection for sex, breed or specific rib involved.

Tumours of the chest wall should be assumed to be malignant until proven otherwise. Large volume biopsy is important for accurate histological diagnosis. Thorough clinical staging should be performed prior to planning definitive treatment. Biological behaviour of osteosarcoma of the thoracic wall parallels that of appendicular osteosarcoma with a reported median survival time of 5-12 weeks following surgery with curative intent. Adjuvant chemotherapy using cisplatin significantly lengthens disease free interval and survival following surgical excision of thoracic wall osteosarcoma. Chondrosarcoma is associated with a more favourable prognosis, with reported median survival times of up to 3 years (Veterinary Co-operative Oncology Group, 1993; Pirkey-Ehrhart et al, 1995).

Definitive surgery involves wide surgical resection of the involved chest wall. As much of the rib as possible should be removed dorsal and ventral to the lesion. Overlying soft tissues and biopsy tracts must be included in the excision. At least one rib cranial and one rib caudal to the lesion should be included in the excision.

RECONSTRUCTIVE TECHNIQUES FOR CHEST WALL DEFECTS

There are several goals which must be met to achieve successful reconstruction of the chest wall. The reconstruction must:

- result in an air-tight seal of the pleural space from the external environment
- provide rigid enough stability to prevent paradoxical movement
- be durable enough to protect internal organs from trauma.

Ideally, thoracic wall reconstruction will also result in a cosmetically acceptable appearance. Primary clo-

sure techniques, mobilization of autogenous tissues and implantation of synthetic materials have all been used for reconstruction of the chest wall. It is generally accepted that the maximum number of ribs which may be resected successfully in the dog and cat is six.

Primary closure of chest wall defects

Primary closure may be considered when the ribs cranial and caudal to the excised segment can be brought into apposition without undue tension (see Figure 31.3). Encircling sutures are passed around the rib cranial and caudal to the defect and tied to maintain approximation of the ribs. Suture sizes ranging from 3.0 to 4.0 should be used, depending on the patient's weight. Intercostal, latissimus dorsi, pectoral and/or external abdominal oblique muscles may be mobilized and sutured to further protect and seal the defect. Primary closure is generally difficult to achieve following resection of more than one rib. Other reconstructive techniques are recommended in resections involving three or more ribs.

Closure of chest wall defects using prosthetic materials

Many synthetic materials have been evaluated and recommended for chest wall reconstruction (Bright, 1981; Runnels and Trampel, 1986). Materials used should be durable enough to prevent paradoxical movement and protect underlying lung, should be well tolerated by the host and induce minimal inflammatory

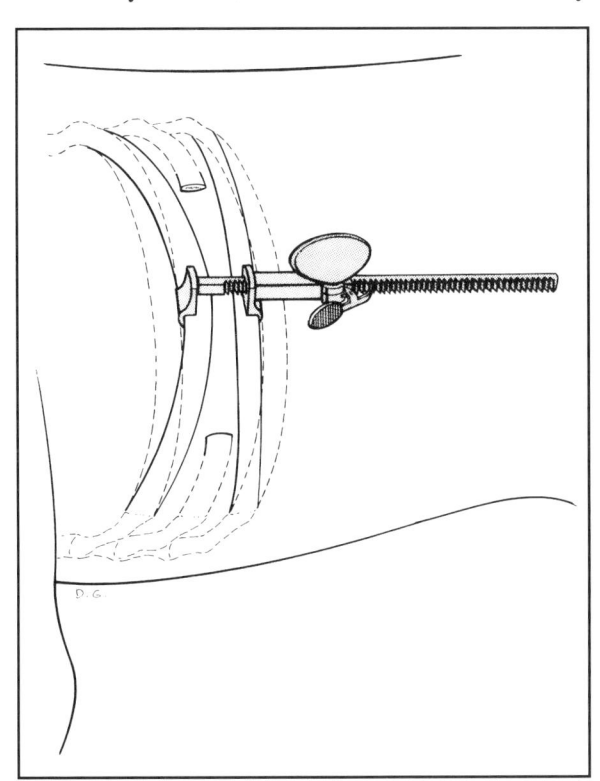

Figure 31.3: The chest wall can generally be reconstructed by advancement of adjacent ribs following excision of one or two ribs. A rib approximator is useful to appose ribs during suture placement.

reaction and should be relatively easy to work with. Non-absorbable materials such as silastic sheeting, polytetrafluoroethylene, carbon/polycaprolactone composites, and polypropylene mesh have been used successfully. More recently interest has developed in evaluating absorbable materials, such as polydioxanone-band grids, which are eventually replaced by host tissue (Puma *et al.*, 1992).

The prosthetic material is placed intrapleurally to initially bridge the defect following chest wall resection (see Figure 31.4). The material is cut to overlap adjacent ribs and fit snugly within the defect. Edges of the prosthetic material should be folded back on themselves to avoid exposure of rough or irritating edges to pulmonary parenchyma. Multiple mattress sutures placed around ribs and through intercostal musculature are used to stabilize the prosthetic material within the defect. The material should be sutured under moderate tension. Good soft tissue coverage of the pros-

thetic material is important to prevent extrusion of the material, contamination and infection. An omental flap or regional musculature, such as the latissimus dorsi or external abdominal oblique muscles, is elevated and transposed over the defect. Skin is closed directly whenever possible. If cutaneous excision precludes direct closure, an axial pattern skin flap based on the thoracodorsal artery and vein may be used.

Advantages of prosthetic reconstruction include ready access to reconstructive materials and relatively simple technique. The primary disadvantage is predisposition to infection, necessitating strict aseptic technique. As a large, non-vascularized foreign substance the prosthetic material may harbour bacteria and serve as a nidus for infection. Infected prosthetic materials must be removed and the defect subsequently reconstructed with vascularized tissue. Prosthetic materials should not be used for chest wall reconstruction in the presence of contamination or established infection.

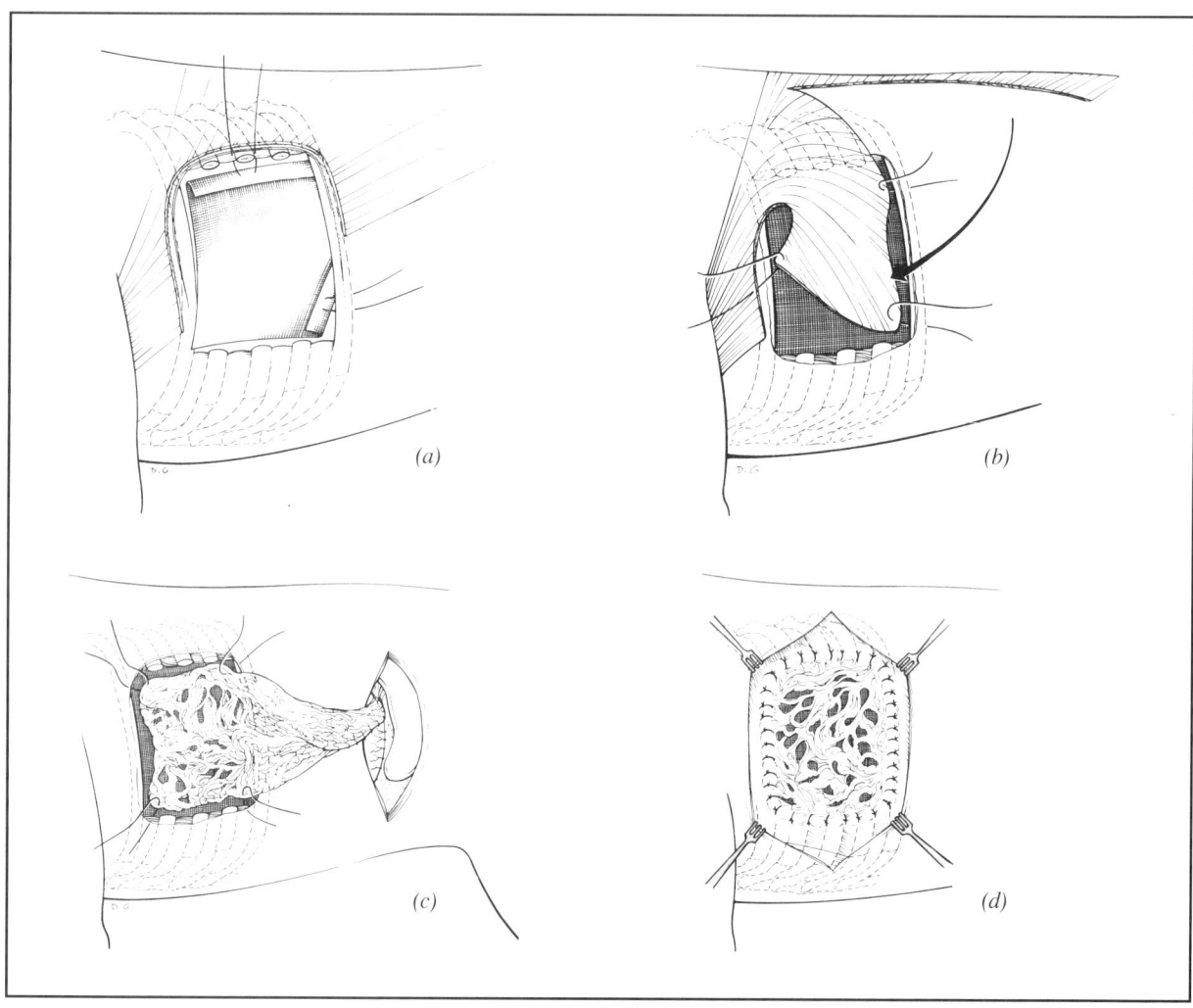

Figure 31.4: *(a) Non-absorbable prosthetic mesh may be used to reconstruct large thoracic wall defects. The mesh is placed intrapleurally and is trimmed to fit snugly in the defect. Mesh edges are turned outward to protect underlying lung parenchyma. The mesh is sutured using mattress sutures placed around adjacent ribs and intercostal musculature. (b) The latissimus dorsi muscle may be elevated and rotated to provide a vascular soft tissue cover. Extensive loss of the latissimus dorsi muscle with the initial dissection precludes use of this technique in many instances of tumour excision. (c), (d) An omental pedicle flap based on either the right or left gastroepiploic artery and vein may be harvested through a paracostal incision. The omentum is advanced to the thoracic wall defect through a generous subcutaneous tunnel and may be used to provide a vascular cover to the thoracic wall repair.*

Closure of chest wall defects using autogenous tissues

Vascularized autogenous tissues are ideal for chest wall reconstruction. An improved knowledge of vascular angiosomes (composites of tissue supplied by a single source artery and vein) along with the advent and increased clinical application of more advanced surgical techniques involving use of pedicled tissue flaps or microvascular transfer of tissues has facilitated the use of appropriate autogenous tissues for reconstruction. The surgeon is no longer necessarily limited to autogenous tissues in the immediate vicinity of the resection for reconstructive application.

Regional muscles, most notably the latissimus dorsi and external abdominal oblique muscles, may be elevated on a vascular pedicle and sutured into chest wall defects (Pavletic *et al.*, 1987; Alexander *et al.*, 1991). Use of muscle alone for reconstruction may provide inadequate stability in defects involving more than three ribs.

Osteomyocutaneous flaps

Skin, latissimus dorsi muscle and underlying split rib elevation has been described in people as an osteomyocutaneous flap for reconstruction of particularly large defects (Hirase *et al.*, 1991). Rigidity is provided through the provision of autogenous vascularized bone within the flap. A latissimus dorsi myocutaneous flap which could have application in thoracic reconstruction has been described in dogs (Pavletic *et al.*, 1987).

Advancement of the diaphragm

Defects of the caudal chest wall may be reconstructed by advancement of the diaphragm (Aronsohn, 1984) (see Figure 31.5). The diaphragmatic attachments to the costal arch are severed and the diaphragm is advanced and sutured to the last rib cranial to the defect. Although not generally necessary, the caudal lung lobe on the affected side may be resected to facilitate diaphragmatic advancement. The resulting abdominal wall defect is closed using local muscle flaps.

Omental pedicle flaps

These may also be used in chest wall reconstruction (Bright *et al.*, 1982). The omentum actively contributes a neovascular supply to the reconstructed area, but does little to directly improve immediate stability or durability of the reconstruction. Omentum is therefore most often used in conjunction with prosthetic reconstruction, when excision of regional musculature precludes adequate soft tissue coverage of the prosthetic material. Omentum is harvested through a paracostal incision as a pedicle flap, based on either the right or left gastroepiploic artery and vein. Alternatively, one layer of omentum may be opened near the gastric attachment and the omentum 'unfolded' to achieve adequate length. It is then exteriorized and passed through a generous subcutaneous tunnel to the defect. Care should be taken during flap elevation and transposition to avoid kinking or compression of omental vasculature.

Diaphragmatic defects

Repair of traumatic diaphragmatic rupture and congenital diaphragmatic defects is described in Chapter 30. For large defects, a transversus abdominus muscle flap has been described for reconstruction (Helphrey, 1982).

REFERENCES

Alexander LG, Pavletic MM and Engler SJ (1991) Abdominal wall reconstruction with a vascular external abdominal oblique myofascial flap. *Veterinary Surgery* **20**, 379-384

Aronsohn M (1984) Diaphragmatic advancement for defects of the caudal thoracic wall of the dog. *Veterinary Surgery* **13**, 26-28

Boudrieau RJ and Muir WW (1987) Pathophysiology of traumatic diaphragmatic hernia in dogs. *Compendium of Continuing Education for the Practicing Veterinarian* **9**, 379-384

Bright RM (1981) Reconstruction of thoracic wall defects using Marlex mesh. *Journal of the American Animal Hospital Association* **17**, 415-420

Bright RM, Birchard SJ and Long GG (1982) Repair of thoracic wall defects in the dog with an omental pedicle flap. *Journal of the American Animal Hospital Association* **18**, 277-282

Evans SM and Biery DN (1980) Congenital peritoneopericardial diaphragmatic hernia in the dog and cat. a literature review and 17 additional case histories. *Veterinary Radiology* **21**, 108-111

Helphrey ML (1982) Abdominal flap graft for repair of chronic diaphragmatic hernia in the dog. *Journal of the American Veterinary Medical Association* **181**, 791-793

Hirase Y, Kojima T, Kinoshita Y, Bang H-H, Sakaguchi T and Kijima M (1991) Composite reconstruction for chest wall and scalp using multiple ribs -- latissimus dorsi osteomyocutaneous flaps as pedicled and free flaps. *Plastic and Reconstructive Surgery* **87**, 555-561

Kolata RJ (1981). Management of thoracic trauma. *Veterinary Clinics of North America* **11**, 103-112

McKiernan BC, Adams WM and Huse DC (1984) Thoracic bite wounds and associated internal injury in 11 dogs and 1 cat. *Journal of the American Veterinary Medical Association* **184**, 959-964

Pavletic MM, Kostolich M, Loblik P and Engle S (1987) A comparison of the cutaneous trunci myocutaneous flap and latissimus dorsi

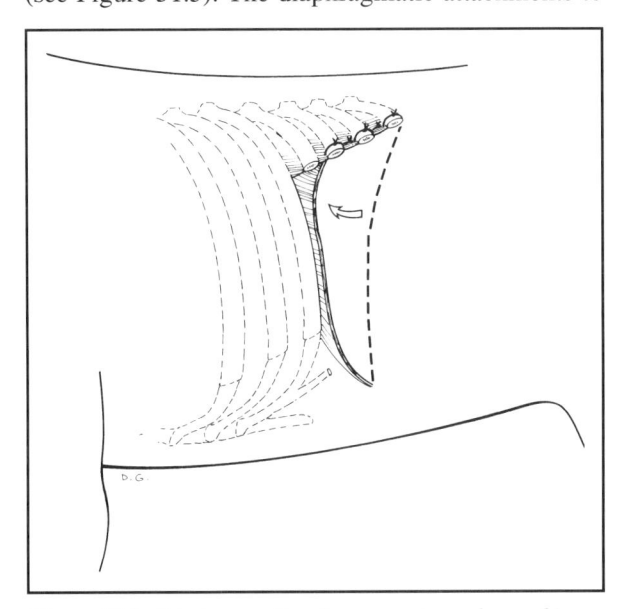

Figure 31.5: Diaphragmatic advancement may be used in the reconstruction of caudal thoracic wall defects. The diaphragmatic edge is elevated from its normal attachment and advanced cranially.

myocutaneous flap in the dog. *Veterinary Surgery* **16**, 283–293

Pirkey-Ehrhart N, Withrow SJ, Straw RC *et al.* (1995) Primary rib tumors in 54 dogs. *Journal of the American Animal Hospital Association* **31**, 65–69

Puma F, Ragusa M and Daddi G (1992) Chest wall stabilization with synthetic reabsorbable material. *Annals of Thoracic Surgery* **53**, 408–411

Rudolphy VJ, Tukkie R and Klopper PJ (1991) Chest wall reconstruction with degradable processed sheep dermal collagen in dogs. *Annals of Thoracic Surgery* 52, 821–825

Runnels CM and Trampel DW (1986) Full-thickness thoracic and abdominal wall reconstruction in dogs using carbon/polycaprolactone composite. *Veterinary Surgery* **15**, 363–368

Veterinary Cooperative Oncology Group (1993) Retrospective study of 26 primary tumors of the osseous thoracic wall in dogs. *Journal of the American Animal Hospital Association* **29**, 68–72

Index